P9-BXZ-315

What People Are Saying About the *Natural Health Bible* and TNP.com

"The *Natural Health Bible* is a rigorous, comprehensive, up-to-date, and refreshingly accessible overview of the rapidly changing landscape of natural medicine and its applications for promoting health and treating disease. As a neurologist/neuroscientist who studies the mechanisms of actions of natural antioxidants and herbs, and who treats patients with Alzheimer's Disease, migraine headaches, and a host of other neurological conditions, I have found the book and the Web site to be indispensable resources."

—*Rajiv R. Ratan M.D., Ph.D.*
Harvard Institutes of Medicine

"An impressive book that answers my skepticism about the way "natural" remedies are sometimes marketed. Instead of relying on hype and testimonials, *The Natural Pharmacist: Natural Health Bible* presents a critical analysis of the available science supporting the health promoting effects of various vitamins and herbs—it's more objective than anything I've read on the subject."

—*Jan Fawcett, M.D.*
Professor and Chairman,
Department of Psychiatry,
Rush-Presbyterian–St.Luke's Medical Center, Chicago

"The *Natural Health Bible* is a wonderful resource providing comprehensive and easy-to-understand information about supplements and natural medicine."

—*Ray Sahelian, M.D.*
Author of Mind Boosters: A Guide to Natural Supplements
That Enhance Your Mind, Memory, and Mood

"This book is excellent in that it appeals to both professionals and lay persons. A good book to have for everyday reference."

—*Gordon Weesner, R.Ph.*
El Dorado Hills, CA

"The *Natural Health Bible* is a useful and readable guide to nutritional and herbal therapies edited by two respected authorities in the field. It is not just a collection of monographs, but a well-referenced compilation organized by health condition and by supplement ingredients."

—*Rob McCaleb, President*
Herb Research Foundation

"Our first priority is to offer our visitors the most accurate and in-depth health, medical, and nutrition information possible. By licensing TNP.com's exceptional content, we provide consumers with scientifically-based research on natural products that responds to their needs."

—*Robin Broitman*
SVP and General Manager,
DiscoveryHealth.com

"This excellent reference should be on everyone's bookshelf."

—*Jackie V. Davison-Hoepker, Ph.D.*
Former Associate, Psychohormonal Research
Johns Hopkins University

"The *Natural Health Bible* is a well-researched, easy-to-use reference loaded with valuable, useful information."

—*Dan Labriola, N.D.*
Voted one of the top physicians in Seattle
by Seattle Magazine
Author of Complementary Cancer Therapies

"The *Natural Health Bible* is a valuable and comprehensive resource for the health care professional and layman alike. It provides useful information on neutraceuticals that anyone can easily use."

—*Burt Berkson M.D., M.S., Ph.D.*
The Integrative Medical Center of New Mexico
Author of The Alpha Lipoic Acid Breakthrough

"THE NATURAL PHARMACIST provides AccentHealth.com with trustworthy, independent, science-based information about herbs, supplements and other complementary treatments, which helps us empower consumers to take an active role in managing their health care."

—*Karen-Lee Ryan, Editor in Chief*
AccentHealth.com

"Millions of health plan members turn to the Internet every day to obtain information about alternative medicine, herbs, and supplements. By offering THE NATURAL PHARMACIST'S Herb Index, we are confident that the information our clients' members are receiving is accurate, reliable, and comes from respected sources."

—*Patrick Irvine, Medical Director*
Consumer Health Interactive

"The *Natural Health Bible* is an excellent resource of comprehensive yet concise information about the myriad dietary supplements currently available. While not closing the door on certain claims that are presently unsubstantiated, it simply presents the current state of knowledge and suggests a reasonable interpretation of the evidence."

—*Jerry Cott, Ph.D.*
Scientific Director and Chief Science Officer
Scientific Herbal Products, Inc.

"As a doctor and educator of dentistry, I am a skeptic until evidence is provided. The information in this book has been thoroughly investigated and is supported by research, so I can use it on a regular basis with confidence."

—*Ben Dykes, D.D.S.*
Folsom, CA

"I was very happy to find THE NATURAL PHARMACIST Web site and book. As a first-year intern and alternative medicine enthusiast, it is nice to have such a complete resource with research support. Your work is much appreciated and has been direly needed."

—*John Rickelman Jr., D.O.*
Northeast Regional Medical Center
Kirksville, MO

"I constantly get e-mails from consumers asking health questions...whenever I receive a question about supplements, herbs, etc., I point them to your site. You have some great information. Also the *Natural Health Bible*, is an excellent resource for consumers and health professionals to learn more about herbs, supplements, and vitamins. So much information about these topics in one place is a rare find!"

—*Jeffrey Werner, M.S., R.D., L.D.*
Founder of Foundhealth.com

"In my work as a Medicines Information pharmacist, I am using the TNP site more and more. I find it well organized; relevant sections are easy to find. The information given is useful and, most importantly, referenced."

—*Dorothy Browne, M. Ed.*
New Zealand Pharmaceutical Society

"I've been searching for years to find bona fide scientific information on herbal medicine. Objective sources like the *Natural Health Bible* are crucial indeed."

—*Neuland Collier*
Certified Pharmacy Technician

From acne to weight loss and from aloe to zinc, this book has it all!

—*Robyn Huff*
Dallas, TX

"My wife and I have definitely saved money since buying this book. It has allowed us to make wise decisions based on our individual needs before purchasing herbs or supplements."

—*Steve and Diane Carmell*
Burlington, VT

"My health-conscious daughter introduced me to THE NATURAL PHARMACIST, and now I'm hooked. I use the Web site and the book regularly to answer my health questions."

—*Joe Cornejo*
Kaneohe, Oahu, HI

THE NATURAL PHARMACIST
Board of Advisors:

Steven Bratman, M.D.

Andrea M. Girman, M.D., M.P.H.

David J. Kroll, Ph.D.

Richard Harkness, Pharm., FASCP

James W. Cooper, Jr., Ph.D., B.C.P.S., C.G.P.

Melvyn R. Werbach, M.D.

Michael Springer

Stephen G. Gillespie, Ph.D., R.Ph.

Mary L. Chavez, Pharm.D.

Contributors:

Anna M. Barton

Marian Broida, R.N.

Angelo DePalma, Ph.D.

Ann Eastman, Ph.D.

Lisa Fleige, R.D.

Julie Leigh, R.N.

Deborah Lieberman

Candice Mohr

Catherine Monahan

Carol Poole

Sibylle Preuschat

Natasha Senjanovic

Other Books
in THE NATURAL PHARMACIST Series

The Natural Pharmacist Guide to Arthritis

The Natural Pharmacist Guide to Diabetes

The Natural Pharmacist Guide to Echinacea and Immunity

The Natural Pharmacist Guide to Feverfew and Migraines

The Natural Pharmacist Guide to Garlic and Cholesterol

The Natural Pharmacist Guide to Ginkgo and Memory

The Natural Pharmacist Guide to Heart Disease Prevention

The Natural Pharmacist Guide to Kava and Anxiety

The Natural Pharmacist Guide to Menopause

The Natural Pharmacist Guide to PMS

The Natural Pharmacist Guide to Reducing Cancer Risk

The Natural Pharmacist Guide to Saw Palmetto and the Prostate

The Natural Pharmacist Guide to St. John's Wort and Depression

The Natural Pharmacist Guide to Preventing Osteoporosis with Ipriflavone

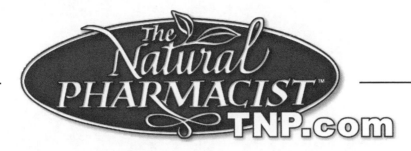

The Natural PHARMACIST™ TNP.com

Natural Health Bible

Revised and Expanded, 2nd Edition

**From the Most Trusted Alternative Health Site in the World—
Your A–Z Guide to Over 300 Conditions,
Herbs, Vitamins, and Supplements**

Steven Bratman, M.D.
with David Kroll, Ph.D.

Prima
HEALTH

A Division of Prima Publishing

Visit us online at www.TNP.com

© 2000 by Prima Publishing

All rights reserved. No part of this book may be reproduced or transmitted in any form or by any means, electronic or mechanical, including photocopying, recording, or by any information storage or retrieval system, without written permission from Prima Publishing, except for the inclusion of quotations in a review.

Warning—Disclaimer
This book is not intended to provide medical advice and is sold with the understanding that the publisher and the author are not liable for the misconception or misuse of information provided. The author and Prima Publishing shall have neither liability nor responsibility to any person or entity with respect to any loss, damage, or injury caused or alleged to be caused directly or indirectly by the information contained in this book or the use of any products mentioned. Readers should not use any of the products discussed in this book without the advice of a medical professional.

The Food and Drug Administration has not approved the use of any of the natural treatments discussed in this book. This book, and the information contained herein, has not been approved by the Food and Drug Administration.

PRIMA HEALTH and colophon are trademarks of Prima Communications, Inc.
THE NATURAL PHARMACIST™, TNP.com, and THENATURALPHARMACIST.com are trademarks of Prima Communications, Inc.

All products mentioned in this book are trademarks of their respective companies.

Library of Congress Cataloging-in-Publication Data on file

ISBN 0-7615-2448-7
00 01 02 DD 10 9 8 7 6 5 4 3 2 1
Printed in the United States of America

Visit us online at www.TNP.com and www.primahealth.com

CONTENTS

PART TWO:
HERBS AND SUPPLEMENTS

Contents

WHAT MAKES THIS BOOK DIFFERENT?

The interest in natural medicine has never been greater. According to the National Association of Chain Drug Stores, 65 million Americans are using natural supplements, and the number is growing! Yet it is hard for the consumer to find trustworthy sources for balanced information about this emerging field. Why? Frankly, natural medicine has had a checkered history. From snake oil potions sold at the turn of the century to those books, magazines, and product catalogs that hype miracle cures today, this is a field where exaggerated claims have been the norm. Proponents of natural medicine have tended to abuse science, treating it more as a marketing tool than a means of discovering the truth.

But there is truth to be found. Studies of vitamins, minerals, and other food supplements have been with us since these nutritional substances were first discovered, and the level and quality of this science has grown dramatically in the last 20 years. Herbal medicine has been neglected in the United States, but in Europe, this, the oldest of all healing arts, has been the subject of tremendous and ongoing scientific interest.

At present, for a number of herbs and supplements, it is possible to give reasonably scientific answers to the following questions: How well does this work? How safe is it? What types of conditions is it best used for?

THE NATURAL PHARMACIST series is designed to cut through the hype and tell you what we know and what remains to be researched regarding popular natural treatments. These books are more conservative than any others available, more honest about the weaknesses of natural approaches, more fair in their comparisons of natural and conventional treatments. You won't find any miracle cures here, but you will discover useful options that can help you become healthier.

WHY CHOOSE NATURAL TREATMENTS?

Although the science behind natural medicine continues to grow, this is still a much less scientifically validated field than conventional medicine. You might ask, "Why should I resort to an herb that is only partly proven, when I could take a drug with solid science behind it?" There are at least three good reasons to consider natural alternatives.

First, some herbs and supplements offer benefits that are not matched by any conventional drug. Echinacea is a good example. If you have a cold and take echinacea, you'll recover faster. No standard medication can do the same.

Another example is glucosamine sulfate for arthritis. Glucosamine seems to slow the progression of arthritis, meaning that it protects your joints from getting worse over time. There is no pill or tablet your doctor can prescribe that offers the same benefit.

In many cases, the science behind natural treatments is very strong. For example, there is more evidence for the herb St. John's wort than there was for Prozac when it was first approved as a drug. The science behind other natural treatments is less than perfect, but when the risks are low and the possible benefit high, a natural treatment may be worth trying. It is a little-known fact that for many conventional treatments the science is less than perfect as well, and physicians must balance uncertain benefits against incompletely understood risks.

A second reason to consider natural therapies is that some may offer benefits comparable to those of drugs with fewer side effects. Again, the herb St. John's wort is a good example. Scientific evidence suggests that this herb is just as effective for mild to moderate depression as standard drugs, while producing fewer side effects. Saw palmetto for benign enlargement of the prostate, ginkgo for relieving symptoms and perhaps slowing the progression of Alzheimer's disease, and chondroitin for osteoarthritis are other examples. This is not to say that herbs and supplements are completely harmless—they're not—but for most the level of risk is quite low. The biggest potential problems are interactions between drugs and herbs, and we cover these thoroughly in our books.

Finally, there is a philosophical point to consider. For many people, it "feels" better to use a treatment that comes from nature instead of from a laboratory. Just as you might rather wear all-cotton clothing than polyester or look at a mountain landscape rather than the skyscrapers of a downtown city, natural treatments may simply feel more compatible with your view of life. We can quibble endlessly about just what "natural" means and whether a certain treatment is "actually" natural or not, but such arguments are beside the point. The difference is in the feeling, and feelings matter. In fact, having a good feeling about taking an herb may lead you to use it more consistently than you would a prescription drug.

Of course, at times synthetic drugs may be necessary and even lifesaving. But on many other occasions it may be quite reasonable to turn to an herb or supplement instead of a drug.

To make good decisions you need good information. Unfortunately, while hundreds of books on alternative medicine are published every year, many are highly misleading. The phrase "studies prove" is often used when the studies in question are so small or so badly conducted that they prove nothing at all. You may even find that the "data" from other books comes from studies with petri dishes and not real people!

You can't even assume that books written by well-known authors are scientifically sound. Many of these authors rely on secondary writers, leading to a game of "telephone," where misconceptions are passed around from book to book. And there's a strong tendency to exaggerate the power of natural remedies, whitewashing them with selective reporting.

THE NATURAL PHARMACIST series gives you the balanced information you need to make informed decisions about your health needs. Setting a new, high standard of accuracy and objectivity, these books take a realistic look at the herbs and supplements you read about in the news. You will encounter both favorable and unfavorable studies in these pages and will learn about both the benefits and the risks of natural treatments.

THE NATURAL PHARMACIST series is the source you can trust.

Steven Bratman, M.D.
David Kroll, Ph.D.

WHAT'S NEW IN THIS EDITION?

Research in the field of natural medicine is growing exponentially. For this revised second edition of our best-selling *The Natural Pharmacist: Natural Health Bible*, we've added thousands of new studies. We've also translated over 100 non-English studies to report them accurately and scoured the research databases of the world to find older but meaningful studies that had been forgotten. This book is now based on a research database that includes over 3,500 full-text studies. We've added 50 new chapters to Part One, Conditions, 49 new chapters to Part Two, Herbs and Supplements, and expanded and updated existing chapters. The *Natural Health Bible, Revised and Expanded 2nd Edition* is truly the most comprehensive and up-to-date book on the science-based use of herbs and supplements.

INTRODUCTION

So that you can easily access the information you need, the *Natural Health Bible* is divided into two parts. Part One, Conditions, contains information on over 100 illnesses and health problems, from acne to varicose veins. In each entry, you will find a description of the condition, as well as the various conventional treatments, herbs, supplements, and lifestyle changes that might help. Treatments that have fairly good evidence behind them or are widely used are called *Principal Proposed Treatments*; the remainder are called *Other Proposed Treatments*.

If you're interested primarily in herbs, vitamins, minerals, and other supplements, then turn to Part Two, Herbs and Supplements. This section covers over 200 of today's popular natural substances, from acidophilus to zinc. For each herb or supplement, we discuss its various uses, the scientific evidence behind those uses, and dosage information, as well as safety issues of which you should be aware. If there is considerable evidence for a substance's effectiveness for a given condition, or if it is widely used for that purpose, that condition is listed under *Principal Proposed Uses*. Otherwise, it falls in the category of *Other Proposed Uses*.

RESOURCES USED

The *Natural Health Bible, Revised and Expanded 2nd Edition* is based on science, not opinion, anecdote, or folk wisdom. To a considerable extent, it turns to European sources of scientific information, where the study of herbs and supplements is a part of mainstream medicine. For example, this book often quotes the opinions of Germany's Commission E, a branch of the German Federal Health Agency charged with evaluating the safety and efficacy of medicinal herbs. It also reports the conclusions of the European Scientific Cooperative on Phytotherapy (ESCOP). But even more than that, this book is based on a comprehensive survey of all the scientific evidence in world literature regarding the use of natural treatments. If there is evidence to report you will find it here; also, if there is little to no evidence backing a given treatment, that will be pointed out as well.

DOSAGE INFORMATION FOR SUPPLEMENTS

There are two ways to take supplements: at a nutritional dose or a therapeutic dose. Because this is an issue that doesn't arise with standard medications (or with herbs), we want to take a moment to explain it here.

Your body needs a certain amount of various vitamins and minerals to maintain health. If you don't get enough in your diet, you may need supplements to avoid a form of malnutrition. When you take just enough of a nutrient to supply your body's needs, you are taking it at a nutritional dose. The exact quantity you need depends on your age, sex, and which authority you ask.

In the United States, the most important standard is the Dietary Reference Intake (DRI). For some supplements, however, it has been impossible to determine the optimum intake, and a looser standard is used instead, the Estimated Safe and Adequate Daily Dietary Intake (ESADDI). To make matters more confusing, in Canada, the prevailing standard is the Recommended Nutrient Intake (RNI), and these figures often disagree with the U.S. RDA levels. Other standards have been set by the Food and Agricultural Organization and the World Health Organization of the United Nations, as well as by other individual countries, and again there is significant variation.

This book provides the U.S. DRI guidelines when they're available; otherwise it uses the ESADDI guidelines.

But there is another, entirely different way of taking supplements. You can take them at a level that greatly exceeds your nutritional needs. This is described as a "therapeutic dosage" and it is listed under a heading separate from that for nutritional requirements.

For example, the estimated dietary requirement of vitamin E is about 10 to 15 IU (international units) daily. But when used as an antioxidant supplement, the typical recommended dosage is 400 to 800 IU daily—25 to 80 times higher than nutritional needs. There is simply no way you could reasonably get this much from food. This is a therapeutic dose, not a nutritional dose.

It's hard to get too worried about the safety of supplements taken at or near your nutritional needs. However, when they are used in gigantic doses, it is always possible that new health risks are created. In this book, we carefully distinguish between nutritional and high-dose use of all supplements described. Each one has its own heading.

Terms You Should Know

Throughout this book we refer to the various types of scientific studies used to evaluate the effectiveness of medical treatments. So that you will understand the nature of each one, and the level of confidence you can place in its results, we briefly describe these research methods here.

Double-Blind Studies

The best and most reliable form of research is the double-blind placebo-controlled study. A treatment cannot really be said to be proven effective unless it has been examined in properly designed and sufficiently large double-blind studies.

In these experiments, one group of subjects receives the "real thing"—the active substance being tested. The other half receives a placebo designed to appear, as much as possible, like the real thing. The purpose of this kind of study is to eliminate the power of suggestion. It is true, although hard to believe, that placebo (fake) treatments can produce dramatic and long-lasting results in a majority of the people who are given them. The double-blind study keeps both doctors and participants in the dark as to who is receiving the placebo and who is receiving the real treatment. If the people in the real treatment group fare significantly better, it is a strong indication that the treatment really works.

A good double-blind study should enroll at least 100 people, preferably as much as 300. Dramatically effective treatments can prove themselves in somewhat smaller trials; however, research involving 30 or fewer people generally doesn't prove anything at all.

Single-Blind Studies

If only the participants are kept in the dark, but the doctors know which group is which, the study is called single-blind. This type of study is a bit questionable as it allows for bias on the part of the doctors conducting the study. (Doctors can subtly convey confidence or a lack of it if they know who is receiving real treatment and who is not; they can also unconsciously bias their evaluation of the results.)

Open Studies

If both the doctors and the participants know who is receiving a treatment and who is not, the procedure is called an open study. The results have to be taken with a handful of salt: Open studies are not at all reliable.

Uncontrolled Studies

Sometimes a group of people are given a treatment and simply followed for a period of time to see if they improve. The results of such studies mean practically nothing at all. Due to the placebo effect, one can be sure from the outset that they will mostly improve; it is impossible to tell how much (if any) of this improvement is due to the effect of the treatment itself.

Observational Trials Versus Intervention Trials

All of the studies just described involve giving participants a treatment; in other words, "intervening" in their lives. They all fall in the category of an "intervention trial."

Observational studies, on the other hand, simply follow large (sometimes gigantic) groups of people for years and keep track of a great deal of information about them, including diet. Researchers do not do anything to them; they just examine the collected data closely and try to identify which dietary and lifestyle factors are associated with better health and longer life.

Observational studies are often the only practical way to gain information about the long-term health effects of nutrition and lifestyle. Unfortunately, the results can be misleading. For example, if an observational study finds that people who drink green tea develop less cancer, it is not necessarily the green tea that deserves the credit. Green tea drinkers may also tend to exercise more and to eat more healthful foods in general. Maybe it is those habits, and not the tea, that plays the most important role. Researchers try to look closely at the data and eliminate such factors, but it can be very tricky to do so properly.

In Vitro Studies

An in vitro study is a trial that tests a substance in a test tube. Such studies are really only spurs for further research, as they don't prove that a treatment is effective in real life. An herb or supplement taken by mouth must be absorbed into the bloodstream, survive processing by the liver, and still manage to be effective when diluted by the fluids of the body. It's a long leap from a test tube to a treatment that actually works.

Animal Studies

Evidence from studies enrolling animals means more than evidence from in vitro studies. However, because animals may process nutrients and even herbs differently than we do, the results can't be taken as completely reliable.

Statistical Significance

For nearly all types of studies, there is one more step to take that is necessary to interpret the results. A mathematical analysis must be made to see if the results are meaningful.

It is always possible that an apparent result can be just due to chance. For example, if you flip a coin 20 times, and it comes up heads 14 times, does these mean that the coin is biased? Probably not. But if you flip it 4,000 times and it comes up heads 3,500 times, it probably is a trick coin.

Likewise, if a study only enrolls 20 people, the results might be due to chance alone. But results seen in larger studies are more likely to mean something.

Researchers use various statistical methods to analyze the outcome of a study and determine whether the results are meaningful. This analysis is called a test for statistical significance. You can't draw any conclusions from a study if the results are not statistically significant. In this book, unless stated otherwise, all results mentioned were found to be statistically significant according to the mathematical methods used by the researchers.

The Limitations of This Book

Remember that no book can substitute for individualized medical care from a physician. Every person is different and has specific health needs only a doctor can assess. Furthermore, in many cases it is possible to use combinations of treatments—both natural and pharmaceutical—in sophisticated ways that cannot be described in a book of this type. The information contained in the following text should be regarded as an introduction, a suggestion for where to start.

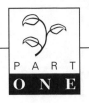

Conditions

ACNE

Principal Proposed Treatments   There are no well-established natural treatments for acne.

Other Proposed Treatments   Zinc, Chromium, Vitamin E, Selenium, Burdock, Red Clover, Tea Tree Oil

---

The blackheads and sometimes painful pimples that we know as acne occur most commonly during adolescence, but they may persist into later life as well. There is much we still don't understand about what causes acne. We do know that during adolescence and other times of hormonal imbalance, such as around menopause, the oil-secreting glands in the skin increase their level of secretions. A combination of naturally occurring yeast and bacteria then breaks down these secretions, causing the skin to become inflamed and the pimples to eventually rupture. In severe cases, acne can lead to permanent scars.

Conventional treatment, which usually is quite successful, consists primarily of antibiotics, cleansing agents, and chemically modified versions of **vitamin A** (see page 432).

PROPOSED TREATMENTS

While there are no dramatically effective alternative treatments for acne, there are a few options that may provide some help.

Warning: Do not rely on any of the treatments discussed in this section to treat severe acne where scarring is a consideration.

Zinc

People with acne have been shown to have lower-than-normal levels of zinc in their bodies.[1–4] However, this doesn't prove that taking zinc supplements will help acne. For example, it is possible that the factors that cause acne also affect zinc levels.

Double-blind studies involving a total of more than 300 people have tried to discover whether taking extra zinc can relieve the symptoms of acne. The results have been generally positive, indicating a definite but somewhat mild effect.

In one of these studies, 54 people were given either placebo or 135 mg of zinc as zinc sulfate daily. Zinc produced slight but measurable benefits.[5] Similar results have been seen in other studies using 90 to 135 mg of zinc daily.[6–10] In some studies, however, no benefits were seen.[11,12]

Two studies have compared zinc against a standard treatment for acne, the antibiotic tetracycline. One found that zinc was as effective as tetracycline,[13] but another found the antibiotic more effective.[14]

However, fairly high dosages of zinc (more than is completely safe) seem to be required to produce these benefits. See the chapter on **zinc** for more information.

Other Herbs and Supplements

Other commonly mentioned natural treatments for acne include **chromium** (see page 251), **vitamin E** (see page 451), **selenium** (see page 407), **burdock** (see page 232), and **red clover** (see page 397). **Tea tree** (see page 421) oil has antiseptic properties and has been suggested as an alternative to benzoyl peroxide for direct application to the skin. There haven't been any solid studies examining these treatments, however.

ALLERGIES

Related Terms   Hay Fever

Principal Proposed Treatments   There are no well-established natural treatments for allergies.

Other Proposed Treatments   Nettle Leaf, Quercetin, OPCs, Other Flavonoids, Vitamin C, Spirulina, Vitamin B$_6$, Vitamin B$_{12}$, Cat's Claw, *Coleus forskohlii*, GLA (Gamma-Linolenic Acid), Fish Oil, MSM, Betaine Hydrochloride, Bee Pollen

*For other types of allergies, see **Asthma** and **Eczema***

About 7% of all Americans suffer from hay fever, an allergic condition that can cause runny nose, sneezing, and teary eyes. It is known officially as *allergic rhinitis, allergic sinusitis,* or *allergic* **conjunctivitis** (see page 55), depending on whether symptoms manifest mainly in the nose, sinuses, or eyes, respectively. Hay fever usually peaks when particular plants are pollinating or when molds are flourishing. People who suffer from year-round hay fever may be allergic to ever-present allergens such as dust mites.

Here's how hay fever works. In response to the triggers noted above, an individual prone to allergies develops an exaggerated immune response. Substances known as IgEs flood the nasal passages, white blood cells called eosinophils arrive by the millions and billions, and inflammatory substances such as histamine, prostaglandins, and leukotrienes are released in massive amounts. The overall effect is the familiar one of swelling, dripping, itching, and aching.

The mechanism of allergic response is fairly well understood. Why allergic people react so excessively to innocent bits of pollen, however, remains a complete mystery.

Conventional treatment for hay fever consists of antihistamines (now available in forms that don't make you sleepy); decongestants, nasal steroids, or cromolyn sodium; and occasionally allergic desensitization ("allergy shots"). For most people, some combination of these treatments will be successful.

PROPOSED TREATMENTS

The following treatments are widely recommended for allergies, but they have not been scientifically proven effective at this time.

Nettle Leaf

According to one preliminary double-blind placebo-controlled study, freeze-dried extract of stinging **nettle leaf** (see page 369) can at least slightly improve allergy symptoms.[1]

A typical dosage is two to three 300 mg capsules of nettle leaf. Nettle leaf has an extensive history of use in food and is believed to be safe. However, safety in young children, pregnant or nursing women, and those with severe liver or kidney disease has not been established.

For theoretical reasons, some researchers suggest that nettle may interact with conventional medications for diabetes and high blood pressure, but no actual problems of this type have been officially reported.

Quercetin, OPCs, and Other Flavonoids

Test tube studies suggest that flavonoids—biologically active compounds found in many plants—may help reduce allergy symptoms.[2–5] A particular flavonoid, **quercetin** (see page 396), seems to be one of the most active.[6–11] Many texts on natural medicine claim that quercetin works like the drug cromolyn (Intal) by stopping the release of allergenic substances in the body. However, while we have direct evidence that cromolyn is effective, there have not been any published studies in which people were given quercetin and their allergic symptoms decreased. It is a long way from test-tube studies to real people. If you do wish to take quercetin, a particular form of the substance, *quercetin chalcone,* may be better absorbed than other forms.

OPCs (see page 373) from grape seed or pine bark are also often said to be effective. But at the present time, we don't really know whether any of these treatments are really helpful for allergies.

Vitamin C

Vitamin C (see page 444) is often suggested as a treatment for allergies, but the research results are very preliminary and somewhat contradictory.[12,13,14]

Other Treatments

Highly preliminary evidence suggests **spirulina** (see page 413) may counter allergic reactions.[15,16]

Vitamin B$_6$ (see page 439), **vitamin B$_{12}$** (see page 442), **cat's claw** (see page 242), *Coleus forskohlii* (see page 259), **GLA** (see page 304), **fish oil** (see page 282), **MSM** (see page 364), and **betaine hydrochloride** (see page 219) are sometimes recommended for hay fever, but there is as yet no significant evidence that they are effective. **Bee pollen** (see page 215) is sometimes suggested for treating hay fever on the theory it might help the body build up resistance to local pollens. However, there is no evidence that it works. In some cases, severe allergic reactions to the bee pollen itself might occur.

ALOPECIA AREATA

Related Terms   Baldness

Principal Proposed Treatments   Essential Oils (Combination of Thyme, Lavender, Rosemary, and Cedarwood)

Other Proposed Treatments   Khellin, Biotin, Zinc, Nickel Sulfate, *Primula obconica*

Baldness (alopecia) that occurs suddenly in a specific area is referred to as alopecia areata. It can strike both men and women at any age, but usually starts during childhood. Unlike male-pattern or female-pattern baldness, which cause hair to thin on the sides, front, and crown of the head, alopecia areata starts with one or more small, round, smooth patches in the scalp or beard area. Rarely, it causes total body hair loss, a condition called alopecia universalis.

Like most types of baldness, alopecia areata has no cure. However, in many cases, hair grows back on its own without treatment. Widespread hair loss is less likely to reverse itself. Corticosteroids injected under the skin may promote some hair growth, but the results usually don't last.

An interesting approach to the treatment of alopecia involves inducing mild allergic reactions using either nickel sulfate or the leaves of the plant *Primula obconica*.[1,2] It appears that when these substances irritate the skin they trigger new hair growth, but larger studies are needed to confirm the findings.

PRINCIPAL PROPOSED TREATMENTS
Essential Oils

One study suggests that a combination of essential oils applied topically may stimulate hair growth in people with alopecia areata.

What Is the Scientific Evidence for Essential Oils?

A double-blind placebo-controlled trial enrolled 84 individuals who massaged either essential oils or a non-treatment oil into their scalps each night for 7 months.[3] The results showed that 44% of those in the treatment group experienced new hair growth compared to only 15% of the control group. The treatment oil contained essential oils of thyme, rosemary, lavender, and cedarwood.

Dosage

In this study, 2 to 3 drops of each essential oil were added to a mixture of grape seed and jojoba oil.

Safety Issues

Although there are no reported side effects associated with using thyme, rosemary, lavender, and cedarwood oils topically, essential oils can be toxic if taken internally. They can also cause allergic reactions, which may be severe, when applied topically.

OTHER PROPOSED TREATMENTS

Very preliminary evidence suggests that topical khellin, an extract of the fruit of the Mediterranean plant khella (*Ammi visnaga*), may promote new hair growth when combined with ultraviolet light (UVA) therapy. Khellin selectively sensitizes the skin to UVA and is related to drugs used to treat **psoriasis** (see page 148).[4]

The supplements **zinc** (see page 463) aspartate and **biotin** (see page 221), taken together in high (and possibly dangerous) doses, have been tried for alopecia areata in children.[5]

Hypnotherapy has also been proposed as a treatment for alopecia areata, but a very small study found it had no effect.[6]

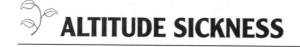

ALTITUDE SICKNESS

Related Terms   Acute Mountain Sickness, High-Altitude Sickness

Principal Proposed Treatments   There are no well-established natural treatments for altitude sickness.

Other Proposed Treatments   *Ginkgo biloba,* High-Carbohydrate Diet, Magnesium, Glutamine, Vitamin C, Vitamin E, Silymarin

Altitude sickness is a set of symptoms caused by the lower pressure and reduced amount of oxygen at high altitudes (above 7,000 feet). The symptoms are headache, fatigue, and nausea, or, in serious cases, extreme fatigue, impaired motor control, and fluid accumulation in the brain and lungs. In general, the greater the altitude and the more rapid the ascent, the greater the likelihood of severe symptoms. Many deaths on Mt. Everest and other high mountains can be attributed to the effects of altitude sickness. However, in most cases, altitude sickness is a benign condition that afflicts people from sea level when they go on a ski vacation or hiking in the mountains.

The best treatment for altitude sickness is prevention. Individuals planning an ascent of high mountains such as Mt. Everest should take as much time as possible to acclimate to the starting elevation. Keep in mind that full adjustment to the reduced oxygen content of the air may take several weeks. In general, ascents should be gradual: one recommendation suggests 2 days for an 8,000-foot elevation gain plus 1 day for each 1,000 to 2,000 feet afterwards.[1]

However, such recommendations are not practical for people who fly to a vacation destination such as a ski resort and must deal with the effects of reduced oxygen all at once. To prevent or treat mild cases of altitude sickness, you should drink plenty of water and avoid alcohol, caffeine, and salty foods. If severe symptoms develop, the best response is to descend as rapidly as possible.

Conventional treatments include acetazolamide or dexamethasone for prevention or treatment of mild altitude sickness, and nifedipine for people prone to pulmonary edema.[2] Ibuprofen and related drugs may help with headache.

PROPOSED TREATMENTS

While there are no well-documented natural treatments for altitude sickness, there are a few options that may provide some help.

Ginkgo biloba

A double-blind placebo-controlled study of 44 mountaineers on a Himalayan expedition found that 80 mg twice daily of standardized **ginkgo** (see page 298) extract prevented symptoms of mountain sickness as well as symptoms related to cold extremities.[3]

Ginkgo appears to be safe. Extremely high doses have been given to animals for long periods of time without serious consequences.[4] Safety in young children, pregnant or nursing women, or those with severe liver or kidney disease, however, has not been established.

However, ginkgo "thins" the blood and might cause bleeding problems.[5,6] For this reason, it should not be used before surgery or labor and delivery; it also should not be combined with blood-thinning drugs such as Coumadin (warfarin), heparin, aspirin, and Trental (pentoxifylline). It is also possible that ginkgo could cause bleeding problems if combined with natural blood thinners, such as garlic and high-dose vitamin E.

High-Carbohydrate Diet

High-carbohydrate meals are often recommended for preventing altitude sickness. The reasoning is that carbohydrate ingestion increases carbon dioxide production, which in turn stimulates an increased rate of breathing.[7] However, studies on the subject have produced somewhat contradictory results.[8,9,10]

Other Treatments

Very weak evidence suggests that **magnesium** (see page 351), **glutamine** (see page 310), **vitamin C** (see page 444), **vitamin E** (see page 451), and **silymarin** (see page 361), alone or in combination, may be helpful in preventing altitude sickness. However, there is no real evidence as yet that any of these treatments are effective.

ALZHEIMER'S DISEASE, NON-ALZHEIMER'S DEMENTIA, AND NORMAL AGE-RELATED MEMORY LOSS

Principal Proposed Treatments Ginkgo, Phosphatidylserine, Acetyl-L-Carnitine, Huperzine A, Vinpocetine

Other Proposed Treatments Vitamin E, DHEA (Dehydroepiandrosterone), DMAE, Inositol, Magnesium, NADH, Phosphatidylcholine, Lecithin, Choline, Pregnenolone, Vitamin B$_1$, Vitamin B$_{12}$, Vitamin C, Zinc, Bee Pollen

Most people over the age of 40 experience some memory loss. We don't know what causes this normal experience, and there is no conventional treatment available to treat it. As we shall see in this chapter, there are a few natural treatments that might be helpful.

Alzheimer's disease is much more serious than ordinary forgetfulness. It leads to severe mental deterioration (dementia) in the elderly. It has been estimated that 30 to 50% of people over 85 years old suffer from this disease.

Microscopic examination shows that nerve cells in the thinking parts of the brain have died and disappeared, particularly cells that release a chemical called acetylcholine. However, we do not know exactly what causes Alzheimer's disease.

Alzheimer's begins with subtle symptoms, such as loss of memory for names and recent events. It progresses from difficulty learning new information, to a few eccentric behaviors, to depression, loss of spontaneity, and anxiety. Over the course of the disease, the individual gradually loses the ability to carry out the activities of everyday life. Disorientation, asking questions repeatedly, and an inability to recognize friends are characteristics of moderately severe Alzheimer's. Eventually, virtually all mental functions fail.

Similar symptoms may be caused by conditions other than Alzheimer's disease, such as multiple small strokes (called multi-infarct, or vascular, dementia), alcoholism, and certain rarer causes. It is very important to begin with an examination to discover what is causing the symptoms of mental decline. Various easily treatable conditions, such as depression, can mimic the symptoms of dementia.

Once the diagnosis of Alzheimer's or non-Alzheimer's dementia has been made, treatment may begin with drugs such as Cognex or Aricept. These medications usually produce a modest improvement in mild to moderate Alzheimer's disease by increasing the duration of action of acetylcholine. However, they can cause sometimes severe side effects due to the exaggeration of acetylcholine's action in other parts of the body.

PRINCIPAL PROPOSED TREATMENTS

There are at least three natural treatments for Alzheimer's disease with significant scientific evidence behind them: ginkgo, phosphatidylserine, and acetyl-L-carnitine. Huperzine A and vinpocetine, while not technically natural substances, may also improve mental function. There is some evidence that ginkgo and phosphatidylserine might be helpful for normal age-related memory loss as well.

Ginkgo: Strong Evidence It Improves Memory and Mental Function

The most well-established herbal treatment for Alzheimer's disease (and, indeed, one of the few herbs that probably deserves the description "proven effective") is the ancient herb *Ginkgo biloba*. **Ginkgo** (see page 298), the oldest surviving species of tree, has been traced back 300 million years. Although it died out in Europe during the Ice Age, ginkgo survived in China, Japan, and other parts of East Asia. It has been cultivated extensively for both ceremonial and medical purposes, and some especially revered trees have been lovingly tended for over 1,000 years. Asian herbalists used ginkgo seeds to treat asthma and other conditions.

In Europe, researchers focused on ginkgo leaf, using standardized extracts of it rather than the whole herb. By 1995, ginkgo leaf extract had become the most widely prescribed herb in Germany. Today, German family physicians generally favor it above all drug treatments for dementia.[1]

Ginkgo also appears to be helpful for normal age-related memory loss.

What Is the Scientific Evidence for Ginkgo?

Alzheimer's Disease and Non-Alzheimer's Dementia The scientific record for ginkgo in these conditions is extensive and impressive. According to a 1992 article published in *Lancet,* over 40 double-blind controlled trials had been performed by that date, evaluating the benefits of ginkgo in treating severe age-related mental decline.[2] Of these studies, which involved about 1,000 participants, eight were rated of good quality and all but one produced positive results. Most of these studies were performed prior to a full recognition of the identity of Alzheimer's disease, but they are presumed to have involved both Alzheimer's and non-Alzheimer's cases. The

authors of the *Lancet* article felt that the evidence was strong enough to conclude that ginkgo extract is an effective treatment for severe age-related mental decline.

Studies since 1992 have provided additional evidence for this conclusion.[3,4] Interestingly, German physicians are so certain that ginkgo is effective that they find it difficult to perform scientific studies of the herb. To them, it is unethical to give a placebo to people with Alzheimer's when they could be taking ginkgo instead and have additional months of useful life ahead.[5] This objection does not apply in the United States, where ginkgo is not an approved treatment.

A recent study published in the *Journal of the American Medical Association* reported the results of a year-long, double-blind trial of ginkgo in over 300 people with Alzheimer's or non-Alzheimer's dementia.[6] Participants were given either 40 mg of the ginkgo extract or a placebo 3 times daily. The results showed that 27% of the treated group showed significant improvement on an overall rating scale that evaluates the severity of Alzheimer's disease, compared to only 14% in the placebo group. Also, 40% of those given placebo worsened over the course of the study, whereas only 19% of the treated participants worsened.

The study's authors interpret these statistics to mean that in about 20% of cases, ginkgo may slow the development of Alzheimer's disease by 6 months to 1 year. These results do not make ginkgo out to be a miracle cure, but they do confirm that it is a useful treatment for dementia.

Ordinary Age-Related Memory Loss   The results of four double-blind studies suggest that ginkgo might be useful for ordinary age-related memory loss as well.

In a double-blind placebo-controlled trial, 241 seniors complaining of mildly impaired memory were given either placebo or low-dose or high-dose ginkgo for 24 weeks.[7] The results showed modest improvements in certain types of memory, especially in the low-dose ginkgo group.

A double-blind placebo-controlled trial examined the effects of ginkgo extract in 40 men and women (ages 55 to 86) who did not suffer from any mental impairment.[8] Over a 6-week period, the results showed improvements in measurements of mental function.

Another double-blind trial of 26 individuals found that a single dose of ginkgo extract improved short-term memory, especially in people over 50.[9]

Finally, a fourth trial followed 60 individuals aged 61 to 88 years who suffered from mild to moderate mental impairment.[10] They were divided into three groups: placebo, 120 mg of ginkgo daily, or 240 mg of ginkgo daily. Over a period of 3 months, participants treated with the 120 mg of standardized ginkgo extract showed distinct and significant improvement in mental function as compared to placebo. Interestingly, the higher dose of ginkgo did not prove any better than the placebo.

How Does Ginkgo Work?

In the past, scientists believed that dementia was caused by a reduced blood and oxygen supply to the brain. Because ginkgo appears to improve circulation (as described in the chapter on **intermittent claudication**), European physicians assumed that ginkgo was simply getting more blood to brain cells and thereby making them work better. However, advances in the understanding of age-related mental decline have led scientists to move away from this theory. Ginkgo is now believed to function by directly stimulating nerve cell activity and protecting nerve cells from further injury.[11]

Dosage

The standard dosage of ginkgo is 40 to 80 mg 3 times daily of a 50:1 extract standardized to contain 24% ginkgo-flavone glycosides.

Safety Issues

Ginkgo appears to be very safe. Extremely high doses have been given to animals for long periods of time without serious consequences.[12]

In all the clinical trials of ginkgo up to 1991, which have involved almost 10,000 people, the incidence of side effects produced by ginkgo extract was extremely small. Only 21 cases of gastrointestinal discomfort were reported, and even fewer cases of headaches, dizziness, and allergic skin reactions.[13]

However, ginkgo is known to "thin" the blood, and highly regarded journals have reported cases of bleeding in the skull and the iris chamber associated with ginkgo use.[14,15] For this reason, ginkgo should not be combined with drugs that also thin the blood, such as Coumadin (warfarin), heparin, Trental (pentoxifylline), or even aspirin. In most German studies of ginkgo, participants were not allowed to take any blood thinners. There may conceivably be risks in combining ginkgo with natural substances that thin the blood as well, such as garlic and high-dose vitamin E, although there have been no reports of such problems. Ginkgo should also be used with caution, if at all, by those with bleeding disorders such as hemophilia, or during the periods before or after surgery and prior to labor and delivery.

Safety for pregnant or nursing women and those with severe liver or kidney disease has not been established.

Phosphatidylserine: Good Evidence of Effectiveness

Like ginkgo, the supplement **phosphatidylserine** (PS; see page 387) is widely used in Europe to treat various forms of dementia as well as normal age-related memory loss. Phosphatidylserine is one of the many substances involved in the structure and maintenance of cell membranes. While it is tempting to speculate that phosphatidylserine works by strengthening nerve cells

against damage, we really don't know how this supplement works.

What Is the Scientific Evidence for Phosphatidylserine?

Overall, the evidence for PS in dementia is quite strong. Double-blind studies involving a total of over 1,000 people suggest that phosphatidylserine (at least the type from a cow's brain) is an effective treatment for Alzheimer's disease and other forms of dementia.

The largest of these studies followed 494 elderly subjects in northeastern Italy over a course of 6 months.[16] All suffered from moderate to severe mental decline, as measured by standard tests. Treatment consisted of either 300 mg daily of PS or placebo. The group that took PS did significantly better in both behavior and mental function than the placebo group. Symptoms of depression also improved.

These results agree with those of numerous smaller double-blind studies involving a total of over 500 people with Alzheimer's and other types of age-related dementia.[17–24]

There is some evidence that PS can also help people with ordinary age-related memory loss. In one double-blind study that enrolled 149 individuals with memory loss but not dementia, phosphatidylserine provided significant benefits as compared with placebo.[25] Individuals with the most severe memory loss showed the most improvement.

Dosage

The standard dosage of phosphatidylserine is 100 mg 2 to 3 times daily; however, some studies have used 200 mg twice daily. After full effects are achieved, a lower dosage of 100 mg daily may be sufficient to maintain good results.

Safety Issues

Phosphatidylserine is generally regarded as safe. Side effects are rare and are typically limited to mild gastrointestinal distress. However, there are concerns that phosphatidylserine may interact with the blood-thinning drug heparin.[26] Maximum safe doses in young children, pregnant or nursing women, and those with severe liver or kidney disease have not been established.

Acetyl-L-Carnitine: May Be Slightly Helpful

Carnitine (see page 238) is a vitamin-like substance that is often used for **angina** (see page 10), **congestive heart failure** (see page 54), and other heart conditions. A special form of carnitine, acetyl-L-carnitine, sometimes called L-acetyl-carnitine, appears to be useful in Alzheimer's disease. Although we don't know precisely how it works, it may mimic the effects of the naturally occurring brain chemical acetylcholine, which is found in lower-than-normal levels in the brains of people with Alzheimer's disease.

What Is the Scientific Evidence for Acetyl-L-Carnitine?

Numerous double- or single-blind studies involving a total of more than 1,400 people have evaluated the potential benefits of acetyl-L-carnitine in the treatment of Alzheimer's disease and other forms of dementia.[27–37] Most have found at least mildly positive results. However, the benefits are slight at most, and one of the best-designed studies found no benefit.

One of these studies followed 130 people with the clinical diagnosis of Alzheimer's disease for 1 year.[38] The treated group showed a slower rate of deterioration in 13 of 14 measurements of dementia. However, one recent large study failed to find any statistically significant benefit.[39] The probable explanation is that acetyl-L-carnitine is only slightly effective.

Dosage

A typical dosage of acetyl-L-carnitine is 500 to 1,000 mg 3 times daily.

Safety Issues

Acetyl-L-carnitine appears to be a very safe substance.[40] However, individuals on dialysis should not receive this (or any other supplement) without a physician's supervision. The maximum safe dosages in pregnant or nursing women and those with severe liver or kidney disease have not been established.

Huperzine A: More Like a Drug Than an Herb

Huperzine A (see page 327) is an extremely potent chemical derived from a particular type of club moss (*Huperzia serrata* [Thumb] Trev.). Like caffeine and cocaine, huperzine A is a medicinally active, plant-derived chemical that belongs to the class known as alkaloids. It was first isolated in 1948 by Chinese scientists.[41] This substance is really more a drug than an herb, but it is sold over the counter as a dietary supplement for memory loss and mental impairment.

What Is the Scientific Evidence for Huperzine A?

Many experiments have found that huperzine A can improve memory skills in aged animals as well as in younger animals whose memories have been deliberately impaired.[42–57]

All clinical trials of huperzine to date were performed in China and reported in Chinese.

A double-blind placebo-controlled study evaluated 103 people with Alzheimer's disease who received either huperzine A or placebo twice daily for 8 weeks.[58] About 60% of the treated participants showed improvements in memory, thinking, and behavioral functions compared to 36% of the placebo-treated group, and the difference was significant.

Benefits were also seen in an earlier double-blind trial using injected huperzine in 160 individuals with dementia or other memory disorders.[59]

However, another double-blind trial of 60 individuals with Alzheimer's disease found no significant difference in symptoms between the treated and the placebo groups.[60]

Huperzine is also reportedly helpful for improving memory in healthy individuals. A double-blind trial of 34 matching pairs of junior middle school students reported improvements in memory in the treated group.[61]

Huperzine A inhibits the enzyme acetylcholinesterase. This enzyme breaks down acetylcholine, which seems to play an important role in mental function. When the enzyme that breaks it down is inhibited, acetylcholine levels in the brain tend to rise. Drugs that inhibit acetylcholinesterase (such as tacrine and donepezil) seem to improve memory and mental functioning in people with Alzheimer's and other severe conditions. The research on huperzine A indicates that it works in much the same way.

The chemical action of huperzine A is very precise and specific. It "fits" into a niche on the enzyme where acetylcholine is supposed to attach.[62,63] Because huperzine A is in the way, the enzyme can't grab and destroy acetylcholine. This mechanism has been demonstrated by considerable scientific work, including sophisticated computer modeling of the shape of the molecule.[64]

Although it originally comes from a plant, huperzine A is highly purified in a laboratory and is just a single chemical. It is just not much like an herb. Herbs contain hundreds or thousands of chemicals. In this way, huperzine A resembles drugs such as digoxin, codeine, Sudafed, and vincristine (a chemotherapy drug), which are also highly purified chemicals taken from plants. If we wish to call huperzine A a natural treatment, we need to call these (and dozens of other standard drugs) natural as well.

Dosage

Huperzine A is a highly potent compound with a recommended dose of only 100 to 200 mcg twice a day for age-related memory loss. We recommend using it only under a doctor's supervision.

Safety Issues

Perhaps because it works so specifically, huperzine A appears to have few side effects. However, children, pregnant or nursing women, or those with high blood pressure or severe liver or kidney disease should not take huperzine A except on a doctor's recommendation. We also don't know whether huperzine A interacts adversely with any drugs.

Vinpocetine: Appears to Be Effective, but Is Not a Natural Substance

Vinpocetine (see page 431) is a chemical derived from vincamine, a constituent found in the leaves of common periwinkle (*Vinca minor* L.) as well as the seeds of various African plants. It is used as a treatment for memory loss and mental impairment.

Developed in Hungary over 20 years ago, vinpocetine is sold in Europe as a drug under the name Cavinton. In the United States it is available as a "dietary supplement," although the substance probably doesn't fit that category by any rational definition. Vinpocetine doesn't exist to any significant extent in nature. Producing it requires significant chemical work performed in the laboratory.

What Is the Scientific Evidence for Vinpocetine?

A significant level of evidence supports the idea that vinpocetine can enhance memory and mental function, especially in those with Alzheimer's disease and related conditions. It may also be helpful for those with ordinary age-related memory loss, although this has not been proven.

One 3-month double-blind placebo-controlled study followed 84 individuals with age-related mental impairment.[65] According to several standard rating scales, the severity of the illness improved by a statistically significant margin in the treatment group as compared to the placebo group. Similarly positive results have been seen in many other studies,[66] although at least one study did not find benefit.[67]

We don't know how vinpocetine works, although there are numerous theories. There is some evidence that vinpocetine can safeguard brain cells against damage caused by lack of oxygen.[68] However, whether this effect really has anything to do with vinpocetine's effects on mental function remains unclear.

Dosage

Vinpocetine is available in 10-mg capsules, usually taken 3 times per day. This supplement is probably best taken with meals, as it is better absorbed that way.[69] We recommend that it be used only on physician advice.

Safety Issues

No serious side effects have been reported in any of the clinical trials. However, there are some concerns that vinpocetine might impair the effectiveness of Coumadin (warfarin).[70] Safety in pregnant or nursing women, young children, or those with severe liver or kidney disease has not been established.

OTHER PROPOSED TREATMENTS

Preliminary evidence suggests that **vitamin E** (see page 451) at the high dosage of 2,000 IU (dl-alpha-tocopherol) daily may slow the progression of Alzheimer's disease.[71] A physician's supervision is essential when taking this much vitamin E due to potential risks of bleeding complications.

An observational study suggests that regular use of vitamin E and vitamin C supplements might help prevent vascular dementia, but not Alzheimer's disease.[72] Another study suggests that a diet high in vegetables as well as vitamins E and C from food sources may help prevent Alzheimer's disease and other forms of dementia.[73]

DHEA (see page 268),[74] **DMAE** (see page 270),[75,76] **inositol** (see page 330), **magnesium** (see page 351), **NADH** (see page 368), **pregnenolone** (see page 391), **vitamin B$_1$** (see page 434), **vitamin B$_{12}$** (see page 442), **vitamin C** (see page 444), **zinc** (see page 463), and **bee pollen** (see page 215) have also been suggested as treatments for Alzheimer's disease. However, as yet there is no real scientific evidence to confirm or deny their effectiveness.

The related substances **choline** (see page 248), phosphatidylcholine, and **lecithin** (see page 343) have been studied quite extensively in individuals with Alzheimer's disease and other conditions involving the brain.[77–85] The impetus for this research is the fact that an important neurotransmitter, acetylcholine, is made from choline. However, several studies, some of them double-blind, have not found any benefit from taking these supplements for Alzheimer's disease.[86–90]

AMYOTROPHIC LATERAL SCLEROSIS

Related Terms   Lou Gehrig's Disease, ALS

Principal Proposed Treatments   There are no well-established natural treatments for amyotrophic lateral sclerosis.

Other Proposed Treatments   BCAAs, L-Threonine, Creatine, Vitamin B$_{12}$, CoQ$_{10}$, Genistein, Guanidine

Visit Us at TNP.com

Amyotrophic lateral sclerosis (ALS) is a nerve disorder that causes progressive muscle weakness. It usually begins with weakness in the hands or feet, which then spreads to the rest of the body. Affected muscles become spastic (tight and prone to spasm) and ineffective. As the weakness spreads, speaking, breathing, and swallowing become difficult. ALS is always fatal, and most people die within 3 years of being diagnosed. However, for reasons that are unclear, some individuals (such as the physicist Stephen Hawking) live much longer.

The cause of ALS is unknown and there is no cure for the disorder. Physical therapy can help the muscles maintain strength and flexibility for a time. Drugs such as baclofen may reduce muscle spasms and cramping. Eventually, individuals with ALS must be fed through a tube and sustained on a ventilator.

PROPOSED TREATMENTS

BCAAs: Mixed Results

BCAAs (branched-chain amino acids; see page 213) are most well-known as a **sports supplement** (see page 158), but have also been tried as a treatment for ALS. The theory behind this treatment is that people with ALS might not metabolize the substance glutamate properly. Glutamate plays a major role in nerve function. Since BCAAs help the body to metabolize glutamate, they could be useful for ALS. However, at best, BCAAs have been found only modestly effective in ALS, and study results have been mixed.[1–6]

One very small double-blind placebo-controlled study found that people treated with BCAAs for one year maintained muscle strength and the ability to walk longer than those on placebo.[7] However, other studies found no effect,[8,9] and one actually found a slight in-crease in deaths during the study period among those treated with BCAAs compared to placebo.[10]

L-Threonine

L-threonine, an essential amino acid, has been tried for ALS because, like BCAAs, it affects glutamate metabolism. Open trials and one double-blind study have shown some short-term improvement in symptoms, but in other research the results have not been impressive.[11–14]

Creatine

Another sports supplement, **creatine** (see page 264), has been tried for ALS based on studies showing that it can improve muscle performance in certain situations. Evidence from animal and open human trials suggest that creatine may improve strength and slow the progression of the disease.[15,16,17] However, double-blind human studies are needed to discover whether creatine is truly a useful treatment for ALS.

Other Treatments

Other nutrients that have been tried for ALS with some promising results include **vitamin B$_{12}$** (see page 442), **CoQ$_{10}$** (see page 256), **genistein** (see page 294), and guanidine.[18–22] However, there is no solid evidence as yet that they are effective.

Numerous other nutritional supplements have been tried for ALS that appear to be ineffective. These include multivitamins, **vitamin E** (see page 451), AMP, and octacosanol.[23,24]

One very small trial tested a combination pill containing amino acids, antioxidants, and the calcium channel–blocker nimodipine, finding some evidence that it might slow the progression of the disease.[25]

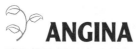

ANGINA

Principal Proposed Treatments   L-Carnitine and L-Propionyl-Carnitine

Other Proposed Treatments   Coenzyme Q$_{10}$ (CoQ$_{10}$), Magnesium, Hawthorn, Khella, *Coleus forskohlii*, Vitamin E

Essentially, angina is a muscle cramp in the heart—the one muscle that cannot take a rest. It develops when the heart muscle does not receive enough oxygen for its needs.

People usually experience angina as a squeezing chest pain, similar to a heavy weight or a tight band, accompanied by sweating, shortness of breath, and possibly pain radiating into the left arm or neck. Usually, angina is brought on by exercise—the more rapidly the heart pumps, the more oxygen it needs. Atherosclerosis (hardening of the arteries) is the most common cause of angina.

Conventional treatment for angina is very effective. Drugs that expand (dilate) the heart's arteries, such as nitroglycerin, can give immediate relief. Other drugs help over the long term by making the heart's work easier. Surgical treatments (such as angioplasty and coronary artery bypass grafting) physically widen the blood vessels that feed the heart.

To prevent heart attacks, current recommendations suggest that most people take daily doses of aspirin, make lifestyle changes such as diet and exercise to lower cholesterol, and reduce other factors that accelerate atherosclerosis.

PRINCIPAL PROPOSED TREATMENTS

Angina is a serious disease that absolutely requires conventional medical evaluation and supervision. No one should self-treat for angina. However, alternative treatments can provide a useful adjunct to standard medical care when monitored by an appropriate health-care professional. We intentionally do not give dosages in this section as they should be individualized by your physician; however, you can find general guidelines in the separate chapters on each substance.

L-Carnitine

Studies suggest that the vitamin-like substance **L-carnitine** (see page 238) can relieve angina symptoms. Carnitine plays a role in the cellular production of energy. Although carnitine does not address the cause of angina, it appears to help the heart produce energy more efficiently, thereby enabling it to get by with less oxygen.

In a controlled study involving 200 participants, carnitine improved angina symptoms in people also taking standard medications.[1] Over the 6 months of the study, the carnitine-treated group showed significant improvement in exercise tolerance and a lower incidence of abnormal electrocardiogram readings. Side effects were negligible. A special form of carnitine known as L-propionyl-carnitine also appears to be effective.[2] Consult with your physician regarding dosage and specific safety issues.

OTHER PROPOSED TREATMENTS

Coenzyme Q$_{10}$ (CoQ$_{10}$; see page 256) is best known as a treatment for congestive heart failure, but it may offer benefits in angina as well.[3] **Magnesium** (see page 351) has also shown some promise.[4] **N-acetyl cysteine** (see page 366) may be helpful when taken along with the drug nitroglycerin, but severe headaches may develop.[5,6,7] The herbs **hawthorn** (see page 320), khella, and **Coleus forskohlii** (see page 259) may also be useful, but as yet there is little evidence that they work. **Vitamin E** (see page 451) has been found only slightly effective, and **beta-carotene** (see page 217) may actually increase angina.[8]

Lifestyle Approaches

In the long term, restoring your heart's arteries back to normal is the best thing you can do for your angina. The famous Lifestyle Heart Trial, conducted by Dr. Dean Ornish, showed that people who adopt a lowfat vegetarian diet and other healthful lifestyle habits can actually reverse the level of blockage in their coronary arteries.[9]

Absolute vegetarianism is not essential for good results. In general, eating a diet low in red meat and high in whole grains and fresh fruits and vegetables seems wise. Olive oil and canola oil appear to be among the healthiest vegetable oils for use in cooking. For additional suggestions, see the chapter on **atherosclerosis.**

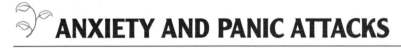

ANXIETY AND PANIC ATTACKS

Principal Proposed Treatments   Kava

Other Proposed Treatments   Valerian, 5-HTP (5-Hydroxytryptophan), Melatonin, Chamomile, Gamma Oryzanol, Hops, Lemon Balm, Passionflower, Skullcap, Suma, Inositol (for Panic Disorder), Selenium, Flaxseed Oil, General Multivitamin, GABA

As Kierkegaard pointed out long ago, we live in the age of anxiety. Most of us suffer from chronic anxiety to some extent because modern life is jagged, fast-paced, and divorced from the natural rhythms that tend to create a harmonious inner life. The calming cycles of farming, the instinctive satisfactions of hunting and gathering, and pure faith in religion gave our ancestors inner resources that few of us possess today.

People who suffer from the emotional illness called anxiety disorder, however, go a step beyond this common feeling. The quality of their lives is significantly diminished by the pervading presence of fear, which is often unrelated to any obvious cause. Even if a cause can be identified, the magnitude of anxiety they experience is greater than the actual degree of stress.

Typical symptoms of anxiety disorder include feelings of tension, irritability, worry, frustration, turmoil, and hopelessness, along with insomnia, restless sleep, grinding of teeth, jaw pain, an inability to sit still, and an incapacity to cope. Physical sensations frequently arise as well, including a characteristic feeling of being unable to take a full, satisfying breath; dry mouth; rapid heartbeat; heart palpitations; a lump in the throat; tightness in the chest; and cramping in the bowels. Anxiety can also give rise to panic attacks. These may be so severe that they are mistaken for heart attacks. The heart pounds and palpitates, the chest feels tight and painful, and the whole body tenses with unreasoning fear. Such attacks can be triggered by anxiety-provoking situations, but they may also come out of nowhere, perhaps even

Anxiety and Panic Attacks

awakening you from sleep. When a person tends to suffer more from panic attacks than generalized anxiety, physicians call the illness *panic disorder.*

The medical treatment of anxiety involves mainly antianxiety drugs. Some, such as Xanax, are effective immediately; others, such as BuSpar, take a week or more to reach full effect. Antidepressant drugs may also be helpful. Panic attacks are generally more difficult to treat than other aspects of anxiety.

Medications are best used in the short term, and it is advisable to seek more permanent help through psychotherapy.

PRINCIPAL PROPOSED TREATMENTS

The herb kava is widely used in Europe as a medical treatment for anxiety.

Kava: Widely Used in Europe for Anxiety

In Europe, the herb **kava** (see page 338) is widely prescribed for anxiety. Kava is a member of the pepper family that has long been cultivated by Pacific Islanders for use as a social and ceremonial drink. The first description of kava came to the West from Captain James Cook on his celebrated voyages through the South Seas. Cook reported that when village elders and chieftains occasionally gathered for significant meetings, they would hold an elaborate kava ceremony at the beginning to break the ice. Typically, each participant would drink two or three bowls of chewed-up kava mixed with coconut milk. They also drank kava in less formal social settings as a mild intoxicant.

When European scientists learned about kava's effects, they set to work trying to isolate its active principles. However, it was not until 1966 that substances named kavalactones were isolated and shown to be effective on their own. One of the most active of these is the chemical dihydrokavain, which has been found to produce a sedative, painkilling, and anticonvulsant action.[1,2,3] Other named kavalactones include kavain, methysticin, and dihydromethysticin.

High doses of kava extracts cause muscular relaxation and, at very high doses, paralysis without loss of consciousness.[4–7] Kava is also a local anesthetic, producing peculiar numbing sensations when held in the mouth.

Germany's Commission E, that country's official herb-regulating body, has authorized the use of kava as a medical treatment for "states of nervous anxiety, tension, and agitation." It is also used for **insomnia** (see page 103).

What Is the Scientific Evidence for Kava?

According to double-blind studies involving a total of about 400 participants, kava appears to be an effective treatment for symptoms of anxiety. The best study was a 6-month, double-blind trial that tested kava's effectiveness in 100 individuals with various forms of anxiety.[8] Over the course of the trial, they were evaluated with a list of questions called the Hamilton Anxiety Scale (HAM-A). The HAM-A assigns a total score based on symptoms such as restlessness, nervousness, heart palpitations, stomach discomfort, dizziness, and chest pain. Lower scores indicate reduced anxiety.

Although it took a while for results to develop, by 8 weeks participants who were given kava showed significantly improved HAM-A scores compared to the placebo group. These good results were sustained throughout the duration of the treatment. Interestingly, previous studies had shown a good response in 1 week, especially in menopause-related anxiety.[9,10,11] How fast does kava really work? We will need additional research to know for sure, but you should probably give it a couple of months before deciding whether it works for you.

Another study compared kava against standard antianxiety drugs. For a period of 6 weeks, 174 people with symptoms of anxiety were given either kava or one of two antianxiety medications (oxazepam or bromazepam).[12] Improvement in HAM-A scores was about the same in both groups. However, for technical reasons this study didn't actually prove that kava is equally effective as those standard medications.

Although we don't know exactly how kava functions in the body, its method of action seems to involve brain receptors for a substance known as gamma-aminobutyric acid (GABA).[13] This would make it similar to benzodiazepine drugs like Valium and Xanax. GABA is believed to play a role in anxiety that is somewhat similar to serotonin's role in depression, although there are many gaps in our knowledge.

Dosage

Kava is usually sold in a standardized form for which the total dose of kavalactones per pill is listed. The dose used should supply about 40 to 70 mg of kavalactones 3 times daily. The total daily dosage should not exceed 300 mg of kavalactones. Be patient, because the benefits may take a while to develop (see What Is the Scientific Evidence for Kava?).

Safety Issues

When used appropriately, kava appears to be safe. Animal studies have shown that doses up to 4 times the normal dose cause no problems at all, and 13 times the normal dose causes only mild problems in rats.[14]

A study of 4,049 participants who took a rather low dose of kava (70 mg of kavalactones daily) for 7 weeks found side effects in 1.5% of cases. These were mostly mild gastrointestinal complaints and allergic rashes.[15] A 4-week study of 3,029 individuals given 240 mg of kavalactones daily showed a 2.3% incidence of basically the same side effects.[16] However, long-term use (months

Visit Us at TNP.com

to years) of kava in excess of 400 mg kavalactones per day can create a distinctive generalized dry, scaly rash called "kava dermopathy."[17] It disappears promptly when the kava use stops.

One case report suggests that a kava product might have caused liver inflammation in a 39-year-old woman.[18] However, because the product was not analyzed, it isn't clear whether kava itself or a contaminant was responsible; the authors also could not rule out other causes of liver inflammation.

Kava does not appear to produce mental cloudiness.[19,20] Nonetheless, we wouldn't recommend driving after using kava until you discover how strongly it affects you. It makes some people quite drowsy.

High doses of kava are known to cause inebriation. For this reason, there is some concern that it could become an herb of abuse. There have been reports of young people trying to get high by taking products they thought contained kava. One of these products, fX, turned out to contain dangerous drugs but no kava at all. European physicians have not reported any problems with kava addiction.[21]

One study suggests that kava does not amplify the effects of alcohol.[22] However, there is a case report indicating that kava can increase the effects of other sedatives.[23] For this reason, kava should not be combined with alcohol, prescription tranquilizers or sedatives, or other depressant drugs. Kava should also not be used by individuals who have had dystonic reactions from antipsychotic drugs, or who have Parkinson's disease, due to the risk of increased problems with movement.[24]

Germany's Commission E warns against the use of kava during pregnancy and nursing. Safety in young children and those with severe liver or kidney disease has also not been established.

Transitioning from Medications to Kava

If you are taking Xanax or other drugs in the benzodiazepine family, switching to kava will be very difficult. You must seek a doctor's supervision because withdrawal symptoms can be severe and even life-threatening. Additionally, if you are taking Xanax on an "as needed" basis to stop acute panic attacks, kava cannot be expected to have the same rapidity of action.

It is easier to make the switch from milder antianxiety drugs, such as BuSpar, and antidepressants. Nonetheless, a doctor's supervision is still strongly advised.

OTHER PROPOSED TREATMENTS

The following natural treatments are widely recommended for anxiety, but they have not been scientifically proven effective at this time.

Valerian: May Provide Calming Effects

The herb **valerian** (see page 428) is best known as a remedy for insomnia. However, according to one preliminary double-blind study, it also produces calming effects in stressful situations.[25] The standard dosage is 2 to 3 g twice daily.

Valerian is generally regarded as safe. However, safety in young children, pregnant or nursing women, and those with severe liver or kidney disease has not been established.

Other Herbs and Supplements

Preliminary evidence suggests that the supplement **5-HTP** (see page 198), more commonly used for depression, might also be helpful for anxiety.[26]

Based on its ability to promote sleep, **melatonin** (see page 357) has been tried as a treatment for reducing anxiety while waiting for surgery to begin. A double-blind placebo-controlled study of 75 women waiting for surgery compared melatonin against a standard treatment[27] and found it somewhat effective. Whether melatonin is effective for other forms of anxiety has not been determined.

Other herbs or supplements that are frequently recommended for anxiety include **chamomile** (see page 244), **gamma oryzanol** (see page 290), **hops** (see page 324), **lemon balm** (see page 359), **passionflower** (see page 382), **skullcap** (see page 410), and **suma** (see page 420), as well as **inositol** (see page 330) for panic disorder.

Supplementation with **selenium** (see page 407) (200 mcg daily), **flaxseed oil** (see page 285) (2 to 6 tablespoons daily), or a general multivitamin are all said to help relieve anxiety symptoms in some people.

GABA: No Evidence That It Is Effective

Because GABA (gamma-aminobutyric acid) is known to play a central role in anxiety, some alternative practitioners suggest simply taking this amino acid as a supplement. However, no scientific evidence suggests that orally ingested GABA gets to where it can do any good.

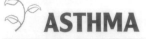

ASTHMA

Principal Proposed Treatments   Tylophora, Boswellia, *Coleus forskohlii,* Vitamin C, Ephedra (Unsafe)

Other Proposed Treatments   Vitamin B$_{12}$, Quercetin, Vitamin B$_6$, Butterbur, Elimination Diet
Antioxidants: Vitamin E, Beta-Carotene, Selenium
Essential Fatty Acids: GLA from Evening Primrose Oil, Fish Oil, Flaxseed Oil
Magnesium, Aloe, Chamomile, Damiana, Elecampane, Garlic, Grindelia, Licorice, Marshmallow, Mullein, Onion, Reishi, Yerba Santa, Betaine Hydrochloride, Lobelia Inflata

Asthma

Visit Us at TNP.com

People who are having an asthma attack have real trouble taking a breath. Many people with stuffy noses from hay fever or colds say, "I can't breathe," but they retain the option of breathing through the mouth. Asthmatics, however, know what "I can't breathe" really means. Instead of their nasal passages, it is the bronchial tubes in their lungs that become swollen and clogged. Breathing can become frighteningly difficult.

Asthma involves two conditions: (1) contraction of the small muscles surrounding the bronchial tubes and (2) swelling of the lining of those tubes. Until recently, treatment usually addressed the first aspect of asthma; but in the last decade, it has become clear that tissue swelling is more fundamental.

Conventional medical treatment for asthma involves bronchodilators, which relax the bronchial muscles, and anti-inflammatory medication, which helps relieve the swelling of tissue. The most effective treatments for reducing this inflammation are steroids, inhalable forms of which have been developed that do not cause as many side effects as oral drugs, such as prednisone. Nonsteroidal drugs, such as cromolyn (Intal), are also available.

The conventional treatment of asthma is highly effective in most cases.

PRINCIPAL PROPOSED TREATMENTS

Perhaps the most promising natural treatment for asthma is the herb tylophora. Another possibility is an herb more famous for rheumatoid arthritis, boswellia. The herb *Coleus forskohlii* may also be helpful, but it is really more like a drug than an herb. Vitamin C also appears to be somewhat helpful. The Chinese herb ma huang is definitely effective for mild asthma, but it isn't safe.

Warning: None of these treatments have been shown to be effective for severe asthma. Do not stop your standard asthma medication except on the advice of a physician.

Tylophora: A Promising Treatment for Asthma

The herb *Tylophora indica* (also called *Tylophora asthmatica;* see page 426) appears to offer considerable promise as a treatment for asthma. It has a long history of use in the traditional Ayurvedic medicine of India.

In a double-blind placebo-controlled study of 195 individuals with asthma, participants who were given 40 mg of a tylophora alcohol extract daily for 6 days showed significant improvement as compared to placebo; the difference was even more marked months after use of the herb was stopped.[1]

Similar results were seen in a double-blind placebo-controlled study of 110 individuals with asthma.[2] The authors noted that it was remarkable that only 6 days of treatment could produce such long-standing benefits.

However, the design of these studies was a bit convoluted, and various pieces of information are missing from the reports, causing some difficulty in evaluating the validity of these trials.

Another double-blind study that enrolled 135 individuals and followed a more straightforward design found no benefit from tylophora.[3] The bottom line: Although tylophora is promising, larger and better studies are necessary to discover whether tylophora is truly effective.

We don't know how tylophora might work in asthma, but it may have anti-inflammatory, antiallergic, adrenal gland–stimulating, and antispasmodic actions.[4–7]

The typical dosage of tylophora leaf is 200 mg twice daily. In the first study mentioned previously, tylophora caused nausea, vomiting, soreness of the mouth, and alterations in taste sensation in more than half of the participants. The other two studies found similar side effects, but far less frequently. The difference may have been because the first study had people chew the whole leaves from the plant, whereas the other studies have used dried leaves or powdered extract in capsule form.

Due to the lack of comprehensive safety studies on tylophora, it should not be used by children, pregnant or nursing women, or those with severe kidney or liver disease. Whether tylophora interacts with any drugs is unknown.

Boswellia: Possibly Helpful

The herb **boswellia** (see page 228) has shown promise as a treatment for rheumatoid arthritis. It is thought to work by inhibiting inflammation. Since asthma involves inflammation as well and can be treated by some of the same drugs that treat rheumatoid arthritis, boswellia has been tried for this purpose too.

One 6-week double-blind placebo-controlled study of 80 individuals with relatively mild asthma found that treatment with boswellia at a dose of 300 mg 3 times daily reduced the frequency of asthma attacks and improved objective measurements of breathing capacity.[8] However, further research needs to be performed to follow up this pilot study before boswellia can be described as a proven treatment for asthma.

Although comprehensive safety testing has not been completed, boswellia appears to be reasonably safe when used as directed. Reported side effects are rare and consist primarily of occasional allergic reactions or mild gastrointestinal distress. Safety in young children, pregnant or nursing women, or those with severe liver or kidney disease has not been established.

Coleus forskohlii: May Be Effective, but More Like a Drug Than an Herb

Another herb sometimes recommended for asthma also comes from India, *Coleus forskohlii* (see page 259). While there is some evidence that it might work,[9,10,11] we cannot give it a wholehearted recommendation. As presently sold, the herb is more like a drug than an herb. Natural *Coleus forskohlii* contains small amounts of a potent substance called forskolin. However, manufacturers deliberately modify the herb to dramatically increase its forskolin content. Forskolin appears to be safe, but more studies need to be undertaken before it can be recommended for self-treatment.

Vitamin C: Appears to Provide Some Benefits

Many studies have been conducted on the effects of vitamin C in treating asthma. When you put all the results together, it appears that the regular use of high-dose vitamin C provides some benefits.[12,13] A typical recommended dosage is 1 to 3 g daily, but taking more than 200 mg a day may not add any extra benefits.

Vitamin C has not been definitely associated with any significant harm. However, high-dose vitamin C can cause copper deficiency, so if you take more than 1 to 2 g per day of vitamin C, you should also take 1 to 3 mg of copper daily. Diarrhea is a common side effect at this dosage, but it usually goes away in a week or so. For other potential safety issues, see the full chapter on **vitamin C.**

Ma Huang: Effective, but Not Safe

The Chinese herb ma huang, also called **ephedra** (see page 277), is definitely effective for mild asthma, because it contains the drug ephedrine. However, we cannot recommend using it because of safety concerns. This Chinese herb is a member of a primitive family of plants that look like thin, branching, connected straws. A related species, *Ephedra nevadensis,* grows wild in the American Southwest and is widely called Mormon tea. However, only the Asian species of ephedra contains the active compounds ephedrine and pseudoephedrine.

Ma huang was traditionally used by Chinese herbalists in the early stages of respiratory infections and for the short-term treatment of certain kinds of asthma, eczema, hay fever, narcolepsy, and edema. However, ma huang was not supposed to be taken for an extended period of time, and people with less than robust constitutions were warned to use only low doses or to avoid ma huang altogether.

Japanese chemists isolated ephedrine from ma huang at the turn of the twentieth century, and it soon became a primary treatment for asthma in the United States and abroad. Ephedra's other major ingredient, pseudoephedrine, became the decongestant Sudafed.

Although ephedrine can still be found in a few over-the-counter asthma drugs, physicians seldom prescribe it today. The problem is that ephedrine mimics the effects of adrenaline and causes symptoms such as rapid heartbeat, high blood pressure, agitation, insomnia, nausea, and loss of appetite. The newer asthma drugs are much safer and easier to tolerate. This is a situation in which synthetic drugs are less dangerous than a natural one. We do not recommend using ma huang for asthma.

OTHER PROPOSED TREATMENTS

The following natural treatments for asthma are often widely recommended, but they have not been scientifically proven effective at this time.

Vitamin B$_{12}$

Supplementation with **vitamin B$_{12}$** (see page 442) is said to be effective for asthma.[14] However, the scientific evidence in its favor consists almost entirely of open studies that did not attempt to eliminate the placebo effect.

Quercetin

The flavonoid **quercetin** (see page 396) is often recommended as a treatment for asthma on the basis of test-tube studies that show it can inhibit the release of inflammatory substances from special cells called mast cells. Because the asthma drugs Intal and Tilade are believed to work in the same way, many natural medicine authorities have often recommended quercetin as an equivalent treatment. However, even though significant direct evidence exists that Tilade and Intal actually work, no such evidence yet exists for quercetin. Interestingly, Intal is derived from a Mediterranean herb named khella.

Vitamin B₆

Vitamin B₆ (see page 439) is often mentioned as a treatment for asthma, but the evidence that it works is weak and contradictory. A double-blind study of 76 asthmatic children found significant benefit from vitamin B₆ after the second month of usage.[15] Children in the treated group were able to reduce their doses of bronchodilators and steroids. However, a recent double-blind study of 31 adults who also used either inhaled or oral steroids did not show any benefit.[16]

The dosages of vitamin B₆ used in these studies were quite high, in the range of 200 to 300 mg daily. Because of the risk of nerve injury, it is not advisable to take this much without medical supervision.

Butterbur

Preliminary evidence suggests that the herb **butterbur** (see page 233) may be helpful for asthma.[17,18]

Elimination Diet

Some people with asthma may also have food allergies. If this is the case, eliminating the offending food from the diet might reduce asthma symptoms.[19] The only reliable way to discover if you are allergic to a certain food is through eliminating potentially allergenic foods from the diet then systematically reintroducing them to see if a reaction occurs. For more information on elimination diets see the chapter on **food allergies.**

Antioxidants

Antioxidants, such as **vitamin E** (see page 451), **beta-carotene** (see page 217), and **selenium** (see page 407), are frequently recommended for asthma on the grounds that they may protect inflamed lung tissue. However, there is little direct scientific evidence that they work at this time.

Essential Fatty Acids

Essential fatty acids, such as **GLA** (see page 304) and those found in **fish oil** (see page 282) and **flaxseed oil** (see page 285), are suspected to inhibit inflammatory responses such as those that occur in asthma. However, most of the studies that tried fish oil as a treatment for asthma found no benefit.[20–27] One study found that fish oil can actually worsen aspirin-related asthma.[28]

Magnesium

Magnesium (see page 351) is frequently mentioned as a treatment for asthma, but no good studies have shown that oral magnesium is helpful. Some evidence exists that intravenous and inhaled magnesium may offer some short-term benefit,[29,30] but the relevance of these findings to taking magnesium supplements by mouth is unclear.

Other Herbs and Supplements

Other commonly recommended asthma treatments include the herbs **aloe** (see page 204), **chamomile** (see page 244), **damiana** (see page 265), **elecampane** (see page 276), **garlic** (see page 291), grindelia, **licorice** (see page 344), **marshmallow** (see page 355), **mullein** (see page 365), onion, **reishi** (see page 400), and **yerba santa** (see page 461), as well as the supplement **betaine hydrochloride** (see page 219). *Lobelia inflata* is a traditional herbal treatment for asthma; but according to traditional directions, it should be taken to the point of vomiting, a process we can hardly recommend.

ATHEROSCLEROSIS AND HEART DISEASE PREVENTION

Principal Proposed Treatments   Vitamin B₆, Folate, Garlic
  Antioxidants: Vitamin E, Vitamin C (in Combination with Vitamin E or Alone), Selenium, OPCs from Grape Seed or Pine Bark, Lipoic Acid, Turmeric, Resveratrol, Coenzyme Q₁₀ (CoQ₁₀)
  Lifestyle Changes

Other Proposed Treatments
  Omega-3 Fatty Acids: Fish Oil, Flaxseed Oil, Flaxseed
  Aortic Glycosaminoglycans, Green Tea, Bilberry Fruit and Leaf, Ginger, Ginkgo, Hawthorn, Magnesium, Genistein, Astragalus, Copper, GLA (Gamma-Linolenic Acid), Grass Pollen, Lutein, TMG (Trimethylglycine)

Not Recommended Treatments   Beta-Carotene

Atherosclerosis, or hardening of the arteries, is the leading cause of death in men over age 35 and all people over 45. Most heart attacks and strokes are due to atherosclerosis. Although the origin of this condition is not completely understood, we know that it is accelerated by factors such as high blood pressure or **hypertension** (see page 98), **high cholesterol** (see page 88), **diabetes** (see page 65), mildly impaired glucose tolerance, smoking, and physical inactivity.

Current theories suggest that atherosclerosis begins with injury to the lining of arteries. High blood pressure physically stresses this lining, while circulating substances such as low-density lipoprotein (LDL) cholesterol, homocysteine, free radicals, and nicotine chemically damage it. White blood cells then attach to the damaged wall and take up residence. Then, for reasons that are not entirely clear, they begin to accumulate cholesterol and other fats. Platelets also latch on, releasing substances that cause the formation of fibrous tissue. The overall effect is a thickening of the artery wall called a fibrous plaque.

Over time, the thickening increases, narrowing the bore of the artery. When blockage reaches 75 to 90%, the person begins to notice **angina** (see page 10) symptoms, specifically heart pain. In the lower legs, blockage of the blood flow leads to leg pain with exercise, a condition called **intermittent claudication** (see page 106).

Blood clots can develop on the irregular surfaces of the artery and may become detached and block downstream blood flow. Fragments of plaque can also detach. Heart attacks are generally caused by such blood clots, whereas strokes are more often caused by plaque fragments or gradual obstruction. Furthermore, atherosclerotic blood vessels are weak and can burst.

With a disease as serious and progressive as atherosclerosis, the best treatment is prevention. Conventional medical approaches focus on lifestyle changes, such as increasing aerobic exercise, reducing the consumption of saturated fats, and quitting smoking. The regular use of aspirin also appears to be quite helpful by preventing platelet attachment and blood clot formation. If necessary, drugs may be used to lower cholesterol levels or blood pressure.

Recently, conventional medicine has also begun to suggest keeping levels of homocysteine low by adding supplemental **folate** (see page 288) and **vitamin B$_6$** (see page 439) to the diet. Consult with your physician for late-breaking information regarding the ideal dose of these supplements. At the time of this writing, recommendations suggest 400 to 800 mcg of folate daily along with 10 to 20 mg of vitamin B$_6$.

Because the following material is so complex, we have summarized this information in the section called Putting It All Together. You can skip to it now if you want just the conclusions.

PRINCIPAL PROPOSED TREATMENTS

In the field of preventing atherosclerosis, conventional and alternative approaches overlap. Natural medicine supports (indeed, it first championed) many of the lifestyle changes now encouraged by conventional medicine, and treatments such as vitamin B$_6$ and folate are now widely recommended by physicians. Many other "alternative" approaches for preventing atherosclerosis are on the verge of acceptance into conventional medicine.

Numerous studies have been performed to determine precisely which nutrients are most helpful in preventing atherosclerosis. However, it is tricky to interpret the results of this research.

The most common and potentially most confusing type of study is the observational study. This type of study follows large groups of people for years and keeps track of a great deal of information about them, including diet. Researchers then examine the data closely and try to identify which dietary factors are associated with better health and longer life.

However, the results can be misleading. For example, if an observational study finds that people who take vitamin supplements live longer, it is not necessarily the vitamins that deserve the credit. Vitamin users also tend to exercise more and to eat more healthful foods, habits that may play a more important role than the vitamins. It is hard to tell.

A more reliable kind of study is the intervention trial. In these studies, some people are given a certain vitamin and then compared to others who are given a placebo (or sometimes no treatment at all). The best intervention trials use a double-blind design. The results of intervention trials are far more conclusive than those of observational studies. Unfortunately, they are very expensive to perform, and relatively few have been completed.

This section details the evidence that is available to date. Because this is such a rapidly changing field, new evidence will likely have been found by the time you read this chapter. Consult a health-care professional for the latest information.

(For other natural treatments that may reduce two important risk factors for atherosclerosis, see the chapters on **cholesterol** and **hypertension.**)

Garlic: Appears to Lower Cholesterol and Blood Pressure, and May Provide Other Benefits

Many, but not all, studies have found that **garlic** (see page 291) can lower cholesterol, and some evidence indicates that it can reduce hypertension as well. These two factors, as well as studies that look at garlic's overall effects on arteries, strongly suggest that garlic can reduce the risk of atherosclerosis.

Garlic preparations have been shown to slow the development of atherosclerosis in rats, rabbits, and human blood vessels, reducing the size of plaque deposits by nearly 50%.[1,2] Furthermore, in a double-blind placebo-controlled study that followed 152 individuals for 4

Atherosclerosis and
Heart Disease Prevention

years, standardized garlic powder at a dosage of 900 mg per day significantly slowed the development of atherosclerosis as measured by ultrasound.[3] While this study suffered from some statistical flaws, it nonetheless provides direct evidence that garlic can protect against hardening of the arteries.

Some of garlic's benefits for the arteries may be independent of its effect on cholesterol and blood pressure. An observational study of 200 individuals suggests that garlic protects the arteries in other ways as well.[4] The study measured the flexibility of the aorta, the main artery exiting the heart. Even in individuals with the same blood pressure and cholesterol levels, those who took garlic showed less evidence of damage to their arteries.

Significantly, there was no difference in cholesterol levels or blood pressure between those who regularly consumed garlic and those who did not. Therefore, it appears that garlic may also reduce atherosclerosis by other means besides affecting these two important risk factors, such as by "thinning" the blood.

Keep in mind that because garlic does produce a blood-thinning effect, it should not be taken by those on blood thinners such as Coumadin (warfarin), heparin, Trental (pentoxifylline), and perhaps even aspirin except under medical supervision. Garlic might also conceivably cause bleeding problems if combined with other natural substances that mildly thin the blood, such as **ginkgo** (see page 298) and high-dose **vitamin E** (see page 451). Do not take garlic supplements immediately prior to or after surgery or labor and delivery.[5]

Antioxidants: Widely Recommended, but Do They Really Work?

The body is engaged in a constant battle against damaging chemicals called free radicals, or pro-oxidants. These highly reactive substances are believed to play a major role in atherosclerosis, cancer, and aging in general.

To counter the harmful effects of free radicals, the body manufactures antioxidants to chemically neutralize them. However, the natural antioxidant system may not always be equal to the task. Sources of free radicals, such as cigarette smoke and smoked meat, may overwhelm this defense mechanism. In the not-too-distant future, tests of "antioxidant status" may join cholesterol and blood pressure as standard components of preventive medicine screening.

Certain dietary nutrients augment the body's natural antioxidants and may be able to help out when the primary system is under stress. Vitamins E and C and beta-carotene are the best known, but many other substances found in fruits and vegetables are also strong antioxidants. For years we've been thinking that individual antioxidant supplements might offer considerable protection against heart disease, especially vitamin E.

However, recent evidence appears to douse these high expectations.

Vitamin E: Not the Magic Bullet We Thought

The latest research findings appear to have turned the tables on our once high hopes for **vitamin E** (see page 451). Now it looks increasingly unlikely that this antioxidant vitamin is a "magic bullet" that by itself can put a dent in heart disease.

The Heart Outcomes Prevention Evaluation (HOPE) trial found that natural vitamin E (d-alpha tocopherol) at a dose of 400 IU daily did not reduce the number of heart attacks, strokes, or deaths from heart disease any more than a placebo.[6] The details of this well-designed double-blind trial were published in the January 20, 2000, issue of *The New England Journal of Medicine*. The trial, lasting an average of 4.5 years, followed over 9,000 men and women who had existing heart disease or were at high risk for it.

We already knew that vitamin E supplements (50 IU synthetic) didn't work for heart disease in smokers,[7,8,9] but that could be readily explained away: Perhaps vitamin E, especially in that relatively small dose, could not overcome the damaging effects of smoking.

The Cambridge Heart Antioxidant Study (CHAOS) trial,[10] published in 1996, is what really had gotten our hopes up. In that trial, people with existing heart disease who took natural vitamin E (400 IU or 800 IU daily) had substantially fewer nonfatal heart attacks compared to the placebo group after about 1.5 years. Even so, and this may resonate with the latest findings, heart-related deaths were not reduced in the vitamin E group. Furthermore, it has been suggested that possible flaws in the design of this trial might make its findings questionable.

Large observational studies in both men and women found substantial benefits for vitamin E (100 IU).[11,12,13] One observational study of 11,178 people, aged 67 to 105 years, found good results from combining vitamins E and C.[14] Those who were taking vitamin E supplements at the beginning of the study had a 34% lower risk of death from heart disease than those who were not. Vitamin C supplements alone did not seem to make a difference, but the combination of vitamins E and C boosted the risk reduction to 53%. Long-term use of vitamin E granted an even stronger risk reduction of 63%. By their nature, though, observational studies cannot fully control for lifestyle factors, so it is possible that people taking vitamin E might also eat better and exercise more, which would influence the results.

So where does all this leave us? Experts uncomfortable with abandoning vitamin E have wondered whether it could be that vitamin E supplements exert a benefit in people who do not already have heart disease or are at low risk for it. Or, perhaps it takes vitamin E longer to exert a clinical benefit than the follow-up period of the studies. Realistically, though, there is no real evidence that this is true.

It might be that we just can't expect vitamin E—or perhaps any other single nutrient—to carry the full burden alone. The antioxidants are a package deal in nature. This group of nutrients, including vitamins E, A, C, selenium, and others, may work best as a team in nature's finely tuned botanical orchestra. The fact that lone vitamin E supplementation appears not to be the magic bullet we had hoped for hints that it might be better to take a balanced, comprehensive array of nutrients rather than depending on high doses of a few key nutrients to carry the load. We will be eagerly awaiting the outcome of ongoing trials of vitamin E combined with other antioxidants.

In addition, vitamin E itself is present in several forms in food, and some researchers believe that this mixture may work best and that perhaps taking too much of one form of vitamin E may blunt the effect of the others.[15]

The optimum dose of vitamin E is not known. A typical recommendation is 400 IU daily. This dosage is generally believed to be safe. Vitamin E is generally regarded as safe when taken at the recommended dosage of 400 to 800 IU daily. However, vitamin E does have a "blood thinning" effect that could lead to problems in certain situations. In one study of 28,519 men, vitamin E supplementation at the low dose of about 50 IU synthetic vitamin E per day caused an increase in fatal hemorrhagic strokes, the kind of stroke caused by bleeding.[16] However, it reduced the risk of a more common type of stroke, and the two effects essentially canceled out.

Based on its blood-thinning effects, there are concerns that vitamin E could cause problems if it is combined with medications that also thin the blood, such as Coumadin (warfarin), heparin, and aspirin. Theoretically, the net result could be to thin the blood *too* much, causing bleeding problems. A study that evaluated vitamin E plus aspirin did in fact find an additive effect.[17] In contrast, the results of a study on vitamin E and Coumadin found no evidence of interaction, but it would still not be advisable to combine these treatments except under a physician's supervision.[18]

There is also at least a remote possibility that vitamin E could interact with herbs that possess a mild blood-thinning effect, such as **garlic** (see page 291) and **ginkgo** (see page 298). Individuals with bleeding disorders such as hemophilia, and those about to undergo surgery or labor and delivery should also approach vitamin E with caution.

Vitamin C: Best with Vitamin E

A combination of **vitamin C** (see page 444) and vitamin E may offer added antioxidant benefits. This makes sense because vitamin E fights free radicals that dissolve in fats while vitamin C fights those that dissolve in water. However, the evidence for a possible enhanced effect of this combination against heart disease comes only from observational studies,[19] and the evidence that vitamin C supplements taken by themselves are helpful for atherosclerosis is also weak.[20,21,22] There have been about as many positive as negative studies. Foods containing vitamin C do appear to be helpful, probably because they contain numerous other healthy substances as well.

Beta-Carotene: Best in Food, Not As a Supplement

The study results involving **beta-carotene** (see page 217) are interesting. Beta-carotene is one member of a large category of substances in foods known as *carotenes,* which are found in high levels in yellow, orange, and dark green vegetables.

Many studies suggest that eating foods high in carotenes can prevent atherosclerosis.[23] However, isolated beta-carotene in supplement form may not help, and could actually increase your risk, especially if you consume too much alcohol.[24]

A huge double-blind intervention trial involving 29,133 Finnish male smokers found 11% *more* deaths from heart disease and 15 to 20% *more* strokes in those participants taking beta-carotene supplements.[25] This certainly does not encourage one to take it.

Similar poor results with beta-carotene were seen in another large double-blind study in smokers.[26] Furthermore, beta-carotene supplementation was also found to increase the incidence of angina in smokers.[27]

What is happening here? Clearly, smoking presents a challenge to antioxidants. However, the question remains: Why should beta-carotene not only fail to help but actually worsen the situation?

One possible explanation is that beta-carotene in the diet always comes along with other naturally occurring carotenes. It is quite likely that other carotenoids in the diet are equally or more important than beta-carotene alone.[28] Taking beta-carotene supplements may actually promote deficiencies of other natural carotenes,[29] and overall that may hurt more than it helps.

The moral of the story is that you should eat your vegetables but maybe not take beta-carotene supplements.

Other Antioxidants: May Be Helpful, but Little Direct Evidence

Many other antioxidant vitamins, supplements, and herbs have been suggested as preventive treatments for atherosclerosis. **Selenium** (see page 407), **OPCs** (see page 373) from grape seed or pine bark, **lipoic acid** (see page 347), **turmeric** (see page 425), **resveratrol** (see page 401) from red wine and grape skins, and

coenzyme Q$_{10}$ (see page 256) are commonly mentioned. However, although a number of interesting studies have suggested that these substances may be beneficial, the state of the evidence is still too preliminary to draw any conclusions.

Lifestyle Approaches

This fact cannot be emphasized enough: The most important way to prevent atherosclerosis involves lifestyle changes such as quitting smoking, increasing exercise, and adopting a diet high in whole grains, fruits, and vegetables and low in animal products.[30] Olive oil and canola oil are probably among the most healthful of vegetable oils. Heating oils to high temperatures (as in fried foods) can oxidize them and make them less healthful.[31]

The moderate use of alcohol, and specifically red wine, appears to help prevent atherosclerosis, although this is controversial as well.[32–35] Coffee may slightly increase cardiovascular risk,[36] although some studies have shown no effect when other factors, such as smoking and diets high in animal fats (often associated with coffee use), are taken into account.[37,38] Coffee probably does not have a significant effect on cholesterol levels, but this is debatable as well. See the chapter on **cholesterol** for further information.

OTHER PROPOSED TREATMENTS

Although the following treatments are widely recommended for atherosclerosis, they cannot be considered scientifically proven at this time.

Omega-3 Fatty Acids

There is some evidence that omega-3 fatty acids, such as those found in **fish oil** (see page 282), can prevent atherosclerosis and reduce risk of heart disease.[39–43] They appear to significantly decrease serum triglycerides (a good effect), leave total cholesterol alone (neutral), and modestly raise high-density lipoprotein or HDL cholesterol (a good effect).[44] Fish oil may also help prevent blood clots, and lower homocysteine levels.[45] Studies contradict one another about whether fish oil can lower blood pressure.[46–52]

Contrary to some reports, fish oil does not seem to increase bleeding or affect blood sugar control in people with diabetes.[53]

Flaxseed oil (see page 285) has been suggested as an alternative to fish oil. While fish oil is much better studied, there is some evidence, including two double-blind studies, that flaxseed oil or whole **flaxseed** (see page 286) may reduce LDL ("bad") cholesterol, perhaps slightly reduce hypertension, and slow down atherosclerosis.[54–60]

Aortic Glycosaminoglycans

Aortic glycosaminoglycans (GAGs; see page 207) are substances obtained from the inside lining of the arteries of cows.

According to a recent study, 200 mg per day of GAGs can significantly slow the rate of thickening of arteries.[61] After 18 months of treatment, the additional layering of the inside vessel lining was 7.5 times less in the group receiving GAGs than in the group that did not receive any treatment. Preliminary evidence suggests that this supplement may work in several ways: supplying material for repair of arteries, "thinning" the blood, and improving cholesterol levels.[62,63]

A typical dosage is 50 to 100 mg twice a day. Glycosaminoglycans are regarded as safe because they commonly occur in foods, although extensive safety studies have not been performed. However, if you are taking drugs that powerfully decrease blood clotting, such as Coumadin (warfarin) or heparin, do not use aortic GAGs except under physician supervision. Aortic GAGs interfere slightly with blood clotting, and there is at least a chance that the combination could cause bleeding problems.

Other Herbs and Supplements

Some but not all observational studies suggest that **green tea** (see page 318) might help prevent heart disease.[64–67]

Many herbs appear to decrease platelet stickiness, including **bilberry** (see page 220), **feverfew** (see page 280), **ginger** (see page 296), **ginkgo** (see page 298), and **hawthorn** (see page 320). Whether this translates into an actual benefit for preventing atherosclerosis remains unknown.

There is also some evidence that **magnesium** (see page 351) may reduce the atherosclerosis risk caused by hydrogenated oils, margarine-like fats found in many "junk" foods.[68]

Indirect evidence suggests that **DHEA** (see page 268) might help prevent heart disease;[69–74] however, it seems likely to be more beneficial for men than for women.

Weak evidence suggests **genistein** (see page 294) may be helpful for preventing heart disease by reducing cholesterol and keeping it from depositing on cell walls.[75,76,77]

Other treatments sometimes mentioned for atherosclerosis include **astragalus** (see page 212), **copper** (see page 262), **GLA** (see page 304), **grass pollen** (see page 317), **lutein** (see page 348), **bilberry** (see page 220) leaf, and **TMG** (see page 423), although there is little evidence as yet that they are helpful.

Atherosclerosis and Heart Disease Prevention

Visit Us at TNP.com

For other natural substances that may help prevent atherosclerosis by lowering its major risk factors, see the chapters on **cholesterol** and **hypertension.**

PUTTING IT ALL TOGETHER

This section is so complicated that we'd like to summarize all the information here in one place.

Little doubt exists that regular exercise and a diet high in fresh fruits and vegetables and low in animal fats can help prevent atherosclerosis. Unheated olive oil and canola oil are probably among the most healthful sources of dietary fat.

The promise of supplemental vitamin E and most other antioxidants has not panned out so far. Supplemental vitamin B_6 (10 to 20 mg daily) and folate (400 to 800 mcg daily) appear to be helpful because of their effects on homocysteine levels. Garlic, too, appears to be beneficial. The evidence for other herbs and supplements is promising but incomplete at present.

Finally, do not forget to take care of your cholesterol and blood pressure.

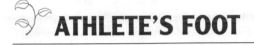

ATHLETE'S FOOT

Related Terms   Ringworm, Onychomycosis, Tinea Pedis

Principal Proposed Treatments   Tea Tree Oil

Other Proposed Treatments   Garlic, Oil of Bitter Orange, Other Essential Oils, Various Tropical/Traditional Medicinal Plants

Athlete's foot is the common name for a fungal infection of the foot, often called ringworm (although there is no worm involved). The three fungi most commonly implicated in athlete's foot, *Trichophyton rubrum, T. mentagrophytes,* and *Epidermophyton floccosum,* favor the warm, moist areas between the toes and tend to flare up during warm weather. Similar infections can occur in the nails, scalp, groin, and beard.

Infection with these fungi generally causes mild scaling between the toes, but it can also cause more severe scaling, an itchy red rash, or blisters that cover the toes and the sides of the feet. Since the fungus may also cause the skin to crack, it can lead to bacterial infections, especially in older people or those with poor circulation in their feet. If the infection takes root under the toenails, it is called onychomycosis, and can be very difficult, if not impossible, to eradicate.

Because the fungi that cause athlete's foot thrive in warm, moist areas, it's important to keep the feet clean and dry. Over-the-counter or prescription topical antifungal treatments containing miconazole, clotrimazole, econazole, or ketoconazole can generally cure athlete's foot, but treatment may have to be continued for a month or more for full results. In severe cases, oral antifungal medications may be necessary.

PRINCIPAL PROPOSED TREATMENTS

Preliminary evidence suggests that tea tree oil might be helpful for athlete's foot.

Tea Tree Oil

Tea tree oil (*Melaleuca alternifolia;* see page 421) has a long traditional use in Australia for the treatment of skin and other infections. This use is supported by evidence that tea tree oil is an effective antiseptic, active against many bacteria and fungi.[1,2] Two preliminary studies suggest it may be helpful for athlete's foot.

What Is the Scientific Evidence for Tea Tree Oil?

A double-blind placebo-controlled trial followed 104 individuals given either a 10% tea tree oil cream, the standard drug tolnaftate, or placebo.[3] The results showed that tea tree oil reduced the symptoms of athlete's foot more effectively than placebo, but less effectively than tolnaftate. Neither treatment cured the infection in 100% of the cases, but each treatment cured many cases.

Another double-blind study followed 112 people with fungal infections of the toenails, comparing 100% tea tree oil to a standard topical antifungal treatment, clotrimazole.[4] The results showed equivalent benefits; however, because topical clotrimazole is not regarded as a particularly effective treatment for this condition, the results mean little.

Dosage

Tea tree preparations contain various percentages of tea tree oil. For treating fungal infections, a 70% to 100% concentration is generally used. It is usually applied 2 to 3 times daily, until symptoms resolve. However, tea tree oil can be irritating to the skin, so start with low concentrations until you know your tolerance.

The best tea tree products contain oil from the *alternifolia* species of *Melaleuca* only, standardized to contain not more than 10% cineole (an irritant) and at least 30% terpinen-4-ol.

Safety Issues

Like other essential oils, tea tree oil can be toxic if taken orally in excessive doses. As the maximum safe dosage has not been determined, we recommend using it only topically, where it is believed to be quite safe. However, don't get it in your eye or it will sting badly.

In addition, an increasing number of cases of skin inflammation caused by allergy to tea tree oil have been reported.[5]

Safety in young children, pregnant or nursing women, or people with severe liver or kidney disease has not been established.

OTHER PROPOSED TREATMENTS

Garlic (see page 291) has known topical antifungal properties,[6,7,8] and there is highly preliminary evidence suggesting that ajoene, a compound derived from garlic, might help treat athlete's foot.[9] However, fresh garlic's strong smell presents practical objections, and the use of garlic or its constituents for athlete's foot has not been tested in double-blind trials.

Very preliminary evidence suggests that oil of bitter orange, a flavoring agent from dried bitter orange peel, might have some effectiveness against athlete's foot when applied topically.[10] Test tube studies indicate that the aromatic constituents of other essential oils such as **peppermint** (see page 384) and eucalyptus also have antifungal activity, but they have yet to be tested on people.[11]

More than 120 plants traditionally used to treat skin diseases in Mexico, Palestine, British Columbia, and Guatemala have demonstrated antifungal properties in test tube studies. Further research is needed to determine if they are safe and effective for athlete's foot or other fungal infections.[12-18]

ATTENTION DEFICIT DISORDER

Related Terms   Attention Deficit and Hyperactivity Disorder, ADHA, Adult Attention Deficit Disorder, AADD, Hyperkinetic Syndrome

Principal Proposed Treatments   There are no well-established natural treatments for attention deficit disorder.

Other Proposed Treatments   DMAE (2-dimethylaminoethanol), Calcium, Zinc, Magnesium, Iron, Inositol, Trace Minerals, Blue-Green Algae, Combined Amino Acids (GABA, Glycine, Taurine, L-Glutamine, L-Phenylalanine, L-Tyrosine), Combined Polysaccharides (Galactose, Glucose, Mannose, N-acetylneuraminic Acid, Fucose, N-acetylgalactosamine, N-acetylglucosamine, Xylose), St. John's Wort

Originally, the term *attention deficit disorder* (ADD) referred to children who seemed incapable of concentrating at school. Today, however, the definition has broadened to include many adults as well. Characteristics of ADD and the related condition ADHD (attention deficit and hyperactivity disorder) include difficulty sustaining attention or completing tasks, easy distractibility, impulsive behavior, and hyperactivity (excessive movement and an inability to sit still). These problems make it difficult to succeed at work or at school.

Conventional treatment focuses on stimulants such as caffeine, Dexedrine, and Ritalin. These drugs produce a paradoxically calming effect in people with ADD, for reasons we don't understand. Certain antidepressants may also be useful.

PROPOSED TREATMENTS
DMAE

There is some evidence that the supplement **DMAE** (see page 270) may be helpful for ADD, according to studies performed in the 1970s. Two such studies were reported in a review article on DMAE.[1] Fifty children aged 6 to 12 years who had been diagnosed with hyperkinesia (their diagnosis today would likely be ADD) participated in a double-blind study comparing DMAE to placebo. The dose was increased from 300 mg daily to 500 mg daily by the third week, and continued for 10 weeks. Evaluations revealed statistically significant test score improvements in the treatment group compared to the placebo group.

Another double-blind study compared DMAE with both methylphenidate (Ritalin) and placebo in 74 children with "learning disabilities" (also probably what we would

Autism

call ADD today).[2] It found significant test score improvement for both treatment groups over a 10-week period. Positive results were also seen in a small open study.[3]

Other Natural Treatments

Two authors sympathetic to natural medicine reviewed all the literature in print on a few other widely recommended options for ADD: supplementation with niacin (or **vitamin B₃**; see page 437), **vitamin B₆** (see page 439), and multivitamin and mineral tablets.[4] They failed to find any evidence of a positive effect.

Other supplements that are sometimes recommended for ADD include **calcium** (see page 234),

zinc (see page 463), **magnesium** (see page 351), **iron** (see page 333), **inositol** (see page 330), trace minerals, blue-green algae, combinations of amino acids (usually GABA, **glycine** [see page 311], **taurine** [see page 420], **L-glutamine** [see page 310], **L-phenylalanine** [see page 385], and **L-tyrosine** [see page 426]), and combinations of the polysaccharides (galactose, glucose, mannose, N-acetylneuraminic acid, fucose, N-acetylgalactosamine, N-acetylglucosamine, and xylose). **St. John's wort** (see page 414) is also sometimes recommended. However, there is little to no evidence for any of these treatments at this time.

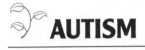

AUTISM

Related Terms   Autistic Disorder, Childhood-Onset Pervasive Developmental Disorder, Infantile Autism, Atypical Autism

Principal Proposed Treatments   Vitamin B₆, Magnesium

Other Proposed Treatments   Vitamin C, Vitamin B₁₂, Folate, Biotin, Avoiding Milk or Gluten, Inositol, Melatonin

Autism is a developmental disorder that typically begins in the first three years of life, although a variant of autism called childhood-onset pervasive developmental disorder may occur in children up to the age of 12. Children with autism are unable to develop normal social relationships, often withdrawing into a world of their own. Other symptoms include ritualistic and compulsive behavior, such as rocking or humming, and an inability or unwillingness to speak. Autistic children may also suffer from other neurological disorders such as seizures, hyperactivity, mental retardation, or obsessive-compulsive disorder.

Perhaps the most famous example of autism is the character Raymond Babbit, played by Dustin Hoffman in the film *Rain Man*. The portrayal of this character is reasonably accurate, although Raymond is "high functioning" for a person with autism, falling on the upper end of the intelligence and behavior scale. Like other autistic individuals, Raymond insists on various rituals such as eating certain foods and watching specific TV programs right on schedule, and becomes highly agitated if this routine is disrupted. He also likes to memorize such things as phone books. In addition, he can perform a few intellectual feats such as calculating difficult arithmetic in his head; most people with autism do not have this ability, but many are surprisingly highly skilled in some specific intellectual areas.

The cause of autism is not known, though it is believed to be at least partially genetic. Its onset may be

related to a viral infection, an enzyme deficiency (phenylketonuria), or the fragile X syndrome (a chromosomal disorder).

Conventional treatments for autism typically target individual symptoms associated with the disorder. Treatments include anticonvulsants for epilepsy, clonidine or imipramine for attention deficit hyperactivity disorder, and certain SSRIs or tricyclic antidepressants for compulsive behaviors.[1] Numerous experimental treatments have been tried, including secretin, as well as various behavioral training programs.

PRINCIPAL PROPOSED TREATMENTS
Vitamin B₆ and Magnesium

A combination of **vitamin B₆** (see page 439) and **magnesium** (see page 351) has shown promising results in lessening the symptoms of autism.[2-12] However, the high doses used require physician supervision.

What Is the Scientific Evidence for Vitamin B₆ and Magnesium?

Six double-blind placebo-controlled trials enrolling a total of about 150 children have evaluated the effects of vitamin B₆ and magnesium combination therapy for autism, with positive results.[13-18] However, the study design used in many of these trials was rather complicated and difficult to evaluate. For example, the largest trial (actually, a series of four closely intertwined trials)

Visit Us at TNP.com

involved multiple groups of participants taking different treatments with inadequate time in between for the vitamins and minerals to wash out.[19] These studies were marked by other flaws as well; in addition, they were all performed by one research group.

For these reasons, until better-designed trials reported by independent laboratories are published, this therapy cannot be considered proven.

Dosage

The dosages used in studies varied, but most of them used 30 mg of vitamin B_6 per kilogram of body weight and 10 to 15 mg of magnesium per kilogram of body weight. These are high doses which present some health risks (see Safety Issues below).

Safety Issues

The doses of B_6 used in these studies are quite high, and might produce toxic effects such as damage to the nervous system. (See the chapter on **vitamin B_6** for more information.) For this reason, physician supervision is necessary.

The dosages of magnesium in these studies are also high. Loose stools are a likely side effect. In addition, there has been one case of death caused by excessive use of magnesium supplements in a developmentally and physically disabled child.[20] This is another reason that physician supervision is mandatory.

In addition, magnesium can interfere with the absorption of some antibiotics including those in the tetracycline and fluoroquinolone families and nitrofurantoin.[21-28] It also may reduce the absorption of penicillamine and digoxin.[29-36] Also, when combined with oral diabetes drugs in the sulfonylurea family (Tolinase, Micronase, Orinase, Glucotrol, Diabinese, DiaBeta), magnesium may cause blood sugar levels to fall more than expected.[37] Finally, potassium-sparing diuretics such as amiloride may reduce magnesium excretion.[38,39] For this reason, if you are taking potassium-sparing diuretics, you should not take magnesium supplements unless under a doctor's supervision.

OTHER PROPOSED TREATMENTS

A 10-week double-blind placebo-controlled study of 18 autistic children found some evidence that **vitamin C** (see page 444) might be helpful.[40]

Various B vitamins including **B_{12}** (see page 442), **folate** (see page 288), and **biotin** (see page 221) have also been suggested for autism,[41,42] but there is no good scientific evidence as yet that they work. A diet free of gluten and milk has also been tried.[43,44] The supplement **inositol** (see page 330) failed to prove effective in a very small double-blind trial.[45]

Melatonin (see page 357) may be useful for autistic children who have sleep disorders.[46]

BENIGN PROSTATIC HYPERPLASIA

Related Terms   Prostate Enlargement

Principal Proposed Treatments   Saw Palmetto, Pygeum, Nettle Root, Sitosterols, Grass Pollen

Other Proposed Treatments   Pumpkin Seeds, Zinc, Flaxseed Oil

If you're a man, and you live long enough, you will almost certainly develop benign prostatic hyperplasia (BPH). Ninety percent of all men show signs of such prostatic enlargement by the age of 80. Symptoms include difficulty in starting urination, a diminished force of urinary stream, a sensation of fullness in the bladder after urination, and the need to urinate many times at night. Ultimately, the obstruction can become so severe that urination is impossible.

The most common treatment for BPH is surgery that removes most of the prostate gland. Although this surgery is fairly safe, it is traumatic. The drugs Cardura, Flomax, Hytrin, and Proscar can relieve symptoms of BPH. In addition, Proscar has been shown to shrink the prostate and cut by half the need for surgery.

PRINCIPAL PROPOSED TREATMENTS

Men who suspect they may suffer from BPH should make sure to see a physician to rule out prostate cancer. After this has been done, many natural options are available that have good scientific backing. Indeed, it's hard to think of another condition for which so many natural therapies have been shown effective.

Saw Palmetto: A Well-Documented Alternative to Prostate Medications

The best-documented herbal treatment for BPH is the oil of the berry of the **saw palmetto** (see page 406) tree. Saw palmetto is a native of North America; although Europeans are the principal consumers of saw palmetto, it is still grown mainly in North America.

Historically, Native Americans used saw palmetto berries for the treatment of various urinary problems in men and for breast disorders in women. European and U.S. physicians took up saw palmetto as a treatment for BPH, but in the United States the herb ultimately fell out of favor.

European interest endured, and in the 1960s French researchers discovered that, by concentrating the oils of the saw palmetto berry, they could maximize the herb's effectiveness. Subsequently, a standardized version of saw palmetto oil became an accepted treatment for prostate enlargement in New Zealand, France, Germany, Austria, Italy, Spain, and other European countries.

This herb is so well accepted in Europe that synthetic pharmaceuticals are considered alternative therapy for BPH. In Germany, saw palmetto is the seventh most common single-herb product prescribed. Studies suggest that benefits will develop after about 4 to 6 weeks of treatment in two-thirds of men who try it.

Saw palmetto offers two potential advantages over conventional drug treatment. The most obvious is that it usually causes no side effects. Another advantage is that saw palmetto does not change protein-specific antigen (PSA) levels. Lab tests that measure PSA are used to screen for prostate cancer. However, the widely used drug Proscar can artificially lower PSA levels, which may have the unintended effect of masking prostate cancer.

Saw palmetto is also sometimes used for chronic prostatitis. However, there is no scientific evidence that it works for this problem.

What Is the Scientific Evidence for Saw Palmetto?

The scientific evidence for saw palmetto in prostate enlargement is quite impressive, although not perfect.

At least seven double-blind studies involving a total of about 500 participants have compared the benefits of saw palmetto against placebo over a period of 1 to 3 months.[1–7] In all but one of these studies, the herb significantly improved urinary flow rate and most other measures of prostate disease.

A double-blind study followed 1,098 men who received either saw palmetto or the drug Proscar over a period of 6 months.[8] According to the results, the two treatments were about equally successful at reducing noticeable symptoms, and neither produced much in the way of side effects. However, Proscar lowered PSA levels, presenting a risk of masking prostate cancer (see the previous discussion under the heading Saw Palmetto). Saw palmetto did not cause this problem. On the other hand, careful measurements showed that Proscar caused men's prostates to shrink by 18%, while saw palmetto only caused a 6% decrease in size. Although prostate size does not correlate well with severity of symptoms, such a de-

crease in size might indicate a reduced likelihood of need for surgery. This is a potential advantage for the drug.

Finally, a 6-month double-blind placebo-controlled trial of 44 men given a saw palmetto herbal blend (containing, in addition, nettle root and pumpkin seed oil) also found shrinkage in prostate tissue.[9] No significant improvement in symptoms was seen, but the authors pointed out that the study size was too small to statistically detect such improvements if they did occur.

Although there are many theories about how saw palmetto works, none have been conclusively established. The best evidence suggests that the herb interferes with male hormones.

Dosage

The standard dosage of saw palmetto is 160 mg twice daily of an extract standardized to contain 85 to 95% fatty acids and sterols. It can also be taken in one daily dose of 320 mg.[10] Taking more than this dose will not give you better results.

Note: Make sure to get a full medical checkup to rule out prostate cancer before you self-treat with saw palmetto. Furthermore, all men over the age of 50 should also continue regular prostate checkups with their physicians.

Safety Issues

Saw palmetto appears to be essentially nontoxic.[11] It's also nearly side-effect free. In a 3-year study involving 435 participants, only 34 complained of side effects, which were mainly the usual mild gastrointestinal distress.[12] No drug interactions are known.

Safety in pregnancy and nursing has not been established. However, because saw palmetto is intended for men only, this is not a terrible drawback. Those with severe liver or kidney disease should not use saw palmetto (or any other herb) except on the advice of a physician.

Pygeum: Another Well-Documented Natural Choice

The **pygeum** (see page 395) tree is a tall evergreen native to central and southern Africa. Its bark has been used since ancient times for urinary problems. In recent years, pygeum has become a popular European treatment for BPH—a use that is supported by good scientific evidence—although it's more widely used in France and Italy than in Germany. Pygeum is expensive and difficult to grow.

Pygeum is also sometimes used for prostatitis, as well as **impotence** (see page 100) and **male infertility**[13,14] (see page 116); however, there is little real evidence that it works.

What Is the Scientific Evidence for Pygeum?

At least 10 double-blind trials of pygeum have been performed, involving a total of over 600 participants and ranging in length from 45 to 90 days.[15-19] Overall, the results make a reasonably strong case that pygeum can reduce symptoms such as nighttime urination, urinary frequency, and residual urine volume. The best of these trials was conducted at 8 sites in Europe and included 263 men between 50 and 85 years of age.[20] Participants received 50 mg of a pygeum extract or placebo twice daily. The results showed significant improvements in residual urine volume, voided volume, urinary flow rate, nighttime urination, and daytime frequency.

We don't really know how pygeum works. Unlike the standard drug finasteride, it does not appear to work by affecting the conversion of testosterone to dihydrotestosterone.[21] Rather it is thought to reduce inflammation in the prostate, and also to inhibit prostate growth factors, substances implicated in inappropriate prostate enlargement.[22,23,24] We don't know whether pygeum can reduce the need for prostate surgery or whether it affects PSA levels.

Dosage

The proper dosage of pygeum is 50 mg twice per day (occasionally 100 mg twice daily) of an extract standardized to contain 14% triterpenes and 0.5% n-docosanol. A dose of 100 mg once daily appears to be as effective as the most common dosage of 50 mg twice daily.[25]

There is some reason to believe that pygeum's effectiveness might be enhanced when it is combined with nettle root.[26,27]

Safety Issues

Pygeum appears to be essentially nontoxic, both in the short and the long term.[28] The most common side effect is mild gastrointestinal distress. However, safety in those with severe liver or kidney disease has not been established.

Nettle Root

Anyone who lives in a locale where **nettle** (see page 369) grows wild will likely discover the powers of this dark green plant. Depending on the species, the fine hairs on its leaves and stem cause burning pain that lasts from hours to weeks. Both its leaves and roots can be used as medicine. The root is a popular European treatment for BPH. Over a period of several months, nettle appears to reduce obstruction of urinary flow and decrease the need for nighttime urination.

Nettle leaf (not the root) is sometimes used for **allergies** (see page 2).

What Is the Scientific Evidence for Nettle Root?

Nettle root has not been as well studied as saw palmetto or pygeum.

In a 4- to 6-week double-blind study of 67 men, treatment with nettle root produced a 14% improvement in urine flow and a 53% decrease in residual urine (urine that was not completely expelled from the bladder).[29]

Another double-blind study of 40 men showed a significant decrease in frequency of urination after 6 months.[30] A double-blind study of 50 men over 9 weeks showed a significant improvement in urination volume.[31]

Dosage

According to Germany's Commission E, the proper dosage of nettle root is 4 to 6 g daily of the whole root or a proportional dose of concentrated extract. As mentioned previously, nettle root might work well in combination with pygeum.

Safety Issues

Nettle root appears to be nearly side-effect free. In one study of 4,087 people who took 600 to 1,200 mg of nettle daily for 6 months, less than 1% reported mild gastrointestinal distress, and only 0.19% experienced allergic reactions (skin rash).[32]

Although detailed safety studies have not been reported, no serious adverse effects have been noted in Germany, where nettle root is widely used. For theoretical reasons, there are some concerns that nettle may interact with conventional medications used for diabetes or high blood pressure, but there are no published reports of such problems occurring.

Safety in those with severe liver or kidney disease has not been established.

Sitosterols

Numerous plants contain cholesterol-like compounds called **sitosterols** (see page 409) and their close relatives sitosterolins. Of these, beta-sitosterol and beta-sitosterolin are considered the most important therapeutically.

A review of the literature, published in 1999, found a total of four randomized, double-blind placebo-controlled studies on sitosterol mixtures (primarily beta-sitosterol, with other sitosterols and sitosterolins as well) for BPH, enrolling a total of 519 men.[33] All these studies found significant benefits in both perceived symptoms and objective measurements, such as urine flow rate. The largest trial followed 200 men with BPH for a period of 6 months.[34] After the study was completed, many of the participants were followed for an additional year, during which the benefits continued.[35]

The daily dosage of beta sitosterol is 60 to 135 mg. Effects usually take 4 weeks to develop.

Detailed safety studies of sitosterols have not been performed, and safety in individuals with severe kidney or liver disease has not been established. However, no significant side effects have been observed.[36]

Grass Pollen

A special extract of **grass pollen** (see page 317) is widely used in Europe for the treatment of BPH. Although a couple of double-blind and other types of studies have found it to be effective,[37–51] the total evidence is weaker than that for the treatments just described.

Grass pollen extract is just beginning to become widely available in the United States. Look for products that contain rye pollen (*Secale cereale*).

OTHER PROPOSED TREATMENTS

There are a few other treatments often recommended for BPH, but they lack any real scientific evidence. Pumpkin seeds are approved for use in BPH by Ger-

many's Commission E. The mineral **zinc** (see page 463) is also commonly recommended in both Europe and the United States as a treatment for prostate disease, as is flaxseed oil. But in the absence of meaningful studies for these treatments we'd suggest sticking with one of the proven herbs previously mentioned.

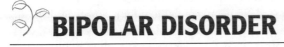

BIPOLAR DISORDER

Related Terms   Manic-Depression, Manic-Depressive Disease

Principal Proposed Treatments   Fish Oil

Other Proposed Treatments   Flaxseed Oil, Lecithin, Choline, Vitamin C, Folate, Inositol, Vitamin B$_{12}$

Previously known as manic-depressive disease, bipolar disorder is a common mental health condition manifested by alternating periods of mania—extreme high energy—and deep depression. In the "up" or manic phase, people may sleep little, talk fast, develop grand and unworkable plans, and sometimes behave bizarrely—for example, giving away all their money overnight. In the "down" phase, they may contemplate suicide.

Bipolar disorder was thought to be untreatable, until the accidental discovery that the mineral lithium can dramatically improve symptoms of mania. Later, various antiseizure medications were also found to help for reasons that are not clear. However, all of these treatments can cause significant side effects, and none is completely effective for everyone.

People with this condition generally require life-long treatment with lithium or other drugs to control manic episodes, and sometimes antidepressants to control depression.

PRINCIPAL PROPOSED TREATMENTS

Fish Oil

One of the newest but most promising natural treatments for bipolar disorder is **fish oil** (see page 282), a substance best known for its possible benefits in preventing heart disease. The results of a small double-blind study were met with considerable scientific interest, and fish oil is currently the subject of ongoing research.

What Is the Scientific Evidence for Fish Oil?

In a double-blind study reported in 1999, 30 people with bipolar disorder took either fish oil capsules containing omega-3 fatty acids or placebo for 4 months, in addition to

their regular medications.[1] The study authors found that those taking the fish oil had longer symptom-free periods than those taking placebo. The researchers used five different standardized tests to measure symptoms, examining levels of depression, mania, and overall progress. The people taking fish oil proved emotionally healthier than those taking placebo on all but one of these tests.

The idea of using fish oil came from test tube studies suggesting that omega-3 fatty acids might dampen overactive nerve signals, thereby stabilizing mood swings.[2] This is similar to one possible explanation of how lithium and antiseizure medications work.[3]

Dosage

In the study reported above, participants took very high dosages of fish oil: 7 capsules twice daily of a specially concentrated omega-3 fatty acid formula containing 440 mg of EPA and 240 mg of DHA per capsule. They also continued their regular medications for bipolar disorder. Most fish oil capsules contain only 300 mg of omega-3 fatty acids at the most. To replicate the dose in the study, you need to find similarly concentrated capsules, or take about 30 fish oil capsules a day.[4] If this seems unwieldy, consider substituting flaxseed oil (see below).

Remember that fish oil is intended to supplement, not replace, other medications for bipolar disorder.

Safety Issues

Fish oil is generally considered safe when taken in usual doses. The worst side effect most people experience is fishy burps. The very large doses in the study caused occasional mild gastrointestinal problems, mostly loose stools, which improved with a lower dose. Fish oil slightly "thins" the blood, and might pose a risk for

Bladder Infection

people on other blood-thinning medications such as Coumadin (warfarin) or heparin. Cod liver oil is not the best source of fish oil, as it might provide too much vitamin A and D to be safe, especially for pregnant women.

OTHER PROPOSED TREATMENTS

A variety of other supplements have been proposed for bipolar disorder. However, the evidence that they work is weak at best.

Flaxseed Oil

The same researchers who conducted the fish oil study have also experimented with **flaxseed oil** (see page 285) for bipolar disorder.[5] Flaxseed oil contains alphalinolenic acid (ALA), an omega-3 fatty acid related to the fatty acids in fish oil. In the researchers' informal observations of 22 people with bipolar disorder, all but 4 appeared to benefit from flaxseed oil. However, lacking a double-blind study, these results can't be taken as reliable. When a double-blind study is finally performed, flaxseed oil may turn out not to be helpful at all.

These researchers reported a dose of 1 tablespoon (15 ml) daily of flaxseed oil, which contains about 7 g of ALA. This dose is a lot more convenient than 14 capsules of concentrated fish oil a day! Like fish oil, flaxseed oil is considered safe in usual doses. But remember, flax oil is not meant as a substitute for standard medications.

Lecithin and Choline

Two related substances, **lecithin** (see page 343) and **choline** (see page 248), have been proposed as remedies for various psychological and neurological diseases, including bipolar disorder. Lecithin contains a substance called phosphatidylcholine (PC) which breaks down into the nutrient choline. Tiny studies of six individuals apiece have found that both lecithin and choline may be helpful in treating symptoms of bipolar disorder, particularly mania.[6,7] While promising, these treatments need to be studied in much larger groups before any real conclusions can be drawn.

Vitamin C

Two rather flawed double-blind studies found that **vitamin C** (see page 444) might help bipolar disorder,[8,9] but it is hard to draw conclusions because of the ways in which the studies were designed: one study used only a single dose of vitamin C.[10]

Folate

According to one study, deficiencies in **folate** (see page 288) may be linked to greater levels of emotional symptoms in people taking lithium long-term.[11] In this study, those who were found to have the highest levels of folate in their blood also did the best on standardized tests of depression and emotional well-being.[12] However, this does not prove that taking extra folate will help.

A double-blind study attempted to answer this question. In it, 75 people on lithium for a variety of disorders were given either folate or placebo for a year.[13] Individuals with bipolar disorder who took folate did no better, on average, than those taking placebo.

Other Possible Treatments

Vitamin B$_{12}$ (see page 442) and **inositol** (see page 330) have also been proposed as treatments for bipolar disease, but there is no real evidence that they work. In addition, caution is advised with inositol (see below).

Risky Combinations

A number of supplements may be risky for those with bipolar disorder. For example, one case report suggests that inositol (mentioned above as a possible treatment for bipolar disorder) may have been responsible for precipitating manic episodes in three people.[14]

Several reports have raised the concern that **SAMe** (see page 403) can trigger manic episodes as well.[15–19] This would not be surprising if true, as SAMe appears to possess antidepressant properties, and antidepressants are well known to trigger manic episodes. This suggests that other natural antidepressant treatments could also cause problems, most notably the herb **St. John's wort** (see page 414), but also **5-HTP** (see page 198) and **phenylalanine** (see page 385). However, there are, as yet, no actual reports of problems.

Finally, there was a case report that high doses of the supplement L-glutamine (more than 2 g per day) may also have triggered episodes of mania in two people without bipolar disorder.[20]

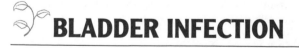

BLADDER INFECTION

Related Terms   Urinary Tract Infection

Principal Proposed Treatments   Cranberry, Uva Ursi

Other Proposed Treatments   Goldenseal, Probiotics, Vitamin C, Zinc, Low-Sugar Diet, Goldenrod, Juniper, Lapacho, Sandalwood, Methionine

Bladder infections are a common problem for women, accounting for more than 6 million office visits each year. Men, because of the greater distance between their bladder and urethral opening, only rarely develop bladder infections.

The primary symptoms of a bladder infection are burning during urination, frequency of urination, and urgency to urinate, possibly accompanied by pain in the lower abdomen and cloudy or bloody urine. Occasionally, the infection spreads upward into the kidneys, producing symptoms such as intense back pain, high fever, chills, nausea, and diarrhea.

Conventional treatment for bladder infections consists of appropriate antibiotic treatment guided by urine culture. Recently, a report was released suggesting that it is appropriate for women with frequent bladder infections to have on hand a prescription for antibiotics for the purpose of self-treatment when symptoms arise. Women who have had extremely frequent bladder infections sometimes take antibiotics continuously to prevent the condition.

PRINCIPAL PROPOSED TREATMENTS

Women who do not want to use antibiotics may be able to find some help through the use of herbs. However, if symptoms do not improve or signs of a kidney infection develop, medical attention is essential to prevent serious complications.

Cranberry: May Help Prevent Infections

Cranberry (see page 263) juice is commonly used to prevent bladder infections as well as to overcome low-level chronic infections. The cranberry plant is a close relative of the common blueberry. Native Americans used it both as food and as a treatment for bladder and kidney diseases. The Pilgrims learned about cranberry from local tribes and quickly adopted it for their own use. Subsequent physicians used it for bladder infections, for "bladder gravel," and to remove "blood toxins."

In the 1920s, researchers observed that drinking cranberry juice makes the urine more acidic. Because common urine infection bacteria such as *E. coli* dislike acid surroundings, physicians concluded that they had discovered a scientific explanation for the traditional uses of cranberry. This discovery led to widespread medical use of cranberry juice for bladder infections. Cranberry fell out of favor after World War II, only to return in the 1960s as a self-treatment for bladder infections.

More recent research has revised the conclusions reached by scientists in the 1920s. It appears that acidification of the urine is not so important as cranberry's ability to interfere with the bacteria establishing a foothold on the bladder wall.[1–4] If the bacteria can't hold on, they will be washed out with the stream of urine. Furthermore, studies suggest that in women who frequently develop bladder infections, bacteria have an especially easy time holding on to the bladder wall.[5]

When taken regularly, cranberry juice may fix this problem and break the cycle of repeated infection. Cranberry juice also seems to be helpful for chronic bladder infections, those that continue for months with few to no symptoms.

What Is the Scientific Evidence for Cranberry?

A 6-month study followed 153 women with an average age of 78.5 years.[6] This study looked at chronic bladder infections rather than acute bladder infections. Chronic bladder infections are relatively common in older women and may cause few or no symptoms. The evidence suggests that cranberry can eliminate continuing infections.

Half of the participants were given a standard supermarket cranberry cocktail, and the other half were given a placebo drink prepared to look and taste the same. Both treatments contained the same amount of vitamin C, which was important because vitamin C itself may have some antibacterial effects.

Commercial cranberry cocktail is mostly sugar and contains little cranberry juice. It is natural to wonder whether straight cranberry juice would have been more effective. Nonetheless, the results suggest that even cranberry juice cocktail can prevent chronic bladder infections, as well as eliminate ones that have already begun.

There was a 58% lower rate of bacteria in the urine of the women treated with cranberry as compared to those given placebo. Also, if a woman had bacteria in the urine at one point in the study, the chance that she would still have it a month later was 73% lower in the cranberry group.

This study has been criticized for several flaws in its design, especially the method used to analyze the urine. It also doesn't tell us whether regular use of cranberry will prevent ordinary acute bladder infections. Nonetheless, it definitely suggests that cranberry juice does have real potential in the treatment of bladder infections.

However, another double-blind placebo-controlled study evaluated the effectiveness of cranberry extract in children with bladder paralysis (neurogenic bladder) who needed to use a catheter.[7] The results showed no benefit.

Dosage

The proper dosage of dry cranberry juice extract is 300 to 400 mg twice daily. For those people who prefer juice, 8 to 16 ounces daily should be enough. For best effect, use true cranberry juice, not sugary cranberry juice cocktail.

Safety Issues

There are no known risks associated with this food for adults, children, and pregnant or nursing women. However, excessive use of cranberry juice may weaken the effect of slightly alkaline drugs, such as many antidepressants and prescription painkillers, by causing them to be excreted more rapidly in the urine.

Uva Ursi: Appears to Be Effective for Acute Bladder Infections

While cranberry is most often used to prevent bladder infections or to treat simmering chronic infections, **uva ursi** (see page 427), also known as bearberry, can be used to treat the classic painful, acute bladder infection. Uva ursi has a long history of use for urinary conditions in both America and Europe. Until the development of sulfa antibiotics, its principal active component, arbutin, was frequently prescribed by physicians as a treatment for bladder and kidney infections.

The uva ursi plant is a low-lying evergreen bush whose berries are a favorite of bears, thus the name bearberry. However, it is the leaves that are used medicinally. We do not know for sure how uva ursi works. It appears that the arbutin contained in uva ursi leaves is broken down in the intestine to another chemical, hydroquinone. This is altered a bit by the liver and then sent to the kidneys for excretion.[8] Hydroquinone then acts as an antiseptic in the bladder.

The European Scientific Cooperative on Phytotherapy (ESCOP) is a scientific organization assigned the task of harmonizing herb policy among European countries. ESCOP recommends uva ursi for "uncomplicated infections of the urinary tract such as cystitis when antibiotic treatment is not considered essential."[9]

Warning: This herb is definitely not appropriate for kidney infections. If you develop symptoms such as high fever, chills, nausea, vomiting, diarrhea, or severe back pain, get medical assistance immediately.

Furthermore, hydroquinone can be toxic (see Safety Issues). For this reason it is not a good idea to take uva ursi for a long period of time.

What Is the Scientific Evidence for Uva Ursi?

Surprisingly little research has been done on uva ursi.[10]

Treatment   No double-blind studies have evaluated the clinical effectiveness of uva ursi. Two studies evaluated the antibacterial power of the urine of people who were taking uva ursi and found activity against most major bacteria that infect the urinary tract.[11,12]

Prevention   One double-blind study followed 57 women for 1 year.[13] Half were given a standardized dose of uva ursi (in combination with dandelion leaf, intended to promote urine flow), while the others received placebo. Over the course of the study, none of the women on uva ursi developed a bladder infection, whereas five of the untreated women did. However, most experts do not believe that continuous treatment with uva ursi is a good idea.

Dosage

The dosage of uva ursi should be adjusted to provide 400 to 800 mg of arbutin daily.[14,15,16] This dosage should not be exceeded. If the herb is not successful within 1 week, you should definitely seek medical attention. No more than 2 weeks of treatment with uva ursi is recommended even under medical supervision, and it should not be used more than five times a year. Uva ursi should be taken with meals to minimize gastrointestinal upset.

Interestingly, research suggests that arbutin's antibiotic activity depends on the presence of alkaline urine. Many women take vitamin C during bladder infections to acidify the urine and, it is hoped, inhibit the bacteria. However, this may tend to block the effect of uva ursi. For this reason, it may be counterproductive to use both uva ursi and vitamin C. Conversely, supplements thought to alkalinize the urine may improve uva ursi's effectiveness. These include calcium citrate, calcium gluconate, and baking soda.

Safety Issues

Unfortunately, hydroquinone is a liver toxin, a carcinogen, and an irritant.[17–20] For this reason, uva ursi is not recommended for young children, pregnant or nursing women, and those with severe liver or kidney disease.

However, significant problems are rare among people using uva ursi products in appropriate dosages for a short period of time. Gastrointestinal distress (ranging from mild nausea and diarrhea to vomiting) can occur, especially with prolonged use.[21]

OTHER PROPOSED TREATMENTS

The following treatments are often proposed as treatments for bladder infections, but there is as yet little to no scientific confirmation of their effectiveness.

Goldenseal

The herb goldenseal is widely recommended for bladder infections, based on the antibiotic properties of its ingredient berberine. However, we don't know for sure if, when goldenseal is taken by mouth, enough berberine accumulates in the bladder to do anything.

In the past, herbalists would instill goldenseal preparations directly into the bladder, a process that we do not recommend trying yourself. However, because berberine has been reported to cause uterine contractions and to increase levels of bilirubin, goldenseal should not be used by pregnant women.[22,23] The safety of goldenseal in young children, nursing women, and those with severe liver or kidney disease has not been established. For other potential safety issues, see the chapter on **goldenseal.**

Probiotics

Probiotics (see page 200), or "friendly bacteria," particularly those found in live yogurt such as *Lactobacillus* *acidophilus, Bifidobacterium bifidum* (bifidus for short), and *Lactobacillus bulgaricus* may also be useful in preventing bladder infections. Many bladder infections are caused by the migration of vaginal and rectal bacteria into the urinary tract. When friendly bacteria are present, pathogenic, or disease-causing, bacteria have a difficult time proliferating. Friendly bacteria may be taken orally or introduced in the form of a douche.

Unfortunately, the quality control of acidophilus supplements seems to be very poor. Unless you have a home microbiology lab, it will be difficult for you to tell whether the acidophilus you are buying is really alive. Live culture yogurt may be preferable, unless your store can supply documentation proving that its acidophilus is still alive at time of purchase.

Other Supplements

Many nutritionally oriented physicians believe that regularly taking **vitamin C** (see page 444) and **zinc** (see page 463) supplements and decreasing sugar in the diet will help improve immunity against bladder infections. Herbs such as **goldenrod** (see page 313), **dandelion** (see page 266), **juniper** (see page 337), cleavers, **parsley** (see page 381), buchu, and **sandalwood** (see page 405) may increase urine flow, which could be helpful for increasing speed of recovery from an infection that has already occurred. The herb **lapacho** (see page 342) and the supplement **methionine** (see page 360) are also sometimes recommended for bladder infections, but there is no real evidence that they work.

🌱 BRITTLE NAILS

Related Terms   Onychoschizia, Onychorrhexis, Onychoschisis

Principal Proposed Treatments   Biotin

Other Proposed Treatments   Calcium, Cysteine, Gelatin-Containing Preparations, Iron, Vitamin A, Zinc, Horsetail (*Equisetum arvense*)

Brittle fingernails are a common condition, occurring in about 20% of people; more women than men develop brittle nails.[1]

Brittle nails usually break or peel off in horizontal layers, starting at the nail's free end. The term "brittle nails" can also refer to a condition in which lengthwise splits appear in the nail. In either case, the nail's structure is faulty.

Brittle nails may be caused by trauma to the nail, including repeated wetting and drying, repeated exposure to detergents and water, and excessive exposure to harsh solvents, such as those found in nail polish remover.[2,3] If your nails are regularly exposed to such stresses, it may be worth trying protective gloves when washing dishes and doing other chores. In the case of nail polish remover, gentler, less toxic brands have recently become available. Check with retailers of natural cosmetic products.

Nail brittleness may also be caused by an underlying medical condition, such as Raynaud's disease, low thyroid function (hypothyroidism), or lung conditions.[4,5] Other possible causes include skin diseases (psoriasis, lichen planus, alopecia areata) as well as endocrine disorders, tuberculosis, Sjögren's syndrome, and malnutrition.[6] Selenium poisoning can also cause brittle nails.[7]

Because of all these possibilities, it is important to rule out a serious underlying problem before trying nutritional or herbal treatments for brittle nails. If a medical cause for this condition is not found, it may be worth considering some of the following approaches.

PRINCIPAL PROPOSED TREATMENTS

Although no herb or supplement has been proven effective for brittle nails, there is some evidence that the B vitamin **biotin** (see page 221) might help.

Animal studies suggest that biotin supplementation can be helpful for deformed hooves in horses and pigs.[8–12] Since animal hooves are made of keratin, the same substance from which human nails are made, these findings have encouraged researchers to study the effects of biotin on brittle nails in humans.

Preliminary evidence from a small controlled study suggests that biotin may increase the thickness of brittle nails, reduce their tendency to split, and improve their microscopic structure.[13] To arrive at their results, the researchers used a scanning electron microscope to examine the effects of biotin in 8 women with brittle nails who were given 2.5 mg of biotin daily over 6- to 9-month periods. (An additional 24 individuals were also studied; 10 served as controls, and the other 14 were examined in a way that makes the interpretation of their results questionable.) Because all nail clippings were examined without the researchers being aware of whose clippings they were looking at, these results have some validity. However, the study was too small to allow definitive conclusions.

Two small open studies also reported benefits with biotin supplementation.[14,15] However, because there was no control group in either study, the results can't be taken as reliable.

Biotin is believed to be safe at the dosage used in these studies: 2.5 mg daily. However, maximum safe dosages for young children, pregnant or nursing women, or those with severe liver or kidney disease have not been established.

OTHER PROPOSED TREATMENTS

A number of other nutritional therapies have been tried for brittle nails, including **calcium** (see page 234), cysteine, gelatin-containing preparations, **iron** (see page 333), **vitamin A** (see page 432), and **zinc** (see page 463). However, as of yet, there is no real evidence that any of these treatments work.[16]

The herb horsetail (*Equisetum arvense*) is also sometimes mentioned as a treatment for brittle nails, again without proof that it works. See the chapter on **horsetail** for more information.

CANCER PREVENTION (Reducing the Risk)

Principal Proposed Treatments   Vitamin E, Selenium, Garlic, Tomatoes (Lycopene), Vitamin C, Green Tea, Soy, Isoflavones, Folate

Other Proposed Treatments   Calcium, Vitamin D, Fiber, Flaxseed (Lignans), Grapes (Resveratrol), Cartilage, Sulforaphane, Quercetin, Conjugated Linoleic Acid, Fish Oil, N-Acetyl Cysteine, Turmeric, Rosemary, Betulin, Bromelain, Citrus Juices, Ellagic Acid, Genistein, Ginseng, Glycine, Grass Pollen, Kelp, Licorice, Melatonin, MSM (Methyl Sulfonyl Methane), Milk Thistle, Nettle, OPCs (Oligomeric Proanthocyanidins), Papaw Tree Bark, Probiotics, Spirulina and Other Forms of Blue-Green Algae

Not Recommended Treatments   Beta-Carotene

Cancer is the second major cause of death (next to heart disease) in the United States. It claims the lives of more than half a million Americans a year out of the nearly 1.4 million who get the disease. The probability of getting cancer increases with age. Two-thirds of all cases are in people older than 65.[1]

According to the American Cancer Society, one in two men and one in three women will face cancer during their lifetimes. However, it appears that you significantly cut your cancer risk by how you choose to lead your life. That is the bright consensus of an international panel convened by the American Institute for Cancer Research and the World Cancer Research Fund.[2]

The panel found four key ways to reduce the odds of getting cancer: eat the right foods, exercise, watch your weight, and do not smoke. The experts reviewed diet and cancer findings from over 4,500 studies to reach this consensus.

What Causes Cancer?

Cancer is believed to begin with a mutation in a single cell. However, a cell doesn't become cancerous overnight. Several mutations in a row are necessary to create all the characteristic features of cancer. Ordinarily, cells have a self-destruct mechanism that causes them to die when their DNA is damaged. However, in developing cancer cells, something interferes with the self-destruct sequence. It may be that the cancer-causing mutations themselves turn off the countdown.

The DNA alterations that create a cancer cell give it a certain independence from the ordinary rules of cell behavior. Normal cells are highly influenced by nearby cells, with the result that they "get along" well with their neighbors. For example, the growth of a healthy cell is ruled by special growth factors given off by surrounding tissues. However, cancer cells either grow without such growth factors or simply make their own. Many types of cancer cells can also trigger the growth of new blood vessels to feed them.

Cancerous mutations appear to be caused mainly by exposure to carcinogenic substances, of which tobacco is the most common. Many carcinogens exist in the diet as well, such as salt-cured and smoked meats.

Free radicals also appear to play a major role in promoting cancer. These chemically unstable substances are produced by many factors, and are believed to affect heart disease and aging (for more information about free radicals in general, see the chapter on **atherosclerosis**). The best-documented natural treatments for preventing cancer have antioxidant properties.

Hormones can also help cancer get a start. For example, a newly formed cancer of the prostate or the breast is stimulated by the hormones that ordinarily control tissue in that part of the body. This is why estrogen-

Cancer Prevention

replacement therapy can increase the risk of breast cancer and why estrogen suppression is often recommended for women with a history of breast cancer.

Substances found in soy may help reduce the incidence of certain cancers by blocking the effects of estrogen and other hormones. However, this is not yet certain, and there is some contradictory evidence.[3]

The key to preventing cancer is to minimize your exposure to carcinogens. Quitting smoking is essential, and reducing your intake of smoked, charred, pickled, and salt-cured meat is also believed to be helpful. Refined grains (such as white flour) may also increase the risk of developing certain types of cancer.[4] Eating a diet that is high in fruits, vegetables, and whole grains and low in saturated fat (found primarily in dairy and meat) also appears to lower your chance of developing various forms of cancer.[5] Vegetables in the broccoli family may be particularly helpful. When it comes to natural cancer prevention, conventional and natural medicine are converging. The dietary suggestions listed previously were originally championed by "alternative" physicians, but they are all presently mainstream. Furthermore, many of the supplements described here are rapidly entering the mainstream as well.

Because the following material is so complex, we have summarized it in the section titled Putting It All Together. You can skip to it now if you want just the conclusions.

PRINCIPAL PROPOSED TREATMENTS

It is rather difficult to prove that taking a certain supplement will reduce the chance of developing cancer. You really need enormous long-term, double-blind studies in which some people are given the supplement while others are given placebo. However, relatively few studies of this type have been performed.

For most supplements, the evidence that they help prevent cancer comes from observational studies, which are much less reliable. Observational studies have found that people who happen to take in high levels of certain vitamins or herbs in their diets develop a lower incidence of specific cancers. However, in such studies it is very difficult to factor out other influences that may play a role. For example, individuals who take vitamins may also exercise more, or take better take care of themselves in other ways. Such "confounding factors" make the results of observational studies somewhat untrustworthy.

Vitamin E: May Reduce the Odds of Several Types of Cancer

In a double-blind trial that involved 29,133 smokers, those who were given 50 mg of synthetic **vitamin E** (see page 451) daily for 5 to 8 years showed a 32% reduction in the incidence of prostate cancer and a 41% drop in prostate cancer deaths.[6] Surprisingly, results were seen soon after the beginning of supplementation. This was unexpected because prostate cancer grows very slowly. A cancer that shows up today actually started to develop many years ago. The fact that vitamin E almost immediately lowered the incidence of prostate cancer suggests that it somehow blocks the step at which a hidden prostate cancer makes the leap to being detectable.

Similarly promising results have been seen in stomach cancer; mouth, throat, and laryngeal cancer; and liver cancer.[7–10] However, vitamin E does not appear to be helpful against lung cancer, and the evidence regarding colon cancer is quite mixed.[11–19]

Vitamin E is typically supplemented at a dose of 400 to 800 IU daily. Realistically, you can't get this much vitamin E in your diet, so supplements are necessary.

Vitamin E is generally believed to be safe at this dosage level. However, vitamin E is known to affect blood clotting and for this reason should not be combined with aspirin or prescription blood thinners except under a physician's supervision.[20] Vitamin E may also present some risk of bleeding on its own. In one study of 28,519 men, vitamin E supplementation at the low dose of about 50 IU synthetic vitamin E per day caused an increase in fatal hemorrhagic strokes, the kind of stroke caused by bleeding. (However, it reduced the risk of a more common type of stroke, and the two effects essentially canceled out.)[21]

Selenium: May Protect Against Lung, Prostate, and Colon Cancer

It has long been known that severe **selenium** (see page 407) deficiency increases the risk of cancer.[22] However, by itself, this does not prove that taking selenium supplements will make a difference if you are not deficient in it.

However, one double-blind study did find that selenium supplements can dramatically reduce the incidence of cancer. The results were so impressive they caught the researchers by surprise. The study was actually designed to detect selenium's effects on skin cancer.[23] It followed 1,312 individuals, half of whom were given 200 mcg of selenium daily. The participants were treated for an average of 2.8 years and were followed for about 6 years. Although no significant effect on skin cancer was found, the researchers were startled when the results showed that people taking selenium had a 50% reduction in overall cancer deaths and significant decreases in cancer of the lung (40%), colon (50%), and prostate (66%). The findings were so remarkable that the researchers felt obliged to break the blind and allow all the participants to take selenium.

While this evidence is very promising, it has one major flaw. The laws of statistics tell us that when researchers start to deviate from the question their research was designed to answer, the results may not be trustworthy. For this reason, further research needs to

Visit Us at TNP.com

be done to truly confirm that selenium actually can help prevent these types of cancer.

The usual recommended therapeutic dosage of selenium is 100 to 200 mcg daily. Of the various sources of selenium, organic forms, such as selenomethionine, selenium-rich yeast, and selenium-enriched garlic, may be preferable to inorganic sodium selenite.[24,25] However, this is a bit controversial.[26,27] When taken at the recommended dosage, selenium is believed to be safe and side-effect free. Long-term use of selenium at a level of 200 mcg daily has been found to be safe in adults, and doses up to 350 mcg daily are believed to be harmless.[28] Toxic effects begin to be seen at levels above 850 mcg daily and include gastrointestinal distress, central nervous system changes, garlic-like breath odor, and loss of hair and fingernails.

Maximum safe dosages in young children, pregnant or nursing women, and those with severe liver or kidney disease have not been established.

Garlic: May Reduce the Risk of Colon Cancer

Evidence from observational studies suggests that **garlic** (see page 291) may help prevent cancer.

In the Iowa Women's Study, a very large and well-conducted observational study (a trial in which researchers observe the participants to try to identify lifestyle factors associated with better health), women who ate significant amounts of garlic were found to be about 30% less likely to develop colon cancer.[29] Similar results were seen in other observational studies performed in China, Italy, and the United States.[30,31]

We do not know for sure how garlic might work to prevent cancer. Like vitamin E, whole garlic possesses antioxidant properties.[32,33] Furthermore, various garlic extracts have also been shown to suppress the known DNA-damaging activity of several drugs and toxins.[34] Finally, garlic contains high levels of selenium, which is thought to reduce the risk of cancer (see the previous discussion under the heading Selenium).[35]

It's unclear how much garlic is needed for a cancer-preventive effect, but one or two cloves daily should probably suffice. Side effects (other than bad breath) are rare, and garlic is on the FDA's list of agents that are generally recognized as safe. However, raw garlic in excessive doses can cause stomach upset, heartburn, nausea and vomiting, diarrhea, facial flushing, rapid heartbeat, and insomnia. Garlic appears to interfere with blood clotting, so it should not be combined with blood-thinning drugs such as Coumadin (warfarin), Trental (pentoxifylline), or even aspirin except under medical supervision, nor should it be taken immediately before or after surgery or labor and delivery.[36] There might also be some risk involved in combining garlic with other blood-thinning herbs or natural supplements, such as

ginkgo (see page 298) and high-dose **vitamin E** (see page 451), although no problems have been reported.

Beta-Carotene: Helpful in the Diet, Harmful As a Supplement?

In the early 1980s, a review of the observational studies clearly showed that people whose diets are high in fruits and vegetables have a significantly decreased risk for cancer.[37,38] Some of the strongest evidence relates to lung cancer, for which a high intake of fruits and vegetables was associated with as much as a 70% reduced risk.

Scientists then set about trying to identify the active principle in fruits and vegetables. One group of substances widely available in these foods is carotenes (named after carrots). A careful examination of the data suggests that the level of carotenes in the diet is strongly connected with protection against lung cancer.[39] Evidence also suggests that carotenes protect against bladder cancer,[40] breast cancer,[41] esophageal cancer,[42] and stomach cancer.[43]

The best-known carotene is **beta-carotene** (see page 217), a strong antioxidant that the body can convert to **vitamin A** (see page 432). It was a natural step to assume that it was the beta-carotene in these foods that was making the difference. In animal studies, beta-carotene supplements seemed to significantly reduce the incidence of cancer.[44] Unfortunately, studies in which people were actually given beta-carotene supplements (rather than foods containing it) have not shown wonderful results.

The anticancer bubble burst for beta-carotene in 1994 when the results of the Alpha-Tocopherol, Beta-Carotene (ATBC) study came in. Apparently, beta-carotene did not prevent but actually *increased* the risk of getting lung cancer by 18%. This intervention trial had followed 29,133 male smokers in Finland who took supplements of either about 50 IU of vitamin E (alpha-tocopherol) or 20 mg of beta-carotene, or both, or a placebo daily for 5 to 8 years.[45] This was the same study mentioned previously in which vitamin E reduced the risk of prostate cancer; however, beta-carotene worked in the opposite direction.

In January 1996, researchers monitoring the Beta-Carotene and Retinol Efficacy Trial (CARET) confirmed this bad news with more of their own: the beta-carotene group had 46% more cases of lung cancer deaths.[46] This study involved smokers, former smokers, and workers exposed to asbestos.

Alarmed, the National Cancer Institute (NCI) pushed the brake pedal on the $42 million trial 21 months before it was finished. At about the same time, the 12-year Physicians' Health Study of 22,000 male physicians was finding that 50 mg of beta-carotene taken every other day had no effect at all—good or bad—on the risk of cancer or heart disease.[47,48] In this study, 11%

of the participants were smokers, and 39% were ex-smokers.

Similarly, another study of beta-carotene supplements failed to find any effect on the risk of cancer or heart disease in women.[49]

Interestingly, in both the ATBC study and the CARET study, higher levels of carotene intake from the diet *were* associated with lower levels of cancer. Apparently, beta-carotene is not effective alone. Other carotenes found in fruits and vegetables appear to be more important for preventing cancer (see, for example, the following discussion on lycopene). It is possible that taking beta-carotene depletes the body of other carotenes, thereby producing an overall harmful effect.[50]

These studies also found that beta-carotene supplements may increase the risk of heart disease and stroke as well. Therefore, we recommend getting your beta-carotene from foods, rather than supplements. The best dietary sources of carotenes are yellow-orange vegetables and dark green vegetables.

Tomatoes (Lycopene): May Be More Important Than Beta-Carotene

Lycopene (see page 349), a carotenoid like beta-carotene, is found in high levels in tomatoes and pink grapefruit. Lycopene appears to exhibit about twice the antioxidant activity of beta-carotene and may be more important for preventing cancer than the better-known vitamin.

In one study, elderly Americans consuming a diet high in tomatoes reduced their risk for cancers by 50%.[51] Men and women who ate at least seven servings of tomatoes weekly developed less stomach and colorectal cancers compared to those who ate only two servings weekly.

In another study, 47,894 men were followed for 4 years in an observational study looking for influences on prostate cancer.[52] Their diets were evaluated on the basis of how often they ate fruits, vegetables, and foods containing fruits and vegetables. High levels of tomatoes, tomato sauce, and pizza in the diet were strongly connected to the prevention of prostate cancer. After an evaluation of known nutritional factors in these foods as compared to other foods, lycopene appeared to be the common denominator. Additional impetus has been given to this idea by the discovery of lycopene in reasonably high levels in the human prostate,[53] as well as evidence that men with higher lycopene levels in the blood have a lower risk of prostate cancer.[54]

Further evidence suggests that lycopene might help prevent numerous other forms of cancer as well, including lung, colon, and breast cancer.[55]

Cooked tomatoes appear to be more bioavailable (more readily used by the body) than raw tomatoes, especially when the tomatoes are cooked in oil. Tomato juice does not seem to be helpful.

Vitamin C: Helpful in the Diet, Not Helpful As a Supplement?

As with beta-carotene, most of the positive studies of **vitamin C** (see page 444) and cancer prevention have looked at the effect of vitamin C in the diet rather than at actual vitamin C supplements. It is possible the other plant substances that come along with vitamin C are equally or more important. Studies involving vitamin C supplements have not produced stellar results.

Several studies have found a strong association between high dietary vitamin C intake and a reduced incidence of stomach cancer.[56,57,58] One way in which vitamin C may work is by preventing the formation of carcinogenic substances known as N-nitroso compounds in the stomach.

Evidence also suggests that vitamin C from food may also provide a protective effect in colon, esophageal, laryngeal, bladder, cervical, rectal, breast, and perhaps lung cancer.[59–63] However, dietary vitamin C intake does not appear to be associated with protection against prostate cancer.[64]

A few studies have used supplemental vitamin C instead of dietary vitamin C. One found that vitamin C supplementation at 500 mg or more daily was associated with a lower incidence of bladder cancer.[65] However, another study found no connection.[66]

Supplemental vitamin C at 1 g daily failed to prevent new colon cancers after one colon cancer had developed.[67] In another large observational study, 500 mg or more of vitamin C daily over a period of 6 years provided no significant protection against breast cancer.[68] Another study found similar results.[69]

Thus, just as with beta-carotene, it may be that the natural dietary substances that come along with vitamin C are more important for cancer prevention than the vitamin alone. In this case, water-soluble flavonoids may be responsible for the benefit. Eat your fruits and vegetables!

Green Tea: May Help Prevent Many Types of Cancer

Both **green tea** (see page 318) and black tea come from the tea plant called *Camellia sinensis*, which has been cultivated in China for centuries. The key difference between the two is in preparation. For black tea, the leaves are allowed to oxidize, a process believed to lessen the potency of therapeutic compounds known as polyphenols. Green tea is made by lightly steaming the freshly cut leaf, a process that prevents oxidation and possibly preserves more of the therapeutic effects.

Laboratory and animal studies suggest that tea consumption protects against cancers of the stomach, lung, esophagus, duodenum, pancreas, liver, breast, and colon.[70,71] A 1994 study of skin cancer in mice found that both black and green teas, even decaffeinated versions, inhibited skin cancer in mice exposed to ultraviolet light and other carcinogens.[72,73] After 31 weeks, mice given the teas brewed at the same concentration humans drink had 72 to 93% fewer skin tumors than mice given only water.

However, results from human studies have not been so clear-cut—some have shown a protective effect, and others have not. Nonetheless, the overall weight of the evidence does lean toward the positive side.[74]

One study followed 8,552 Japanese adults for 9 years.[75] Women who drank more than 10 cups daily had a delay in the onset of cancer and also a 43% lower total rate of cancer occurrence. Males had a 32% lower cancer incidence, but this finding was not statistically significant.

A study in Shanghai, China, found that those who drank green tea had significant reductions in the risk of developing cancers of the rectum and pancreas. No significant decrease in colon cancer was found.[76] A total of 3,818 residents aged 30 to 74 were included in the population study. For men, those who drank the most tea had a 28% lower incidence of rectal cancer and a 37% lower incidence of pancreatic cancer compared to those who did not drink tea regularly. For women, the respective reductions in cancer frequency were even greater: 43% and 47%.

Another study in Shanghai found similar results for stomach cancer. Green tea drinkers were 29% less likely to get stomach cancer than nondrinkers, with those drinking the most tea having the least risk.[77] Interestingly, the risk of stomach cancer did not depend on the person's age at which he or she started drinking green tea. Researchers suggested that green tea may disrupt the cancer process at both the intermediate and the late stage.

However, this is a rapidly evolving field, and new information has been released suggesting that there were significant flaws in the green tea studies just described. Other recent evidence indicates that black tea may be more protective than green tea. We suggest talking to your physician about the latest information.

The active ingredients in green tea are believed to be polyphenols, especially one known as epigallocatechin gallate (EGCG). Like vitamin C, polyphenols may block the formation of nitrosamines and other cancer-causing compounds and may trap or detoxify carcinogens.[78] Green tea may also exert an estrogen-blocking effect that is helpful in preventing breast and uterine cancer,[79] and another study suggests that it might prevent the development of tumors by blocking the growth of new blood vessels.[80]

The optimum dosage of green tea is unknown. However, you might want to use the amount correlated with good results in the observational studies. That would mean either drinking 3 cups of green tea daily or taking 100 to 150 mg 3 times daily of a green tea extract standardized for 80% total polyphenols and 55% epigallocatechin content. No significant side effects are associated with green tea, other than those due to its (rather low) caffeine content.

Soy: May Reduce the Risk of Hormone-Related Cancers

In many animal studies, soybeans, soy protein, or other soy extracts decreased cancer risk, and observational studies show that the same effect may occur in people as well.[81–87] According to the data we have, **soy** (see page 411) may help prevent hormone-related cancers such as prostate, breast, and uterine cancer. However, there is a bit of contradictory evidence, too. One highly preliminary study in humans found changes suggestive of increased breast cancer risk after women took a commercial soy protein product.[88]

Soybeans provide estrogen-like compounds known as **isoflavones** (see page 335), especially genistein and daidzein. These substances bind to the same sites in the body as estrogen, occupying these sites and keeping natural estrogen away. Estrogen stimulates certain forms of cancer, but soy isoflavones exert a milder estrogen-like effect that may not stimulate cancer as much as natural estrogen. This may partially explain soy's apparent protective effect.[89,90] Soy or soy extracts may also affect cancers in other ways, but more remains to be discovered.

However, in observational studies, it is difficult to tell whether the soy is exerting a directly positive effect on its own or whether some of the benefit is due to the fact that people who eat more soy also eat less meat. For more definitive results, we need studies in which soy or soy extracts are added to the diets of a large group of people while another group is given placebo treatment. Unfortunately, this type of research into soy is still in its infancy. It will require more extensive investigation before we can be absolutely sure that soy prevents cancer.

Soy foods are believed to be safe, although high doses of soy can interfere with mineral absorption. There is also some concern that soy may not be advisable for women who have already had breast cancer. In addition, intensive use of soy products by pregnant women could exert a hormonal effect that impacts unborn fetuses.[91,92]

There are some concerns that soy may impair thyroid function or reduce absorption of thyroid medication, at least in children.[93,94,95] For this reason, individuals with impaired thyroid function should use soy with caution.

Folate

Folate (see page 288) deficiency may predispose individuals toward developing cancer of the cervix,[96] colon,[97,98] lung,[99] breast,[100] and mouth.[101] Large observational studies suggest that folate supplements may help prevent colon cancer, especially when taken for many years.[102,103,104] Since deficiency of this essential vitamin is quite common (and quite unhealthy), you really can't go wrong taking extra folate.

A typical dosage is 400 mcg daily. Folate is safe, but because it can mask vitamin B_{12} deficiency, it is wise to get your B_{12} level checked before taking high doses (800 mcg or more).

OTHER PROPOSED TREATMENTS

The substances mentioned in this section have less evidence behind them than the antioxidants discussed previously. However, this is a rapidly growing field. By the time you read this section, new information will undoubtedly be available.

Calcium

Some, but not all, studies have found evidence that **calcium** (see page 234) supplementation might reduce the risk of colon cancer.[105–114]

Vitamin D

Some studies have connected higher **vitamin D** (see page 449) levels with a lower incidence of cancer of the breast, colon, pancreas, and prostate, but overall the research has yielded mixed results.[115–121]

Fiber

Dietary fiber has been thought to help prevent colon cancer.[122,123] However, recent studies have found either little benefit or none at all.[124–130]

Flaxseed (Lignans)

Substances known as lignans are found in several foods and may produce anticancer benefits. They are converted in the digestive tract to estrogen-like substances known as enterolactone and enterodiol.[131,132] Like soy isoflavones (see the previous discussion under the heading Soy), these substances prevent estrogen from attaching to cells and may thereby block its cancer-promoting effects.

Lignans are found most abundantly in **flaxseed** (see page 286) (the whole seed), a high-fiber grain that has been cultivated since ancient Egyptian times. However, contrary to some reports, flaxseed *oil* contains no lignans.[133] **Flaxseed oil** (see page 285) is a rich source of the omega-3 fatty acid: alpha-linolenic acid.

Although flaxseed or flaxseed oil is sometimes recommended as prevention or treatment for cancer, the evidence is still extremely preliminary.[134–141] Weak evidence also suggests that the alpha-linolenic acid in flaxseed oil may act against breast cancer. Low levels of alpha-linolenic acid in breast fatty tissues were associated with an increase in cancer and its spread (metastasis) to other areas of the body.[142] Test tube studies found that flaxseed or one of its lignans inhibited the growth of human breast cancer cells.[143] Other studies suggest that the lignans enterolactone and enterodiol inhibited the growth of human colon tumor cells.[144]

The optimum dose of flaxseed is not known. The typical supplemental dosage of flaxseed recommended by some nutritionists is 1 tablespoon of the whole or bruised seed (not ground) with plenty of liquid 2 to 3 times daily; for flaxseed oil, a typical dose is 1 to 2 tablespoons daily. In some studies, participants took 5, 15, or even 45 g of ground flaxseed per day. Flaxseed oil is easily damaged by heat and light, so do not cook with it. The most palatable way to take it is by adding it to foods, such as using it as a salad dressing.

Flaxseed and its oil appear to be safe nutritional supplements when used as directed. Because of their potential effects on estrogen, however, avoid taking large amounts of either if you are pregnant or breast-feeding. Very sensitive test tube studies suggest large doses of flaxseeds may actually stimulate cancer cells.[145] If you have cancer, particularly breast cancer, talk with your doctor before consuming large amounts of flaxseed or lignans. As with many substances, there have been reports of life-threatening allergic reactions to flaxseed.

Grapes (Resveratrol)

Resveratrol (see page 401) is a phytochemical found in at least 72 different plants, including mulberries and peanuts. Grapes are its richest source. Red wine, which is made from grapes, contains a lot of resveratrol, which may account for some of the beneficial effects attributed to wine in some studies.

Resveratrol is an antioxidant with intriguing anticancer effects as determined in test tube studies.[146,147] However, little direct evidence supports the idea that resveratrol is helpful. The proper dosage is not known, and safety studies have not yet been completed.

Cartilage

Based on the belief that sharks don't get cancer, shark **cartilage** (see page 241) has been heavily marketed as a cure for cancer. While this is a myth (sharks do get cancer), shark cartilage has, in fact, shown some promise. Shark cartilage tends to inhibit the growth of new blood vessels (angiogenesis). Since cancers must build new blood vessels to feed themselves, this effect might be beneficial.

Shark cartilage also inhibits substances called matrix metalloproteases (MMPs).[148] These little-understood enzymes affect the "extracellular matrix," the framework of substances that lie between cells in the body. MMPs are thought to play a role in diseases of the cornea, gums, skin, blood vessels, and joints, as well as cancer and illnesses that involve excessive fibrous tissue.

A number of test tube experiments have found that shark cartilage extracts prevent new blood vessels from forming in chick embryos and other test systems.[149–154] As mentioned previously, this effect could conceivably mean that shark cartilage might fight cancer. These findings have

Visit Us at TNP.com

"Candida"

Visit Us at TNP.com

led to other test tube experiments, animal studies, and preliminary human trials to investigate the possible anticancer effects of shark cartilage. The results suggest that a particular liquid shark cartilage extract might be useful in the treatment of various cancers, including lung, prostate and breast cancer.[155–160] However, not all studies have been positive.[161,162]

Double-blind trials are needed to provide conclusive data. These are now underway in the United States and Canada.

Other Treatments on the Horizon

Provocative evidence suggests that a substance called sulforaphane, found in broccoli and related vegetables, may possess anticancer properties. Recently, broccoli sprouts have been touted as a cancer treatment on the basis of their high content of sulforaphane. However, this recommendation is still highly speculative.

Test-tube and animal research also suggests that the supplements **quercetin**[163–167] (see page 396) and **conjugated linoleic acid**[168] (see page 261) might have anticancer properties.

One study provides preliminary supporting evidence for the notion that **fish oil** (see page 282) reduces the risk of prostate cancer.[169]

A preliminary study suggests that **N-acetyl cysteine** (NAC; see page 366) treatment may help to prevent colon cancer.[170] However, this evidence has not been confirmed by additional studies.

Weak or indirect evidence also suggests some cancer-preventive benefits for the spices **turmeric** (see page 425) and rosemary as well as for betulin (from white birch tree), **bromelain** (see page 229), citrus juices, ellagic acid (from grapes, raspberries, strawberries, apples, walnuts, and pecans), **genistein** (see page 294), **ginseng** (see page 301), **glycine** (see page 311), **grass pollen** (see page 317), **kelp** (see page 340), **licorice** (see page 344), **melatonin** (see page 357), **MSM** (see page 364), **milk thistle** (see page 361), **nettle** (see page 369), **OPCs** (oligomeric proanthocyanidins; see page 373), papaw tree bark, probiotics or "friendly" bacteria such as **acidophilus** (see page 200), and **spirulina** (see page 413) or other types of blue-green algae.[171–188]

PUTTING IT ALL TOGETHER

To prevent cancer, the best thing you can do for yourself is to eat a diet high in fruits and vegetables and whole grains and low in smoked, charred, pickled, and salt-cured meats as well as other animal products. Increasing exercise and losing weight also appears to help significantly, and to stop smoking is essential.

Vitamin E might reduce the incidence of various forms of cancer, particularly prostate cancer, but also cancer of the colon, stomach, mouth, throat, larynx, and liver. A typical dosage is 400 IU daily of alpha-tocopherol.

Selenium supplementation (200 mcg daily) might be helpful for preventing lung, colon, and prostate cancers.

Garlic could help prevent colon cancer.

Purified beta-carotene has not been shown to prevent cancer (and it may even increase the risk), but carotenes in the diet appear to protect against lung cancer as well as cancer of the bladder, breast, stomach, and upper digestive tract.

Folate supplements may help prevent colon cancer and possibly other types of cancer as well.

Tomatoes seem to reduce the occurrence of prostate cancer as well as stomach, lung, breast, and colon cancer, perhaps due to their content of the natural carotene lycopene. Cooked tomatoes appear to be more bioavailable (more readily used by the body) than raw tomatoes, especially when the tomatoes are cooked in oil.

Green tea may help prevent colon cancer, and weaker evidence suggests that it may help prevent cancer of the stomach, small intestine, pancreas, lungs, breast, and uterus.

Soy may help prevent hormone-sensitive cancers, such as those of the breast, prostate, uterus, and colon.

Little direct evidence supports the idea that vitamin C supplements prevent cancer, but foods high in vitamin C seem to lower the incidence of stomach cancer as well as colon, esophageal, laryngeal, bladder, cervical, rectal, and breast cancer.

Please refer to the chapters on these substances to learn about safety issues associated with some of them.

"CANDIDA"/YEAST HYPERSENSITIVITY SYNDROME

Principal Proposed Treatments   There are no well-established natural treatments for "candida"/yeast hypersensitivity syndrome.

Other Proposed Treatments   Probiotics, Capryllic Acid, Grapefruit Seed Extract, Betaine Hydrochloride, Peppermint Oil, Oregano Oil, Lavender Oil, Tea Tree Oil, Barberry, Red Thyme, Lapacho, Garlic, Avoiding Foods with High Mold Content, Low-Sugar Diet

Candida albicans is a naturally occurring yeast that flourishes in moist areas, such as the digestive tract, the vagina, and skin folds. Ordinarily, its population is kept in check by bacteria that live in the same areas. When normal bacteria are disturbed by antibiotics, however, yeast populations can grow to abnormally high levels.

For women, the most common symptom of excess *Candida* is a **vaginal yeast infection** (see page 182), as marked by itchiness, redness, burning on urination, and a yeasty odor. However, *Candida* can also overpopulate in the mouth (thrush), in the warm moist environment under a diaper (diaper rash), and in other areas.

Candida usually confines itself to the surface of mucous membranes and does not penetrate deeply into the body. However, in people whose immune systems are severely depressed, such as those with AIDS or leukemia, candida can become a dangerous, invasive organism. The medical name for this rare and dire condition is *systemic candidiasis.*

Besides this official meaning, systemic candidiasis has another meaning that was coined in the world of alternative medicine. As used there, it is a loose term connoting a whole syndrome of symptoms believed to be related to candida. Equivalent terms are *chronic Candida, yeast syndrome, yeast hypersensitivity syndrome,* or just plain *Candida* for short.

Conventional medicine does not recognize the existence of this alternative syndrome. However, for several years it was practically impossible to walk into an alternative practitioner's office and not walk out with the diagnosis of candida. Fortunately, this excess enthusiasm has cooled in recent years. Among people who believe that they have a candida problem, perhaps 1 in 20 will benefit significantly from treatment for it. *Candida* is more a fad than a reality. Nonetheless, it has some reality behind it as well.

The story of "the yeast syndrome" begins in 1983, when Orion Truss published *The Missing Diagnosis.* This was followed by William Crook's much more famous *The Yeast Connection.* These books claim that a person who is chronically colonized by too much *Candida* may develop an allergy-like hypersensitivity to it. The symptoms of this allergy are said to be similar to those of other allergies, including sinus congestion, fatigue, intestinal gas, difficulty concentrating, depression, muscle aches, and many other common complaints.

The regimen outlined by Dr. Crook consists of two parts: treatments that tend toward diminishing the total body burden of *Candida;* and less convincing recommendations that attempt to lessen allergic reactions toward yeast in general.

To decrease the amount of yeast in the body, Dr. Crook recommends avoiding certain substances, including antibiotics, corticosteroids, birth control pills, sugar, and most sweet foods (it is his contention that dietary sugar "feeds yeast"). He also recommends the use of various supplements and even strong prescription drugs to directly kill yeast or at least interfere with its growth.

Next, Dr. Crook recommends avoiding foods containing yeast of any type, for he believes that those who are allergic to *Candida* will also be allergic to other members of the fungus family. Thus Dr. Crook forbids fermented foods, such as beer, cheese, breads containing baker's yeast, tomato paste (which has a significant mold content), and even mushrooms.

Some of these recommendations seem far-fetched. Although both mushrooms and *Candida* fall into the broad category of fungi, they are not very closely related. Cats and elephants are both mammals, for example, but an allergy to one does not generally imply an allergy to the other. It is difficult to believe that those with sensitivity to *Candida* should also cross-react with food mushrooms, and we have seldom seen it in real life.

Similarly, *Candida* and baker's yeast bear only a distant relationship. Although many people with apparent *Candida* problems do in fact react negatively to bread, it may not be the yeast in the bread that is causing the problem. People with allergies to *Candida* are basically highly allergenic people. They may simply be allergic to the wheat in bread rather than to the yeast. After all, wheat is the second most common food allergen.

There is no conventional medical treatment for yeast hypersensitivity syndrome because conventional medicine does not recognize its existence.

PROPOSED TREATMENTS

There is no scientific evidence that any treatment can reduce the symptoms caused by oversensitivity to *Candida.*

Many treatments can reduce the amount of yeast in the body, and people with a genuine allergy to *Candida* may feel better once this is achieved. Unfortunately, it isn't possible to eliminate *Candida albicans* permanently. No matter how successful a treatment may be, as soon as it is stopped, *Candida* will return. It has to because it is a natural inhabitant of the body. However, we know from other conditions, such as vaginal yeast infections, that sufficient intake of **probiotics** (see page 200), or "friendly" bacteria, can help keep yeast regrowth within reasonable bounds. It is probably best to use a mixture of organisms, including acidophilus, bulgaricus, and bifidus. The daily dose should provide 3 to 10 billion viable organisms.

Agents that may reduce the amount of yeast in the body include capryllic acid, grapefruit seed extract, **betaine hydrochloride** (see page 219), **peppermint** (see page 384) oil, oregano oil, lavender oil, **tea tree** (see page 421) oil, barberry, red thyme, pau d'arco also called **lapacho** (see page 342), and **garlic** (see page 291). However, the scientific foundation for the use of these treatments is weak, and the appropriate dosage of each has not been determined. Some of these treatments may be toxic if taken to excess or for prolonged periods.

Other Treatments

As mentioned earlier, proponents of the candida syndrome further believe that it is important to restrict sugar in the diet, even fruit sugar. This concept is based on the idea that "sugar feeds yeast." However, there is no scientific evidence that dietary sugar increases the growth of *Candida*. They also recommend eliminating all foods with high mold content, such as alcoholic drinks, peanuts, cheeses, bread, and dried fruits. Although these foods cannot increase the amount of *Candida* in your body, they contain yeasts that you could conceivably be allergic to.

CANKER SORES

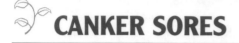

Principal Proposed Treatments   Deglycyrrhizinated Licorice (DGL)

Other Proposed Treatments   Acidophilus, Calendula, Vitamin B$_1$

Canker sores are small ulcers in the mouth caused by an assortment of viruses. A susceptibility to canker sores tends to run in families. No successful conventional treatment is available.

PRINCIPAL PROPOSED TREATMENTS

A chemically altered form of the herb **licorice** (see page 344) known as deglycyrrhizinated licorice (DGL) may be useful in canker sores.

DGL is best known as a useful treatment for **ulcers** (see page 180). One preliminary study suggests that DGL might help relieve the discomfort of canker sores as well.[1] This form of licorice is believed to be safe, although safety has not been established in young children, pregnant or nursing women, and those with severe liver or kidney disease. The main problem with DGL is that it must be sucked to coat the canker sores, and some people find its taste objectionable.

According to one report, whole licorice possesses significant estrogenic activity and, as such, shouldn't be taken by women who have had breast cancer.[2] Licorice may also reduce testosterone levels in men.[3] For this reason, men with impotence, infertility, or decreased libido may want to avoid this herb. It is not clear whether the same potential exists with DGL, but it is less likely.

OTHER PROPOSED TREATMENTS

Other herbs and supplements sometimes recommended for canker sores include **acidophilus** (see page 200), **calendula** (see page 237), and **vitamin B$_1$** (see page 434), but there is little evidence as yet that they are effective.

CARDIOMYOPATHY

Principal Proposed Treatments   Coenzyme Q$_{10}$ (CoQ$_{10}$), Carnitine

Cardiomyopathy is a little understood condition in which the muscle tissue of the heart becomes diseased. There are several distinct forms of cardiomyopathy that may or may not be similar in origin. Medical treatment consists mainly of medications that attempt to compensate for the increasing failure of the heart to function properly. A heart transplant may ultimately be necessary.

PRINCIPAL PROPOSED TREATMENTS

Cardiomyopathy is certainly not a disease that you should treat yourself! For this reason, we deliberately do not discuss dosage or safety issues in this section, although general guidelines can be found in the chapters on these substances. However, in consultation with your physician, you may want to consider adding the following two supplements to your treatment regimen.

Coenzyme Q$_{10}$

There is some evidence that the naturally occurring substance **coenzyme Q$_{10}$** (CoQ$_{10}$; see page 256) can be beneficial in some forms of cardiomyopathy.[1,2,3]

In a 6-year trial, 143 people with moderately severe cardiomyopathy were given CoQ$_{10}$ daily in addition to standard medical care.[4] The results showed a significant improvement in cardiac function (technically, ejection fraction) in 84% of the study participants. Most of them improved by several stages on a scale that measures the severity of heart failure (technically, NYHA class). Furthermore, a comparison with individuals on conventional therapy alone appeared to show a reduction in mortality.

This study was an open trial, meaning that participants knew that they were being treated, so such studies are not fully reliable due to the power of suggestion. However, these results, including objective measurements of heart function, were so impressive that it is hard to believe the power of suggestion alone could explain them. Nonetheless, double-blind studies are more definitive.

There have been a few such studies of CoQ_{10} in cardiomyopathy. One double-blind controlled trial followed 80 people with various forms of cardiomyopathy over a period of 3 years.[5] Of those treated with CoQ_{10}, 89% improved significantly, but when the treatment was stopped, their heart function deteriorated.

No benefit was seen in another double-blind study, but it was a smaller and shorter trial and enrolled only people who had one particular type of cardiomyopathy (idiopathic dilated cardiomyopathy).[6]

However, there are concerns that CoQ_{10}, like many other substances, might interact with the blood-thinning drug Coumadin (warfarin).[7] Individuals taking warfarin should not take CoQ_{10} (or any other supplement) except under physician supervision.

Carnitine

There is a little evidence that the vitamin-like supplement **carnitine** (see page 238) may be useful in cardiomyopathy.[8,9] Carnitine is believed to work well with CoQ_{10}, and the two treatments are often combined.[10]

CARPAL TUNNEL SYNDROME

Principal Proposed Treatments   Vitamin B_6

Other Proposed Treatments   Bromelain, Proteolytic Enzymes

Carpal tunnel syndrome (CTS) is a common and often disabling condition most often associated with data entry and general computer use, but it can affect anyone who performs repetitive hand motions. CTS strikes women more often than men and is a relatively common complication of pregnancy. It also occurs frequently among people with rheumatoid arthritis and diabetes.

CTS is caused by compression of the median nerve. On its way to the hand, the nerve passes through an opening in the wrist called the carpal tunnel. Constant, repetitive hand motion may aggravate the ligaments and tendons encased in the tunnel, causing them to swell. As the tunnel walls close in, they compress the median nerve. This causes tingling and numbness in the thumb, index finger, middle finger, and half of the ring finger. The discomfort of CTS often wakes people during the night and eventually makes it difficult to grasp small objects.

Most instances of CTS are job related. Paying attention to proper ergonomics is essential for preventing CTS. This might involve repositioning a computer keyboard or taking breaks more often. Conventional medical treatment for more stubborn CTS cases is fairly successful. Splinting the affected hand, especially at night, may help reduce symptoms. Nonsteroidal anti-inflammatory medications such as ibuprofen or naproxen may help, as can cortisone injections. When such measures fail, the swollen ligament may be released surgically by cutting it at the base of the wrist, thus freeing the median nerve from pressure. In extreme cases, a person with work-related CTS may have to switch jobs.[1]

PRINCIPAL PROPOSED TREATMENTS

More than 25 years ago, researchers noted that people with CTS seemed to be deficient in **vitamin B_6** (see page 439).[2] This led to widespread use of B_6 as a CTS remedy. However, a recent study found no association between CTS and B_6 deficiency.[3] In any case, even if B_6 deficiency were common in CTS, that by itself wouldn't prove that taking B_6 *supplements* can reduce symptoms.

A few studies have investigated the effectiveness of vitamin B_6 for CTS. Most were poorly designed and involved few people. The two (albeit small) randomized, double-blind placebo-controlled studies that do exist found no evidence that vitamin B_6 effectively treats CTS. The first study, which enrolled only 15 people, found no significant difference after 10 weeks among those taking vitamin B_6, placebo, or nothing at all.[4] The second, involving 32 people, did find some benefits, but these were fairly minor.[5] There was no improvement in nighttime pain, numbness, or tingling, nor in objective measurements of median nerve function. Some benefit, however, was seen in the relatively less important symptoms of finger swelling and discomfort after repetitive motion.

A typical recommended dose of vitamin B_6 for CTS is 200 mg twice daily. However, this far exceeds necessary nutritional requirements and could present some risks.

Visit Us at TNP.com

Cataracts

Taking more than 2,000 mg (2 g) daily may cause nerve damage. Although lower doses of B_6 are usually not harmful, nerve-related symptoms have been reported at doses as low as 200 mg when taken for a long period.[6,7]

The bottom line: Because vitamin B_6 has not been proven effective and may be harmful in high doses, we do not recommend it for carpal tunnel syndrome.

OTHER PROPOSED TREATMENTS

Bromelain (see page 229) and other **proteolytic enzymes** (see page 393) are sometimes recommended for the treatment of carpal tunnel syndrome, but there is no evidence as yet that they work.

Acupuncture has also been tried, but has not been proven effective for CTS.

CATARACTS (Prevention)

Principal Proposed Treatments   Vitamin C, Vitamin E
  Dietary Carotenes: Lutein, Lycopene

Other Proposed Treatments   Bilberry, Ginkgo, OPCs (Oligomeric Proanthocyanidins), Turmeric, Cysteine, Lipoic Acid, Vitamin B_3 (Niacin), Vitamin B_2 (Riboflavin), Selenium, Taurine, Zinc

Cataracts—an opaque buildup of damaged proteins in the lens of the eye—are the leading cause of visual decline in those over 65. In fact, most people in that age group have at least the beginnings of cataract formation. Many factors contribute to the development of cataracts but damage by free radicals is believed to play a major role. (See the chapter on **atherosclerosis** for a description of free radicals.)

Cataracts can be removed surgically. Although this has become a relatively quick, safe, easy, and painless surgery, it does not result in completely normal vision. Clearly, preventing cataracts, if possible, would be preferable.

PRINCIPAL PROPOSED TREATMENTS

Evidence suggests that various antioxidants may help prevent cataracts.

Vitamin C

In an observational study of 50,800 nurses who were followed for 8 years, a history of taking **vitamin C** (see page 444) supplements for more than 10 years was associated with a 45% lower risk of cataracts.[1]

Interestingly, diets high in vitamin C were not found to be protective—only supplemental vitamin C made a difference. This is the opposite of what has been found with vitamin C in the prevention of other diseases (see the chapters on **atherosclerosis** and **cancer**).

Vitamin C is generally believed to be quite safe, at least at dosages up to 500 mg daily. There is some reason for concern that long-term use of vitamin C can cause **kidney stones** (see page 109).[2] However, in large-scale observational studies, individuals who consume large amounts of vitamin C have shown either no change or a decreased risk of kidney stone formation.[3,4,5] Nonetheless, there may be certain individuals who are particularly at risk for vitamin C–induced kidney stones.[6] People with a history of kidney stones and those with kidney failure should probably restrict daily vitamin C intake to about 100 mg daily. Taking more than 1,000 mg daily of vitamin C can deplete the body's **copper** (see page 262) stores, so taking 1 to 3 mg of copper daily as a supplement may be advisable.

Vitamin E

According to observational studies (not as large as the one described under vitamin C), researchers have found that foods high in vitamin E, as well as **vitamin E** (see page 451) supplements, are associated with a reduced risk of cataracts.[7–12] These results are corroborated by a study in animals,[13] but further work needs to be done to establish vitamin E as a treatment for preventing cataracts.

A typical dosage of vitamin E is 400 IU daily. Vitamin E is generally believed to be safe at this dose. However, in one study of 28,519 men, vitamin E supplementation at the low dose of about 50 IU per day caused an increase in fatal hemorrhagic strokes, the kind of stroke caused by bleeding.[14] (On the other hand, it reduced the risk of a more common type of stroke, and the two effects essentially canceled out.) Considering its ability to reduce blood clotting, vitamin E should not be taken by those with bleeding problems, or combined with aspirin or prescription blood thinners, such as Coumadin (warfarin) and Trental (pentoxifylline), except under a physician's supervision.[15] There also might conceivably be potential risks in combining vitamin E with other natural substances known to thin the blood, such as **garlic** (see page 291) and **ginkgo** (see page 298), although no problems have been reported.

Carotenes

Foods high in carotenes (beta-carotene, lutein, lycopene, and others) might protect against cataract formation.[16–19] In studies, **lutein** (see page 348), found in dark-green vegetables, seemed to be especially helpful for women, whereas the carotenes found in carrots were more helpful in men. **Lycopene** (see page 349), a carotene found in tomatoes, was associated with a reduced occurrence of cataracts in both sexes.

However, taking the supplement beta-carotene by itself does not appear to be protective.[20,21] This is one more strike against this antioxidant, which has failed to prove beneficial in other conditions as well (see the discussions of beta-carotene in the chapters on **atherosclerosis** and **cancer**).

If you drink too much alcohol, it might be especially wise to avoid high-dose beta-carotene.[22]

OTHER PROPOSED TREATMENTS

Herbs high in antioxidant flavonoids may also be helpful in protecting against cataracts. The ones most commonly mentioned include **bilberry** (see page 220), **ginkgo** (see page 298), **OPCs** (see page 373), and **turmeric** (see page 425). One double-blind trial found that a combination of bilberry and **vitamin E** (see page 451) could help stop mild cataracts from getting worse.[23]

The supplements cysteine, **lipoic acid** (see page 347), **niacin** (vitamin B$_3$; see page 437), **riboflavin** (vitamin B$_2$; see page 436), **selenium** (see page 407), **taurine** (see page 420), and **zinc** (see page 463) are sometimes mentioned as helpful for preventing cataracts, but the evidence that they really work is not yet strong.

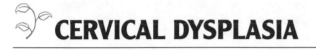

CERVICAL DYSPLASIA

Principal Proposed Treatments There are no well-established natural treatments for cervical dysplasia.

Other Proposed Treatments Folate, Multivitamin and Mineral Supplement, Selenium
  "Emmenagogue Herbs": Squaw Vine, Motherwort, True Unicorn, False Unicorn, Black Cohosh, Blessed Thistle

---

Very few cancers can be identified so far ahead of the danger point as cancer of the cervix. The cells lining the surface of the cervix begin to show changes visible under a microscope a decade or more before invasive cancer develops, in plenty of time for definitive treatment. For this reason, a regular, properly performed and interpreted Pap smear is one of medicine's most effective preventive methods.

The stages of progression from a healthy cervix to cancer begin with what is called mild dysplasia: precancerous alterations in structure and activity. Subsequently, altered cells spread from the surface of the cervix down toward the underlying tissue. In the early stages, cancerous changes may disappear on their own, but once these cells fully penetrate the lining, progression to true cancer usually occurs within 5 to 10 years.

Medical treatment consists of watchful waiting for spontaneous regression during the early stages and more aggressive removal of the cervical lining by laser, freezing, or other techniques if no regression occurs. These options are usually successful; however, they are invasive and frequently uncomfortable.

PROPOSED TREATMENTS

It has been claimed that various natural herbs and supplements can improve the odds of early stages of dysplasia changing back to normal cells. If your physician suggests watchful waiting and a repeat examination, it should be safe to try some of these methods during the waiting period. However, there is no real scientific evidence that these treatments are effective, and in all circumstances close medical supervision is necessary to verify good results or identify failure. Alternative treatment is definitely not advisable for severe cervical dysplasia.

Folate

Folate (see page 288) deficiency appears to increase the ease with which cervical cancer can develop. However, taking extra folate does not appear to reverse cervical dysplasia once it has occurred.[1,2]

General Nutritional Support

Studies have found that women with cervical dysplasia tend to show a high frequency of general nutritional deficiencies, as high as 67% in one survey.[3] For this reason, it probably makes sense to take a multivitamin and mineral supplement. Particular vitamins most commonly associated with cervical dysplasia when deficient include **beta-carotene** (see page 217), **vitamin C** (see page 444), **vitamin B$_6$** (see page 439), **selenium** (see page 407), and, as previously mentioned, folate.[4,5] However, a double-blind placebo-controlled study of 141 women found that neither vitamin C nor beta-carotene supplements taken daily in doses of 500 mg and 30 mg, respectively, could reverse cervical dysplasia.[6]

Visit Us at TNP.com

Emmenagogues

Many practitioners of herbal medicine feel that a class of herbs known as emmenagogues can be helpful in cervi-cal dysplasia. These include squaw vine, **motherwort** (see page 363), true unicorn, false unicorn, **black cohosh** (see page 223), and blessed thistle.

CHRONIC FATIGUE SYNDROME

Related Terms   Myalgic Encephalomyelitis, Post-Viral Fatigue Syndrome

Principal Proposed Treatments   There are no well-established natural treatments for chronic fatigue syndrome.

Other Proposed Treatments   Essential Fatty Acids (GLA and Fish Oil), NADH, Carnitine, Echinacea, Ginseng, Beta-Carotene, DHEA, Licorice, Multivitamin and Mineral Supplementation

Chronic fatigue syndrome (CFS) has been a subject of controversy for many years. Medical authorities were once quite skeptical regarding whether it even existed. However, in 1988, the Centers for Disease Control officially recognized CFS. Today, CFS is defined essentially as follows: Unexplained, persistent, or relapsing fatigue with a definite beginning; it is not the result of exertion; it is not relieved by rest; and it results in significant reduction of activities.

In addition, at least four of the following symptoms persist or recur for 6 or more consecutive months of the illness:

- Impairment in short-term memory or concentration
- Sore throat
- Tender lymph nodes in the neck or armpits
- Muscle pain
- Pain in many joints, without redness or swelling
- Headache of new pattern or severity
- Unrefreshing sleep
- Malaise following exercise, that lasts for more than 24 hours

Frequently, symptoms of CFS follow a viral infection; some individuals with CFS describe their symptoms as a flu that never goes away.

The cause (or causes) of CFS remains unknown. Because its symptoms somewhat resemble those of mononucleosis (caused by the Epstein-Barr virus), for a time the disease was called "Chronic Epstein-Barr Syndrome." However, further investigation disclosed that evidence of past or current Epstein-Barr infection is no more common in individuals with CFS than in the general population. Nonetheless, this erroneous and misleading term still crops up in literature on CFS.

Other syndromes with a similar pattern of symptoms to CFS include **fibromyalgia** (see page 80), multiple chemical sensitivities, and food allergies; some consider these conditions to be closely related to each other, but there is no real evidence to support this hypothesis.

There is no dramatically effective treatment for CFS. Antidepressants (such as Prozac and Zoloft) may improve energy and mood; older antidepressants (such as amitriptyline) may improve sleep; antihistamines and decongestants can help allergic symptoms that frequently occur in CFS; and nonsteroidal anti-inflammatory drugs (such as ibuprofen and naproxen) may help pain. Careful attention to lifestyle issues, such as exercise level and use of caffeine, may also offer benefit.

Other approaches to CFS that have been tried include **magnesium** (see page 351) injections,[1,2,3] corticosteroid treatment,[4–9] and the antidepressant fluoxetine combined with graded exercise.[10–13]

For a time, researchers expressed some excitement over initial findings that deliberately raising blood pressure might help individuals with CFS. However, a double-blind placebo-controlled study of 25 people given a 6-week course of fludrocortisone and increased dietary sodium to raise blood pressure found no improvement in CFS symptoms.[14]

PROPOSED TREATMENTS

There are some promising natural treatments for CFS, but the scientific evidence for them is not yet strong.

Essential Fatty Acids

In a double-blind placebo-controlled study, 63 people were given either a combination of essential fatty acids, containing evening primrose oil (a source of **GLA;** see page 304) and **fish oil** (see page 282), or liquid paraffin placebo over a 3-month period.[15] At 1 and 3 months, participants in the treatment group reported significant improvement in CFS symptoms as compared to the placebo group. The researchers also found that at the beginning of the study many participants had abnormal essential fatty acid levels, and these improved with treatment.

However, in 1999, researchers tried to replicate this study with 50 other people, using more precise means of measuring CFS symptoms.[16] The results showed no difference between individuals given essential fatty acids and those given placebo (sunflower oil). These researchers also found no difference in fatty acid levels between individuals with CFS and individuals without CFS who served as controls.

NADH (Nicotinamide Adenine Dinucleotide)

NADH is a naturally occurring chemical that plays a significant role in cellular energy production. **NADH supplements** (see page 368) have been tried in hopes they might improve energy levels in athletes and in individuals with chronic fatigue.

A double-blind placebo-controlled crossover trial that followed 26 people given 10 mg of NADH for a 4-week period showed some improvement in symptoms during NADH treatment as compared to the period of placebo treatment (31% vs 8%).[17] However, larger studies will have to be performed to actually prove a benefit with this supplement.

Carnitine

Carnitine (see page 238) is a substance the body uses to convert fatty acids to energy. Early studies reported decreased carnitine levels in people with CFS.[18] Based on these, an unblinded crossover trial (8 weeks with each treatment, and a 2-week "washout" period in between) enrolled 30 individuals with CFS to evaluate the potential benefits of carnitine supplements.[19] The results suggest potential benefit with this supplement.

However, this study was severely flawed. One problem was that, rather than using a placebo group for comparison purposes, researchers chose to investigate the antiviral drug amantadine. This drug has no proven efficacy in CFS, and it caused so many side effects that more than half of the participants dropped out during the period they were taking amantadine. This high dropout rate makes statistical interpretation of the results unreliable. In addition, the lack of blinding in the study also impairs the trustworthiness of the results.

Other Herbs and Supplements

A test tube study of **echinacea** (see page 273) and **ginseng** (see page 301) found that both increased cellular immune function in cells taken from people with CFS.[20] However, many herbs and supplements can cause measurable changes in immune function, and such observations do not prove that there will be an actual benefit in people with the disease.

Both **beta-carotene** (see page 217) and **DHEA** (see page 268) have also been suggested as treatments for CFS, but the evidence that they work is highly preliminary.[21,22,23]

Based on the theory mentioned above that CFS might be related to low blood pressure, the herb **licorice** (see page 344) has been recommended for CFS by some herbalists. Licorice raises blood pressure (and causes other potentially harmful effects) when taken in high doses for a long time. However, there is no evidence that it works for CFS, and other treatments to raise blood pressure have proven ineffective for CFS.[24]

Although some authorities have suggested that CFS might be caused by deficiencies of multiple vitamins and minerals, a double-blind placebo-controlled study of 42 people found no significant improvement in CFS symptoms when a vitamin-mineral supplement was given 4 times daily after meals for 3 months.[25]

CHRONIC OBSTRUCTIVE PULMONARY DISEASE

Related Terms   COPD, Chronic Bronchitis, Emphysema

Principal Proposed Treatments   N-Acetyl Cysteine (NAC)

Other Proposed Treatments   L-Carnitine, Essential Oil Monoterpenes, Antioxidant-Rich Diet, Fish Oil, Magnesium, High-Fat Low-Carbohydrate Diet, Coenzyme Q_{10}

Chronic obstructive pulmonary disease (COPD) is a permanent lung condition caused, most often, by cigarette smoking. It starts with a wheezing cough and gradually progresses to a shortness of breath that accompanies even the slightest exertion such as dressing or eating. COPD encompasses both emphysema and chronic bronchitis.

Emphysema consists of the destruction of the tiny air sacs (alveoli) in the lungs and weakening of the support structure around them. This leads to a collapse of the small airways in the lungs, especially on inhalation, and reduces the body's ability to take in oxygen and expel carbon dioxide.

COPD

Visit Us at TNP.com

Chronic bronchitis is a persistent, mucus-producing cough caused by inflammation, scarring the lungs. This inflammation also impairs the body's ability to exchange new air for old. Finally, COPD also involves spasm of the airways similar to what occurs in asthma.

Because cigarette smoking contributes to both emphysema and chronic bronchitis, anyone who has COPD should stop smoking. Quitting smoking won't reverse the condition, but it might stop COPD from getting worse. Airborne irritants such as chemical fumes exacerbate symptoms and should also be avoided. Standard treatment for COPD includes using bronchodilators such as ipratropium and albuterol to reduce muscle spasms, and corticosteroids to control inflammation in the airways. Severe COPD may require continuous oxygen therapy.

Malnutrition is common among people with COPD and seems to correspond to the severity of the condition.[1,2] It's been suggested that the caloric needs of people with COPD increase as the disease progresses.[3] Because malnutrition in turn can worsen lung function and make people more prone to infection, many researchers now recommend that individuals with COPD receive supplemental nutrition as part of their treatment.[4,5]

PRINCIPAL PROPOSED TREATMENTS

N-acetyl cysteine may improve breathing in people with COPD.

N-Acetyl Cysteine

N-acetyl cysteine (NAC; see page 366) is a specially modified form of the dietary amino acid cysteine. NAC has been thought to help break up mucus, which was the original rationale for using it in respiratory conditions. However, continuing research has tended to cast doubt on this explanation of its action. NAC might actually work in some altogether different way that is not as yet clearly defined. In any case, evidence suggests that regular use of NAC is helpful for symptoms of chronic bronchitis.[6]

What Is the Scientific Evidence for NAC?

Regular use of NAC may diminish the number of severe bronchitis attacks. A review and meta-analysis of available research focused on eight reasonably well-designed double-blind placebo-controlled trials of NAC for chronic bronchitis.[7-15] The results of these studies, involving a total of about 1,400 individuals, suggest that NAC taken daily at a dose of 400 to 1,200 mg can reduce the number of acute attacks of severe bronchitis.

Dosage

Optimal dosages of NAC have not been determined. The amount used in studies has varied from 250 to 1,500 mg daily.

Safety Issues

NAC appears to be a very safe supplement when taken alone, although one study in rats suggests that 60 to 100 times the normal dose can cause liver injury.[16]

The combination of the heart drug nitroglycerin and NAC can cause severe headaches.[17,18] Safety in young children, women who are pregnant or nursing, and individuals with severe liver or kidney disease has not been established.

OTHER PROPOSED TREATMENTS

Carnitine

Evidence from three double-blind placebo-controlled studies enrolling a total of 49 individuals suggests that **L-carnitine** (see page 238) can improve exercise tolerance in COPD, presumably by improving muscular efficiency in the lungs and other muscles.[19,20,21]

Essential Oil Monoterpenes

Eucalyptus is a standard ingredient in cough drops and in oils added to humidifiers. A standardized combination of three essential oils has been studied for effectiveness in sinus infections, acute and chronic bronchitis, and other respiratory conditions.[22-26] This essential oil combination may be helpful for preventing flare-ups of chronic bronchitis as well. However, it does not appear to improve breathing ability.

The studied combination includes cineole from eucalyptus, d-limonene from citrus fruit, and alpha-pinene from pine. These oils are all in a chemical family called monoterpenes. A 3-month double-blind trial of 246 individuals with chronic bronchitis found that treatment with essential oil monoterpenes helped prevent the typical worsening of chronic bronchitis that occurs during the winter.[27] However, another study found no improvement in objective measures of lung function during usage of essential oils.[28]

Dietary Factors

Observational studies suggest a correlation between respiratory problems such as bronchitis and emphysema and diets low in antioxidants from food, such as **vitamin A** (see page 432), **vitamin E** (see page 451), **vitamin C** (see page 444), and **beta-carotene** (see page 217).[29-32] Another population study found that high vitamin C intake was associated with better lung function.[33] However, such studies don't prove that taking supplements of such nutrients will help. Indeed, a study of vitamin E and beta-carotene supplementation found no effect on COPD symptoms.[34] The effects of vitamin C supplements on COPD haven't yet been studied. It might be wiser to eat fruits and vegetables rather than take antioxidant supplements.

Results from another observational study suggest that a diet high in **fish oil** (see page 282) may protect cigarette smokers against COPD.[35]

Yet another observational study suggests that dietary **magnesium** (see page 351) intake is closely related to lung function.[36] There is also some indication that diuretic drugs and corticosteroids commonly prescribed for COPD deplete magnesium levels, so taking magnesium supplements might not hurt.[37]

Evidence from several studies suggests that a lowfat, high-carbohydrate diet worsens exercise performance and lung function in people with COPD, whereas a high-fat, low-carbohydrate diet appears to improve COPD symptoms.[38,39,40] The reason is that carbohydrates cause the body to produce increased amounts of carbon dioxide, and individuals with COPD have trouble getting rid of carbon dioxide.

Coenzyme Q_{10}

Finally, slight evidence from a small open trial suggests that **coenzyme Q_{10}** (see page 256) improves lung function in individuals with COPD.[41]

COLDS AND FLUS

Principal Proposed Treatments Echinacea, Andrographis, Zinc, Vitamin C, Ginseng, Essential Oil Monoterpenes

Other Proposed Treatments Vitamin E, Probiotics, Elderberry, Arginine, Glutamine, Thymus Extract, Kelp, Ashwagandha, Astragalus, Garlic, Maitake, Reishi, Suma, Ginger, Kudzu, Osha, Yarrow, Marshmallow, Mullein, Peppermint

A cold is a respiratory infection caused by one of hundreds of possible viruses. However, because these viruses are so widespread, it is perhaps more accurate to say that colds are caused by a decrease in immunity that allows one of these viruses to take hold.

Colds occur more frequently in winter, but no one knows exactly why. Nearly everyone catches colds occasionally, but some people catch colds quite frequently, and others tend to stay sick an unusually long time.

Conventional medicine can neither cure nor prevent the common cold. Furthermore, none of the over-the-counter treatments have been found to shorten the duration of a cold or even provide significant temporary relief. Some of the natural treatments described in this section may be able to do better.

People often want to take antibiotics for colds, and many physicians will prescribe them—even though antibiotics have no effect on viruses. Many believe that when the mucus turns yellow, it means that a bacterial infection has occurred for which antibiotic treatment is indicated. However, viruses can also produce yellow mucus; and even if bacteria have made a home in the excess mucus, they may be only innocent bystanders and produce no symptoms.

Colds, however, can be complicated by bacterial infections. In such cases antibiotic treatment may be indicated. Decongestants and other symptomatic treatments have not been shown to be dramatically effective.

PRINCIPAL PROPOSED TREATMENTS

Remember the old saying "a cold lasts seven days, but if you treat it properly you will get over it in a week"?

Actually, it may be possible to prove folk wisdom wrong by using the right natural supplement. A significant body of research suggests that the herb echinacea can significantly shorten colds and make them less severe. The herb andrographis and the nutritional supplements zinc and vitamin C also seem to help. In addition, there are two treatments that might help prevent colds as well: the herbs andrographis and ginseng.

Echinacea: Reduces Cold and Flu Symptoms and Helps Recovery

Until the 1930s, **echinacea** (see page 273) was the number-one cold and flu remedy in the United States. It lost its popularity with the arrival of sulfa antibiotics. Ironically, sulfa antibiotics are as ineffective against colds as any other antibiotic, while echinacea does seem to be at least somewhat helpful. In Germany, echinacea remains the main remedy for minor respiratory infections.

This herb is thought to be an immune stimulant, a type of treatment not found in conventional medicine. Drugs attack infections, but echinacea appears to activate the body's infection-fighting capacity. However, there is no evidence that echinacea strengthens or "nourishes" the immune system when taken over the long term. It probably just stimulates it into action in the short term. Indeed, long-term use of echinacea has not proved effective.

There are three main species of echinacea: *Echinacea purpurea*, *Echinacea angustifolia*, and *Echinacea pallida*. *E. purpurea* is the most widely used, but the other two are also available. It isn't clear if any one type is better than the others.

What Is the Scientific Evidence for Echinacea?

Reasonably large and well-designed double-blind placebo-controlled studies, involving a total of about 650 individuals, have found echinacea effective for reducing the symptoms and duration of colds. These studies have used all three species of the herb. We don't know which one is better, or whether they are all equivalent.

Reducing the Symptoms and Duration of Colds   Clinical studies with various species of echinacea have found benefits in lessening the symptoms and duration of colds. One double-blind study of 100 individuals with acute flu-like illnesses found that echinacea could significantly reduce cold symptoms.[1] Half of the group received a combination herb product containing *E. angustifolia,* the other half took placebo. The participants rated the severity of symptoms of headache, lethargy, cough, and limb pain. In the treated group, symptoms were significantly less severe.

Another double-blind study of echinacea's effect on flu-like illnesses followed 180 people who were given either 450 mg or 900 mg of *E. purpurea* daily or placebo.[2] By about the third day, those participants receiving the higher dose of echinacea (900 mg) were doing significantly better than those in the placebo or low-dose echinacea groups. Reduction of symptoms was also seen in another double-blind study of *E. purpurea* involving about 200 participants.[3] Echinacea has also been found to reduce the time needed to get well. A double-blind placebo-controlled study using the *E. pallida* species followed 160 adults with recent onset of cold-like illnesses.[4] The results showed that treatment reduced the average period of illness from 13 days to about 9.5 days, compared to placebo. (These must have been bad colds to last so long!) Evidence from a double-blind study involving 120 people tells us that *E. purpurea* can cut in half the time it takes for your cold to "turn the corner" and start to get better. This study is described in the next section, "Aborting" a Cold.

Finally, a double-blind study of 263 individuals with colds found that a particular combination herbal treatment containing echinacea, wild indigo, and wormwood significantly relieved cold symptoms and reduced the time to recovery.[5] **Note:** Do not attempt to mix these ingredients yourself. Wild indigo and wormwood can be dangerous if used improperly.

"Aborting" a Cold   A double-blind study suggests that echinacea can not only make colds shorter and less severe, it can sometimes stop a cold that is just starting.[6] In this study, 120 people were given *E. purpurea* or placebo as soon as they started showing signs of getting a cold.

Participants took either echinacea or placebo at a dosage of 20 drops every 2 hours for 1 day, then 20 drops 3 times a day for 9 more days. The results over the 10-day study period were promising. Fewer people in the echinacea group felt that their initial symptoms actually developed into "real" colds (40% of those taking echinacea versus 60% taking the placebo actually became ill). Also, among those who did come down with "real" colds, improvement in the symptoms started sooner in the echinacea group (4 days instead of 8 days). Both of these results were statistically significant. However, echinacea's ability to shorten the duration of colds was more dramatic.

Preventing Colds   Several studies have attempted to discover whether the daily use of echinacea can prevent colds from even starting, but the results have not been promising.

In one double-blind placebo-controlled trial, 302 healthy volunteers were given an alcohol tincture containing either *E. purpurea* root, *E. angustifolia* root, or placebo for 12 weeks.[7] The results showed that *E. purpurea* was associated with perhaps a 20% decrease in the number of people who got sick, and *E. angustifolia* with a 10% decrease. However, the difference was not statistically significant. This means that the benefit, if any, was so small that it could have been due to chance alone.

Another double-blind placebo-controlled study enrolled 109 individuals with a history of four or more colds during the previous year, and gave them either *E. purpurea* juice or placebo for a period of 8 weeks.[8] No benefits were seen in the frequency, duration, or severity of colds. (Note: this paper is actually a more detailed look at a 1992 study widely misreported as providing evidence of benefit.)[9]

Another study, not yet published, found indications that regular use of echinacea might actually increase the risk of colds.[10] For a period of 6 months, 200 people were given either echinacea or placebo. Use of the herb was associated with a 20% higher incidence of sore throat, runny nose, and sinusitis. This suggests that long-term use of echinacea might actually slightly impair immune function.

Another double-blind placebo-controlled trial followed 117 individuals, each given echinacea for 14 days and then inoculated with a cold virus.[11] No difference in rate or severity of infection was seen.

One double-blind placebo-controlled study did find that long-term use of echinacea offered some help, but only for those especially prone to colds.[12] The study involved 609 students at the University of Cologne. Half of the participants were treated with a German product containing *E. angustifolia* for at least 8 weeks; the other half received placebo.

In the group as a whole, echinacea did not significantly decrease the number of colds. However, of the 609 participants, 363 students were rated as particularly prone to infection, based on the number of colds each had developed the winter before. This relatively high-risk group did show a reduction in the number of colds they caught, compared to the control group: the infection-prone students developed on average 20% fewer colds (a statistically significant, although small, improvement).

The bottom line: echinacea is probably not worth using as a long-term preventive treatment. It is better used directly at the onset of a cold to reduce its severity and duration.

Dosage

The three species of echinacea are used interchangeably. The typical dosage of echinacea powdered extract is 300 mg 3 times daily. Alcohol tincture (1:5) is usually taken at a dosage of 3 to 4 ml 3 times daily, echinacea juice at 2 to 3 ml 3 times daily, and whole dried root at 1 to 2 g 3 times daily. Echinacea is usually taken at the first sign of a cold and continued for 7 to 14 days.

There is no broad agreement on which ingredients should be standardized in echinacea tinctures and solid extracts.

Many herbalists feel that liquid forms of echinacea are more effective than tablets or capsules because they believe that part of echinacea's benefit is due to direct contact with the tonsils and other lymphatic tissues at the back of the throat.[13] These tissues act as an early warning system for infections. By stimulating them, echinacea may encourage the body to fight a cold more promptly.

Finally, **goldenseal** (see page 314) is frequently combined with echinacea in cold preparations. However, there is no evidence that oral goldenseal stimulates immunity, nor did traditional herbalists use it for this purpose.[14]

Safety Issues

Echinacea appears to be very safe. Even when taken in very high doses, it does not appear to cause any toxic effects.[15,16] Side effects are also rare and usually limited to minor gastrointestinal symptoms, increased urination, and allergic reactions.[17] However, severe allergic reactions have occurred occasionally, some of them life threatening.[18]

Germany's Commission E warns against using echinacea if you have an autoimmune disorder such as multiple sclerosis, lupus, or rheumatoid arthritis, as well as tuberculosis or leukocytosis. Rumors say that echinacea should not be used if you have AIDS. These warnings are purely theoretical, being based on fears that echinacea might actually activate immunity in the wrong way. While no evidence shows that echinacea use has actually harmed anyone with these diseases, caution is advisable.

Germany's Commission E also recommends against using echinacea for more than 8 weeks. Since there is no evidence that echinacea is effective when taken long term, this is probably sensible. The safety of echinacea in pregnant or nursing women and those with severe kidney or liver disease has not been established. In German studies from the 1950s and 60s, more than 1,000 children were given injected forms of echinacea, with no apparent harm.[19] Given these findings, it seems likely that oral echinacea is safe for children, but we don't know this for sure.

Andrographis: A Promising Treatment for Colds

Andrographis (see page 205) is a shrub found throughout India and other Asian countries, sometimes called "Indian echinacea" because it is believed to provide much the same benefits. It was widely used during the terrible influenza epidemics that occurred in the early 1900s. Recently, it has become popular in Scandinavia as a treatment for colds.

Although we don't know how andrographis might work for colds, some evidence suggests that it might stimulate immunity.[20] Interestingly, the ingredient of andrographis used for standardization purposes, andrographolide, does not appear to affect the immune system as much as the whole plant extract.

What Is the Scientific Evidence for Andrographis?

According to a few well-designed studies, andrographis can reduce the symptoms of colds and possibly prevent colds as well.

Reducing Cold Symptoms   A 4-day double-blind placebo-controlled trial of 158 adults with colds found that treatment with andrographis significantly reduced cold symptoms.[21] Participants were given either placebo or 1,200 mg daily of an andrographis extract standardized to contain 5% andrographolide. The results showed that by day 2 of treatment, and even more by day 4, individuals given the actual treatment experienced significant improvements in symptoms as compared to participants in the placebo group. The greatest response was seen in earache, sleeplessness, nasal drainage, and sore throat, but other cold symptoms improved as well.

Good results were seen in two other double-blind placebo-controlled studies involving a total of over 100 participants.[22,23]

Another double-blind study, which involved 152 adults, compared the effectiveness of andrographis (at either 3 g per day or 6 g per day) versus acetaminophen for sore throat and fever.[24] The higher dose of andrographis (6 g) decreased symptoms of fever and throat pain, as did acetaminophen, while the lower dose of andrographis (3 g) did not. There were no significant side effects in either group.

Preventing Colds   According to one double-blind placebo-controlled study, andrographis may increase resistance to colds.[25] A total of 107 students, all 18 years old, participated in this 3-month trial that used a dried extract of andrographis. Fifty-four of the participants took two 100-mg tablets standardized to 5.6% andrographolide daily—considerably less than the 1,200 to 6,000 mg per day that has been used in studies on treatment of colds. The other 53 students were given placebo tablets with a coating identical to the treatment. Then, once a week throughout the study, a clinician evaluated all the participants for cold symptoms.

By the end of the trial, only 16 people in the group using andrographis had experienced colds, compared to 33 of the placebo-group participants. This difference was statistically significant, indicating that andrographis reduces the risk of catching a cold by a factor of two as compared to placebo.

Dosage

A typical dosage of andrographis is 400 mg 3 times daily, taken with lots of liquids at mealtimes. Andrographis is typically standardized to its andrographolide content, usually 4 to 6% in many commercial products.

Safety Issues

No significant adverse effects have been reported in human studies of andrographis. In one study, researchers tracked participant reports of side effects, in addition to monitoring lab tests for liver function, complete blood counts, kidney function, and some other laboratory measures of toxicity.[26] All of their tests were within the normal limits for both the placebo and the andrographis groups.

However, full formal safety studies have not been completed. This means that the herb is not recommended for young children, pregnant or nursing women, or those with severe liver or kidney disease.

There are some concerns from animal studies that andrographis may impair fertility. One study showed that male rats became infertile when fed 20 mg of andrographis powder per day.[27] In this case, the rats stopped producing sperm and exhibited physical changes in some of the testicular cells involved in sperm production. Researchers also detected evidence of degeneration of structures in the testicles. However, another study showed no evidence of testicular toxicity in male rats that were given up to 1 g per kilogram of body weight per day for 60 days, so this issue remains unclear.[28]

One group of female mice also did not fare well on andrographis.[29] When fed 2 g per kilogram body weight daily for 6 weeks (thousands of times higher than the usual human dose), all female mice failed to get pregnant when mated with males of proven fertility. Meanwhile, of the control females, 95.2% got pregnant when mated with a similar group of male mice.

While andrographis is probably not a useful form of birth control, these animal studies are somewhat worrisome and warrant further investigation.

Also, because andrographis may stimulate gallbladder contraction, it should not be used by individuals with gallbladder disease except under physician supervision.[30]

Zinc: Appears Effective If You Use the Right Form

Another famous alternative treatment for colds is the use of **zinc** (see page 463) lozenges. In cases of zinc deficiency, the immune system does not function properly.[31,32] Because zinc is commonly deficient in the diet, especially among senior citizens,[33] nutritional zinc supplementation may certainly be useful for those who get sick easily. Indeed, a recent 2-year double-blind study suggests that zinc and selenium taken together in nutritional doses can reduce the number of infections in nursing home residents.[34] Ten other studies performed in third world countries have found that zinc supplements at nutritional doses can increase resistance to infection.[35,36]

However, zinc is most commonly recommended to be used in a different way: sucking on high doses of zinc lozenges at the onset of cold symptoms. This method may work by directly killing viruses in the throat rather than improving the nutritional status of the body. At press time, a large study reported that zinc nasal spray might be even more effective.

What Is the Scientific Evidence for Zinc?

A double-blind study concluded that proper use of zinc lozenges can cause many cold symptoms to go away faster than they would otherwise.[37] In this trial, 100 people who were experiencing the early symptoms of a cold were given a lozenge that either contained 13.3 mg of zinc from zinc gluconate or was just a placebo. Participants took the lozenges several times daily until their cold symptoms subsided. The results were impressive. Coughing disappeared within 2.2 days in the treated group versus 4 days in the placebo group. Sore throat disappeared after 1 day versus 3 days in the placebo group, nasal drainage in 4 days (versus 7 days), and headache in 2 days (versus 3 days).

Positive results have also been seen in double-blind studies of zinc acetate.[38,39]

Not all studies have shown such positive results.[40] However, the overall results appear to be favorable.[41] It has been suggested that the exact formulation of the zinc lozenge plays a significant role. Flavoring agents, such as citric acid and tartaric acid, appear to prevent zinc from killing viruses, and chemical forms of zinc other than zinc gluconate or zinc acetate may not work.[42] Sweeteners such as sorbitol, sucrose, dextrose, and mannitol are fine, but the information on glycine as a flavoring agent is equivocal.

One recent trial with the right form of zinc lozenge found no benefit, but this may have been due to a cherry flavoring that was added to the lozenges.[43] The bottom line is that certain forms of zinc are probably helpful for colds.

Dosage

The typical dosage is 13 to 23 mg of zinc as zinc glu-conate or zinc acetate, taken every 2 hours at the earliest signs of a cold and continued for no more than a week or two. Lozenges should not contain any other flavorings besides carbohydrate sweeteners such as sorbitol, su-crose, dextrose, and mannitol. Glycine also might be an acceptable flavoring.

For long-term nutritional supplementation of zinc, 10 to 25 mg daily is typically recommended. Zinc can cause **copper** (see page 262) deficiency, so it should be com-bined with 1 to 3 mg of copper daily.

Safety Issues

The short-term use of zinc every 2 hours is believed to be safe. However, high doses of zinc should not be kept up for more than a week or two because such doses can actually depress the immune system and cause other symptoms if taken for too long. As mentioned previously, zinc can also deplete the body of copper.

Vitamin C: Not a Cure, but It Helps

As the most famous of all natural treatments for colds, **vitamin C** (see page 444) has been subjected to irre-sponsible hype from both proponents and opponents. Enthusiasts claim that if you take vitamin C daily, you will never get sick, while critics of the treatment insist that vitamin C has no benefit at all.

However, a cool-headed evaluation of the research in-dicates something in between. Numerous studies have found that vitamin C supplements taken at a dose of 1,000 mg daily or more *can* significantly reduce symp-toms of colds and help you get over a cold faster.[44,45,46] Benefits appear to be greater for children than for adults, and the exact amount of the benefit varies widely between studies.

In most of these studies, participants took vitamin C supplements on a daily basis throughout the period of the study.[47] However, a few studies evaluated the benefits of taking vitamin C only at the onset of cold symptoms. This method, which is perhaps the most popular way of using vitamin C for colds, appears to be just as effective.

There is no real evidence that vitamin C can prevent colds in general. However, there are two exceptions to this. One is the "post-marathon sniffle." Heavy en-durance exercise temporarily weakens the immune sys-tem, leading to a high incidence of infection following marathons and triathlons. There is some evidence that vitamin C can prevent such colds.[48,49]

The other situation in which vitamin C might help prevent colds is when you are *deficient* in the vitamin. In such cases, making sure to get your dietary allowance might help keep you healthier.[50]

We don't know the exact dose of vitamin C to use for colds. A typical recommendation is 500 to 1,000 mg 3 to 6 times daily while cold symptoms last. The short-term use of high doses of vitamin C is believed to be safe, al-though diarrhea may occur.

Ginseng: May Actually Prevent Colds

Although most people in the West think of **ginseng** (see page 301) as a stimulant, in Eastern Europe ginseng is widely believed to improve overall immunity to illness. As we have seen, echinacea does not seem to prevent colds. But it appears that regular use of ginseng may be able to provide this important benefit.

There are actually three different herbs commonly called ginseng: Asian or Korean ginseng *(Panax ginseng)*, American ginseng *(Panax quinquefolius)*, and Siberian "ginseng" *(Eleutherococcus senticosus)*. The latter herb is actually not ginseng at all, but some herbalists believe that it functions identically.

What Is the Scientific Evidence for Ginseng?

A double-blind placebo-controlled study looked at the potential immune-stimulating effects of *Panax ginseng*.[51] This trial enrolled 227 individuals at three medical of-fices in Milan, Italy. Half were given ginseng at a dose of 100 mg daily, and the other half took placebo. Four weeks into the study, all participants received influenza vaccine.

The results showed a significant decline in the fre-quency of colds and flus in the treated group compared to the placebo group (15 versus 42 cases). Also, antibody measurements in response to the vaccination rose higher in the treated group than in the placebo group.

While more research is needed, this study suggests that ginseng may be able to do what echinacea, zinc lozenges, and vitamin C cannot: prevent colds.

Dosage

The typical recommended daily dose of *Panax ginseng* is 1 to 2 g of raw herb, or 200 mg daily of an extract stan-dardized to contain 4 to 7% ginsenosides. *Eleutherococ-cus* is taken at a dosage of 2 to 3 g whole herb or 300 to 400 mg of extract daily.

Ordinarily, a 2- to 3-week period of using ginseng is recommended, followed by a 1- to 2-week "rest" period. Russian tradition suggests that ginseng should not be used by those under 40 years old.

Safety Issues

The various forms of ginseng appear to be nontoxic, both in the short and long term, according to the results of studies in mice, rats, chickens, and dwarf pigs.[52–55] Gin-seng also does not seem to be carcinogenic.

Side effects are rare. Occasionally women report menstrual abnormalities and/or breast tenderness when they take ginseng. However, a large double-blind trial found no estrogen-like effects.[56] Unconfirmed reports suggest that highly excessive dosages of ginseng can cause insomnia, raise blood pressure, increase heart rate, and possibly cause other significant effects. Whether some of these cases were actually caused by caffeine mixed in with ginseng remains unclear. Ginseng allergy can also occur, as can allergy to any other substance.

In 1979, an article was published in the *Journal of the American Medical Association* claiming that people can become addicted to ginseng and develop blood pressure elevation, nervousness, sleeplessness, diarrhea, and hypersexuality. This report has since been thoroughly discredited and should no longer be taken seriously.[57,58]

However, an unpublished report suggests that ginseng can interfere with drug metabolism, specifically drugs processed by an enzyme called "CYP 3A4." Ask your physician or pharmacist whether you are taking any medications of this type. There have also been specific reports of ginseng interacting with MAO inhibitor drugs[59] and with a test for digitalis,[60] although again it is not clear whether it was the ginseng or a contaminant that caused the problem.

Safety in young children, pregnant or nursing women, or those with severe liver or kidney disease has not been established. Interestingly, Chinese tradition suggests that ginseng should not be used during pregnancy or lactation.

Essential Oil Monoterpenes: May Reduce Symptoms

Eucalyptus is a standard ingredient in cough drops and in oils meant to be added to humidifiers. A standardized combination of three essential oils, including oils derived from eucalyptus, has been tested for its usefulness in respiratory conditions. The studied combination includes cineole from eucalyptus, d-limonene from citrus fruit, and alpha-pinene from pine. Numerous double-blind trials have found them effective for sinus infections, acute and chronic bronchitis, and other respiratory conditions, in both adults and children.[61–65] These oils are all in a chemical family called monoterpenes.

Dosage

In studies, this essential oil combination was taken at a dose of 300 mg 3 to 4 times daily.

Safety Issues

Other than minor gastrointestinal complaints, no side effects have been reported with this essential oil combination. However, be advised that essential oils can be toxic if taken to excess. Maximum safe doses in young children, women who are pregnant or nursing, and individu-

als with severe liver or kidney disease have not been established.

OTHER PROPOSED TREATMENTS

There is some evidence that **vitamin E** (see page 451) may improve immune function, but whether this translates into an effect on colds has not been determined.[66] The same may be said of various **probiotics** (see page 200), such as acidophilus.[67,68]

A recent study suggests that the herb **elderberry** (see page 276) can significantly reduce the length and severity of flu symptoms.[69] Elderberry-flower tea is made by steeping 3 to 5 g of dried flowers in one cup of boiling water for 10 to 15 minutes. A typical dosage is 1 cup 3 times daily. Standardized extracts should be taken according to the directions on the product's label.

Elderberry flower is generally regarded as safe. Side effects are rare and consist primarily of occasional mild gastrointestinal distress or allergic reactions. Nonetheless, safety in young children, pregnant or nursing women, or those with severe liver or kidney disease is not established.

Based on a small double-blind study, the supplement **arginine** (see page 208) might also be helpful for preventing colds.[70]

There is some evidence that the supplement **glutamine** (see page 310) may, like vitamin C, help prevent post-exercise infections.[71,72]

The thymus gland plays a role in immunity. Highly preliminary evidence suggests that an extract made from the thymus glands of calves may help break up the cycle of recurrent respiratory infections.[73]

There is some evidence that elements in **kelp** (see page 340) might help to prevent infection with several kinds of viruses, including influenza.[74] However the evidence is very preliminary at this time.

Various herbs are said to work like ginseng and enhance immunity over the long term, including **ashwagandha** (see page 212), **astragalus** (see page 212), **garlic** (see page 291), **maitake** (see page 354), **reishi** (see page 400), and **suma** (see page 420). However, there is as yet no good evidence that they really work.

Several herbs, including **ginger** (see page 296), **kudzu** (see page 341), **osha** (see page 376), and **yarrow** (see page 460), are said to help avert colds when taken at the first sign of infection; but again, there is no scientific evidence that they are effective. Other herbs sometimes recommended to reduce cold symptoms include **marshmallow** (see page 355), **mullein** (see page 365), and **peppermint** (see page 384).

COLIC

Related Terms Infantile Colic

Principal Proposed Treatments There are no well-established natural treatments for colic.

Other Proposed Treatments Dietary Changes, Counseling, Herbal Combinations, Chiropractic Spinal Manipulation

The mere thought of a colicky baby is often enough to strike fear in the heart of the parents of a newborn child. A baby with colic may cry for hours despite the parents' attempts at consolation; although the colicky phase will eventually end, it may seem like an eternity while it continues.

Colic is often defined as excessive (frequently inconsolable) crying that lasts for more than 3 hours on at least 3 days per week, continuing for at least 3 weeks; additionally, there must be no medical problem causing the crying. Other symptoms frequently associated with colic include pulling the knees up towards the stomach, a hard and/or swollen stomach, and excessive gas. Crying occurs most often in the evening. Colic typically ends by the age of 4 to 5 months.

Colicky babies may be at an increased risk of abuse at the hands of exhausted and frustrated parents. Additionally, the parent may not properly bond with the child because of feelings of inadequacy and anger, leading to the child developing behavioral problems as he or she grows.

No one knows for sure what causes colic, although there are many theories. One view attributes it to painful digestive cramps and/or excessive gas caused by allergic reaction to foods (such as milk). Another theory suggests that some babies may simply have a sensitive temperament, possibly compounded by a parental inability to respond to the infant's needs. Finally, what we call colic may just be an extreme version of normal infant crying, or an increased perception of normal crying by parents with less tolerance for it.

The antispasmodic and sedating drugs dicyclomine and dicycloverine appear to be effective for colic,[1] but they can have dangerous side effects in infants and are not recommended. The gas-relieving drug dimethicone is also sometimes recommended, but evidence suggests that it does not work for colic.[2]

PROPOSED TREATMENTS

A number of natural approaches to colic have been tried, but none can be considered scientifically proven at this time.

Dietary Changes

Cow's milk is thought to be a highly **allergenic food** (see page 82). Not only can infant formula—which con-tains cow's milk—produce allergic reactions, but even breast-fed infants may be exposed to cow's milk proteins if the mother consumes milk. [3–7]

Numerous small, open and double-blind studies have evaluated the effects of cow's milk in the diet of infants with colic.[8–23] Most of these found an improvement in crying when cow's milk protein was removed from the diet of formula-fed infants, or from the diet of the mothers in breast-fed infants.[24–31] However, not all studies had positive results.[32,33,34]

Many researchers recommend eliminating cow's milk from the infant's or the mother's diet for 2 to 3 days to see if symptoms improve. If eliminating this milk protein works, and if formula is preferred to breast-feeding, it might be better to try a hypoallergenic milk formula rather than soy formula, since it is possible to develop allergies to soy.[35,36,37]

If no improvement is seen through eliminating cow's milk, it might be worthwhile searching in the breast-feeding mother's diet for other potential food allergens, such as wheat, soy, or eggs.[38,39,40] However, it is important to keep nutritional needs in mind: the nursing mother who eliminates certain foods needs to maintain an adequate intake of calcium, protein, and other nutrients.

It should be noted that most infants with colic are able to tolerate cow's milk protein as they get older, so neither the mother nor the baby are doomed to life without milk. Researchers propose that this might be the result of an immature digestive system; according to this theory, maturation of the digestive tract is the reason that colic usually disappears on its own in time.

Milk also contains lactose, a form of sugar that many adults can't digest. However, reducing the lactose content of infant formula has not been found helpful in treating colic.[41]

Behavioral Counseling

Many doctors believe that the cause of colic is not physical; rather, that it results from a child's oversensitivity to stimuli in the environment.[42–46] Overanxious parents might contribute to the problem by adding more stimulation in an attempt to calm their child. Other parents might under-react in the belief that paying too much attention to the infant's cries will "spoil" him. Either response could set up a vicious cycle leading to long periods of inconsolable crying.

Based on these theories, some authorities recommend counseling the parents of a colicky infant on appropriate coping strategies, including building a personal support system and occasionally leaving the child with a different caregiver to provide a respite.

Studies evaluating the effects of carrying a colicky child more, or using a motion-simulation device, have not found benefit.[47,48]

Other Treatments

One small double-blind placebo-controlled study found that an herbal tea eliminated colic in 57% of 33 infants in the treatment group, as opposed to only 26% in the placebo group (a significant difference).[49] The tea contained extracts of **chamomile** (see page 244), vervain, **licorice** (see page 344), fennel, and **lemon balm** (see page 359), herbs with an antispasmodic reputation. However, the safety of this herbal combination in infants has not been established.

Chiropractic spinal manipulation has also been tried for colic.[50] One controlled study compared chiropractic treatments with the drug dimethicone (found ineffective in this study for colic). Fifty infants were randomly assigned one of the treatments for 2 weeks. By the sixth day of treatment, the spinal manipulation group cried significantly less than those on dimethicone. Whether this was a specific effect of the manipulation or a general response to attention and touch has not been determined.

In Britain, a preparation called "gripe water" is widely sold for the treatment of colic.[51] Varying formulations exist; however, all include aromatic oils such as dill, spearmint, or caraway, combined with alcohol, sucrose (sugar), and sodium bicarbonate. There is no scientific evidence to show whether or not gripe water works. It should be noted that at the recommended dosage, the infant would receive the equivalent of five shots of whiskey. That would be enough to calm anyone down.

Other herbs sometimes recommended for colic include cardamom, angelica, **peppermint** (see page 384), lemon balm, and **yarrow** (see page 460). However, no scientific evidence as yet supports their use.

The use of salt substitutes containing potassium have also been recommended, but they can be dangerous.[52]

CONGESTIVE HEART FAILURE

Principal Proposed Treatments   Coenzyme Q_{10} (CoQ_{10}), Hawthorn, Vitamin B_1
Other Proposed Treatments   Taurine, L-Carnitine, Arginine, Creatine, Magnesium

When the heart sustains injury that weakens its pumping ability, a complicated physiological state called congestive heart failure (CHF) can develop. Fluid builds up in the lungs and lower extremities, the heart enlarges, and many symptoms develop, including severe fatigue, difficulty breathing while lying down, and altered brain function.

Medical treatment for this condition is quite effective and sophisticated and consists of several drugs used in combination.

PRINCIPAL PROPOSED TREATMENTS

CHF is too serious a condition for self-treatment. The supervision of a qualified health-care professional is essential. For this reason, we deliberately do not provide detailed dosage information in this section (but you can find general guidelines in the chapters on each individual substance). However, given medical supervision, some of the following treatments may be quite useful. In Japan and Europe, coenzyme Q_{10} is frequently added to standard treatment for added benefit. The herb hawthorn alone may be effective for mild CHF. The supplement vitamin B_1 (thiamin) may be helpful for individuals who use certain medications for CHF: loop diuretics.

Coenzyme Q_{10}: Can Be Taken with Standard Medical Treatment

The substance known as **coenzyme Q_{10}** (CoQ_{10}; see page 256) appears to be quite helpful when combined with standard treatment for CHF. CoQ_{10} occurs naturally in the energy-producing subunits of all plant and animal cells (the mitochondria). This safe supplement is widely used in Europe, Israel, and Japan as an approved treatment for a variety of cardiovascular conditions.

One double-blind study followed 80 people with CHF and found that adding CoQ_{10} to standard treatment significantly improved heart function.[1] Another study tracked 641 individuals for 1 full year and found both improved symptoms and a reduced need for hospitalization.[2]

However, one 6-month double-blind study of 45 individuals with congestive heart failure found no benefit.[3]

CoQ_{10} appears to be essentially nontoxic and side-effect free.[4] However, there are concerns that CoQ_{10}, like many other substances, might interact with the blood-thinning drug Coumadin (warfarin).[5] Individuals taking

Coumadin should not take CoQ_{10} (or any other supplement) except under physician supervision.

Hawthorn: Approved in Germany for Mild CHF

The name **hawthorn** (see page 320) is derived from "hedgethorn," reflecting this spiny tree's use as a living fence in much of Europe. During the Middle Ages, hawthorn was used to treat dropsy, a condition that we now call CHF. It was also used for other heart ailments and for sore throat.

Hawthorn is widely regarded in modern Europe as a safe and effective treatment for the early stages of CHF. Although not as potent as that other famous heart herb of the Middle Ages, foxglove (digitalis), hawthorn is much safer. The active ingredients in foxglove are the drugs digoxin and digitoxin. However, hawthorn does not appear to have any single active ingredient. This has prevented it from being turned into a drug.

Like digitalis, hawthorn speeds up the heart and increases its force of contraction. However, it may offer one very important advantage. Digitalis and other medications that increase the power of the heart also make it more irritable and liable to dangerous irregularities of rhythm. In contrast, hawthorn appears to have the unique property of both strengthening the heart and stabilizing it against arrhythmias.[6,7,8] Also, with digitalis the difference between the proper dose and the toxic dose is very small. Hawthorn has an enormous range of safe dosing.[9]

Between 1981 and 1994, 14 controlled clinical studies of hawthorn were conducted, most of them double-blind.[10] A total of 741 people participated in these trials. The collective results strongly suggest that hawthorn is an effective treatment for early stages of CHF. Comparative studies suggest that hawthorn is about as effective as a low dose of the conventional drug captopril.

Note: Although captopril and other standard drugs in the same family have been shown to reduce mortality associated with CHF, there is no similar evidence for hawthorn.

Hawthorn appears to be quite safe. Germany's Commission E lists no known risks, contraindications, or drug interactions with hawthorn, and mice and rats have been given phenomenal doses without showing significant toxicity.[11] However, because hawthorn obviously affects the heart, it should not be combined with other heart drugs without a physician's supervision.

Side effects are also rare and consist mainly of mild stomach upset and occasional allergic reactions (skin rash). Safety in young children, pregnant or nursing women, and those with severe kidney or liver disease has not been established.

Vitamin B₁: Depleted by Loop Diuretics

Evidence suggests that individuals with congestive heart failure are commonly deficient in **vitamin B_1** (thiamin; see page 434), due to their use of loop diuretics (such as Lasix).[12] Since the heart depends on B_1 for proper function, taking a B_1 supplement may be advisable.

A small double-blind study found that intravenous administration of thiamin could improve heart function in individuals with CHF.[13] Similar results were seen in an earlier uncontrolled study.[14]

It is likely that oral vitamin B_1 would be helpful, too.

OTHER PROPOSED TREATMENTS

Several studies suggest that the amino acid **taurine** (see page 420) may be useful in CHF[15–21] and may be more effective than CoQ_{10}.[22] Taurine is believed to be safe.

Another treatment for CHF that has some evidence is the expensive supplement **L-carnitine** (see page 238), especially when given in the special form called L-propionyl-carnitine.[23–27] Carnitine is frequently combined with CoQ_{10}.

Three small double-blind studies enrolling a total of about 70 individuals with congestive heart failure found that oral **arginine** (see page 208) at a dose of 5 to 15 g daily could significantly improve symptoms as well as objective measurements of heart function.[28,29,30]

Recent evidence suggests that the sports supplement **creatine** (see page 264) may offer some help too, especially for the sensation of fatigue that often accompanies CHF.[31,32,33]

Additionally, there is also some evidence that supplementing with **magnesium** (see page 351) may be useful.

Finally, it is important to pay attention to all the general considerations that bring health to the heart, such as those described in the chapter on **atherosclerosis**.

CONJUNCTIVITIS

Principal Proposed Treatments   There are no well-established natural treatments for conjunctivitis.

Other Proposed Treatments   Eyebright, Barberry, Oregon Grape, Goldenseal, Calendula, Chamomile, Vitamin A, Bee Propolis

Constipation

Also called "pinkeye," conjunctivitis is an inflammation of the conjunctiva, which is the clear membrane that covers the eyeball. Symptoms in the affected eye include a bloodshot appearance, crusty discharge, and discomfort that may feel like something has gotten in the eye. Conjunctivitis is frequently caused by a viral infection, sometimes of the same viruses that cause **colds** (see page 47). In such cases, conjunctivitis could be called "a cold in the eye" and is really no more serious than any other cold. Other causes of conjunctivitis include bacterial infections, **allergies** (see page 2), environmental irritants such as smoke or pollution, exposure to chemicals such as chlorine or contact lens solution, or injuries to the eye.

Medical treatment varies depending on the cause of the inflammation. Common viral conjunctivitis does not require treatment—but if conjunctivitis is due to the **herpes** (see page 86) virus, urgent treatment is necessary. For bacterial eye infections, antibiotic ointment or oral antibiotics are usually prescribed; for allergic conjunctivitis, prescription eye drops and/or antihistamines may be used.

PROPOSED TREATMENTS
Herbal Teas

Traditionally, herbal teas have been applied to the eyes directly, or in compress or poultice form. **Note**: We do not recommend this method because, if absolute sterility is not assured, further serious infection may occur. Furthermore, allergic reactions to herbal products are relatively common, and may themselves cause eye irritation.

As the name indicates, **eyebright** (see page 279) is a traditional herbal treatment for eye conditions; however, this recommendation may be based more on the bloodshot appearance of its petals rather than any actual medicinal effect.

The herbs barberry, **Oregon grape** (see page 375), and **goldenseal** (see page 314) contain berberine, a substance with antimicrobial and antibacterial properties. A special berberine preparation is used as a pharmaceutical treatment for conjunctivitis in Germany, but is not used widely elsewhere.

The herb **calendula** (see page 237) is thought to possess anti-inflammatory and antiseptic properties, and has been used traditionally as an eye compress.

Chamomile (see page 244) tea has also traditionally been used to soothe conjunctivitis symptoms.

Vitamin A

There is some evidence that individuals with chronic conjunctivitis may have a **vitamin A** (see page 432) deficiency.[1] However, this does not prove that taking vitamin A supplements would be helpful in treating or preventing conjunctivitis.

Bee Propolis

Preliminary studies suggest **bee propolis** (see page 216) may be helpful for treating conjunctivitis. However, because it was applied topically to the eye in these trials, we do not recommend this treatment out of concerns regarding sterility.[2]

CONSTIPATION

Principal Proposed Treatments
> **Increased Dietary Fiber:** Psyllium Husks, Debittered Fenugreek Seeds, Flaxseed
> Increased Water Intake, Cascara Sagrada, Dandelion, He Shou Wu, MSM (Methyl Sulfonyl Methane)

In the nineteenth century, a naturopathic concept came into being whose influence persists today: namely, that regular, frequent, and complete bowel movements are necessary for optimum health. William Harvey Kellogg, of Kellogg's cereal fame, wrote extensively of the dangers of "auto-intoxication" purportedly caused by inadequate elimination. He and others claimed that a concrete-like sludge builds up on the wall of the colon, increasing in thickness over time and destroying the health of the body.

However, in modern times physicians have performed millions of direct examinations of the colon, using the procedure known as colonoscopy, without finding any evidence of such a coating. Caked colons are a myth.

Furthermore, conventional medicine has never observed any connection between elimination and overall health. Many people eliminate only once a week or so, and their health appears to be no worse than that of the population at large. Nonetheless, most people find constipation unpleasant, and for some it becomes a severe chronic problem.

Conventional treatment for constipation involves mainly increasing exercise and intake of dietary fiber and water while reserving laxatives, suppositories, and enemas for emergencies.

Visit Us at TNP.com

PRINCIPAL PROPOSED TREATMENTS

Occasional constipation can be safely self-treated. However, if constipation becomes a chronic problem, it should be evaluated by a physician.

Increasing dietary fiber and water intake is the first treatment to try for chronic constipation. Some of the most useful forms of fiber are psyllium husks, debittered **fenugreek** (see page 279) seeds, and **flaxseed** (see page 286). A typical dosage is 5 to 10 g 1 to 3 times daily, with at least 16 ounces of liquid. Start with the lower doses and work up gradually, as too much fiber all at once can actually worsen constipation.

The herb cascara sagrada is an approved over-the-counter treatment for constipation. However, when taken by itself, it can occasionally cause dependence. It is often combined in small amounts with other herbs, including barberry, turkey rhubarb, **dandelion** (see page 266), **red raspberry** (see page 398), **goldenseal** (see page 314), and **cayenne** (see page 243), that gently affect the digestive tract. However, the safety and efficacy of these combinations have not been proven. Dandelion used alone and the Chinese herb **He shou wu** (see page 322) are also reputed to be effective. The supplement **MSM** (see page 364) is sometimes suggested for constipation, although no real evidence exists supporting this use.

A final point about constipation: Like sleep, elimination is inhibited by thinking too much about it. Part of the key to solving chronic constipation problems is to decrease the sense of worry and anxiety that surrounds the issue. Although constipation is certainly unpleasant, its evils have been greatly exaggerated. Thinking less about it will often go a long way toward solving the problem.

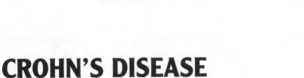

CROHN'S DISEASE

Related Terms   Inflammatory Bowel Disease (Ulcerative Colitis)

Principal Proposed Treatments   Nutritional Support

Other Proposed Treatments   Fish Oil, Glutamine, Probiotics, Avoidance of Allergenic Foods

Crohn's disease is a disease of the bowel that is closely related to **ulcerative colitis** (see page 179). The two are grouped in a category called inflammatory bowel disease (IBD), because they both involve inflammation of the digestive tract.

The major symptoms of Crohn's disease include fever, non-bloody or (less frequently) bloody diarrhea, abdominal pain, and fatigue. The rectum may be severely affected, leading to fissures, abscesses, and fistulas (hollow passages). Intestinal obstruction can occur, and over time fistulas may develop in the small bowel. Other complications include gallstones, increased risk of cancer in the small bowel and colon, and pain in or just below the stomach that mimics the pain of an ulcer. Arthritis, skin sores, and liver problems may develop as well.

Crohn's disease tends to wax and wane, with periods of remission punctuated by severe flare-ups. Medical treatment aims at reducing symptoms and inducing and maintaining remission.

Sulfasalazine is one of the most commonly used medications for Crohn's disease. Given either orally or as an enema, it can both decrease symptoms and prevent recurrences. Corticosteroids such as prednisone are used similarly, sometimes combined with immunosuppressive drugs such as azathioprine. In severe cases, partial removal of the bowel may be necessary.

Another approach involves putting individuals with Crohn's disease on an *elemental* diet. This involves special formulas consisting of required nutrients but no whole foods. Sometimes, after a period on such a diet, whole foods can be restarted one at a time.

PRINCIPAL PROPOSED TREATMENTS

Individuals with Crohn's disease can easily develop deficiencies in numerous nutrients. Malabsorption, decreased appetite, drug side effects, and increased nutrient loss through the stool may lead to mild or profound deficiencies of protein, **vitamins A** (see page 432), **B$_{12}$** (see page 442), **C** (see page 444), **D** (see page 449), **E** (see page 451), and **K** (see page 456), **folate** (see page 288), **calcium** (see page 234), **copper** (see page 262), **magnesium** (see page 351), **selenium** (see page 407), and **zinc** (see page 463).[1–10] Supplementation to restore adequate body supplies of these nutrients is highly advisable, and may improve specific symptoms as well as overall health. We recommend working closely with your physician to identify any nutrient deficiencies and to evaluate the success of supplementation to correct them.

Visit Us at TNP.com

OTHER PROPOSED TREATMENTS

A 1-year double-blind trial involving 78 participants with Crohn's disease in remission who were at high risk for relapse found that **fish oil** (see page 282) supplements helped keep the disease from flaring up.[11] However, a double-blind placebo-controlled trial that followed 120 individuals for 1 year found that fish oil did not reduce the relapse rate as compared to placebo.[12] Negative results were also seen in a smaller double-blind trial.[13]

Glutamine (see page 310) has been suggested as a treatment for Crohn's disease,[14,15,16] as have **probiotics** (see page 200),[17] but as yet the evidence that either works is highly preliminary at best.

Finally, **food allergies** (see page 82) might play a role in Crohn's disease.[18,19]

CYCLIC MASTALGIA

Related Terms   Cyclic Mastitis, Fibrocystic Breast Disease

Principal Proposed Treatments   Evening Primrose Oil (GLA), Ginkgo, Chasteberry, Iodine

Some women's breasts are unusually tender and lumpy, with symptoms of pain and dull heaviness that vary with the menstrual cycle. This condition is called cyclic mastalgia or mastitis and is often associated with premenstrual stress syndrome (PMS). When the lumps become significant enough to be called cysts, this condition is sometimes called fibrocystic breast disease.

Besides discomfort, perhaps the worst problem of this condition is that it can mimic the appearance of breast cancer on mammograms, leading to false alarms. To make matters worse, fibrocystic changes can also hide true cancers, and women with fibrocystic breast disease may also have a greater tendency toward breast cancer (although this is controversial).

Conventional treatment of cyclic mastalgia has incorporated many staples of alternative medicine. After screening carefully for breast cancer, physicians typically recommend reducing animal fats, avoiding chocolate and caffeine, and supplementing with vitamin E (400 IU daily) and vitamin B_6 (50 mg daily). Some physicians have begun to use evening primrose oil as well. These treatments are more likely to be successful in cases that involve pain but no cysts. Even so, the response to therapy is slow, often requiring over 6 months for full results.

If these natural methods don't work, physicians may prescribe various hormone or hormone-like medications.

PRINCIPAL PROPOSED TREATMENTS

Cyclic mastalgia often occurs in connection with **PMS**. (See the chapter on PMS for information on related treatments.)

Evening Primrose Oil (Source of GLA)

European physicians commonly use evening primrose oil to treat cyclic mastalgia, and the practice has come to be popular among some physicians in the United States as well. Evening primrose contains relatively high concentrations of the essential fatty acid **gamma-linolenic acid** (GLA; see page 304). Fatty acid metabolism is known to be disturbed in women with cyclic mastalgia, and abnormalities in essential fatty acid levels have been found in women with PMS and with nonmalignant breast disease.[1] It appears that supplementation with evening primrose oil may be able to correct this imbalance.

What Is the Scientific Evidence for Evening Primrose Oil?

In uncontrolled studies, evening primrose oil has been found to produce significant benefits in about 44% of women with cyclic mastalgia.[2]

Improvement was also seen in a double-blind placebo-controlled study of 73 women suffering from cyclic breast pain.[3] Discomfort was significantly reduced in the group taking evening primrose oil, whereas no significant improvement was seen in the placebo group.

However, evening primrose oil does not seem to be helpful when there are breast cysts rather than just pain. In a 1-year, double-blind study of 200 women with breast cysts, evening primrose oil did not prove effective.[4,5]

Dosage

A typical dosage of evening primrose oil for cyclic mastalgia is 3 g daily. It must be taken for at least 4 to 6 weeks for noticeable effect, and maximum benefits may require 4 to 8 months to develop. Borage oil and black currant oil contain GLA and are sometimes used instead.

Safety Issues

Animal studies suggest that evening primrose oil is completely nontoxic and noncarcinogenic.[6] Over 4,000 people have taken GLA or evening primrose oil in scientific studies, and no significant adverse effects have ever been noted.

Cyclic Mastalgia

Visit Us at TNP.com

The maximum safe dosage for young children, pregnant or nursing women, or those with severe liver or kidney disease has not been established.

Ginkgo

Although the herb **ginkgo** (see page 298) is primarily used to enhance memory and mental function (see the chapter on **Alzheimer's disease**), it may be helpful for breast tenderness as well. A double-blind placebo-controlled study evaluated 143 women with PMS symptoms, 18 to 45 years of age, and followed them for two menstrual cycles.[7] Each woman received either the ginkgo extract (80 mg twice daily) or placebo on day 16 of the first cycle. Treatment was continued until day 5 of the next cycle, and resumed again on day 16 of that cycle.

The results were impressive. As compared to placebo, ginkgo significantly relieved major symptoms of PMS, especially breast pain.

Dosage

The form of ginkgo used in the study we just described and in all other scientific trials is a highly concentrated extract, in which 50 pounds of the leaf must be used to create 1 pound of product. Such extracts are standardized to contain 24% by weight substances known as ginkgo flavonol glycosides. The proper dosage of ginkgo is 40 to 80 mg 3 times daily. It should be taken from about 2 weeks prior to your menstrual period until bleeding stops.

Safety Issues

Ginkgo extract appears to be quite safe. A review of nearly 10,000 participants taking ginkgo extract showed that less than 1% experienced side effects, and those that did occur were minor.[8] In another study, overall side effects were no greater in the ginkgo group than in the placebo group.[9] When a medication produces no more side effects than the placebo, we can reasonably regard it as essentially side-effect free. Furthermore, according to animal studies, ginkgo is safe even when taken in massive overdose.[10]

However, taking ginkgo presents one potential concern. The herb possesses a mild blood-thinning effect that could conceivably cause bleeding problems in certain situations. For this reason, people with hemophilia should not take ginkgo except on a physician's advice. Using ginkgo in the weeks prior to or just after major surgery or labor and delivery is also not advisable. Finally, ginkgo should not be combined with blood-thinning drugs such as Coumadin (warfarin), heparin, aspirin, and Trental (pentoxifylline) except under medical supervision. Ginkgo might also conceivably interact with natural products that slightly thin the blood as well, such as **garlic** (see page 291) and high-dose **vitamin E** (see page 451).

The safety of ginkgo for young children, pregnant or nursing women, and people with kidney or liver disease has not been established.

Chasteberry

In Germany, the herb chasteberry is frequently used to treat cyclic mastalgia and other symptoms of PMS because of its effect on the pituitary gland to suppress the release of prolactin.[11,12,13] For a more detailed discussion about **chasteberry** use and safety issues, please see the corresponding chapter.

Additional Treatments

Like chasteberry, the herb **bugleweed** (see page 231) appears to reduce prolactin levels, and for this reason has also been tried for the treatment of cyclic mastalgia. However, this herb affects the thyroid gland, and we do not recommend it.

The supplement **iodine** (see page 331) may also be helpful for cyclic mastalgia in some cases.

DEPRESSION (Mild to Moderate)

Principal Proposed Treatments   St. John's Wort

Other Proposed Treatments   Phenylalanine, 5-HTP (5-Hydroxytryptophan), Ginkgo, Phosphatidylserine, SAMe (S-Adenosylmethionine), Inositol, Acetyl-L-Carnitine, Vitamin B_6, Vitamin B_{12}, Folate, Fish Oil, Beta-Carotene, Damiana, NADH, Pregnenolone, Tyrosine

Not Recommended Treatments   Yohimbe, DHEA (Dehydroepiandrosterone)

Depression is a common emotional illness that varies widely in its intensity from person to person. The natural treatments described in this section are useful only for mild to moderate depressive symptoms consisting mainly of depressed mood, fatigue, insomnia, irritability, and difficulty concentrating.

More severe depression includes markedly depressed mood complicated by symptoms such as slowed speech,

Depression

slowed (or agitated) responses, markedly impaired memory and concentration, excessive (or diminished) sleep, significant weight loss (or weight gain), intense feelings of worthlessness and guilt, recurrent thoughts of suicide, and lack of interest in pleasurable activities.

Severe clinical depression is a dangerous and excruciating illness. The emotional structure of the brain has frozen into a pattern of misery that cannot be altered by willpower, a change of scenery, or the most earnest efforts of friends. In a sense, the brain has locked up like a crashed computer. No alternative treatment is especially successful when depression gets this bad.

One of the earliest successful treatments for major depression was shock therapy. This technique is almost the exact equivalent of rebooting a computer, and in cases of major depression its effects were revolutionary. For the first time, a reliable way was available to bring people out of the depths of severe major depression. However, shock treatment was overused at first and became unpopular.

The accidental discovery of antidepressant drugs provided a less interventive route. The original antidepressants, known as MAO inhibitors, could bring people out from the depths of major depression as successfully as shock treatment. However, MAO inhibitors can cause serious and even fatal side effects. No one would ever think of using MAO inhibitors to treat mild to moderate depression.

Subsequently, antidepressants with progressively fewer side effects came on the market, but it was not until the appearance of selective serotonin-reuptake inhibitors (SSRIs), such as Prozac and related drugs, that antidepressants became a viable option for depression that was less than catastrophic. Practically overnight, enormous numbers of people began taking Prozac and similar antidepressants for mild to moderate depression.

The big advantage of the SSRIs is that they don't cause fatigue. Many people find them to be entirely side-effect free. However, side effects are not uncommon and include nausea, insomnia, and sexual disturbances (such as the loss of the ability to experience an orgasm).

PRINCIPAL PROPOSED TREATMENTS

Alternative medicine offers one solidly proven treatment for depression: the herb St. John's wort. The evidence for this herb's effectiveness is nearly as comprehensive as what is required of a drug prior to approval. St. John's wort is only useful for mild to moderate depression, but for this purpose, it may be superior to standard treatments. However, for severe depression, conventional antidepressant drugs are necessary and may be lifesaving.

St. John's Wort: A Well-Established Treatment for Mild to Moderate Depression

St. John's wort (*Hypericum perforatum*) (see page 414) is a common perennial herb, with many branches and bright yellow flowers, that grows wild in much of the world. Its name derives from the herb's tendency to flower around the feast of St. John (wort simply means "plant" in Old English). The species name *perforatum* derives from the watermarking of translucent dots that can be seen when a leaf of the plant is held up to the sun.

St. John's wort has a long history of use in emotional disorders. It began to be considered as a treatment for depression early in the twentieth century, and when pharmaceutical antidepressants were invented, German researchers looked for similar properties in St. John's wort.

Today, St. John's wort is one of the best-documented herbal treatments, with a scientific record approaching that of many prescription drugs. Indeed, this herb is a prescription antidepressant in Germany. It is covered by that country's national health-care system and is prescribed more frequently than any synthetic drug.

St. John's wort is used for mild to moderate depression. Typical symptoms include depressed mood, lack of energy, sleep problems, anxiety, appetite disturbance, difficulty concentrating, and poor stress tolerance. Irritability can also be a sign of depression.

St. John's wort appears to be effective in about 55% of cases. As with other antidepressants, the full benefit takes about 4 to 6 weeks to develop. The most common reported effects are brightened mood, increased energy, and improved sleep.

The big advantage of St. John's wort over standard medications is that it rarely, if ever, causes side effects. However, St. John's wort should never be relied on to treat severe depression. If you or a loved one is feeling suicidal, unable to cope with daily life, paralyzed by anxiety, incapable of getting out of bed, unable to sleep, or uninterested in eating, see a physician at once. Drug therapy may save your life.

Like other antidepressants, St. John's wort can also be used to treat chronic insomnia and anxiety when they are related to depression. It may be effective in seasonal affective disorder (SAD) as well.

St. John's wort appears to be reasonably safe when taken alone. However, there is good reason to believe that it may interfere with the effectiveness of numerous medications, including treatments for HIV infection. (See Drug Interactions for details.)

What Is the Scientific Evidence for St. John's Wort?

All together, at least 17 double-blind studies comparing St. John's wort to placebo have been reported at the time of this writing.[1–4] The results show clearly that St. John's wort is an effective treatment for mild to moderate depression. Good evidence from head to head trials tells us that it is at least as effective as fluoxetine (Prozac)[5,6] and sertraline (Zoloft)[7] for this condition, and causes fewer and less severe side effects.

Visit Us at TNP.com

How Does St. John's Wort Work?

We do not really know how St. John's wort acts. Early research suggested that it works like the oldest class of antidepressants, the MAO inhibitors.[8] However, later research essentially discredited this idea.[9,10] More recent research suggests that St. John's wort inhibits the reuptake of serotonin, dopamine, and norepinephrine.[11,12] The substance hyperforin may be a major active ingredient in St. John's wort.[13]

Dosage

The standard dosage of St. John's wort is 300 mg 3 times daily of an extract standardized to contain 0.3% hypericin. Recently, a new form of the herb has come on the market standardized to 2 to 3% hyperforin instead; however, the dosage amount is the same. Some people take 600 mg of St. John's wort in the morning and 300 mg at night, or 500 mg twice daily.

Yet another form of St. John's wort has also passed double-blind studies. This form contains little hyperforin, and is taken at a dose of 250 mg twice daily.[14,15]

This dosage should not be exceeded, as it is not clear that higher doses produce any better effects, and the chance of side effects might increase.

If the herb bothers your stomach, take it with food.

Remember that the full effect takes 4 weeks to develop, so don't give up too soon!

Warning: Various systemic diseases, such as hypothyroidism, chronic hepatitis, and anemia, may masquerade as depression. Make sure to find out whether you have an undiagnosed medical illness before treating yourself with St. John's wort.

Also, it can sometimes be difficult to assess the true intensity of your own depression. A physician's evaluation is essential. If you suffer from severe major depression, you should take medications rather than St. John's wort.

Safety Issues

St. John's wort is essentially side-effect free. Strangely, this good news has an unfortunate consequence: Some people who try St. John's wort decide that it must not be very powerful because it doesn't make them feel ill, so they quit. Be patient!

In a study designed to look for side effects, 3,250 people took St. John's wort for 4 weeks.[16] Overall, about 2.4% experienced side effects. The most common were mild stomach discomfort (0.6%); allergic reactions, mainly rash (0.5%); tiredness (0.4%); and restlessness (0.3%).

In the extensive German experience with St. John's wort as a treatment for depression, no reports of serious adverse consequences from taking the herb alone have been published.[17] Animal studies involving enormous doses for 26 weeks have not shown any serious toxicity.[18]

Cows and sheep grazing on St. John's wort have sometimes developed severe and even fatal sensitivity to the sun. However, this has never occurred in humans taking St. John's wort at normal doses.[19] In one study, highly sun-sensitive people were given twice the normal dose of the herb.[20] The results showed a mild but measurable increase in reaction to ultraviolet radiation. The moral of the story is, if you are especially sensitive to the sun, do not exceed the recommended dosage of St. John's wort, and continue to take your usual precautions against burning. Nonetheless, there might be problems if you combine St. John's wort with other medications. (See Drug Interactions below for more information.) A recent report also suggests that regular use of St. John's wort might increase the risk of cataracts.[21] Although this is preliminary information, it might make sense to wear sunglasses when outdoors if you are taking this herb on a long-term basis.

Older reports suggested that St. John's wort works like the class of drugs known as MAO inhibitors.[22] This led to a number of warnings, including avoiding cheese and decongestants while taking St. John's wort. However, St. John's wort is no longer believed to act like an MAO inhibitor, and these warnings are now thought to be groundless.[23,24]

Safety in young children, pregnant or nursing women, and those with severe liver or kidney disease has not been established.

Drug Interactions

Herbal experts have warned for some time that combining St. John's wort with drugs in the Prozac family (SSRIs) might raise serotonin too much and cause a number of serious problems. Recently, case reports of such events have begun to trickle in.[25,26] This is a potentially serious risk. Do not combine St. John's wort with prescription antidepressants except on the specific advice of a physician. Since some antidepressants, such as Prozac, linger in the blood for quite some time, you also need to exercise caution when switching from a drug to St. John's wort. If you stop Prozac, you may need to wait 3 weeks or more before starting St. John's wort.

The antimigraine drug sumatriptan (Imitrex) and the pain-killing drug tramadol also raise serotonin levels and might interact similarly with St. John's wort.[27,28]

Perhaps the biggest concern with St. John's wort is the possibility that it may decrease the effectiveness of various medications, including protease inhibitors (for HIV infection), cyclosporine (for organ transplants), digoxin (for heart disease), warfarin (a blood thinner), oral contraceptives, chemotherapy drugs, olanzapine or clozapine (for schizophrenia), and theophylline (for asthma).[29–37] Furthermore, if you are taking St. John's wort and one of these medications at the same time and then stop taking the herb, blood levels of the drug may rise. This rise in drug level could be dangerous in certain circumstances.

Depression

These interactions could lead to catastrophic consequences. Indeed, St. John's wort appears to have caused two cases of heart transplant rejection by interfering with the action of cyclosporine. Also, many people with HIV take St. John's wort in the false belief that the herb will fight the AIDS virus. The unintended result may be to reduce the potency of standard AIDS drugs. In addition, the herb might decrease the effectiveness of oral contraceptives, presenting a risk of pregnancy.[38]

Given all this information, we recommend that individuals taking any critical medication should avoid using St. John's wort until more is known.

Additionally, St. John's wort may interact with drugs that cause increased sun sensitivity such as sulfa drugs and the anti-inflammatory medication Feldene (piroxicam), causing greater risk of sunburn. The medications Prilosec (omeprazole) and Prevacid (lansoprazole) may also intensify the tendency of St. John's wort to cause sun sensitivity.[39]

Finally, it is probably advisable on general principles to discontinue all herbs and supplements prior to surgery and anesthesia, due to the possibility of unpredictable interactions. However, there does not appear to be any specific foundation to publicized claims that St. John's wort interacts with anesthetic drugs.

OTHER PROPOSED TREATMENTS

There are a number of other herbs and supplements that may be helpful in depression, although the evidence for them is not as strong as that for St. John's wort.

Phenylalanine: A Promising Treatment for Depression

Phenylalanine (see page 385) is a naturally occurring amino acid that we all consume in our daily diets. There is some evidence that phenylalanine supplements may help reduce symptoms of depression.

What Is the Scientific Evidence for Phenylalanine?

Phenylalanine occurs in a right-hand and a left-hand form, known as D- and L-phenylalanine, respectively. Some studies have evaluated the D- form and others the L- form, and still others have evaluated mixtures of both. All forms seem to be able to provide some measure of relief for symptoms of depression. The mixed form (DLPA) is the one most commonly available in stores.

A 1978 study compared the effectiveness of D-phenylalanine against the antidepressant drug imipramine (taken in daily doses of 100 mg) and found them to be equally effective.[40] A total of 60 individuals were randomly assigned to either one group or the other and followed for 30 days. D-phenylalanine worked more rapidly, producing significant improvement in only 15 days.

Another double-blind study followed 27 people, half of whom received DL-phenylalanine and the other half imipramine in higher doses of 150 to 200 mg daily.[41,42] When the participants were reevaluated in 30 days, the two groups had improved by the same amount.

Unfortunately, there do not seem to have been any properly designed studies that compared phenylalanine to placebo. Until these are performed, phenylalanine cannot be considered a proven treatment for depression, but it is certainly promising.

Dosage

When used as a treatment for depression, L-phenylalanine is typically started at a dosage of 500 mg daily and then gradually increased to 3 to 4 g daily.[43] However, side effects may develop at dosages above 1,500 mg daily (see Safety Issues).

D- or DL-phenylalanine may be used for depression as well, but the typical dosage is much lower: 100 to 400 mg daily.[44]

Safety Issues

Although most people do not report side effects from any type of phenylalanine, daily doses near or above 1,500 mg of L-phenylalanine can reportedly cause anxiety, headache, and even mildly elevated blood pressure.[45]

The long-term safety of phenylalanine in any of its forms is not known.

Both L- and D-phenylalanine must be avoided by those with the rare metabolic disease phenylketonuria (PKU). The safety of high dosages of L-phenylalanine, or any dosage of D-phenylalanine, has not been established for young children, pregnant or nursing women, or those with severe liver or kidney disease.

There are some indications that combining phenylalanine with antipsychotic drugs might increase the risk of developing the long-term side effect known as tardive dyskinesia, or worsen symptoms in those who already have it.[46,47] We also don't know if it is safe to combine phenylalanine with standard antidepressants.

5-HTP: May Be Effective, but Use Caution

A new, up-and-coming treatment for depression is **5-HTP** (5-hydroxytryptophan; see page 198). When the body sets about manufacturing serotonin, it first makes 5-HTP. The theory behind taking 5-HTP as a supplement is that providing the one-step-removed raw ingredient might raise serotonin levels. However, this plausible idea has not been proven.

The amino acid tryptophan used to be recommended as a treatment for depression on the same basis. It is one step back in the chain, being turned by the body into 5-HTP and then to serotonin. However, tryptophan was

Visit Us at TNP.com

Depression

Visit Us at TNP.com

removed from the market several years ago when a contaminant caused a terrible and often permanent illness in many people who took the supplement. Because 5-HTP is made by a completely different manufacturing process (starting from a plant rather than bacteria), one would not expect the same contaminant to be present. Disturbingly, however, recent reports suggest otherwise (see Safety Issues).

Like St. John's wort, 5-HTP is used mainly in Europe, where many physicians find it an effective treatment for both depression and insomnia.

What Is the Scientific Evidence for 5-HTP?

There have been several preliminary studies of 5-HTP.[48] The best of these trials was a 6-week study of 63 people given either 5-HTP (100 mg 3 times daily) or an antidepressant in the Prozac family (fluvoxamine, 50 mg 3 times daily).[49] The results showed equal benefit between the supplement and the drug. Actually, 5-HTP worked a little better, but from a mathematical perspective, the difference was not statistically significant.

5-HTP caused fewer and less severe side effects than fluvoxamine. The only real complaint was occasional mild digestive distress.

Dosage

The typical dosage of 5-HTP is 100 to 200 mg 3 times daily.

Safety Issues

5-HTP seldom causes noticeable side effects other than occasional digestive distress. However, comprehensive safety studies have not been performed, and an FDA report has raised some questions about this supplement. As we mentioned earlier, the amino acid tryptophan was removed from the stores several years ago when a contaminant caused a terrible and often permanently disabling or fatal illness in many people who took the supplement. Alarmingly, on September 7, 1998, the FDA released a report stating that some commercial 5-HTP preparations had been found to contain a similar contaminant. We suggest you check with your physician for the most recent information.

Another safety issue with 5-HTP involves an interaction with a medication used for Parkinson's disease: carbidopa. Several reports suggest that the combination can create skin changes similar to those that occur in the disease scleroderma.[50,51,52]

According to one report, 5-HTP may cause seizures in children with Down's syndrome.[53]

Like St. John's wort, 5-HTP probably should not be combined with conventional antidepressants. Although safety in children has not been proven, children have been given 5-HTP in studies without any apparent harmful effects.[54,55,56] Safety in pregnant or nursing women and those with severe liver or kidney disease has not been established.

Ginkgo: Improves Mental Function, but May Help Depression, Too

Ginkgo (see page 298) is used mainly for age-related mental decline such as that from **Alzheimer's disease** (see page 5). However, during the studies on impaired mental function, researchers frequently observed improvements in mood and relief from symptoms of depression. This incidental discovery led scientists to investigate whether ginkgo might be useful as an antidepressant treatment.

One study, published in 1990, evaluated this effect in 60 people who suffered from depressive symptoms along with other signs of dementia.[57] The results showed significant improvements among participants given ginkgo extract instead of placebo.

Another study followed 40 depressed individuals over the age of 50 who had not responded successfully to antidepressant treatment.[58] Those who were given ginkgo showed an average drop of 50% in scores on the Hamilton Depression scale, whereas the placebo group showed only a 10% improvement.

In 1994 an interesting piece of research was reported that may shed light on the mechanism by which ginkgo could reduce depression.[59] This study examined levels of serotonin receptors in rats of various ages. When older rats were given ginkgo, the level of serotonin-binding sites increased. However, the same effect was not observed in younger rats. The researchers theorized that ginkgo may block an age-related loss of serotonin receptors.

Reduced receptors for serotonin may mean that the body needs more serotonin to produce a normal effect. Instead of raising the level of serotonin, like Prozac does, ginkgo may thus improve the brain's ability to respond to serotonin (at least in older people). However, this is still highly speculative. More experimentation is needed to clarify the mechanism of ginkgo's action and to better quantify its effectiveness in depression.

The proper dose of ginkgo is 40 to 80 mg of a 24% extract taken 3 times daily. As is the case with conventional antidepressants, the full benefit takes up to 6 weeks to develop.

Ginkgo appears to be very safe. Extremely high doses have been given to animals without serious consequences.[60] In all the clinical trials of ginkgo up to 1991, involving a total of almost 10,000 people, only a small number of participants reported side effects produced by ginkgo extract. There were 21 cases of gastrointestinal discomfort and even fewer cases of headaches, dizziness, and allergic skin reactions.[61]

Depression

However, because ginkgo slightly thins the blood, it should not be combined with anticoagulant drugs or even aspirin. (For more information on this potential risk, see the chapter on ginkgo.)

Safety in young children, pregnant or nursing women, and those with severe liver or kidney disease has not been established.

Phosphatidylserine: Good for Mental Function, May Also Help Depression

Phosphatidylserine (see page 387) is another treatment used mainly for mental decline in the elderly that may also offer antidepressant benefits.[62]

The proper dosage is 100 mg 3 times daily. Full results take anywhere from 4 weeks to 6 months to manifest. Although no side effects have been reported, this rather expensive supplement usually costs from $50 to $75 per month. Safety in young children, pregnant or nursing women, and those with severe liver or kidney disease has not been established.

SAMe: May Be Effective, but Very Expensive

Another European supplement treatment for depression now arrived in the United States is **SAMe** (S-adenosylmethionine; see page 403). SAMe is a very important biological molecule that occurs throughout the body. Its job is to hand over a chemical fragment called a methyl group to other chemicals that need it.

Although several small double-blind studies have found SAMe effective in relieving depression, the sum total of evidence for SAMe as an antidepressant remains small and is flawed by the fact that most studies used an intravenous form of the supplement.[63]

In addition to a lack of reliable evidence, SAMe is extremely expensive. The proper dosage is 400 mg 3 to 4 times daily and can cost over $200 per month, although the price is dropping.

To minimize stomach distress, most physicians recommend starting at a low dose of perhaps 200 mg twice daily and then gradually working up from there. Then, when you reach the full dose, stay at it for a month or so. Once you are feeling better, you can try reducing the dose again.

Recently, SAMe has come on the U.S. market at a recommended dosage of 200 mg twice daily. While this dosage labeling makes SAMe appear more affordable (if you're only taking 400 mg per day, you'll spend only about a third of what you'd pay for the proper dosage), it is unlikely that SAMe will actually work when taken at such a low dosage.

SAMe appears to be quite safe, according to both human and animal studies.[64–67] The most common side effect is mild digestive distress. However, SAMe does not actually damage the stomach.[68]

Like other substances with antidepressant activity, SAMe might trigger a manic episode in those with bipolar disease (manic-depressive illness).[69,70,71]

Safety in young children, pregnant or nursing women, or those with severe liver or kidney disease has not been established.

SAMe might interfere with the action of the Parkinson's drug levodopa.[72] In addition, there may also be risks involved in combining SAMe with standard antidepressants.[73] For this reason, you shouldn't try either combination except under physician supervision.

Other Herbs and Supplements

Weak evidence suggests that the nutritional substance **inositol** (see page 330) might be helpful in depression when taken in extremely high doses (12 g daily).[74] Although this is a nutritional substance, when taken in such enormous doses, its safety cannot be assured.

Preliminary evidence suggests that the substance **acetyl-L-carnitine** (see page 238) may be useful for depression in the elderly.[75,76]

Diets low in **vitamin B$_6$** (see page 439), **vitamin B$_{12}$** (see page 442), or **folate** (see page 288) have been associated with symptoms of depression.[77,78,79] While there is little direct evidence that taking B$_6$ or B$_{12}$ supplements can help depression, an intriguing body of evidence suggests that folate supplements really help.[80–87] In any case, as deficiencies of B$_6$ and folate are common and B$_{12}$ deficiencies occur more often with advancing age, there is a lot to be said for taking these vitamins on general principle. For depression, typical daily doses are 25 to 50 mg of B$_6$, 400 mcg of folate, and 10 to 100 mcg of B$_{12}$. These supplements are safe when taken at these doses.

Intriguing, but highly preliminary, evidence suggests that deficiencies in essential fatty acids may increase the risk of depression; it is possible that **fish oil** (see page 282) supplements could therefore help prevent depression.[88]

The herbs and supplements **beta-carotene** (see page 217), **damiana** (see page 265), **NADH** (see page 368), **pregnenolone** (see page 391), and **tyrosine** (see page 426) are also sometimes recommended for depression, but there is little evidence as yet that they really work.

NOT RECOMMENDED TREATMENTS

The herb **yohimbe** (see page 461) and the hormone **DHEA** (see page 268) are sometimes suggested for depression,[89] but because of potential risks we do not suggest using them except under the supervision of a qualified health-care professional (if at all).

Visit Us at TNP.com

❧ DIABETES

Principal Proposed Treatments

Blood Sugar Control: Chromium, Fenugreek, Gymnema, Ginseng, Aloe, Bilberry Leaf, Bitter Melon, *Coccinia indica*, Garlic, Holy Basil, Nopal Cactus, Onion, Pterocarpus, Salt Bush, CLA, Glucomannan, Vanadium, Vitamin E, Niacinamide, Biotin, Carnitine, Coenzyme Q_{10} (CoQ_{10}), Lipoic Acid

Treatment of Complications: Lipoic Acid, Evening Primrose Oil (GLA), Fish Oil, Vitamin E, Carnitine, Selenium, Inositol, Bilberry, OPCs (Oligomeric Proanthocyanidins), Ginkgo, Vitamin C, Oxerutins, Biotin

To Correct Nutritional Deficiencies: Magnesium, Zinc, Vitamin C, Taurine, Manganese

Preventing Diabetes: Niacinamide

Diabetes has two forms. In the type that develops early in childhood (type 1), the insulin-secreting cells of the pancreas are destroyed (probably by a viral infection), and blood levels of insulin drop nearly to zero. However, in the adult-onset form (type 2), insulin is often plentiful, but the body does not respond normally to it. (This is only an approximate description of the difference between the two types.) In both forms of diabetes, blood sugar reaches toxic levels, causing injury to many organs and tissues.

Conventional treatment for childhood-onset diabetes includes insulin injections and careful dietary monitoring. The adult-onset form may respond to lifestyle changes alone, such as increasing exercise, losing weight, and improving diet. Various oral medications are also often effective for adult-onset diabetes, although insulin injections may be necessary in some cases.

PRINCIPAL PROPOSED TREATMENTS

Several alternative methods may be helpful when used under medical supervision as an addition to standard treatment. They may help stabilize, reduce, or eliminate medication requirements; reduce the symptoms of diabetic complications; or correct nutritional deficiencies associated with diabetes. However, because diabetes is a dangerous disease with many potential complications, alternative treatment for diabetes should not be attempted as a substitute for conventional medical care.

Treatments for Improving Blood Sugar Control

The following treatments may be able to improve blood sugar control in type 1 and/or type 2 diabetes.

Note: Keep in mind that if these treatments work, you will need to reduce your medications to avoid hypoglycemia. For this reason, medical supervision is essential.

Chromium: Helpful in Type 2 Diabetes

Chromium (see page 251) is an essential trace mineral that plays a significant role in sugar metabolism. Reasonably good evidence suggests that chromium supplemen-

tation may help bring blood sugar levels under control in type 2 diabetes. It may also be helpful for pregnancy-related diabetes.

A 4-month study reported in 1997 followed 180 Chinese men and women with type 2 diabetes, comparing the effects of 1,000 mcg chromium, 200 mcg chromium, and placebo.[1] The results showed that HbA1c values (a measure of long-term blood sugar control) improved significantly after 2 months in the group receiving 1,000 mcg, and in both chromium groups after 4 months. Fasting glucose was also lower in the group taking the higher dose of chromium.

Similarly positive results were seen in other small studies.[2,3] However, there have also been negative results.[4,5]

One placebo-controlled study of 30 women with pregnancy-related diabetes found that supplementation with chromium (at a dosage of 4 or 8 mcg chromium picolinate for each kilogram of body weight) significantly improved blood sugar control.[6]

Chromium might also be helpful for treating diabetes caused by corticosteroid treatment.[7,8]

The optimum dosage of chromium is not known. The usual recommended therapeutic dosage is 200 to 400 mcg daily (as chromium picolinate). However, one of the recent studies just described used a higher dose.

Since there have been a few worrisome case reports of toxic effects when chromium has been taken at daily doses ranging from 600 to 2,400 mcg,[9,10] you should consult with your physician on what might be the appropriate dosage for you. Pregnant women should keep in mind that there are also concerns, still fairly theoretical, that chromium picolinate could cause adverse effects on DNA.[11]

Fenugreek: Appears to Be Helpful

The food spice **fenugreek** (see page 279) may also help control blood sugar. For millennia, fenugreek has been used both as a medicine and as a spice in Egypt, India, and the Middle East. Numerous animal studies, as well as small-scale trials in humans (none of which were double-blind) involving a total of about 100 people, have found that fenugreek can reduce blood sugar and serum

Visit Us at TNP.com

cholesterol levels in people with diabetes.[12,13,14] It seems to be helpful in both type 1 and type 2 diabetes.

Dosage   Because the seeds of fenugreek are somewhat bitter, fenugreek is best taken in capsule form. The typical dosage is 5 to 30 g 3 times a day with meals, taken indefinitely.

Safety Issues   As a commonly eaten food, fenugreek is generally regarded as safe. The only common side effect is mild gastrointestinal distress when it is taken in high doses.

Extracts made from fenugreek have been shown to cause uterine contractions in guinea pigs.[15] For this reason, pregnant women should not take fenugreek in doses higher than is commonly used as a spice, perhaps 5 g daily. Safety in young children, nursing women, or those with severe liver or kidney disease has also not been established.

Gymnema: Preliminary Evidence Suggests It Is Effective

A few preliminary studies suggest that the Ayurvedic (Indian) herb **gymnema** (see page 320) may help improve blood sugar control.[16,17,18] In practice, many clinicians report that gymnema is more powerful than the other treatments described in this section. It might be helpful for mild cases of adult-onset diabetes, taken alone or in combination with standard treatment (under a doctor's supervision in either case).

The usual dose of gymnema ranges from 400 to 600 mg daily of an extract standardized to contain 24% gymnemic acids. Because no formal safety studies have been conducted, gymnema should not be taken by young children, pregnant or nursing women, or those with severe kidney or liver disease.

Ginseng: Promising New Evidence

A double-blind study evaluated the effects of ginseng in 36 people newly diagnosed with adult-onset diabetes over an 8-week period.[19] The results showed a reduction in glucose levels, improved glycosylated hemoglobin (a measure of long-term blood sugar control), and improved physical capacity. The authors believed that it was the increased activity that improved blood sugar.

Improved blood sugar control was also seen in two small double-blind placebo-controlled trials using American ginseng (*Panax quinquefolius*).[20,21]

Although ginseng is generally believed to be safe, safety in young children, pregnant or nursing women, and those with severe kidney or liver disease has not been established. (See the chapter on **ginseng** for a more detailed discussion of the potential safety issues associated with this herb.)

Aloe: More Famous for Burns

The succulent aloe plant has been valued since prehistoric times for the treatment of burns, wound infections,

and other skin problems. However, recent evidence suggests that oral **aloe** (see page 204) might be useful for type 2 diabetes.

Evidence from some but not all animal and human studies suggests that aloe gel can improve blood sugar control.[22–27]

For example, a single-blind placebo-controlled trial evaluated the potential benefits of aloe in either 72 or 40 individuals with diabetes (the study report appears to contradict itself).[28] The results showed significantly greater improvements in blood sugar levels among those given aloe over the 2-week treatment period.

Another single-blind placebo-controlled trial evaluated the benefits of aloe in individuals who had failed to respond to the oral diabetes drug glibenclamide.[29] Of the 36 individuals who completed the study, those taking glibenclamide and aloe showed definite improvements in blood sugar levels over 42 days as compared to those taking glibenclamide and placebo.

While these are promising results, large studies that are double- rather than single-blind will be needed to establish aloe as an effective treatment for hypoglycemia.

For the treatment of diabetes, a dosage of 1 tablespoon of aloe vera juice twice daily has been used in studies.

Other than occasional allergic reactions, no serious problems have been reported with aloe gel, whether used internally or externally. However, comprehensive safety studies are lacking. Safety in young children, pregnant or nursing women, or individuals with severe liver or kidney disease has not been established.

Other Treatments That May Help Control Blood Sugar

Preliminary evidence suggests that the herbs **bilberry leaf** (see page 220), **bitter melon** (see page 222), *Coccinia indica,* **garlic** (see page 291), holy basil (*Ocimum sanctum*), nopal cactus (*Opuntia streptacantha*), onion, pterocarpus, and **salt bush** (see page 402) and the supplements **CLA** (conjugated linoleic acid; see page 261), **glucomannan** (see page 307), and **vanadium** (see page 430) might be helpful for diabetes.[30–56] Other herbs traditionally used for diabetes that might offer some benefit include *Cuminum cyminum* (cumin), *Azadirachta indica* (**neem;** see page 368), *Musa sapientum* L. (banana), *Anemarrhena asphodeloides, Catharanthus roseus, Cucumis sativus, Cucurbita ficifolia, Euphorbia prostrata, Guaiacum coulteri, Guazuma ulmifolia, Lepechinia caulescens, Medicago sativa* (**alfalfa;** see page 202), *Phaseolus vulgaris, Psacalium peltatum, Rhizophora mangle, Spinacea oleracea, Tournefortia hirsutissima,* and *Turnera diffusa.*[57–65]

Preliminary studies indicate that vitamin E may also slightly improve blood sugar control in type 2 diabetes.[66,67] (For a discussion of the safety issues and the proper dosage amounts, see the chapter on **vitamin E.**)

The supplements **carnitine** (see page 238), **coenzyme Q₁₀** (see page 256), and lipoic acid (better known as a treatment for complications of diabetes as described under the heading Treating Complications of Diabetes) might also be helpful.[68,69,70]

If your child has just developed diabetes, the supplement niacinamide—a form of niacin, also called **vitamin B₃** (see page 437)—may prolong what is called the honeymoon period.[71] This is the interval during which the pancreas can still make some insulin, and insulin needs are low. By giving your child niacinamide, you may be able to buy some time to allow him or her to adjust to a life of insulin injections.

When used as therapy for a specific disease, niacinamide is taken in dosages much higher than nutritional needs, about 1 to 4 g daily. Because there is a risk of liver inflammation at these dosages, medical supervision is essential.

The supplement **biotin** (see page 221) is also sometimes said to be helpful in diabetes, for both blood sugar control and reduction of complications, but there is as yet little direct evidence that it works.

Warning: Recent animal studies and case reports have raised concerns that the supplement **glucosamine** (see page 308) might *raise* blood sugar levels in individuals with diabetes.[72–76]

Treating Complications of Diabetes

Several supplements may help prevent or treat some of the common complications of diabetes.

Because atherosclerosis is one of the worst problems associated with diabetes, all the suggestions discussed in the chapter on **atherosclerosis** may be useful.

Other herbs and supplements may be helpful for diabetic neuropathy, diabetic retinopathy, and diabetic cataracts, so the treatments discussed in the chapter on **cataracts** may also be of use.

Lipoic Acid: Standard German Treatment for Diabetic Neuropathy

Lipoic acid (see page 347) has been widely used in Germany for decades to treat diabetic peripheral neuropathy, a painful nerve condition that often develops after many years of diabetes. However, most of the evidence of its effectiveness for this condition is limited to studies that used the intravenous form of lipoic acid.

This naturally occurring antioxidant may also help prevent and treat cardiac autonomic neuropathy (injury to the nerves controlling the heart).

Lipoic acid is a vitamin-like substance that plays a role in the body's utilization of energy. Because lipoic acid can be synthesized from other substances, it is not considered an essential nutrient. However, in people with diabetes, levels of lipoic acid are reduced,[77] which suggests (but definitely does not prove) that supplementation would be helpful.

According to some preliminary evidence, lipoic acid may be more effective if it is combined with GLA (gamma-linolenic acid), another supplement used for diabetic neuropathy.[78,79]

What Is the Scientific Evidence for Lipoic Acid? There is some evidence that intravenous lipoic acid can reduce symptoms of diabetic peripheral neuropathy, at least in the short term. Oral lipoic acid has not been well evaluated, and the best study of oral lipoic acid found it ineffective for long-term use.

A randomized double-blind placebo-controlled study that enrolled 503 individuals with diabetic neuropathy found that intravenous lipoic acid helped reduce symptoms over a 3-week period, but long-term oral supplementation was not effective.[80]

A previous double-blind placebo-controlled trial also found short-term benefit with intravenous lipoic acid.[81,82]

Warning: Do not inject lipoic acid products intended for oral use.

The positive evidence for oral lipoic acid in diabetic peripheral neuropathy is limited to open studies or trials that were too small upon which to base conclusions.[83–87]

The DEKAN (Deutsche Kardiale Autonome Neuropathie) study followed 73 people with diabetes, who had symptoms of cardiac autonomic neuropathy, for 4 months.[88] Treatment with 800 mg of oral lipoic acid daily showed significant improvement compared to placebo and no important side effects.

Dosage The typical dosage of oral lipoic acid for diabetic peripheral neuropathy is 300 to 600 mg daily, divided into 2 or 3 doses. For cardiac autonomic neuropathy, a higher dosage of 800 mg daily has been used in studies.

Because lipoic acid occasionally improves the body's response to insulin, it may be necessary to start with lower doses and gradually increase while monitoring blood sugar levels under a physician's supervision.

Safety Issues Lipoic acid appears to have no significant side effects at dosages up to 1,800 mg daily.[89]

Safety for young children, women who are pregnant or nursing, or those with severe liver or kidney disease has not been established. It is also possible that lipoic acid might improve blood sugar control in some cases, and therefore require a reduction in diabetes medications.[90]

GLA (from Evening Primrose): Probably Helpful, but Slow-Acting

The evening primrose is a native American wildflower, named for the late-afternoon opening of its delicate flowers. Perhaps it should be described as a food supplement rather than an herb, for evening primrose oil has been popularized mainly as a source of **GLA** (gamma-linolenic

Diabetes

acid; see page 304), an essential fatty acid also found in black currant and borage oil.

Although many other kinds of fat are unhealthy, essential fatty acids (EFAs) are as necessary as vitamins. The two main kinds of EFAs are called omega-3 and omega-6 fatty acids. The GLA in evening primrose oil is an omega-6 fatty acid. A growing body of scientific evidence suggests that supplementation with GLA may help relieve symptoms of diabetic neuropathy. **Fish oil** (see page 282) may be helpful as well.[91]

What Is the Scientific Evidence for GLA?   Many studies in animals have shown that evening primrose oil can protect nerves from diabetes-induced injury.[92,93] Good results were also seen in a double-blind study that followed 111 people with diabetes from seven medical centers for a period of 1 year.[94] The results showed an improvement in subjective symptoms such as pain and numbness as well as objective signs of nerve injury. Individuals with good blood sugar control improved the most. Another double-blind study also reported positive results.[95]

Dosage   A typical dosage of evening primrose oil for diabetic neuropathy is 4 to 6 g daily. It should be taken with food. Keep in mind that full results may take over 6 months to develop.

Safety Issues   Animal studies suggest that evening primrose oil is nontoxic and noncarcinogenic.[96] Over 4,000 people have taken GLA or evening primrose oil in scientific studies, and no significant adverse effects have ever been noted.

Early reports suggested the possibility that GLA might worsen temporal lobe epilepsy, but this has not been confirmed.[97]

Maximum safe dosages in young children, pregnant or nursing women, and those with severe kidney or liver disease have not been established.

Other Treatments to Help Treat Complications of Diabetes

According to a 52-week double-blind trial of 19 individuals with diabetes, **acetyl-L-carnitine** (see page 238) may help prevent or slow down cardiac autonomic neuropathy (injury to the nerves of the heart caused by diabetes).[98]

Intriguing evidence suggests that **vitamin E** (see page 451) may help protect people with diabetes from developing damage to their eyes and kidneys.[99] There is also some evidence that vitamin E as well as **selenium** (see page 407) might be beneficial for diabetic peripheral neuropathy.[100,101] The supplement **inositol** (see page 330) has also been tried as a treatment for complications of diabetes, but the results have been mixed.[102,103]

Weak evidence suggests that the herb bilberry (120 to 240 mg twice daily of an extract standardized to contain 25%

anthocyanosides) may help prevent eye damage caused by diabetes.[104,105] (For a more complete discussion of **bilberry** use and safety issues, see the chapter on this herb.)

OPCs and **ginkgo** are said to provide similar benefits, although the evidence for these is weaker than that for bilberry. (See the chapters on these substances for more complete discussions.)

Vitamin C (see page 444) is believed to help prevent cataracts in general.[106,107] It is not known for sure whether vitamin C produces the same benefit in people with diabetes. However, it has been suggested that vitamin C may actually be especially useful because of its relationship to sorbitol, a sugar-like substance that tends to accumulate in the cells of people with diabetes. Sorbitol is believed to play a role in the development of diabetic cataracts, and vitamin C appears to help reduce sorbitol buildup.[108] However, the evidence that vitamin C provides significant benefits by this route is at present indirect and far from conclusive. A daily dose of 500 mg should be safe and sufficient.

Preliminary evidence suggests that **oxerutins** (see page 377) might also be helpful for reducing foot and ankle swelling in people with diabetes.[109] In these trials, oxerutin therapy did not affect blood sugar control.

Warning: There is some evidence that the substance **glucosamine** (see page 308), used for arthritis, may increase the risk of diabetic cataracts.[110]

Treating Nutritional Deficiencies in Diabetes

Both diabetes and the medications used to treat it can cause people to fall short of various nutrients. Making up for these deficiencies (either through diet or the use of supplements) may not help your diabetes, but it should make you a healthier person overall.

Magnesium (see page 351) appears to be the most common mineral deficiency in type 1 diabetes.[111,112] People with either type 1 or type 2 diabetes may also be deficient in the mineral **zinc** (see page 463).[113,114,115] **Vitamin C** (see page 444) levels have been found to be low in many diabetics on insulin, even though they were consuming seemingly adequate amounts in their diets.[116,117,118] Some people with type 1 diabetes appear to be deficient in the amino acid **taurine** (see page 420).[119] Finally, **manganese** (see page 354) deficiency reportedly can occur.[120]

Dosage and Safety Issues

So that you do not take unnecessary supplements, you may want to undergo testing to determine whether you are actually deficient in any of these nutrients. However, such testing is expensive. Because these are safe supplements, you may want to take them simply as insurance.

Typical dosages for nutritional correction in diabetes are as follows: magnesium, 350 to 450 mg daily; zinc, 15

Visit Us at TNP.com

to 30 mg daily (combined with 1 to 3 mg daily of **copper** [see page 262]); vitamin C, 500 mg daily; taurine, 2 to 6 g daily; and manganese, 2 to 5 mg daily. A general multivitamin and mineral may not be a bad idea, either, for there may be many other marginal deficiencies in diabetes. However, if you suffer from diabetic kidney disease, you should not take any supplements except on the advice of a physician.

Preventing Diabetes

Exciting evidence from a huge study conducted in New Zealand suggests that the supplement niacinamide—a form of niacin, also known as **vitamin B$_3$** (see page 437)—might be able to reduce the risk of diabetes in children at high risk.[121] In this study, more than 20,000 children were screened for diabetes risk by measuring certain antibodies in the blood (ICA antibodies, believed to indicate risk of developing diabetes). It turned out that 185 of these children had detectable levels. About 170 of these children were then given niacinamide for 7 years (not all parents agreed to give their children niacinamide or stay in the study for that long). About 10,000 other children were not screened, but they were followed to see whether they developed diabetes.

The results were very impressive. In the group in which children were screened and given niacinamide if they were positive for ICA antibodies, the incidence of diabetes was reduced by as much as 60%.

These findings suggest that niacinamide is a very effective treatment for preventing diabetes. (It also shows that tests for ICA antibodies can very accurately identify children at risk for diabetes.)

At present, an enormous-scale, long-term trial called the European Nicotinamide Diabetes Intervention Trial is being conducted to definitively determine whether regular use of niacinamide can prevent diabetes. Results from the German portion of the study have been released, and they were not positive;[122] however, until the entire study is complete, it is not possible to draw conclusions.

For prevention of diabetes in children, the usual dosage of niacinamide is 25 mg per kilogram body weight per day. There are 2.2 pounds in a kilogram, so a 40-pound child would get about 450 mg daily. For safety information, see the chapter on vitamin B$_3$.

Warning: Medical supervision is essential before giving your child long-term niacinamide treatment.

DUPUYTREN'S CONTRACTURE

Principal Proposed Treatments   There are no well-established natural treatments for Dupuytren's contracture.

Other Proposed Treatments   Vitamin E

Named after a nineteenth-century French baron, Dupuytren's contracture is a thickening of tissue in the palm that causes an inability to straighten one or more fingers, usually the ring finger or little finger. The involved tissue hardens and shrinks forming a small lump or "cord" in the palm. Discomfort is unusual. The condition can involve both hands or even the toes, and tends to progress slowly.

If you have Dupuytren's contracture, you may wonder if you injured your hand in some way, but if injury plays any role it is probably not a major one. Although the exact cause of the condition is unknown, the disorder appears to be at least partially inherited.

If the contracture becomes very troublesome, surgery may be useful.

PROPOSED TREATMENTS

There are no well-documented natural treatments for Dupuytren's contracture. However, based on weak and conflicting studies dating back half a century, some natural medicine experts recommend oral vitamin E.

Vitamin E

In the 1940s, a number of physicians reported attempts to treat the condition with **vitamin E** (see page 451).[1,2] Most reported some success; however, their reports were incomplete and highly subjective, leading others to question their findings.

In 1952, two different researchers added an objective measure to their investigations by examining plaster casts of patients' hands before and after treatment, but their results were conflicting.

One researcher treated a group of 19 people with 300 mg daily of oral vitamin E for 300 days and reported moderate improvement in the amount of contraction.[3] In contrast, the other researcher found no improvement among 46 people receiving 200 mg of vitamin E daily for 3 months.[4]

However, since neither of these studies used a control group, the results are not particularly meaningful. Further clinical trials using double-blind placebo-controlled techniques would provide more valuable information.

Dosage

Many of these treatment attempts used the equivalent of 200 to 300 IU of vitamin E daily.

Safety Issues

Vitamin E is generally regarded as safe at these doses. However, vitamin E does have a blood-thinning effect that could lead to problems in certain situations. It's safest not to combine vitamin E with Coumadin (warfarin), aspirin, or other blood-thinning medications except on a physician's advice.

There is also at least a remote possibility that vitamin E could interact with herbs that possess a mild blood-thinning effect, such as garlic and ginkgo. Individuals with bleeding disorders such as hemophilia, and those about to undergo surgery or childbirth, should also approach vitamin E with caution.

DYSMENORRHEA (Painful Menstruation)

Principal Proposed Treatments   Fish Oil, Magnesium

Other Proposed Treatments   Cramp Bark, Bromelain, Turmeric, White Willow, Black Cohosh, *Coleus forskohlii,* Dong Quai, Manganese

We do not know why menstruation is uncomfortable at all, or why it is much more painful for some women than for others and varies so much from month to month.

Occasionally, severe menstrual pain indicates the presence of endometriosis (a condition in which uterine tissue is growing in places other than the uterus) or uterine fibroids (benign tumors in the uterus), but in most cases no such identifiable abnormality can be found. Natural substances known as prostaglandins seem to play a central role in menstrual pain, but the details of the many interactions are scarcely understood, and the available treatments are not specific in their action.

Anti-inflammatory drugs such as ibuprofen usually relieve menstrual pain substantially. However, their blood-thinning effects can increase menstrual flow. Oral contraceptive treatment can also help over the long term, although its success is not guaranteed.

PRINCIPAL PROPOSED TREATMENTS

There is some evidence that the supplements fish oil and magnesium may help reduce menstrual pain.

Fish Oil: Appears to Relieve Cramps

It is believed that the omega-3 fatty acids in **fish oil** (see page 282) may help relieve dysmenorrhea by affecting the metabolism of prostaglandins and other factors involved in pain and inflammation.[1]

In a 4-month study of 42 young women aged 15 to 18, half the participants received a daily dose of 6 g of fish oil, providing 1,080 mg of EPA and 720 mg of DHA daily.[2] After 2 months, they were switched to placebo for another 2 months. The other group received the same treatments in reverse order. The results showed that these young women experienced significantly less menstrual pain while they were taking fish oil.

Another double-blind study followed 78 women, who received either fish oil, seal oil, fish oil with vitamin B_{12} (7.5 mcg daily), or placebo for three full menstrual periods.[3] Significant improvements were seen in all treatment groups, but the fish oil plus B_{12} proved most effective, and its benefits continued for the longest time after treatment was stopped (3 months). The researchers offered no explanation why B_{12} should be helpful.

There are many different types of fish oil products available. A typical daily dose should supply about 1,800 mg of EPA and 900 mg of DHA. Cod liver oil is probably not the best choice due to the potential for excessive intake of **vitamin A** (see page 432) and **vitamin D** (see page 449). **Flaxseed oil** (see page 285) has been proposed as a less smelly alternative to fish oil, but it has not been proven effective.

Because fish oil has a mild "blood-thinning" effect, it should not be combined with powerful blood-thinning medications, such as Coumadin (warfarin) or heparin, except on a physician's advice. However, contrary to some reports, fish oil does not seem to cause bleeding problems when it is taken by itself.[4]

Also, fish oil does not appear to raise blood sugar levels in people with diabetes.[5] Nonetheless, if you have diabetes, you should not take any supplement except on the advice of a physician.

Fish oil may temporarily raise the level of LDL ("bad") cholesterol; but this effect seems to be short-lived, and levels return to normal with continued use.[6,7]

If you decide to use cod liver oil as your fish oil supplement, make sure you do not exceed the safe maximum intake of vitamin A and vitamin D. These vitamins are fat-soluble, which means that excess amounts tend to build up in your body, possibly reaching toxic levels. Pregnant women should not take more than 2,667 IU of vitamin A daily because of the risk of birth defects; 5,000 IU per day is a reasonable upper limit for other individuals. Look at the bottle label to determine how much vitamin A you are receiving. (It is less likely that you will get enough vitamin D to produce toxic effects.)

Magnesium

Preliminary studies suggest that magnesium supplementation may be helpful for dysmenorrhea. A 6-month double-blind placebo-controlled study of 50 women with menstrual pain found that treatment with magnesium significantly improved symptoms.[8] The researchers reported evidence of reduced levels of prostaglandin F_2 alpha, a hormone-like substance involved in pain and inflammation.

Similarly positive results were seen in a double-blind placebo-controlled study of 21 women.[9]

A typical dosage is 250 to 600 mg daily throughout the cycle, or 500 to 1,000 mg for 3 to 5 days prior to the onset of cramps. Some practitioners believe that magnesium works best when combined with vitamin B_6. For a more detailed discussion about other uses and safety issues, see the chapter on **magnesium.**

OTHER PROPOSED TREATMENTS

The herb cramp bark has traditionally been used to relieve menstrual pain. Unfortunately, it has not received any significant scientific attention.

Herbs with possible anti-inflammatory properties may be helpful as well, including **bromelain** (see page 229), **turmeric** (see page 425), and **white willow** (see page 457). Other potentially helpful treatments include **black cohosh** (see page 223), *Coleus forskohlii* (see page 259), **dong quai** (see page 272), and **manganese** (see page 354).

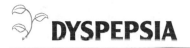

DYSPEPSIA

Related Terms   Gas, Indigestion

Principal Proposed Treatments   There are no well-established natural treatments for dyspepsia.

Other Proposed Treatments   Turmeric, Artichoke Leaf, Boldo, Carminative Herbs, Banana Powder, Chamomile, Valerian, Lemon Balm

Dyspepsia is a catchall term that includes a variety of digestive problems such as stomach discomfort, gas, bloating, belching, appetite loss, and nausea. Although many serious medical conditions can cause digestive distress, the term "dyspepsia" is most often used when no identifiable medical cause can be detected. In this way, dyspepsia is like a stomach version of the symptoms in the intestines and colon called **irritable bowel syndrome** (see page 108).

The standard medical approach to dyspepsia involves looking for a treatable cause and addressing it if one can be identified. Failing that, various treatments are often suggested on a trial-and-error basis, including medications that reduce stomach acid as well as those that decrease spasm in the digestive tract. The drugs cisapride (Propulsid) and metoclopramide (Reglan) increase stomach emptying, and have also been tried for dyspepsia. However, cisapride has been taken off the market, and metoclopramide causes many side effects.

It's thought that stress plays a role in dyspepsia, as it does with irritable bowel syndrome. Interestingly, one study of 30 people with dyspepsia found that after 8 weeks of treatment with placebo, 80% reported their symptoms

had improved.[1] This unusually high placebo response emphasizes the emotional aspect of this condition.

PROPOSED TREATMENTS

In Europe, dyspepsia is commonly attributed to inadequate bile flow from the gallbladder. However, there is little real proof that gallbladder dysfunction is truly the cause of dyspepsia; people who have had their gallbladders removed aren't particularly prone to digestive distress. Nevertheless, many herbal remedies that stimulate gallbladder function are recommended for dyspepsia, and some may be effective.

Herbs that stimulate the passing of gas (carminative herbs) might also help.

Turmeric

The spice **turmeric** (see page 425) contains a substance, curcumin, that stimulates gallbladder contractions.[2,3] There is some evidence that curcumin might be effective for dyspepsia.

A double-blind placebo-controlled study including 106 people compared the effects of 500 mg of curcumin

4 times daily against placebo (as well as against a locally popular over the counter treatment). After 7 days, 87% percent of the curcumin group experienced full or partial symptom relief from dyspepsia as compared to 53% of the placebo group.[4]

Turmeric is on the FDA's GRAS (generally recognized as safe) list, and curcumin, too, is believed to be nontoxic.[5,6]

Reported side effects of turmeric or curcumin are rare and are generally limited to mild stomach distress. However, safety in young children, pregnant or nursing women, or people with severe liver or kidney disease has not been established.

Note: Due to curcumin's effects on the gallbladder, individuals with gallbladder disease should use curcumin only on the advice of a physician.

Combination Herbal Treatments

Other herbs beside turmeric are thought to stimulate the gallbladder, including **artichoke leaf** (see page 210), **boldo** (see page 226), and celandine. Combinations of these herbs are frequently used in Germany for the treatment of dyspepsia.

A double-blind trial of 60 individuals given either an artichoke leaf/boldo/celandine combination or placebo found improvements in symptoms of indigestion after 14 days of treatment.[7] Similarly positive effects were seen in a double-blind trial of 76 individuals given a combination treatment containing turmeric and celandine.[8] However, reports have raised concerns that celandine can damage the liver.[9,10,11]

Carminative Herbs

Various carminative (gas-relieving) herbs have traditionally been used to relieve indigestion, especially when indigestion is accompanied by excessive gas. Typical carminatives include caraway, **chamomile** (see page 244), dill, fennel, **peppermint** (see page 384), spearmint, and turmeric.

Of the many carminatives that are sometimes recommended, peppermint and caraway are the only ones with any real evidence behind them; but even this is highly preliminary.

A double-blind placebo-controlled study including 39 individuals found that an enteric-coated peppermint-caraway oil combination taken 3 times daily for 4 weeks significantly reduced dyspepsia pain as compared to placebo.[12] Of the treatment group, 63.2% was pain free after 4 weeks, compared to 25% of the placebo group.

Results from a double-blind comparative study including 118 individuals suggest that the combination of peppermint and caraway oil is comparably effective to the no-longer-available drug cisapride.[13] After 4 weeks, the herbal combination reduced dyspepsia pain by 69.7%, whereas the conventional treatment reduced pain by 70.2%.

A preparation of peppermint, caraway, fennel, and wormwood oils was compared to metoclopramide in another double-blind study enrolling 60 individuals.[14] After 7 days, 43.3% of the treatment group was pain free compared to 13.3% of the metoclopramide group.

Note: Essential oils of herbs can present health risks. In particular, wormwood is dangerous when taken long term. Physician supervision is recommended.

Other Herbs and Supplements

A controlled (but not blinded) study of 46 people suggests that banana powder, a traditional Indian food, may help treat dyspepsia. After 8 weeks of treatment, 75% of the people taking banana powder reported complete or partial symptom relief compared to 20% of those who received no treatment.[15]

Herbs with a reputation for relaxing a nervous stomach, such as **chamomile** (see page 244), **valerian** (see page 428), and **lemon balm** (see page 359), are also sometimes recommended for dyspepsia. Numerous other herbs that have been recommended for dyspepsia include angelica root, anise seed, bitter orange peel, blessed thistle, cardamom, centaury, chicory, **dandelion** (see page 266) root, **cinnamon** (see page 254), cloves, coriander, **devil's claw** (see page 267), dill, **gentian** (see page 296), **ginger** (see page 296), horehound, **juniper** (see page 337), **milk thistle** (see page 361), radish, rosemary, sage, **St. John's wort** (see page 414), star anise, and **yarrow** (see page 460).

Digestive enzymes (see page 393) are often recommended for indigestion; however, one placebo-controlled crossover study enrolling 37 individuals found no significant difference between the effects of enzymes and placebo on dyspepsia symptoms.[16]

Capsaicin, the active ingredient in **cayenne** (see page 243) pepper, is sometimes recommended for indigestion; however, results from a small crossover placebo-controlled study of 11 individuals suggest that 5 mg capsaicin taken before a high-fat meal did not affect gastric function or dyspepsia symptoms.[17]

A tea made from the "fruits" or seeds of **parsley** (see page 381) is a traditional remedy for colic, indigestion, and intestinal gas.[18,19]

EAR INFECTIONS

Related Terms   Middle Ear Infection, Otitis Media

Principal Proposed Treatments   Xylitol, Breast-Feeding, Avoiding Passive Smoke Inhalation

Other Proposed Treatments   Food Allergen Elimination, Echinacea, Zinc, Vitamin C, Andrographis, Arginine, Ginseng, Thymus Extract

Acute otitis media (AOM) is a painful infection of the middle ear, the portion of the ear behind the eardrum. (Another form of ear infection, otitis externa or swimmer's ear, is entirely different, and is not covered here.) AOM often follows a cold, sore throat, or other respiratory illness. Although it can affect adults, this occurs primarily in infants and young children. It's estimated that by age 7, up to 95% of all U.S. children will have experienced at least one bout of AOM—it's the most common reason parents take a child to the doctor.

When the Eustachian tube connecting the upper part of the throat to the middle ear is blocked by a cold's mucus and swelling, fluids pool behind the eardrum, providing an ideal place for bacteria to grow; an infection may set in, generating even more fluid. The pressure this exerts on the eardrum can be intensely painful. The eardrum turns red and bulges. Children too young to explain their discomfort cry, fuss, and pull at their ears. They might also appear unresponsive because they can't hear well—fluid buildup in the middle ear prevents the eardrum and small bones in the ear from moving, causing temporary hearing loss.

Most hearing loss associated with AOM ends when the infection is treated. However, recurring ear infections and their accompanying short-term hearing losses may affect a child's speech and language development. In addition, a complication called secretory otitis media (fluid build-up in the middle ear) may develop and cause continuous hearing loss for months. Other possible complications of AOM include mastoiditis (an infection of the bone behind the ear) and, occasionally, spinal meningitis.

Without treatment, most middle ear infections resolve on their own, often through a harmless rupture of the eardrum.[1] In the Netherlands, pediatricians take a conservative approach, generally waiting 24 to 72 hours until they are certain an ear infection warrants antibiotics.[2]

However, U.S. doctors tend to initiate treatment early. This practice has been criticized on several grounds. First, antibiotic treatment has not been found effective in preventing complications such as serous otitis[3] or pneumococcal meningitis.[4]

In addition, antibiotic treatment does not even appear to help AOM itself very much. For example, a double-blind placebo-controlled trial of 240 children ages 6 months to 2 years found so little benefit with antibiotic treatment that the authors recommended physician-supervised watchful waiting rather than immediate treatment.[5] In other published reviews, the benefits of antibiotics for AOM have also been found less than impressive. A review of 33 randomized trials involving 5,400 children concluded that antibiotics modestly improved the rate of recovery.[6] An evaluation of six randomized, controlled studies concluded that early antibiotic use had only slight benefit, reducing pain and fever in a small percentage of children and helping to prevent the development of infection in the other ear, but not significantly speeding up recovery of hearing.[7] Finally, children with recurrent ear infections do not appear to benefit from preventive antibiotic treatment.[8]

However, another criticism, that early antibiotic treatment causes an increased rate of ear infection recurrence, does not appear to be correct.[9]

Note: Despite the issues raised above, simply withholding antibiotic treatment can be dangerous. Any child who appears to have an ear infection should be seen by a physician.

When ear infections do reoccur frequently, a physician may insert a tube into the infected ear to drain fluids and relieve pressure, a procedure called tympanostomy. Nearly 1 million U.S. children undergo this procedure each year; however, its usefulness is somewhat controversial.[10,11,12]

PRINCIPAL PROPOSED TREATMENTS

Although there is as yet no natural treatment for AOM, there are several promising approaches parents can take which may help prevent children from developing ear infections.

Xylitol

A natural sugar found in plums, strawberries, and raspberries, xylitol is used as a sweetener in some "sugarless" gums and candies. One of its advantages is that it inhibits the growth of *Streptococcus mutans*, a type of bacteria that causes dental cavities.[13] Xylitol also inhibits the growth of a related bacteria species, *Streptococcus pneumoniae*, implicated in ear infections.[14] Additionally, xylitol acts against *Haemophilus influenza*, another bacteria that frequently causes ear infections.[15]

Visit Us at TNP.com

Based on this evidence, xylitol has been tried as a preventive treatment for middle ear infections with some success. Two well-designed studies enrolling a total of 1,163 children found that chewing gum and syrup sweetened with xylitol helped prevent middle ear infections and decreased the need for antibiotics. Although xylitol clearly did not absolutely prevent ear infections, it significantly decreased the rate at which they occurred.

A large double-blind placebo-controlled trial of 857 children investigated how well xylitol (in chewing gum, syrup, and lozenges) could prevent AOM.[16] The gum was most effective, reducing the risk of developing AOM by a full 40%. Xylitol syrup was also effective, but less so. The lozenges weren't effective: researchers speculated that children got tired of sucking on the large candies and didn't get the proper dose of xylitol. (In addition, the children were able to distinguish between the xylitol and placebo lozenges by taste, making that portion of the study single blind.)

Similarly positive results had been seen in an earlier double-blind study by the same researchers, evaluating about 300 children.[17]

Dosage

In the studies described above, children given xylitol-sweetened gum received 8.4 g of xylitol daily. Those who took syrup received 10 g daily. Xylitol is believed to be safe, but high dosages can cause stomach discomfort and possibly diarrhea.

Breast-Feeding

Breast-feeding may help prevent AOM. Numerous studies tracking ear infection frequency in large groups of infants found that the infants breast-fed exclusively had significantly fewer middle ear infections than those fed formula.[18,19,20] Such observational studies aren't as reliable as placebo-controlled or double-blind designs, but the results do suggest that breast-feeding is a good preventive measure.

Researchers aren't sure how breast milk protects infants from ear infections. Studies attempting to determine if breast milk inhibits bacteria associated with AOM have had mixed results.[21,22]

Avoidance of Cigarette Smoke

Environmental conditions may predispose a child to middle ear infections. A study of 132 daycare students found that the 45 children exposed to cigarette smoke at home had a 38% higher risk of middle ear infections than the 87 children whose parents didn't smoke.[23]

OTHER PROPOSED TREATMENTS
Allergies

Allergies (see page 2) may contribute to ear infections, possibly by increasing the amount of fluid in the middle ear. There is some evidence that children allergic to pollens, dust, molds, and **foods** (see page 82) may be more likely to develop AOM.[24,25,26] Weak evidence suggests that a food allergen elimination diet might help prevent middle ear infections.[27,28]

Other Herbs and Supplements

Numerous herbs and supplements have been proposed for preventing or treating ear infections. These include all herbs and supplements used for **colds** (see page 47), including **echinacea** (see page 273), **zinc** (see page 463), **vitamin C** (see page 444), **andrographis** (see page 205), **arginine** (see page 208), **thymus extract** (see page 422), and **ginseng** (see page 301). There is no evidence as yet that they work for AOM, but it is certainly logical to think they might.

EASY BRUISING

Related Terms   Contusions, Hematomas, Ecchymoses, Bruising

Principal Proposed Treatments   Citrus Bioflavonoids, OPCs (Oligomeric Proanthocyanidins), Bilberry, Vitamin C, Trypsin and Chymotrypsin, Escin (Topical)

Other Proposed Treatments   Bromelain, Comfrey (Topical), Arnica (Topical), Sweet Clover (Topical)

Bruising and bleeding both occur because of damage to blood vessels. When a vein, artery, or capillary is torn or cut, blood flows out into the vessel's surroundings; if the escaped blood is contained within the tissues directly under the skin, we see a bruise.

While all of us bruise from time to time, some people bruise particularly easily. A number of factors, besides being accident-prone, can make this occur.

One factor contributing to easy bruising is thinning skin, caused by aging or by medications such as corticosteroids. Easy bruising can also be due to fragile blood vessel walls. Finally, difficulties with blood clotting, including problems with platelets or clotting factors, can also increase bruising. For this reason, strong blood-thinning drugs such as heparin and warfarin (Coumadin) can lead to excessive bruising. **Warning**: if you're taking these or other anticoagulant drugs and notice increased bruising, contact your doctor, as this situation could be dangerous.

Aspirin or even natural remedies such as high-dose **vitamin E** (see page 451), **ginkgo** (see page 298), and **garlic** (see page 291) may also thin the blood, possibly raising the risk of bruising and other bleeding problems; and if you combine two blood-thinning substances, these effects might multiply. Rarely, severe bruising from minor or unnoticed injuries can be a sign of leukemia or another serious health problem. Especially if this is a new development, discuss your symptoms with a doctor.

However, in most cases, there is no identifiable medical cause for easy bruising, and no conventional treatment. Furthermore, once you have a bruise, there is no conventional therapy to help speed its resolution.

PRINCIPAL PROPOSED TREATMENTS

A number of natural substances might be helpful for easy bruising, including citrus bioflavonoids, the related substances OPCs and bilberry, and vitamin C. In addition, if you already are bruised, you may found some help with a combination of two proteolytic enzymes, trypsin and chymotrypsin or a topical preparation of escin (an extract of horse chestnut).

Citrus Bioflavonoids and Related Substances

Bioflavonoids (or flavonoids) are plant substances that bring color to many fruits and vegetables. Citrus fruits are a rich source of bioflavonoids, including diosmin, hesperidin, rutin, and naringen; studies have found that bioflavonoids contained in citrus fruits can help decrease bruising. Two types of natural compounds related to bioflavonoids, **OPCs** (oligomeric proanthocyanidins; see page 373) and anthocyanosides, may also be able to decrease bruising.

What Is the Scientific Evidence for Citrus Bioflavonoids?

A double-blind study of 96 people with fragile capillaries found that a combination of the bioflavonoids diosmin and hesperidin decreased the tendency to bruise.[1] Participants took 2 tablets daily of these bioflavonoids or placebo for 6 weeks, while researchers used a suction cup to measure their capillaries' tendency to rupture and also looked for spontaneous bruising and other symptoms of fragile capillaries. Those individuals who received bioflavonoids had significantly greater improvements in both capillary strength and symptoms compared to those taking placebo.

Two rather poorly designed studies from the 1960s found benefits with a combination of vitamin C and citrus bioflavonoids for decreasing bruising in collegiate athletes. In a single-blind study of 27 wrestlers, 71% of those taking placebo were injured, with bruises making up more than half their injuries; in contrast, only 38% of those taking the supplement were injured, none of whom sustained bruises.[2] In a follow-up double-blind study of 40 football players, the treated group received fewer severe bruises than the group taking placebo.[3]

Test tube studies have found that OPCs protect collagen, partly by inhibiting an enzyme that breaks it down.[4] One rather poorly designed double-blind study of 37 people—most of whom had fragile capillaries—found that OPCs were more effective than placebo in decreasing capillary fragility[5]; however, the authors of this study left many questions unanswered in their report, making it hard to determine how seriously to take their results.

Anthocyanosides, which are present in high concentrations in **bilberry** (see page 220), may also strengthen capillaries through their effects on collagen. Some European physicians believe that these vessel-stabilizing properties make bilberry useful as a treatment for easy bruising, but the evidence as yet is only suggestive.

Dosage

A typical dosage of citrus bioflavonoids is 500 mg twice daily.

The double-blind study of OPCs used a 100-mg dose daily for 15 days, although the authors felt some people would do better with 150 mg per day.[6]

For bilberry, the standard dosage is 120 to 240 mg twice daily of an extract standardized to contain 25% anthocyanosides.

Safety Issues

Citrus bioflavonoids, as well as OPCs and bilberry, appear to be quite safe. In the study of people taking diosmin and hesperidin, the treatment caused no more side effects than placebo.[7] However, bioflavonoids may have some anticoagulant properties when taken in high doses, and therefore should be used only under medical supervision by individuals on blood-thinning drugs such as Coumadin (warfarin) and heparin. Although safety in pregnancy is not assured, citrus bioflavonoids and bilberry have been studied in pregnant women with no apparent harm.[8,9] Safety in nursing women or individuals with severe liver or kidney disease has not been established, although there are no known risks in these groups.

Vitamin C

Vitamin C (see page 444) is essential for healthy collagen; severe vitamin C deficiency, called scurvy, can lead to easy bruising. Fortunately, scurvy is extremely rare in Western countries today—but marginal vitamin C deficiency is not rare, and might lead to increased risk of bruising.

A 2-month double-blind study of 94 elderly people with marginal vitamin C deficiency found that vitamin C supplements decreased their tendency to bruise.[10]

If your diet is low in fresh fruits and vegetables, you may wish to supplement it with vitamin C. In the study mentioned above, bruising in elderly people decreased significantly with 1 g of oral vitamin C given daily for 2 months.

This dosage of vitamin C should be safe for most people. However, regular use of vitamin C in this dosage range might cause **copper** (see page 262) deficiency and excessive **iron** (see page 333) absorption. Furthermore, people with a history of kidney stones and those with kidney failure who have a defect in metabolizing vitamin C or oxalate should probably restrict vitamin C intake to approximately 100 mg daily, because higher doses may increase their risk of developing stones. People who have glucose-6-phosphate dehydrogenase deficiency, iron overload, kidney failure, or a history of intestinal surgery should also avoid high-dose vitamin C.

The maximum safe dosages of vitamin C for individuals with severe liver or kidney disease have not been determined.

Trypsin and Chymotrypsin

Trypsin and chymotrypsin, naturally produced in the body to help digest protein, are often called **proteolytic enzymes** (see page 393). (Bromelain, discussed below, is a proteolytic enzyme from a plant source.) It is theorized that trypsin and chymotrypsin reduce swelling by breaking down protein fibers that trap fluids in the tissues after an injury, thereby restoring normal circulation in the area.[11] Three small double-blind studies, involving a total of about 80 athletes, found that treatment with proteolytic enzymes significantly speeded healing of bruises and other mild athletic injuries as compared to placebo.[12,13,14]

Unfortunately, it is almost impossible to define a "typical" dose of trypsin and chymotrypsin in treating bruising because different products use different systems for measuring potency, and many studies used forms of these supplements that are no longer on the market. The best approach is to follow the recommended dose on the bottle. Unless you're taking proteolytic enzymes specifically as a digestive aid, it's important to take them on an empty stomach, preferably 30 to 60 minutes before a meal; otherwise, a considerable amount of their activity will simply be taken up in digesting your food.[15]

Proteolytic enzymes are believed to be quite safe. However, if you have ulcers, you should probably avoid them.

Escin

An extract of **horse chestnut** (see page 325) called escin may also help with bruising. Horse chestnut has been traditionally used to treat varicose veins and other problems involving blood vessels and swelling. One double-blind study of 70 people found that about 10 g of 2% escin gel, applied externally to bruises in a single dose 5 minutes after they were induced, reduced bruise tenderness.[16]

No side effects were reported in the study just described. Although some safety concerns have been noted with whole horse chestnut, properly prepared horse chestnut products appear to be quite safe.[17] The safety of topical escin for pregnant women, young children, or those with severe liver or kidney disease has not been established.

OTHER PROPOSED TREATMENTS

Bromelain

Like trypsin and chymotrypsin, bromelain is thought to decrease bruising by breaking down proteins that trap fluids in the tissues after an injury,[18] and it is sometimes used in Europe to speed recovery from injuries. However, better-quality studies are needed before bromelain can be said to be effective.

In one controlled study, 74 boxers with bruises on their faces and upper bodies were given bromelain until all signs of bruising had disappeared;[19] another 72 boxers were given placebo. Fifty-eight of the group taking bromelain had lost all signs of bruising within 4 days, compared to only 10 taking placebo. Unfortunately, this study was apparently not double-blind, meaning that some of its results may have been due to the power of suggestion.

Another study—this one without any type of control group—found that bromelain reduced swelling, pain at rest, and tenderness among 59 patients with blunt injuries, including bruising.[20]

As is the case with other proteolytic enzymes, it is not possible to give a single recommended dose for bromelain because different manufacturers use different methods to describe their products' strength. Be aware that bromelain, like ginkgo and garlic, may thin the blood, and should be avoided by people who have clotting problems or take other blood-thinning medications. Refer to the **bromelain** chapter for dosage and additional safety information.

Easy Bruising

Visit Us at TNP.com

Other Herbs Used for Bruising

The herbs comfrey, arnica, and sweet clover are widely used externally on bruises and other minor injuries, but despite this traditional use, there is no real scientific evidence that they work. A homeopathic preparation of arnica, quite distinct from the herb arnica, is also popular for treating bruises.

Note: There are various safety concerns involved in using comfrey, arnica, and sweet clover internally. For the treatment of bruising, they are used as topical ointments and salves.

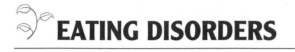

EATING DISORDERS

Related Terms   Bulimia Nervosa, Anorexia Nervosa, Binge Eating Disorder

Principal Proposed Treatments   There are no well-established natural treatments for eating disorders.

Other Proposed Treatments   Zinc, 5-Hydroxytryptophan, St. John's Wort

There are three types of eating disorders: anorexia nervosa, bulimia nervosa, and binge eating disorder. Anorexia nervosa involves compulsive dieting and exercise to reduce weight, leading to dangerous weight loss and, in women, the absence of menstrual periods. Bulimia nervosa is characterized by binge eating followed by purging. The recently identified binge eating disorder is marked by binge eating that isn't followed by purging.

Nearly all the people affected by eating disorders are teen girls and young adult women from the middle and upper socioeconomic classes. The causes of the various disorders aren't known, but it seems indisputable that the current Western emphasis on slimness as a mark of feminine attractiveness contributes greatly.

Because severe anorexia can be life threatening, treatment generally combines a weight-gain program with psychotherapy and, sometimes, antidepressant drugs. Bulimia nervosa and binge eating disorder are both treated with psychotherapy, antidepressants, or appetite suppressants to help control binge eating.

PROPOSED TREATMENTS

While there are no well-established natural treatments for eating disorders, there is some evidence that zinc supplements, when used in conjunction with conventional medical treatments, may help individuals with anorexia to gain weight. Preliminary attempts to treat bulimia by altering serotonin levels are also promising.

Zinc

The relationship between anorexia nervosa and **zinc** (see page 463) deficiency is controversial and the subject of many studies.

Symptoms of zinc deficiency (weight loss, appetite loss, and behavior changes) resemble those of anorexia nervosa to some extent. This has led some researchers to theorize that low zinc levels may be related to the onset of the eating disorder.[1,2]

Several studies have indeed found a correlation between zinc deficiency and anorexia nervosa.[3,4,5] However, it is quite likely that rather than zinc deficiency causing anorexia, the extreme diet of people with anorexia probably causes the zinc deficiency.[6,7,8]

It is possible that zinc deficiency might aggravate symptoms of anorexia by causing weight loss and behavior changes.[9,10,11] However, some evidence contradicts this idea.[12,13]

Once an individual does have anorexia, however, zinc supplements may be helpful. A double-blind placebo-controlled trial of 35 individuals with anorexia found that zinc supplementation enhanced weight recovery.[14,15] However, a smaller double-blind placebo-controlled study found no significant difference between the effects of zinc and placebo on weight gain.[16]

Perhaps, rather than simply supplementing with zinc, a general multivitamin/mineral supplement is a better option to offset the malnutrition that goes along with anorexia.

Other Treatments

Animal and human studies suggest that when levels of the brain chemical serotonin rise, hunger decreases. Individuals who engage in binge eating may have a different response to changes in serotonin levels.[17] In an attempt to change binge eating behavior, some researchers have tried to alter serotonin levels.

Standard antidepressant drugs are most often used for this purpose. However, it might be possible to achieve similar results with tryptophan and related supplements.

The body uses the amino acid L-tryptophan to make serotonin. Preliminary evidence from a small double-blind placebo-controlled study suggests that a combination of L-tryptophan and vitamin B_6 significantly reduced binge eating among individuals with bulimia.[18] This evidence, however, is contradicted by results of another small study that found no significant difference between the effects of L-tryptophan and placebo on binge eating.[19]

Note: L-tryptophan is no longer sold as a supplement due to safety concerns. **5-Hydroxytryptophan** (5-HTP; see page 198) might be a safer option; however, it has not been studied in eating disorders.

The antidepressant herb **St. John's wort** (see page 414) might also raise serotonin levels.

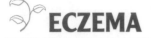

ECZEMA

Principal Proposed Treatments   Evening Primrose Oil (GLA)

Other Proposed Treatments
Topical Herbal Creams: Calendula, Chamomile, Licorice
Burdock, Red Clover, Zinc, *Coleus forskohlii,* Quercetin

Eczema is an allergic reaction shown in the skin. It consists mainly of itchy, inflamed patches on the face, elbows, knees, and wrists. Eczema is most commonly found in infants and young children, and many children with eczema also develop hay fever and asthma.

Medical treatment for eczema consists mainly of topical steroid creams.

PRINCIPAL PROPOSED TREATMENTS

Evening primrose oil, a source of the essential fatty acid **GLA** (gamma-linolenic acid; see page 304), is widely used in Europe for eczema; however, the evidence that it really works is mixed, and more recent studies have not found it to be effective.

Evening Primrose Oil: Standard Treatment for Eczema in Europe

A review of all studies reported up to 1989 found that evening primrose oil frequently reduced the symptoms of eczema after several months of use, with the greatest improvement noticeable in the level of itching.[1] However, this review has been sharply criticized for including poorly designed studies and possibly misinterpreting study results.[2]

A recent, properly designed, double-blind study that followed 58 children with eczema for 16 weeks found no difference between the treated and placebo groups.[3] A 24-week double-blind study of 160 adults with eczema, who were given either placebo or GLA from borage oil, also found no benefit.[4] In addition, negative results were also seen in a 16-week double-blind placebo-controlled study of 102 individuals with eczema.[5] Another double-blind trial followed 39 people with hand dermatitis for 24 weeks. Evening primrose oil at a dosage of 6 g daily produced no significant improvement as compared to placebo.[6]

One recent double-blind trial did find a therapeutic benefit with evening primrose oil, but not for itching.[7]

This information is a bit confusing, and at the present time it isn't clear whether evening primrose oil is effective for treating eczema.

The typical dosage of evening primrose oil is 2 to 4 g daily, taken with food. Full results are said to take over 6 months to develop. Combinations of fish oil and evening primrose oil may be more effective. See the chapter on **GLA** for further details.

OTHER PROPOSED TREATMENTS

The following natural treatments are widely recommended for eczema, but they have not been scientifically proven effective at this time.

Topical Herbal Creams

Topical creams made from **chamomile** (see page 244), **licorice** (see page 344), or **calendula** (see page 237), alone or in combination, are also widely used in Europe to treat eczema. One double-blind study of 161 individuals found chamomile cream equally effective as 0.25% hydrocortisone cream for the treatment of eczema.[8] However, the report didn't state whether doctors or patients were blinded as to which treatment was which, so it isn't clear how reliable the results may be.

Another double-blind placebo-controlled trial by the same authors, involving 72 individuals with eczema, found somewhat odd results: In this trial, chamomile was not significantly more effective than placebo, but both were better than 0.5% hydrocortisone cream.[9] It is difficult to interpret what these results actually mean, but they certainly cannot be taken as proof that chamomile cream is effective.

Burdock and Red Clover

The herbs **burdock** and **red clover** are traditionally drunk as tea to treat eczema. For more information on these herbs, see the corresponding chapters.

Zinc

Zinc (see page 463) supplementation is said to be effective for eczema in some children. The usual dosage is 10 mg of zinc picolinate daily in children under 10, balanced with 1 mg of **copper** (see page 262). For older individuals, the dosage is 15 to 30 mg taken daily, balanced with 1 to 3 mg of copper daily. Too much zinc can be toxic, so dosages should not exceed 30 mg daily.

Other Treatments

The herb *Coleus forskohlii* (see page 259) and the supplement **quercetin** (see page 396) have also been recommended for eczema, but there is as yet little evidence that they really work.

In some individuals, eczema may be related to **food allergies** (see page 82) or sensitivities.[10]

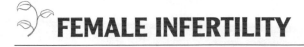

FEMALE INFERTILITY

Principal Proposed Treatments   There are no well-established natural treatments for female infertility.

Other Proposed Treatments   Chasteberry, Multivitamins, Reducing Stress, Ashwagandha, Beta-Carotene, Calcium, Vitamin D

There are many possible causes of female infertility. Tubal disease and endometriosis (a condition in which uterine tissue begins to grow where it shouldn't) account for 50% of female infertility; failure of ovulation is the cause of about 30%; and cervical factors cause another 10%.

An immense industry has sprung up around correcting female infertility, using techniques that range from hormone therapy to in vitro (test-tube) babies. Although these methods have their occasional stunning successes, there is considerable controversy about the high cost and low rate of effectiveness of fertility treatments in general. The good news is that apparently infertile women often eventually become pregnant with no medical intervention at all.

PROPOSED TREATMENTS

The following natural treatments are widely recommended for female infertility, but they have not been scientifically proven effective at this time.

Chasteberry

Because of its effects on the hormone prolactin, the herb chasteberry has been tried as a fertility treatment.[1] However, the only properly designed study of this potential use was too small to return conclusive results.[2]

The typical dose of chasteberry extract is 20 to 40 mg given once a day. Chasteberry is sold often as a liquid extract to be taken at a dosage of 40 drops each morning. However, highly concentrated extracts are also available that require much lower dosing. Chasteberry's safety has not been adequately evaluated. (See the chapter on **chasteberry** for a further discussion of uses and safety issues involving this herb.)

Multivitamins

According to one study, general supplementation with multivitamins may improve female fertility.[3]

Other Treatments

Stress may lead to infertility, and treatments for reducing **stress** (see page 167) might help increase fertility.[4–8]

Other treatments sometimes recommended include **ashwagandha** (see page 212) and **beta-carotene** (see page 217), but there is as yet little real evidence that they work.

One cause of infertility in women is named polycystic ovary syndrome. According to a preliminary study, supplementation with **vitamin D** (see page 449) and **calcium** (see page 234) may be helpful for women with this condition.[9]

Caffeine avoidance has also been recommended for improving fertility, but it has not been shown effective at this time.[10]

FIBROMYALGIA

Related Terms   Fibrositis

Principal Proposed Treatments   SAMe (S-Adenosylmethionine), 5-HTP (5-Hydroxytryptophan), Capsaicin

Other Proposed Treatments   Malic Acid Plus Magnesium, Vitamin B_1, Vitamin E, Selenium, Spirulina

Fibromyalgia is a common chronic condition whose main symptoms are specific tender points on various parts of the body, widespread musculoskeletal discomfort, morning stiffness, fatigue, and disturbed sleep. The cause of the condition is unknown, but it occurs most often in women aged 30 to 50. Other symptoms commonly believed to be associated with fibromyalgia are irritable bowel syndrome, urinary frequency, anxiety, headache, and numbness or tingling.

Apart from tender points on the body, physical exams and lab tests for people with fibromyalgia are usually normal. Because of this, some physicians are inclined to believe that the condition is "all in the patient's head." One researcher has noted that many of the symptoms of fibromyalgia, including certain tender points, are common in the general population, and goes so far as to question whether it is a real condition.[1]

However, the general consensus is that fibromyalgia is real, and the American College of Rheumatologists has given it an official medical definition. It involves the presence of widespread chronic pain and the existence of pain in at least 11 of 18 specific points on the body when pressure is applied. Although the cause of fibromyalgia is not known, it may be related to poor sleeping with incomplete muscular relaxation.

Conventional treatment for fibromyalgia may include antidepressants (particularly those that help induce sleep), anti-inflammatory drugs, muscle relaxants, sleeping pills, and antianxiety medications.

Low-dose antidepressants have been shown to help chronic pain from many causes,[2] and have been found to be effective in reducing fibromyalgia symptoms, even when given in doses too low to treat depression.[3] It may be that antidepressants work for fibromyalgia by improving sleep.

Aerobic exercise may also be helpful for individuals with fibromyalgia.[4]

PRINCIPAL PROPOSED TREATMENTS

There are three natural treatments that might be helpful for fibromyalgia, although the evidence is not yet strong: SAMe (pronounced "sam-ee"), 5-HTP, and capsaicin.

SAMe

SAMe (see page 403), short for S-adenosylmethionine, is a chemical derived from a combination of the amino acid methionine and the main molecule for energy in the body, adenosine triphosphate (ATP). More well known as a treatment for depression and also osteoarthritis, preliminary research suggests that it may be helpful for fibromyalgia as well.

What Is the Scientific Evidence for SAMe?

Four double-blind trials have studied the use of SAMe for fibromyalgia,[5–8] three of them finding it to be helpful. Unfortunately, most of these studies gave SAMe either intravenously or as an injection into the muscles, sometimes in combination with oral doses. When you inject a medication, the effects can be quite different than when you take it orally. For that reason, these studies are of questionable relevance.

However, the one double-blind study that used only oral SAMe did find positive results.[9] In this trial, 44 people with fibromyalgia took 800 mg of SAMe or placebo for 6 weeks. Compared to the group taking placebo, those taking SAMe had improvements in disease activity, pain at rest, fatigue, and morning stiffness, and in one measurement of mood. In other respects, such as the amount of tenderness in their tender points, the group taking SAMe did no better than those taking the placebo.

It isn't clear whether SAMe is helping fibromyalgia through antidepressant effects or some other mechanism.

Dosage

In the double-blind study of oral SAMe, people took 400 mg twice a day—a regimen that can cost upward of $100 a month.

Safety Issues

SAMe appears to be quite safe, according to both human and animal studies. The most common side effect is mild digestive distress. Like other substances with antidepressant activity, SAMe might trigger a manic episode in those with bipolar disease (manic-depression). Its safety in young children, pregnant or nursing women, or those with severe liver or kidney disease has not been established. There may be some risks involved in combining SAMe with standard antidepressants; it also should not be combined with the drug levodopa, used for Parkinson's disease. Consult your doctor before doing so.

5-HTP

5-HTP (see page 198), short for 5-hydroxytryptophan, is most commonly used as a treatment for depression. It is thought to work by increasing the amount of serotonin in the brain. However, evidence that it helps fibromyalgia is still preliminary.

What Is the Scientific Evidence for 5-HTP?

One double-blind study of 50 people with fibromyalgia found that those taking 300 mg of 5-HTP for 30 days reported significant decreases in the number of tender points and the amount of pain they experienced, compared to those taking placebo.[10] They also noted improvements in sleep patterns, morning stiffness, anxiety, and fatigue. Interestingly, the people taking placebo also noted significant improvements in pain and sleep, although less marked than those experienced with 5-HTP. More studies are needed to determine how much 5-HTP really helps.

Dosage

A typical dosage of 5-HTP is 100 or 200 mg three times daily. Once 5-HTP begins to work, it may be possible to reduce the dosage significantly and still maintain good results.

Safety Issues

No significant adverse effects have been reported in clinical studies of 5-HTP. Side effects appear to be limited to occasional mild digestive distress and possible allergic reactions. However, there is a potentially serious concern noted by the FDA: Some batches of 5-HTP have been found to contain a substance that was linked to an untreatable blood disorder among people taking a different supplement, tryptophan. At this time, there is no other information from the FDA regarding specific cautions on using 5-HTP, but you should pay close attention to reports that may follow up on this finding.

Safety in young children, pregnant or nursing women, and those with liver or kidney disease has not been established.

If you are taking prescription antidepressants, do not take 5-HTP in addition except on a physician's advice. There is a chance you might raise serotonin levels too high. Similar risks may occur with other medications that raise serotonin levels, such as tramadol (Ultram), sumatriptan, and zolpidem (Ambien). Also, taking 5-HTP at the same time as the Parkinson's disease medication carbidopa might cause skin changes similar to those that develop in the disease scleroderma.[11,12,13]

Capsaicin

Capsaicin (see page 243), the "hot" in hot chili peppers, is widely used as a treatment for various painful conditions, such as shingles and arthritis. One double-blind study of 45 people found that it may be beneficial for fibromyalgia as well.[14] In this study, participants used either the capsaicin cream or a placebo four times a day for four weeks, rubbing it into the tender points on one side of their body. Those who used the real treatment reported less tenderness in their tender points than those using the placebo. Interestingly, the points on their untreated sides were also less tender. There was no difference between those using capsaicin or placebo in the amount of overall pain or sleep quality. It must be noted, however, that it's hard to believe the study was really double blind, since it's impossible to hide the burning sensation caused by capsaicin!

Dosage

Capsaicin-containing creams are widely available in pharmacies. The cream used in this study contained 0.025% capsaicin, but the researchers suggested that better results might occur with 0.075% capsaicin.

When you start out, use only a little cream, as it will produce a burning sensation. After several applications, the burning will begin to diminish. You can then increase the amount of cream you use. When you no longer feel the burning, you know that you have reached the right dose.

Safety Issues

Capsaicin creams appear to be safe. The only reported side effect is the initial uncomfortable burning sensation, which stops after a few moments. Of course, you will want to avoid getting capsaicin into your eyes or onto other sensitive tissues. The pain can be quite excruciating, although no real harm should result. Take care to wear a glove when applying it, and to wash your hands afterwards.

OTHER PROPOSED TREATMENTS

A natural substance present in apple juice and other plant foods, malic acid is widely marketed as a treatment for fibromyalgia, often in combination with magnesium. However, it has not been proven effective.

A mixture of malic acid and magnesium has been the subject of preliminary studies. In one double-blind study of 24 people, 1,200 mg of malic acid and 300 mg of magnesium taken daily for 4 weeks were no more effective than placebo.[15] Good results have been seen in open trials,[16,17] but such studies cannot eliminate the placebo effect and for that reason are not reliable.

Other proposed natural treatments include **vitamin B₁** (see page 434), **vitamin E** (see page 451), **selenium** (see page 407), and **spirulina** (see page 413), but there is no real evidence that they work.[18]

Food Allergies and Sensitivities

FOOD ALLERGIES AND SENSITIVITIES

Principal Proposed Treatments   Elimination Diet

Other Proposed Treatments   Proteolytic Enzymes, Thymus Extract

A food allergy is defined as an abnormal immune reaction caused by the ingestion of a food or food additive. The most dramatic form of food allergy reaction occurs within minutes, usually in response to certain foods such as shellfish, peanuts, or strawberries. The effects are similar to those of a bee sting allergy, involving hives, itching, swelling in the throat, and difficulty breathing; this immediate type of allergic reaction can be life-threatening.

Other food allergy reactions are more delayed, causing relatively subtle symptoms over days or weeks.[1] These include gastrointestinal problems (constipation, diarrhea, gas, cramping, and bloating), rashes, and headaches. However, because such delayed reactions are relatively vague and can have other causes, it has remained a controversial subject in medicine.

Some food allergy-like reactions do not actually involve the immune system. These are termed food sensitivities (or food intolerance). In most cases, the cause of such sensitivities is unknown.

Delayed-type food allergies and sensitivities might play a role in many diseases, including **asthma** (see page 14), **attention deficit disorder** (see page 22), **rheumatoid arthritis** (see page 151), **vaginal yeast infections** (see page 182), **canker sores** (see page 40), **colic** (see page 53), chronic **ear infections** (see page 73), **eczema** (see page 78), **irritable bowel syndrome** (see page 108), **migraine headaches** (see page 120), **psoriasis** (see page 148), chronic sinus infections, **ulcerative colitis** (see page 179), **Crohn's disease** (see page 57), and celiac disease.[2–9] However, not all experts agree; practitioners of natural medicine tend to be more enthusiastic about the food allergy theory of disease than conventional practitioners.

Conventional treatment for immediate-type food allergy reactions includes desensitization ("allergy shots"), emergency epinephrine (adrenaline) kits for self-injection, and the antihistamine diphenhydramine (Benadryl).

Delayed-type food allergies are much more difficult to identify and treat. Although skin and blood tests are sometimes used, they are probably not reliable.[10–16] The elimination diet and food challenge (described later) may be the only effective approach to identifying or treating this type of food allergy.

Another conventional approach for delayed-type food allergies is oral cromolyn (a drug sometimes used in treating asthma and other allergic illnesses).[17] A double-blind placebo-controlled study of 14 children with milk and other food allergies found that cromolyn was effective in preventing allergic reactions in 11 of 13 cases, whereas placebo was effective in only 3 of 9 cases.[18] In another study, 32 individuals were given cromolyn one half hour before meals and at bedtime.[19] If their food allergy symptoms were prevented, the participants were entered into a double-blind placebo-controlled crossover study using cromoglycate. Of the 31 people who completed the study, 24 experienced relief of gastrointestinal symptoms when taking cromolyn as compared to 2 when taking placebo. In addition, systemic allergic reactions were also blocked with the cromolyn. Unfortunately, the drug also had many side effects.

PRINCIPAL PROPOSED TREATMENTS

There are no well-documented natural treatments for food allergies. The best approach may be the most direct: eliminating allergenic foods from the diet.

Unfortunately, there don't seem to be any foolproof ways of identifying allergenic foods in advance. As mentioned above, food allergy testing appears to be rather unreliable. For this reason, some authorities recommend the use of an elimination diet. This method involves starting with a highly restricted diet consisting only of foods that are seldom allergenic, such as rice, yams, and turkey. Another approach involves eliminating only highly allergenic foods. In either case, if dietary restriction leads to resolution or improvement of symptoms, foods are then reintroduced one by one to see which, if any, will trigger reactions.[20]

There is some evidence that the elimination diet may be effective for chronic or recurrent hives;[21,22,23] it has been tried for many other conditions as well, including irritable bowel syndrome,[24–31] asthma,[32] reflux esophagitis,[33] and Crohn's disease.[34,35]

Cow's milk protein intolerance is thought to be the most common childhood allergy,[36] followed by allergies to eggs, peanuts, nuts, and fish.

There is some evidence that eliminating cow's milk from the diets of infants and their nursing mothers might reduce symptoms of infantile colic,[37–46] although not all studies have found benefit.[47,48,49] Elimination diets in children might also help treat eczema, asthma, hay fever, and ear infections.[50,51]

In hopes of *preventing* food allergies and diseases related to them, some authorities recommend that pregnant and breast-feeding mothers as well as their children should avoid allergenic foods.[52–56] However, it is not clear if this method actually helps. For example, one study evaluated 165 children at high risk of developing allergic symptoms.[57] Careful avoidance of allergenic foods in the diets of the mothers and infants did not reduce the later development of eczema, asthma, hay fever, or food allergy symptoms.

OTHER PROPOSED TREATMENTS

Digestive enzymes such as **bromelain** (see page 229) and other **proteolytic enzymes** (see page 393) have been proposed as a treatment for food allergies, based on the reasonable idea that digesting offending proteins will reduce allergic reactions to them. However, there is no real evidence as yet that they are effective against food allergies.

Thymus (see page 422) extract is a supplement derived from the thymus gland of cows. Highly preliminary evidence suggests that by normalizing immune function, thymus extracts may be helpful for food allergies.[58] However, there are significant safety issues with thymus extract (see the chapter for details), and this study did not prove thymus extract to be effective.

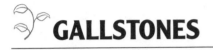

GALLSTONES

Principal Proposed Treatments   There are no well-established natural treatments for gallstones.

Other Proposed Treatments   Peppermint, Milk Thistle, Artichoke Leaf, Boldo, Dandelion Root, Fumitory, Greater Celandine, Turmeric, Betaine Hydrochloride, Coffee (for Prevention), Vitamin C

The job of the gallbladder is to store the bile produced by the liver and to release it on an as-needed basis for digestive purposes. However, it isn't easy to keep this complex mixture of chemicals in liquid form. The various elements of bile have a natural tendency to form sludge, lumps, and hard deposits called gallstones. The body uses several biochemical methods to prevent such condensation from occurring, but this natural chemistry does not always succeed. More than 20% of women and 8% of men develop gallstones at some time in their lives.

You could have gallstones in your body for many years without experiencing any problems. According to current medical guidelines, no treatment is necessary unless pain or other problems begin to develop. However, when a gallstone plugs the duct that leads out of the gallbladder, the organ becomes inflamed and often infected, creating a condition known as cholecystitis.

Generally, gallbladder pain begins with occasional minor attacks that subside rapidly. Perhaps the stones are blocking the duct temporarily and then moving out of the way. However, when full obstruction occurs, the pain often becomes severe and recurrent.

The most reliable symptom of cholecystitis is intense pain beneath the right lower rib cage, often occurring from midnight to 3 A.M. Typically, pain radiates to the right shoulder and is accompanied by a loss of appetite and sometimes nausea. Frequently, fatty meals seem to bring on the pain with particular force.

Techniques for removing the gallbladder have become quite sophisticated. Today, the gallbladder can be removed quickly and usually without complications, bringing full relief of symptoms.

Living without a gallbladder does not seem to bring any long-term consequences. However, many people are opposed on general principle to removing an organ that nature has placed there. The medication Actigall may be able to dissolve gallstones when it is taken for many months.

PROPOSED TREATMENTS

The only time it is appropriate to use alternative treatments for gallstones is before acute cholecystitis develops. Once the gallbladder has become completely blocked, there is a real danger of imminent rupture. Another risk is that a stone may escape the gallbladder and obstruct the common bile duct. When this happens, the liver cannot unload the bile it produces, putting it at risk of permanent injury and creating a true surgical emergency.

However, during the period in which pain is only occasional or intermittent, the risks incurred by postponing surgery are slight. During the same interval when the medication Actigall might be tried, some of the agents described here could be considered as possibilities. Unfortunately, none are well established as effective. Medical supervision is definitely essential.

Peppermint

Preliminary clinical trials suggest that formulas containing **peppermint** (see page 384) and related terpenes (fragrant substances found in plants) can dissolve gallstones.[1]

The proper dosage is not clear, but a typical recommendation is 1 or 2 capsules containing 0.2 ml of peppermint oil 3 times daily. The label should say "enteric coated," meaning that it remains intact until it has passed the stomach. Excessive doses of peppermint oil can cause severe gastrointestinal distress and other symptoms, so do not take more than this amount.

Milk Thistle

Milk thistle, standardized to its silymarin content, has been shown to improve the liquidity of bile,[2] although its actual effects on gallstones in real life are unknown. The standard dosage of milk thistle is 200 mg 2 to 3 times a day of an extract standardized to contain 70% silymarin. (For more information on milk thistle use and safety issues, see the chapter on **milk thistle.**)

Other Herbs and Supplements

Herbs that are widely prescribed in Germany for gallbladder pain include artichoke leaf, **boldo** (see page 226), **dandelion** (see page 266) root, fumitory, greater celandine, and **turmeric** (see page 425).[3] The supplement **betaine hydrochloride** (see page 219) is also sometimes recommended for gallbladder problems, although there is no real evidence as yet that it works.

Warning: Consult a qualified physician before using these substances, as they can cause increased pain and may present other risks.

There is some evidence that regular coffee drinking can reduce the risk of developing gallstones, at least in men aged 40 to 75. In an observational study that tracked about 46,000 male physicians for a period of 10 years, those who drank 2 to 3 cups of caffeinated coffee daily had a 40% reduced risk of developing gallstone disease.[4] Those who drank more coffee had an even greater reduction of risk.

It may be the caffeine in coffee that helps, as other sources of caffeine were also associated with reduced risk of gallstones, while decaffeinated coffee didn't seem to help. Caffeine is known to increase the flow of bile, so this connection makes sense. However, observational studies can be misleading, so these findings can't be taken as absolutely reliable.

Similar evidence suggests that regular use of **vitamin C** (see page 444) supplements might help prevent gallstones in women.[5]

GOUT

Principal Proposed Treatments   There are no well-established natural treatments for gout.

Other Proposed Treatments   Folate, Devil's Claw, Fish Oil, Vitamin E, Selenium, Bromelain, Vitamin A, Aspartic Acid, Cherry Juice, Celery Juice

---

Gout is an inflammatory condition that is caused by the deposit of uric acid crystals in joints (most famously the big toe) as well as other tissues. Typically, attacks of fierce pain, redness, swelling, and heat punctuate pain-free intervals.

Medical treatment consists of anti-inflammatory drugs for acute attacks and of uric acid-lowering drugs for prevention.

PROPOSED TREATMENTS

The following herbs and supplements are widely recommended for gout, but they have not yet been scientifically proven effective.

Folate

Folate (see page 288) has been recommended as a preventive treatment for gout for at least 20 years. Some clinicians report that it can be highly effective. However, what little scientific evidence we have on the method is contradictory.[1,2,3] It has been suggested that a contaminant found in folate, pterin-6-aldehyde, may actually be responsible for the positive effects observed by some clinicians.

A typical dosage of folate for gout is 10 mg daily. However, because folate can mask **vitamin B$_{12}$** (see page 442) deficiency, it is important to consult with a qualified health-care practitioner before using this method. High doses of folate can also cause digestive distress and may worsen seizures in epileptics. The safety of high doses of folate in young children, pregnant or nursing women, and those with severe kidney or liver disease has not been established.

Devil's Claw

The herb **devil's claw** (see page 267) is sometimes recommended as a pain-relieving treatment for gout based on evidence for its effectiveness in various forms of arthritis.[4] A typical dosage is 750 mg 3 times daily of a preparation standardized to contain 3% iridoid glycosides.

Devil's claw appears to be quite safe, and there is no evidence of toxicity at dosages many times higher than recommended. However, safety in pregnant or nursing women and those with severe liver or kidney disease has not been established. It is not recommended for use by those with ulcers, as it can sometimes cause stomach irritation.

Other Supplements

On the basis of interesting reasoning but no concrete evidence of effectiveness, **fish oil** (see page 282), **vitamin E** (see page 451), **selenium** (see page 407), **bromelain** (see page 229), **vitamin A** (see page 432), and aspartic acid have also been recommended for both prevention and treatment of gout.[5]

Folk Remedies

A traditional remedy for gout (with negligible scientific evidence) calls for ½ to 1 pound of cherries a day.[6] You can also buy tablets containing concentrated cherry juice.

Celery juice is another folk remedy for gout that is said to be widely used in Australia.

HEMORRHOIDS

Principal Proposed Treatments   Citrus Bioflavonoids, Oxerutins

Other Proposed Treatments   Horse Chestnut, OPCs (Oligomeric Proanthocyanidins), Gotu Kola, Butcher's Broom, Bilberry, Aortic Glycosaminoglycans, Collinsonia, Slippery Elm, Calendula

Hemorrhoids are swollen, inflamed veins in the rectum that can ache and bleed. They are very common and are usually caused by constipation, a low-fiber diet, a sedentary lifestyle, or pregnancy.

The most important interventions for hemorrhoids aim at reversing their causes. Adopting a high-fiber diet, sitting down less, getting plenty of exercise, and maintaining regular bowel habits can make a significant difference.

Medical treatment consists mainly of stool softeners and moist heat. In more severe cases, surgical procedures may be used.

PRINCIPAL PROPOSED TREATMENTS

Besides the treatments described in this section, the natural treatments used for varicose veins are also often recommended for hemorrhoids because a hemorrhoid is actually a special kind of varicose vein. These include **horse chestnut** (see page 325), **OPCs** (see page 373), **gotu kola** (see page 315), **butcher's broom** (see page 232), and **bilberry** (see page 220).

Bioflavonoids

Bioflavonoids are colorful substances that occur widely in the plant kingdom. A fixed combination of the **citrus bioflavonoids** (see page 254) diosmin and hesperidin has been investigated as a treatment for hemorrhoids with positive results; related semisynthetic bioflavonoids called **oxerutins** (see page 377) also appear to be effective.

Reasonably good evidence suggests that the citrus bioflavonoids diosmin and hesperidin (in a special micronized combination preparation) may be helpful for hemorrhoids. A 2-month double-blind placebo-controlled trial of 120 individuals with recurrent hemorrhoid flare-ups found that treatment with combined **diosmin** (see page 254) and **hesperidin** (see page 254) significantly reduced the frequency and severity of hemorrhoid attacks.[1] Another double-blind placebo-controlled trial of 100 individuals had positive results with the same bioflavonoids in relieving symptoms once a flare-up of hemorrhoid pain had begun.[2] A 90-day double-blind trial of 100 individuals with bleeding hemorrhoids also found significant benefits for both treatment of acute attacks and prevention of new ones.[3] Finally, this bioflavonoid combination was found to compare favorably with surgical treatment of hemorrhoids.[4] However, less impressive results were seen in a double-blind placebo-controlled study in which all participants were given a fiber laxative with either combined diosmin and hesperidin or placebo.[5]

Moderate-size double-blind studies also support the use of oxerutins, including the hemorrhoids that occur during pregnancy, although there have been negative studies as well.[6,7]

Bioflavonoids and oxerutins are considered very safe. The typical dosage of citrus bioflavonoids is 500 mg twice daily; oxerutins are taken at 500 to 1,000 mg 2 or 3 times daily.

Although it is not known precisely how flavonoids work, it is thought that they stabilize the walls of blood vessels, making them less susceptible to injury.

OTHER PROPOSED TREATMENTS

The following natural treatments are widely recommended for hemorrhoids, but they have not been scientifically proven effective at this time.

Preliminary evidence suggests that an extract made from the inner lining of cow aortas called aortic glycosaminoglycans (GAGs) can improve the symptoms of hemorrhoids.[8,9] The recommended dosage is 50 mg twice daily. See the chapter on **aortic glycosaminoglycans** for detailed safety information.

Collinsonia root (also known as stone root) is a traditional remedy for hemorrhoids. The proper dosage varies according to the preparation and is usually listed on the label. Safety studies have not been performed.

The herb **slippery elm** (see page 411) is also sometimes used orally for hemorrhoids; topical **calendula** (see page 237) cream is also a popular treatment. However, there is as yet no real evidence that they work.

HERPES

Related Terms   Genital Herpes, Cold Sores

Principal Proposed Treatments   Melissa (Prevention and Treatment), L-Lysine (Prevention)

Other Proposed Treatments   Eleutherococcus, Vitamin C, Bee Propolis, Sandalwood, Astragalus, Cat's Claw, Elderberry, Licorice

The common virus known as herpes can cause painful blister-like lesions around the mouth and in the genitalia. Slightly different strains of herpes predominate in each of these two locations, but the infections are essentially identical. In both areas, the herpes virus has the devious habit of hiding out deep in the DNA of nerve ganglia, where it remains inactive for months or years. From time to time the virus reactivates, travels down the nerve, and starts an eruption. Common triggers include **stress** (see page 167), dental procedures, infections, and trauma. Flare-ups usually become less severe over time.

Conventional medical treatment consists of antiviral drugs, such as Zovirax. Such medications can shorten the length and intensity of a herpes outbreak or, when taken consistently at lower dosages, reduce the frequency of flare-ups. However, they are not dramatically effective.

PRINCIPAL PROPOSED TREATMENTS

Melissa officinalis (Lemon Balm)

More commonly known in the United States as lemon balm, *Melissa officinalis* (see page 359) is widely sold in Europe as a topical cream for the treatment of genital and oral herpes. This herb is a native of southern Europe and is widely planted in gardens for the purpose of attracting bees. Its leaves give off a delicate lemon odor when bruised.

Melissa cream appears to be helpful in the treatment of genital and oral herpes. It can be applied only at the first sign of blisters or on a regular basis for the prevention of flare-ups. However, there is no evidence that melissa will stop you from infecting another person.

What Is the Scientific Evidence for Melissa?

Early studies of melissa ointments showed a significant reduction in the duration and severity of herpes symptoms (both genital and oral) and, when the cream was used regularly, a marked reduction in the frequency of recurrences.[1] In one study, the melissa-treated participants recovered in 5 days, while participants receiving nonspecific creams required 10 days.[2] Researchers also described a "tremendous reduction" in the frequency of recurrence. However, because these studies weren't double-blind, the results can't be taken as reliable.

A subsequent double-blind study followed 116 individuals with oral or genital herpes at two dermatology centers.[3] Treated subjects showed a significantly better rate of recovery than those on placebo, according to physician and patient ratings.

A recent double-blind placebo-controlled study followed 66 individuals who were just starting to develop a cold sore (oral herpes).[4] Treatment with melissa cream produced significant benefits on day 2, reducing intensity of discomfort, number of blisters, and the size of the lesion. The researchers specifically looked at day 2 because, according to them, that is when symptoms are most pronounced. Furthermore, long-term follow-up suggested that use of melissa can prolong the interval before the next herpes flare-up.

The most commonly used European melissa product is manufactured using a method that tests the herb's activity against the herpes virus. Here's how it's designed: Human or animal cells are grown in a petri dish and then infected with herpes virus. Left alone, the virus would gradually spread throughout the dish, killing all the cells. However, in this test, standard paper disks containing melissa extract are inserted into the petri dish. The commercial extract is standardized so that a dose of 200 mcg per disk forms a 20 to 30 mm zone of protection from the virus.[5]

We don't really know how melissa works. The leading theory is that the herb makes it more difficult for the herpes virus to attach to cells.

Dosage

For treatment of an active flare-up of herpes, the proper dosage is four thick daily applications of a standard melissa 70:1 extract cream. This can be reduced to twice daily for preventive purposes.

Pregnant women should not regard melissa as effective prevention against transmission to the newborn. It also will not prevent spread of the disease in sexually active individuals.

Safety Issues

Topical melissa is not associated with any significant side effects, although allergic reactions are always possible. Safety in young children, pregnant or nursing women, and those with severe liver or kidney disease has not been established.

L-Lysine

Another famous treatment for herpes involves the amino acid **L-lysine** (see page 350). Although study results have been somewhat contradictory, overall the evidence suggests that taking L-lysine on a regular basis might make herpes flare-ups milder and less frequent.[6] L-lysine has also been proposed as a treatment to take at the onset of a herpes attack, but at least one study has found it to be ineffective for this purpose.[7] (Consider using melissa for this latter situation.) L-lysine probably works best when it is combined with dietary changes that restrict levels of another amino acid, **arginine** (see page 208). (To do this, cut down on gelatin, chocolate, peanuts, almonds and other nuts, seeds, and to a lesser extent wheat.)

A double-blind placebo-controlled trial tested the efficacy of L-lysine in preventing recurring herpes simplex.[8] Twenty-seven individuals were given 1,000 mg of L-lysine 3 times a day for 6 months, while 25 subjects received placebo. Those treated with L-lysine experienced, on average, 2.4 fewer herpes flare-ups than the placebo group, a significant result. The L-lysine group also experienced significantly less severe flare-ups and shorter healing time.

Another placebo-controlled double-blind study on 41 subjects found that 1,250 mg of L-lysine per day re-duced the frequency of attacks, but 624 mg did not.[9] However, other studies, including one that enrolled 79 individuals, found no benefit at all.[10,11]

Foods high in L-lysine include vegetables, beans, fish, turkey, and chicken. When taken as a supplement, a typical daily dose is 1,000 mg.

Although L-lysine is an essential part of the diet, the safety of concentrated lysine supplements has not been well studied. In animal studies, high dosages have caused gallstones and elevated cholesterol levels,[12,13] so you may want to use caution when using L-lysine if you have either of these problems. Maximum safe dosages for young children, pregnant or nursing women, or those with severe liver or kidney disease have not been established.

OTHER PROPOSED TREATMENTS

The following natural treatments are widely recommended for herpes, but they have not been scientifically proven effective at this time.

Other Herbs and Supplements

Eleutherococcus (see page 301), incorrectly called Russian or Siberian ginseng, has shown promise for the treatment of herpes. A 6-month double-blind trial of 93 men and women with recurrent herpes infections found that treatment with the herb *Eleutherococcus* (2 g daily) reduced the frequency of infections by almost 50%.[14]

One study suggests that topical treatment with a **vitamin C** (see page 444) solution may speed healing of herpes outbreaks.[15]

Oral vitamin C may also be useful, especially when combined with bioflavonoids.[16] A typical dose is 200 mg of vitamin C combined with 200 mg of mixed bioflavonoids, taken 5 times daily at the very first signs of an impending outbreak. Short-term use of these substances has not been associated with any significant risks.

The results of a small controlled study suggests that the honeybee product **propolis** (see page 216) cream might cause attacks of genital herpes to heal faster.[17]

There is some evidence that elements in **kelp** (see page 340) might help to prevent infection with several kinds of viruses, including herpes simplex.[18] However the evidence is very preliminary at this time.

In test tube studies, **sandalwood** (see page 405) was found to slow the growth of herpes virus.[19]

The herbs **astragalus** (see page 212), **cat's claw** (see page 242), **elderberry** (see page 276), and **licorice** (see page 344) are sometimes recommended for herpes as well, but there is little solid evidence as yet that they really work.

Herpes

Visit Us at TNP.com

HIGH CHOLESTEROL

Principal Proposed Treatments   Garlic, Red Yeast Rice, Stanols, Vitamin B$_3$ (Niacin), Fiber, Soy, Policosanol, Guggul, Artichoke Leaf

Other Proposed Treatments   Pantethine, L-Carnitine, Chitosan, Fish Oil, Flaxseed Oil, Flaxseed, Creatine, Aortic Glycosaminoglycans, Chromium, Calcium, Probiotics, Genistein, Spirulina, Alfalfa, Ashwagandha, Bilberry Leaf, Chondroitin, Copper, Fenugreek, Gamma Oryzanol, Grass Pollen, He Shou Wu, Lecithin, Maitake, Multivitamin/Mineral, Lifestyle Changes

One of the most significant discoveries in preventive medicine is that elevated levels of cholesterol in the blood accelerate atherosclerosis, or hardening of the arteries (see the discussion about cholesterol in the chapter on **atherosclerosis**). Along with high blood pressure, inactivity, smoking, and diabetes, high cholesterol has proven to be one of the most important promoters of heart disease, strokes, and peripheral vascular disease (blockage of circulation to the extremities, usually the legs).

Cholesterol does not directly clog arteries like grease clogs pipes. The current theory is that elevated levels of cholesterol irritate the walls of blood vessels and cause them to undergo harmful changes. Because most cholesterol is manufactured by the body itself, dietary sources of cholesterol (such as eggs) are not usually the most important problem. The relative proportion of unsaturated fats (from plants) and saturated fats (mainly from animal products) in the diet is more significant. The former lower cholesterol levels, whereas the latter raise them.

There is no question that increasing exercise and improving diet are the most important steps to take when cholesterol is high. These fundamental lifestyle changes are frequently effective and produce many benefits that go beyond simply lowering cholesterol levels.

. However, if your cholesterol remains high despite your best efforts, you may need specific cholesterol-lowering treatments. There are a variety of effective drugs to choose from, and some, such as Pravachol (pravastatin), have been shown to prevent heart attacks and reduce mortality. While there are known and suspected risks associated with these medications, the benefits of these medications undoubtedly exceed the risks for those with significantly elevated cholesterol levels. In milder cases, however, some of the options described below might be better first choices.

PRINCIPAL PROPOSED TREATMENTS

There are several herbs and supplements that appear to help lower cholesterol levels. However, before trying them, consult with your physician to find out whether you have time to experiment. If your cholesterol levels are very high and your arteries are already in bad condition, it might be wiser to turn to proven drug treatments.

However, if your physician says that you can safely spend some time exploring your options, the treatments described in this section may be worth trying.

Garlic: Probably Reduces Total Cholesterol

The most well-established herbal treatment for high cholesterol is the kitchen herb **garlic** (see page 291). As far back as the first century A.D., Dioscorides wrote of garlic's ability to "clear the arteries." Today, Germany's Commission E authorizes the use of garlic "as an adjunct to dietary measures in patients with elevated blood lipids (cholesterol) and for the prevention of age-related vascular (blood vessel) changes." However, although the research evidence that garlic really works is impressive, it is not airtight.

The effectiveness of garlic appears to depend heavily on the formulation used. A relatively odorless substance, alliin, is one of the most important compounds in garlic and is believed by many researchers to be a prime active ingredient (or, technically, source of active ingredients). When garlic is crushed or cut, an enzyme called allinase is brought into contact with alliin, turning the latter into allicin. Allicin is most responsible for garlic's strong odor and may also play a major role in lowering cholesterol. The allicin itself then rapidly breaks down into entirely different compounds.

When you powder garlic to put it into a capsule, it acts like cutting the bulb. The chain reaction starts: alliin contacts allinase, yielding allicin, which then breaks down. Unless something is done to prevent this process, garlic powder will not have any alliin left that can be turned into allicin by the time you buy it.

Some garlic producers declare that alliin and allicin have nothing to do with garlic's effectiveness and simply sell products without either one, such as aged powdered garlic and garlic oil. However, there are serious doubts about the effectiveness of these products. Garlic oil, in particular, seems to be entirely ineffective (see What Is the Scientific Evidence for Garlic?).

Raw garlic is the most reliable source of alliin, but its strong odor keeps many people from using it. To solve this problem, manufacturers have devised ways to produce relatively odor-free garlic that still contains a standardized level of alliin. Such products are sold as powdered garlic with a guaranteed alliin content and, often, an "allicin potential" or "allicin yield."

What Is the Scientific Evidence for Garlic?

At least 28 controlled clinical studies of using garlic to treat elevated cholesterol were published between 1985 and 1995. Together, they suggest that garlic can lower cholesterol by about 9 to 12%.[1,2] Virtually all of these studies used garlic standardized to alliin content (see the discussion under Dosage). Garlic oil does not seem to be effective.

One of the best of these studies was conducted in Germany and published in 1990.[3] A total of 261 individuals at 30 medical centers were given either 800 mg of standardized garlic daily or placebo. Over the course of 16 weeks, patients in the treated group experienced a 12% drop in total cholesterol and a 17% decrease in triglyceride levels. The greatest benefits occurred in patients with initial cholesterol levels of 250 to 300 mg/dL.

Another double-blind study, reported in 1996, followed 41 men with cholesterol readings of 220 to 290 mg/dL.[4] The men received either placebo or 7.2 g of aged garlic extract daily for 6 months; then their treatments were switched for 4 months. The results showed a 7% decrease in total serum cholesterol and a 4% decrease in LDL cholesterol in the garlic-treated group. There was also a 5.5% decrease in blood pressure.

One widely quoted study compared garlic to the standard cholesterol-lowering drug bezafibrate.[5] Although the results showed them to be equally effective, the study was not designed properly, so the results mean little. Both groups in the study were asked to improve their diets. The effects of the dietary change could have easily overshadowed real differences between the treatments.

In contrast to these positive results, a couple of other studies have shown no benefit with garlic powder. One study, published in 1996, followed 115 individuals with total cholesterol concentrations of 231 to 328 mg/dL, half of whom received 900 mg daily of a standard garlic extract standardized to contain 1.3% allicin.[6] The results showed no significant difference between the treated and placebo groups. Other studies have also found no benefit.[7,8,9]

However, just as in the bezafibrate study, all participants in these two studies were asked to make dietary changes, which may have overwhelmed garlic's antihypercholesterolemic effects.

It can be said with some certainty that garlic oil is not effective for lowering cholesterol.[10]

Garlic also might modestly reduce blood pressure, making it potentially useful for **hypertension** (see page 98). Furthermore, evidence suggests that it may soften artery walls through mechanisms other than lowering cholesterol and blood pressure,[11] perhaps by protecting against free radicals and hindering blood clotting.[12–19] Because of this multifaceted effect, garlic may be a useful all-around treatment for the prevention of heart disease.[20]

Dosage

In most of the studies that demonstrated the cholesterol-lowering powers of garlic, the daily dosage supplied at least 10 mg of alliin. This is sometimes stated in terms of how much allicin will be created from that alliin. The number you should look for is 4 to 5 mg of "allicin potential." You must allow at least 1 to 4 months of treatment for full effects.

Aged garlic without alliin may also offer some benefit, but don't bother with garlic oil.

Safety Issues

As a commonly used food, garlic is on the FDA's GRAS (generally recognized as safe) list. Rats have been fed gigantic doses of aged garlic (2,000 mg per kilogram body weight) for 6 months without any signs of negative effects.[21] Unfortunately, there is no safety information from animal studies on garlic powder standardized to alliin content, which is by far the most commonly used form of garlic.

The only common side effect of garlic is unpleasant breath odor. Even so-called odorless garlic produces an offensive smell in up to 50% of those who use it.[22]

Other side effects occur only rarely. For example, a study that followed 1,997 people who were given a normal dose of deodorized garlic daily over a 16-week period showed a 6% incidence of nausea, a 1.3% incidence of dizziness on standing (perhaps a sign of low blood pressure), and a 1.1% incidence of allergic reactions.[23] A few reports of bloating, headaches, sweating, and dizziness were also noted.

Raw garlic taken in excessive doses can cause many symptoms, including stomach upset, heartburn, nausea and vomiting, diarrhea, flatulence, facial flushing, rapid pulse, and insomnia.

Because garlic appears to possess blood-thinning effects, it might not be safe to combine garlic with blood thinners, such as Coumadin (warfarin), Trental (pentoxifylline), or aspirin, or with other natural blood-thinning substances like **ginkgo** (see page 298) and **vitamin E** (see page 451). High doses of garlic should not be taken before or after surgery or labor and delivery.[24]

Maximum safe doses in young children, pregnant or nursing women, and those with severe kidney or liver disease have not been established.

Red Yeast Rice: May Be Similar to Standard Drugs

Red yeast rice (see page 399) has recently arrived on the market as a treatment for lowering cholesterol.

However, because of potential risks, it should only be used under physician supervision.

Red yeast rice is a traditional Chinese substance that is made by fermenting a type of yeast called *Monascus purpureus* over rice. This product (called Hong Qu) has been used in China since at least 800 A.D. as a food and also as a medicinal substance. Recently, it has been discovered that this ancient Chinese preparation contains at least 11 naturally occurring substances similar to prescription drugs in the "statin" family, such as Mevacor and Pravachol.

What Is the Scientific Evidence for Red Yeast Rice?

A recent, major U.S. study on red yeast rice was conducted at the UCLA School of Medicine.[25] This was a 12-week double-blind placebo-controlled trial involving 83 healthy participants (46 men and 37 women, aged 34 to 78 years) with high cholesterol levels. One group was given the recommended dose of red yeast rice, while the other group received placebo. Both groups were instructed to consume a lowfat diet similar to the American Heart Association Step 1 diet.

The results showed that red yeast rice was significantly more effective than placebo. In the treated group, average total cholesterol (mg/dL) fell by about 18% by 8 weeks. During the same time period, LDL ("bad") cholesterol decreased by 22% and triglycerides by 11%. There was little to no improvement in the placebo group. HDL ("good") cholesterol did not change in either group during the study.

Similar or even better results have been seen in other U.S. and Chinese studies using various forms of red yeast rice.[26,27]

Dosage

Because red yeast rice products can vary widely in their strength, please refer to the labeling for appropriate dosage.

Safety Issues

While there have been no serious adverse reactions reported in the studies of red yeast rice, some minor side effects have been reported. In a large open trial in which 324 people received red yeast rice, heartburn (1.8%), bloating (0.9%), and dizziness (0.3%) were all mentioned.[28] Formal toxicity studies in rats and mice, giving doses up to 125 times the normal human dose for 3 months, showed no toxic effects, according to information provided by one of the manufacturers of red yeast rice.[29]

However, because red yeast rice contains ingredients similar to the statin drugs, there is a theoretical risk of the same side effects and risks that are seen with those drugs. These include elevated liver enzymes, damage to skeletal muscle, and increased risk of cancer. Also, red yeast rice

should not be combined with erythromycin, other statin drugs, the class of drugs called "fibrates," or high-dose niacin. Serious side effects have occurred when statin drugs were combined with these medications.

Additionally, like statin drugs, red yeast rice may deplete the body of a substance called **coenzyme Q_{10}** (CoQ_{10}; see page 256).[30–33] Taking extra CoQ_{10} might be helpful.

Grapefruit juice can cause a significant and possibly dangerous increase in blood levels of statin drugs. For this reason, grapefruit juice should be avoided when taking red yeast rice.

This product should not be used by pregnant or nursing mothers, or those with severe liver or kidney disease except on a physician's advice.

Stanols

Stanols (see page 418) are substances that occur naturally in various plants. Their cholesterol-lowering effects were first observed in animals in the 1950s. Since then, a substantial amount of research suggests that plant stanols (modified into stanol esters) can help to lower cholesterol in individuals with normal or mildly to moderately elevated cholesterol levels. Stanols are available in margarine spreads, salad dressings, and dietary supplement tablets.

What Is the Scientific Evidence for Stanols?

Plant stanol esters reduce serum cholesterol levels by inhibiting cholesterol absorption.[34] Because they are structurally similar to cholesterol, stanols can displace cholesterol from the "packages" that deliver cholesterol for absorption from the intestines to the bloodstream.[35] The displaced cholesterol is not absorbed and is excreted from the body; the stanols themselves are ultimately not absorbed either.

At least 13 double-blind placebo-controlled studies, ranging in length from 30 days to 12 months and involving a total of more than 935 individuals, have found stanols effective for improving cholesterol levels.[36–48] The combined results suggest that stanols can reduce total cholesterol and LDL ("bad") cholesterol by about 10 to 15%. Stanols did not have any significant effect on HDL ("good") cholesterol or triglycerides in most of these studies.[49]

In one of the best of the double-blind placebo-controlled studies, 153 individuals with mildly elevated cholesterol were given sitostanol ester in margarine (at 1.8 or 2.6 g of sitostanol per day), or margarine without sitostanol ester, for a total of 1 year.[50] The results in the treated group receiving 2.6 g per day showed improvements in total cholesterol by 10.2% and LDL cholesterol by 14.1%—significantly better than the results in the control group. Neither triglycerides nor HDL cholesterol levels were affected.

Two studies found stanols to be helpful for lowering cholesterol levels in individuals with type 2 (adult-onset) diabetes.[51,52] One of these studies examined two treatments: pravastatin (a cholesterol-lowering drug) versus pravastatin along with sitostanol. The combination treatment was more effective at lowering total cholesterol and LDL cholesterol levels than the drug treatment alone.[53] Additive benefits were also seen in a study of nondiabetics taking statin drugs who began taking stanols as well.[54]

Dosage

Typical dosages of stanol esters to lower cholesterol levels range from 3.4 to 5.1 g per day.[55] One manufacturer of a commercially prepared margarine spread recommends taking 3 teaspoons (1.5 g of sitostanol ester per teaspoon) per day. The suggested use varies depending on the product and the quantity of sitostanol ester per serving. It may take up to 3 months to show a substantial decrease in total cholesterol values.[56]

Safety Issues

Stanols are considered safe because they are not absorbed.[57,58] No adverse effects have been reported in any of the studies on lowering cholesterol, with the exception of one study that reported mild gastrointestinal complaints in a few preschool children.[59] In addition, no toxic signs were observed in rats given stanol esters for 13 weeks at levels comparable to or exceeding those recommended for lowering cholesterol.[60]

Although concerns have been expressed that stanols might impair absorption of the fat-soluble **vitamins A** (see page 432), **D** (see page 449), and **E** (see page 451), this does not seem to occur at the dosages of stanols required to lower cholesterol.[61] Stanols might, however, interfere with absorption of alpha- and **beta-carotene** (see page 217),[62,63] although some studies have found no such effect.[64,65] Until more is learned, it may be reasonable for individuals using stanol products to make sure to consume carotenoid-rich vegetables (yellow/orange and dark green vegetables).[66]

Niacin (Vitamin B₃): A Treatment Accepted by Conventional Medicine

The common vitamin niacin, also called **vitamin B₃** (see page 437), is an accepted medical treatment for elevated cholesterol with solid science behind it. According to numerous studies, niacin can lower total cholesterol and LDL ("bad") cholesterol by 15 to 25%, lower triglycerides by 2 to 50%, and raise HDL ("good") cholesterol by 15 to 25%.[67–70] A double-blind study of 140 individuals found extended-release niacin (2,000 mg per day) increased levels of HDL cholesterol from baseline twice as much as did the cholesterol-lowering drug gemfibrozil (1,200 mg per day).[71] Unfortunately, niacin, if taken in sufficient quantities to lower cholesterol, can cause an annoying flushing reaction and occasionally liver inflammation.[72] Close medical supervision is essential when using niacin to lower cholesterol.

To partially counter some of these problems, a special form of niacin has been developed in Europe: inositol hexaniacinate, or "flushless" niacin.[73] The term *flushless* is not quite accurate—some people do flush with inositol hexaniacinate, but the flush is neither as common nor as severe as with ordinary niacin. It is still necessary to check the liver periodically, so a physician's supervision remains essential.

The proper dosage of inositol hexaniacinate is 500 to 1,000 mg 2 to 3 times daily, taken with food. The usual recommendation is to start with the lower dose and raise it only if the cholesterol doesn't fall sufficiently after about 6 weeks.

Ordinary niacin can be used as well, and there are slow-release forms of niacin available by prescription. However, liver inflammation is a real possibility with all forms of niacin.

Fiber: Considered "Heart-Healthy" by the FDA

Water-soluble fiber supplements appear to lower cholesterol, and the FDA has permitted products containing this form of fiber to carry a "heart-healthy" label.[74] Many forms are available, ranging from oat bran to expensive fiber products sold through multilevel marketing firms. A good dose of oat bran is 5 to 10 g with each meal and at bedtime, and psyllium is taken at 10 g with each meal. However, eating a diet high in fresh fruits and vegetables and whole grains may be even better because of the many healthful nutrients such a diet contains.

Soy Protein: Also Labeled "Heart-Healthy"

Soy protein (see page 411) appears to lower total cholesterol by about 9%, LDL ("bad") cholesterol by 13%, and triglycerides by 10%.[75] The FDA has allowed foods containing soy protein to make the "heart-healthy" claim on the label. One study suggests that substituting as little as 20 g daily of soy protein for animal protein can significantly improve cholesterol levels.[76] About this amount can be found in ½ pound of tofu or 2½ cups of soy milk.

Soy **isoflavones** (see page 335) may be the active cholesterol-lowering ingredient in soy protein,[77] although some studies disagree with this assertion.[78,79]

Soy may not be safe for women with a previous history of breast cancer. Evidence from one highly preliminary study in humans found changes suggestive of increased breast cancer risk after women took a commercial soy protein product.[80] There are also concerns that intensive use of soy products by pregnant women could exert a hormonal effect that impacts unborn fetuses.[81,82]

Visit Us at TNP.com

In addition, soy may impair thyroid function or reduce absorption of thyroid medication, at least in children.[83,84,85] For this reason, individuals with impaired thyroid function should use soy with caution.

Policicosanol

Policosanol is a mixture of related substances that includes **octacosanol** (see page 372), and is manufactured from sugar cane.

Octacosanol and policosanol appear to slow down cholesterol synthesis in the liver and also to increase liver reabsorption of LDL cholesterol.[86,87]

Ten double-blind placebo-controlled studies, involving a total of more than 400 individuals and ranging in length from 6 weeks to 12 months, have found policosanol effective for improving cholesterol levels.[88–97] The results suggest that policosanol treatment can reduce total cholesterol and LDL cholesterol by about 20%. Some studies found improvements in HDL cholesterol, but most did not. Interestingly, nine out of ten of these studies enrolled only individuals whose cholesterol levels had not previously improved with diet alone.

In one of the best of these double-blind studies, 74 men and women with elevated cholesterol were given policosanol or placebo for a total of 12 months.[98] The results in the treated group showed improvements in total cholesterol by 17%, LDL cholesterol by 26%, and HDL cholesterol by 14%, a significantly better result than was seen in the placebo group.

One study found policosanol to be safe and effective for reducing cholesterol levels in individuals with type 2 (adult-onset) diabetes.[99] However, individuals with any form of diabetes should seek medical advice before taking policosanol.

Typical dosages of policosanol to lower elevated cholesterol levels range from 5 to 10 mg twice daily. Results may require 2 months to develop.[100,101]

Policosanol appears to be safe at the maximum recommended dose. A few side effects were observed in clinical trials using policosanol or octacosanol. These effects were short-term and mild, and mainly included nervousness, headache, diarrhea, and insomnia.[102]

However, for theoretical reasons, these supplements should not be combined with standard cholesterol-lowering medications except on the advice of a physician.

Guggul: Traditional Indian Herb

Guggul (see page 319), the sticky gum resin from the mukul myrrh tree, may be an effective treatment for high cholesterol. According to preliminary studies, it appears that guggul can lower cholesterol by about 11 to 12% and triglycerides by 12.5 to 17%.[103–106] The full benefits may take several months to develop.

Guggul is manufactured in a standardized form that provides a fixed amount of guggulsterones, the presumed active ingredients in guggul. The typical daily dose should provide 100 mg of guggulsterones.

In clinical trials of standardized guggul extract, no significant side effects other than occasional mild gastrointestinal distress have been seen.[107,108,109] Laboratory tests conducted in the course of these trials did not reveal any alterations in liver or kidney function, blood cell numbers and appearance, heart function, or blood chemistry. However, safety in young children, pregnant or nursing women, or those with severe liver or kidney disease has not been established.

Artichoke (*Cynara scolymus*): A New Treatment

Although primarily used to stimulate gallbladder function, **artichoke leaf** (see page 210) may be helpful for high cholesterol as well.

According to a double-blind placebo-controlled study of 143 individuals with elevated cholesterol, artichoke leaf extract significantly improved cholesterol readings.[110] Total cholesterol fell by 18.5% as compared to 8.6% in the placebo group; LDL cholesterol fell by 23% versus 6%; and the LDL to HDL ratio decreased by 20% versus 7%.

Artichoke leaf may work by interfering with cholesterol synthesis.[111] A compound in artichoke called luteolin may play a role in reducing cholesterol.[112]

Germany's Commission E recommends 6 g of the dried artichoke leaf (or an amount of extract equivalent to it) per day, usually divided into 3 doses.

Artichoke leaf has not been associated with significant side effects in studies so far, but full safety testing has not been completed. For this reason, it should not be used by pregnant or nursing women. Safety in young children or in people with severe liver or kidney disease has also not been established.

In addition, because artichoke leaf is believed to stimulate gallbladder contraction, individuals with gallstones or other forms of gallbladder disease could be put at risk by using this herb. Such individuals should use artichoke leaf only under the supervision of a physician. It is possible that increased gallbladder contraction could lead to obstruction of ducts or even rupture of the gallbladder.

Individuals with known allergies to artichokes or related plants in the Asteraceae family, such as arnica or chrysanthemums, should avoid using artichoke.

OTHER PROPOSED TREATMENTS

There are several other promising alternative treatments for high cholesterol.

A special form of the vitamin pantothenic acid, known as **pantethine** (see page 380), might significantly lower total blood triglycerides as well as cholesterol, but not all studies agree.[113–116] Further research is necessary to prove the safety and effectiveness of this expensive supplement.

L-carnitine (see page 238) is another expensive supplement that might be able to improve cholesterol levels.[117]

Evidence from animal studies and preliminary trials in humans suggests that **chitosan** (see page 247), a type of fiber derived from crustacean shells, can lower cholesterol levels.[118–125] In addition, it may raise levels of high-density lipoprotein, or HDL cholesterol.

The supplement **fish oil** (see page 282) also appears to lower total blood triglycerides, and might raise HDL cholesterol as well.[126]

Although fish oil is much better studied, there is some evidence that **flaxseed oil** (see page 285) or whole **flaxseed** (see page 286) may reduce LDL cholesterol, perhaps slightly reduce hypertension, and, overall, slow down atherosclerosis.[127–133]

Preliminary evidence suggests that **creatine** (see page 264) supplements may also be able to reduce triglycerides.[134]

Preliminary studies suggest that an extract from the lining of the aortas of cows, known as **aortic glycosaminoglycans** (GAGs; see page 207), can improve cholesterol levels.[135,136,137] The typical dosage is 50 mg 2 times daily.

Aortic GAGs are considered safe, as similar substances are widely found in foods. However, if you are taking drugs that powerfully decrease blood clotting, such as Coumadin (warfarin) or heparin, do not use aortic GAGs except under a physician's supervision. Aortic GAGs interfere slightly with blood clotting, and there is at least a chance that the combination could cause bleeding problems.

Supplemental **chromium** (see page 251) may improve blood cholesterol in some people.[138,139] In people taking beta-blockers, it may raise levels of HDL cholesterol.[140] A typical nutritional dosage is 200 mcg of chromium picolinate daily. **Calcium** (see page 234) supplements might slightly improve cholesterol levels.[141,142] A typical nutritional dosage is 1,000 to 1,200 mg daily.

Some but not all studies suggest that "friendly bacteria" (**probiotics;** see page 200) might be able to reduce cholesterol levels.[143–147]

Weak evidence suggests **genistein** (see page 294) may be helpful for reducing cholesterol and keeping it from depositing on cell walls.[148,149,150]

Evidence from animal studies and one small controlled (but not blinded) study in humans suggests that **spirulina** (see page 413) might help lower cholesterol.[151,152,153]

Animal and preliminary human trials suggest that the herb **alfalfa** (see page 202) may be helpful for high cholesterol as well.[154–166]

Other herbs and supplements commonly recommended for high cholesterol include **ashwagandha** (see page 212), **bilberry** (see page 220) leaf, **chondroitin** (see page 250), **copper** (see page 262), **fenugreek** (see page 279), **gamma oryzanol** (see page 290), **grass pollen** (see page 317), **He shou wu** (see page 322), **lecithin** (see page 343), and **maitake** (see page 354), but there is as yet little solid evidence that they really work. Finally, because general nutrient deficiencies can alter cholesterol levels, a basic multivitamin and mineral may be useful.

Lifestyle Approaches

The dietary influence on cholesterol levels is enormous but not entirely understood. Clearly, saturated fats from animal sources raise cholesterol levels, whereas polyunsaturated fats (from plants) lower them.

Much discussion has taken place over precisely which types of nonanimal fats are best. Some studies point toward monounsaturated fats, such as those found in olive oil. Nuts also contain monounsaturated fats, and a growing body of evidence suggests that increased consumption of nuts such as almonds, walnuts, pecans, and macadamia nuts may help lower cholesterol and prevent heart disease.[167–174]

Margarine, long thought to be "better than butter," now appears to be generally unhealthful. The hydrogenated or partially hydrogenated oils that make up margarine are found in other foods as well. However, at the time of this writing a special form of margarine from Finland is touted as being heart-healthy. In addition, taking magnesium may help reduce the risks created by margarine.[175]

Some observational studies have found an association between coffee intake and elevated cholesterol. However, because coffee use is typically associated with other bad habits, such as smoking and a diet high in animal fat, it is difficult to know for sure whether coffee is really causing the problem.[176]

This is a rapidly evolving field, and anything we write here may be outdated by the time you read this. Consult a qualified health professional for the latest information.

Finally, other treatments that may help prevent or reverse **atherosclerosis** should be considered as well.

HIV SUPPORT

Related Terms   Human Immunodeficiency Virus, Acquired Immunodeficiency Syndrome, AIDS

Principal Proposed Treatments   There are no well-established natural treatments for HIV infection.

Other Proposed Treatments

For Inhibiting Viral Replication: Boxwood Extract, Bacailin, Curcumin, Elderberry, Aloe, Schisandra, Spirulina, Reishi, Propolis, Astragalus

For Fighting Weight Loss: MCTs, Glutamine, Whey Protein

For Enhancing the Immune System: N-Acetyl Cysteine, Glutathione, Andrographis, Trichosanthin (Compound Q), Lipoate, Coenzyme Q_{10}, Maitake, Glycyrrhizin, *Momordica charantia*, Echinacea, Ginseng, Omega-6 Fatty Acids, Carnitine, DHEA, Proteolytic Enzymes, Fish Oil

For Treating Symptoms (Such As Diarrhea or Thrush): Bovine Colostrum, Tea Tree Oil, Cinnamon, DHEA, Chinese Herb Combinations

For Treating Medication Side Effects: Zinc, Carnitine, Vitamin B_{12}

For General Nutritional Support: Vitamin A, Beta-Carotene, Vitamin B_1, Vitamin B_2, Vitamin B_6, Niacin, Vitamin B_{12}, Vitamin C, Vitamin E, Choline, Iron, Selenium, Zinc, Multivitamins

Treatments to Avoid: St. John's Wort, Garlic

Note: None of these treatments has been proven effective as yet for the uses cited above.

HIV, or human immunodeficiency virus, is the virus responsible for AIDS (acquired immunodeficiency syndrome). First identified in 1983, this virus progressively destroys or damages cells in the immune system, making its host vulnerable to certain cancers and infections. So-called "opportunistic infections"—caused by microorganisms that do not ordinarily cause illness in healthy people—can have serious or even fatal effects on those with HIV.

Within a month or two of exposure, HIV may cause short-term flu-like symptoms, followed by a symptom-free period lasting months to years during which the virus continues to multiply. After this stage, people with HIV may develop swollen lymph nodes, recurrent herpes sores, diarrhea, weight loss, and/or chronic yeast infections (oral or vaginal)—a state previously called "AIDS-related complex" or ARC. Children may experience delayed development or fail to thrive. The infection is called AIDS when the number of immune cells known as CD4+ or helper t-cells drops below a certain level, or when opportunistic diseases such as *Pneumocystis carinii* pneumonia develop. Today, both ARC and AIDS are sometimes collectively called "symptomatic HIV infection."

HIV is spread most commonly through unsafe sexual practices or by intravenous drug abuse. Mothers can infect their babies before or during birth, or later through breast-feeding.

New hope in treatment for HIV occurred with the discovery of two groups of drugs called *reverse transcriptase inhibitors* and *protease inhibitors*. Both help keep the virus from multiplying. Taken together, they can help slow the spread of the virus and delay the onset of AIDS.

However, they can't prevent people from transmitting the virus to others. (One exception: Pregnant women who take one of these drugs, AZT, may have a much lower chance of passing the virus to their unborn babies.) Although powerful, these treatments do not eradicate the virus, and therefore aren't truly cures for the disease.

Surveys have shown that people with HIV often take natural remedies in addition to multiple medications. If you have HIV, it is particularly important to talk with your doctors about any natural substances you're taking and to be alert to possible interactions. Most importantly, individuals with HIV should not use St. John's wort (see Herbs to Avoid).

PROPOSED TREATMENTS

Among the many proposed natural treatments for HIV, none has more than preliminary evidence.

Inhibiting Viral Replication

Currently, no natural remedies rival the effectiveness of antiretroviral drugs for inhibiting HIV replication in the body. However, preliminary research suggests that an extract of the leaves and stems of the boxwood shrub may delay the progression of HIV disease.[1] Many other herbs and supplements have been proposed as well, but there is little evidence as yet that they work.

Boxwood

In a double-blind placebo-controlled study of 145 people with HIV, French researchers studied the effects of two doses of a preparation made from the evergreen boxwood (*Buxus sempervirens*).[2] The preparation was given in doses of 990 mg and 1,980 mg per day for periods ranging from 4 to 64 weeks.

When participants started the study, they had no symptoms of HIV and had never taken antiretroviral drugs. They were kept off anti-HIV drugs during the study (this was before the use of anti-HIV drugs became widespread). At the end, researchers found that among those taking the lower dose, fewer people developed AIDS, symptomatic HIV, or CD4+ counts below 200 compared to those taking the higher dose or placebo. Additionally, by the end of their treatment period, fewer people in the low-dose group had a large increase in the amount of HIV virus they carried compared to the other two groups.

The researchers had originally planned the study to continue for 18 months (78 weeks). However, as the study progressed, a review committee decided to halt the study early when the average participant had taken boxwood or placebo for only 37 weeks. They felt it was unethical to continue to have some people take placebo, given the positive results among those taking the extract. Nonetheless, further research is necessary to confirm the effectiveness of boxwood extract for HIV, particularly in combination with proven anti-viral drugs which have now become the standard of care for HIV infection.

No severe side effects were reported in this study, and the people taking boxwood had the same overall rate of side effects as those taking placebo.[3]

However, there are some safety concerns with this herb. A substance called cycloprotobuxine is believed to be one of the active ingredients in boxwood.[4] High doses of this substance can cause vomiting, diarrhea, muscular spasms, and paralysis. **Warning**: For this reason, the herb should only be taken under medical supervision! Safety in pregnant or nursing women, young children, or people with liver or kidney disease has not been established. In addition, touching fresh boxwood leaves can occasionally cause skin irritation.[5]

Note: Only a special boxwood extract has been studied as a treatment for HIV infection. Do not try to use raw boxwood leaf, as it might not be safe.

Other Herbs and Supplements

Other substances that have been investigated for possible HIV suppression include bacailin, curcumin, **elderberry** (see page 276), **aloe** (see page 204), schisandra, **spirulina** (see page 413), **reishi** (see page 400), **bee propolis** (see page 216), and **astragalus** (see page 212). However, the evidence that they work is primarily limited to test tube and animal studies; whether these results translate into real improvement among people with HIV has yet to be determined.

The herb St. John's wort contains a substance called hypericin which has been investigated for possible anti-HIV effects. However, contrary to popular belief neither hypericin nor St. John's wort are at all useful for treating HIV.[6] In addition, St. John's wort seriously impairs the activity of standard HIV medications, and might lead to treatment failure. (See Herbs to Avoid.)

Fighting Weight Loss

Weight loss is a frequent symptom of HIV and AIDS. Sometimes weight loss is so extreme that the person seems to "waste away"—hence the name "AIDS wasting syndrome," which is technically defined as the loss of more than 10% of body weight combined with either chronic diarrhea or weakness and fever. Many factors can contribute to this weight loss, including loss of appetite, nausea, malabsorption of nutrients, and mouth sores.

Supplemental MCTs and glutamine, as well as whey protein, may be helpful for this symptom, although there is no definitive evidence as yet that they work.

MCTs: More Research Is Needed

Fat malabsorption is particularly common in HIV infection, and can lead to both diarrhea and weight loss. A particular type of fat known as **MCTs** (medium-chain triglycerides; see page 356) is more easily absorbed than ordinary fats (long-chain triglycerides) and may help decrease diarrhea and wasting. Two small double-blind studies have found that MCTs are more easily absorbed than long chain triglycerides in people with HIV or AIDS.[7,8] However, there is no direct evidence as yet that MCTs actually help people gain weight.

In both of the studies described above, participants consumed nothing but a special nutritional formula containing MCTs. Taking MCTs in this way requires medical supervision to determine the dose.

MCTs are thought to be quite safe, but the safety of long-term use as a general fat substitute has not been established. Some people who consume MCTs, especially on an empty stomach, experience annoying (but not severe) abdominal cramps and bloating. People with HIV or diabetes should not use MCTs (or any other supplement) without a doctor's supervision. The safety of MCTs in young children, pregnant or nursing women, or people with serious kidney or liver disease has not been established.

Glutamine: May Help When Combined With Other Nutrients

Another promising treatment for wasting is the amino acid **glutamine** (see page 310), a substance that plays a role in maintaining the health of the immune system, digestive tract, and muscle cells. Although research is still preliminary, one double-blind placebo-controlled study found that a combination of glutamine and antioxidants

HIV Support

(vitamins C and E, beta-carotene, selenium, and N-acetyl cysteine) led to significant weight gain in people with HIV who had lost weight.[9]

Another small double-blind trial found that combination treatment with glutamine, **arginine** (see page 208), and **beta-hydroxy beta-methylbutyrate** (HMB; see page 323) could increase muscle mass and possibly improve immune status.[10]

Other Herbs and Supplements for Weight Gain

Whey protein is sometimes recommended for weight gain in HIV, but evidence that it works is very preliminary.[11] **Fish oil** (see page 282) may be helpful as well.[12]

Enhancing the Immune System

In test tube studies, a number of substances have been found to improve measures of immunity in HIV infection, for example, by elevating CD4+ counts, changing the ratio between CD4+ cells and other immune cells, increasing amounts of other immune chemicals, or enhancing the body's ability to attack invading substances. However, there is relatively little information on whether they can actually help people with HIV infection.

NAC: Might Support Immune Function

One of the natural substances most widely used by people with HIV in hopes of enhancing immune system function is the antioxidant **NAC** (short for N-acetyl cysteine; see page 366), but evidence that it helps is somewhat conflicting.

NAC is a specially modified form of the dietary amino acid cysteine. In the body, it helps make the important antioxidant enzyme glutathione, which is sometimes used as a supplement itself. Early human trials, including a double-blind study of 45 people, suggest that NAC may increase levels of CD4+ cells in healthy people and slow CD4+ cell decline in people with HIV.[13,14] Another study of NAC combined with selenium had mixed results, affecting t-cell counts in some people but not others.[15] However, preliminary results of yet another study found that NAC had no effect on CD4+ counts or the amount of HIV virus in the blood.[16]

Other Proposed Herbs and Supplements for Enhancing the Immune System

Other natural treatments that are sometimes recommended to boost immunity in HIV include: andrographis, trichosanthin (compound Q), lipoate, coenzyme Q$_{10}$, maitake, a component of **licorice** (see page 344) known as glycyrrhizin, the herb *Momordica charantia* (also called bitter melon), echinacea, ginseng, omega-6 fatty acids, carnitine, DHEA, and proteolytic enzymes. However, there is no real evidence as yet that these treatments actually work. Garlic is sometimes recommended as well; however for safety reasons it should be avoided in HIV infection. (See Herbs to Avoid.)

Fish oil is also sometimes recommended for enhancing immunity in HIV infection. However, one 6-month double-blind study found that a combination of the omega-3 fatty acids in fish oil plus the amino acid arginine was no more effective than placebo in improving immune function in people with HIV.[17]

Treating Symptoms or Opportunistic Infections

Besides the treatments mentioned earlier, a number of natural remedies have been proposed for symptoms of HIV or common opportunistic infections.

Bovine colostrum (see page 260) has been suggested as a treatment for the chronic diarrhea that commonly occurs in people with HIV or AIDS, but the evidence that it works is weak at best.[18,19,20]

Tea tree oil (see page 421) and **cinnamon** (see page 254) have been suggested as treatments for thrush (oral *Candida* infection).[21,22]

Dehydroepiandrosterone (**DHEA**) (see page 268) is a hormone that seems to decrease in people with AIDS, possibly because of malnutrition[23] and/or stress.[24] A trial examining whether supplemental DHEA can improve mood and fatigue among people with HIV returned inconclusive results.[25]

A standardized mixture of Chinese herbs including **astragalus** (see page 212), **andrographis** (see page 205), and more than 30 other herbs was no more effective than placebo in reducing HIV symptoms in a pilot study, or in a larger double-blind study.[26,27]

Treating Medication Side Effects

Several natural treatments have been proposed to treat side effects from two drugs used in HIV: AZT, an antiretroviral drug; and TMP-SMX, a commonly prescribed antibiotic.

Zinc, Carnitine, and Vitamin B$_{12}$: Might Be Helpful With AZT

Taking AZT can lead to **zinc** (see page 463) deficiency, which may interfere with immune function.[28] One partially blinded study found that zinc supplements may benefit people on AZT.[29] In the zinc-treated group, body weight increased or stabilized, CD4+ count rose, and participants had significantly fewer opportunistic infections.

Carnitine (see page 238) has also been proposed as a treatment for AZT side effects, based on very early evidence that it may keep AZT from damaging muscle cells.[30,31]

Based on highly preliminary evidence, **vitamin B$_{12}$** (see page 442) has been suggested as a preventive for blood abnormalities caused by AZT.[32]

Visit Us at TNP.com

NAC: Proposed for Side Effects of TMP-SMX

It has been suggested that the supplement **NAC** (see page 366) might help prevent side effects from the antibiotic TMP-SMX (trimethoprim-sulfamethoxazole). However, two controlled studies found that NAC did not significantly decrease adverse reactions to TMP-SMX.[33,34]

General Nutritional Support

People infected with HIV may be particularly vulnerable to malnutrition because of decreased appetite, poor absorption, or possibly increased requirements for specific nutrients. Studies have found deficiencies of vitamins A, B_1, B_6, B_{12}, E, beta-carotene, choline, folate, selenium, and zinc to be common among people with HIV infection.[35–49] Many deficiencies become more common as the disease worsens. This suggests, but does not prove, that taking supplements of these nutrients may be helpful.

Vitamin A/Beta-Carotene

Vitamin A (see page 432) and **beta-carotene** (see page 217) are described together here because the body uses beta-carotene to produce vitamin A.

Vitamin A deficiency may be linked to lower CD4+ counts as well as higher death rates among people infected with HIV.[50] A few preliminary studies have raised hopes that beta-carotene supplements might increase or preserve immune function or decrease symptoms among people with HIV.[51–54] One small double-blind study suggested that taking beta-carotene might raise white blood cell count in people with HIV.[55] However, two subsequent larger controlled trials found no significant differences between those taking beta-carotene or placebo in white blood cell count, CD4+ count, or other measures of immune function.[56,57]

Two observational studies lasting 6 to 8 years suggest that higher intakes of vitamin A or beta-carotene may be helpful, but they also found that caution is in order with regard to dosage.[58,59] This group of researchers generally linked higher intake of vitamin A or beta-carotene to lower risk of AIDS and lower death rates, with an important exception: people with the highest intake of either nutrient (more than 11,179 IU per day of beta-carotene; or more than 20,268 IU per day of vitamin A) did worse than those who took somewhat less.

Note: Keep in mind also that excessive dosages of vitamin A can be toxic to the liver. Consult with your physician on the right dose for you.

Despite hopes that vitamin A given to pregnant, HIV-positive women might decrease the infection rate of their babies, two double-blind studies have found no significant differences between babies whose mothers took vitamin A compared to those whose mothers took placebo.[60,61] In any case, vitamin A is not considered safe in pregnancy; beta-carotene is preferred.

B-Vitamins

An observational study found that HIV-positive men with the highest intakes of **vitamin B_1** (see page 434), **B_2** (see page 436), **B_6** (see page 439), and **niacin** (see page 437) had significantly longer survival rates, while a similar study found that those taking the most B_1 or niacin had a significantly lower rate of developing AIDS.[62,63]

Vitamin B_{12} (see page 442) deficiencies in people infected with HIV have been linked to neurological symptoms, including slower processing of information in studies of cognitive functioning; early research suggests that restoring B_{12} levels to normal may decrease these symptoms.[64,65] B_{12} deficiency has also been linked to lower CD4+ counts and more rapid development of AIDS.[66]

Vitamin B_6 deficiency has been linked to impaired immune function in one study of people with HIV infection.[67]

Note: Excessive intake of vitamin B_6 can cause neurological problems. Consult with your physician on the right dose for you.

Vitamins C and E

Massive doses of **vitamin C** (see page 444) have at times been popular among people with HIV infection based on highly preliminary evidence.[68,69] An observational study linked high doses of vitamin C with slower progression to AIDS.[70] High intake of **vitamin E** (see page 451) was also linked to decreased risk of progression to AIDS in a different observational study.[71]

However, a double-blind study of 49 people with HIV who took combined vitamins C and E or placebo for 3 months did not show any significant effects on the amount of HIV virus detected or the number of opportunistic infections.[72] It has been suggested that vitamin E may enhance the antiviral effects of AZT, but evidence for this is minimal.[73]

Choline

The substance **choline** (see page 248) has been newly added to the list of essential nutrients. Evidence suggests that individuals with HIV who are low in choline may experience more rapid disease progression.[74]

Iron

A study of 71 HIV-positive children noted a high rate of **iron** (see page 333) deficiency.[75] One observational study of 296 men with HIV infection linked high intake of iron to a decreased risk of AIDS 6 years later.[76]

Note: Do not take iron supplements unless you know that you are iron-deficient.

Selenium

Selenium (see page 407) is required for a well-functioning immune system.[77] Observational studies have linked higher levels of selenium in the blood with higher CD4+ counts[78] and reduced risk of mortality from HIV disease.[79,80]

One open study suggested that selenium supplements might raise blood levels of selenium in people with serious HIV disease.[81] However, in a controlled study of 52 people with HIV, selenium did not improve the clinical conditions or raise CD4+ counts any more than no treatment.[82] A study of selenium combined with NAC had mixed results, affecting t-cell counts in some people but not others.[83]

Selenium has also been proposed as a preventive or treatment for cardiomyopathy, a disorder of the heart muscle that can affect people with AIDS, but evidence so far is weak.[84,85]

Zinc

Some, but not all, studies have found that HIV-positive individuals tend to be deficient in **zinc** (see page 463), with levels dropping lower in more severe disease.[86–91] But does this mean that taking zinc will help? The answer is not clear.

Higher zinc levels have been linked to better immune function and higher CD4+ cell counts, whereas zinc deficiency has been linked to increased risk of dying from HIV.[92,93,94] One preliminary study among people taking AZT found that 30 days of zinc supplementation led to decreased rates of opportunistic infection over the following 2 years.[95]

However, other research has linked higher zinc intake to more rapid development of AIDS.[96] In another study of HIV-positive individuals, those with higher zinc intake or those taking zinc supplements in any dosage had a greater risk of death within the following 8 years.[97]

Multivitamins

Because so many nutrients are affected by HIV infection and treatments, multivitamin supplements are a logical choice.

Researchers interviewed 296 men with HIV but not AIDS about their diets and multivitamin use, then followed their progress for 6 years.[98] Those who took a daily multivitamin had a significantly lower risk of developing AIDS during the study. In a similar study, HIV-positive men who took supplements of vitamin B_1, B_2, or B_6, at levels higher than the Recommended Dietary Allowance, early in the course of their disease had lower death rates 8 years later.[99]

HERBS TO AVOID

Combination of St. John's wort and protease inhibitors is highly dangerous and should be avoided. In a study of healthy volunteers, St. John's wort was found to decrease the blood concentration of indinavir, one of the most widely used protease inhibitors, by 49% to 99%![100] This could lead to treatment failure as well as the emergence of resistant strains of the HIV virus.

Garlic, also, may combine poorly with certain HIV medications. Two people with HIV experienced severe gastrointestinal toxicity from the HIV drug ritonavir after taking garlic supplements.[101]

If you have HIV, talk with your doctor before using any herb or supplement, no matter how harmless it may seem. A number of common herbs may cause interactions with medications. Given the large numbers of drugs, herbs, and supplements taken by many people with HIV, the possibility of interactions is high.

HYPERTENSION (High Blood Pressure)

Principal Proposed Treatments   Garlic, Coenzyme Q_{10} (CoQ_{10})

Other Proposed Treatments   Fish Oil, Calcium, Magnesium, Potassium, Hawthorn, Vitamin C, Glucomannan, Hibiscus, Kelp, Astragalus, *Coleus forskohlii,* Maitake, Beta-Carotene, Flaxseed Oil, Taurine

Most people can't tell when their blood pressure is high, which is why hypertension is called the "silent killer." In this case, what you don't know can hurt you. Elevated blood pressure can lead to a greatly increased risk of heart attack, stroke, and many other serious illnesses. Along with high cholesterol and smoking, hypertension is one of the most important causes of atherosclerosis. In turn, atherosclerosis causes heart attacks, strokes, and other diseases of impaired circulation.

The mechanism by which high blood pressure produces atherosclerosis is similar to a hose fitted with a high-pressure nozzle. All such nozzles come with a warning label that states, "Make sure to discharge pressure in hose after using." Unfortunately, many people frequently fail to pay attention to the warning and leave the hose puffed up with full pressure overnight.

This rather common practice does not produce any immediate consequences. The hose doesn't develop leaks at the seams or burst outright on the first occasion you leave it untended. However, a garden hose that is frequently left under pressure will begin to age more rapidly than it would otherwise. Its lining will begin to crack, its flexibility will diminish, and within a season or two the hose will be sprouting leaks in all directions.

When blood vessels are exposed to constantly high pressure, a similar process is set in motion. Blood pressures as elevated as 220/170 (systolic pressure/diastolic pressure), quite common during activities such as weight lifting, do no harm. Only when excessive pressure is sustained day and night do blood vessel linings begin to be injured and undergo those unhealthy changes known as hardening of the arteries, or atherosclerosis (see the chapter on **atherosclerosis** for more information).

Thus, although it is important to lower blood pressure with all deliberate speed, only rarely does it need to be lowered instantly. In most situations, you have plenty of time to work on bringing down your blood pressure. However, that doesn't mean that you should ignore it. Over time, high blood pressure can damage nearly every organ in the body.

The best way to determine your blood pressure is to take several readings at different times during the day and on different days of the week. Blood pressure readings will vary quite a bit from moment to moment; what matters most is the average blood pressure. Thus, if many low readings balance out a few high readings, the net result may be satisfactory.

However, it is essential not to ignore a high value by saying, "I was just stressed then." Stress is part of life, and if it raises your blood pressure once, it will do so again. To come up with an accurate number, you must include every measurement in your calculations.

In most cases, the cause of hypertension is unknown. The kidneys play an important role in controlling blood pressure, and the level of squeezing tension in the blood vessels makes a large contribution as well.

Lifestyle changes can dramatically reduce blood pressure. Increasing exercise, not smoking, and losing weight can all be highly effective. For many years doctors advised patients with hypertension to cut down on salt in the diet. Today, however, the value of this difficult dietary change has undergone significant questioning. Considering how rapidly our knowledge is evolving, we suggest consulting your physician to find the latest recommendations.

If lifestyle changes fail to reduce blood pressure, or if you can't make these alterations, many effective drugs are available. Sometimes you need to experiment with a few to find one that agrees with you.

PRINCIPAL PROPOSED TREATMENTS

Although there are no well-documented natural treatments for hypertension, garlic and coenzyme Q_{10} have some evidence behind them and are reportedly quite effective. Keep in mind that when blood pressure is consistently higher than 160/110, nondrug treatments (other than lifestyle changes) are seldom enough to bring it down.

Garlic: Appears to Reduce Blood Pressure by 5 to 10%

At least 12 studies have examined the effects of **garlic** (see page 291) on blood pressure, although only two of these involved people with hypertension.[1] Overall, it appears that garlic can reduce blood pressure levels by about 5 to 10%.

One of the best of these trials followed 47 subjects with average blood pressures of 171/101.[2] Over a period of 12 weeks, half were given placebo and the other half received 600 mg of garlic powder daily, standardized to 1.3% alliin. This is the most common form of medicinal garlic powder and is used for lowering cholesterol as well.

Compared to the placebo group, garlic reduced systolic blood pressure by 6% and diastolic pressure by 9%. Although this is not a dramatic improvement, it can definitely be useful.

A typical dosage of garlic is 900 mg daily of a garlic powder extract standardized to contain 1.3% alliin, providing about 12,000 mcg of alliin daily. Garlic is generally regarded as safe; however, because it appears to thin the blood it should not be combined with prescription anticoagulants, such as Coumadin (warfarin) or Trental (pentoxifylline). It also might not be a good idea to take garlic in the weeks before or after surgery or labor and delivery, or combine it with blood-thinning natural supplements such as **ginkgo** (see page 298) or high-dose **vitamin E** (see page 451).

Coenzyme Q_{10}: Appears Effective, but Needs More Study

The supplement coenzyme Q_{10} (CoQ_{10}) is commonly recommended as a treatment for high blood pressure, but the evidence that it works is not yet strong.

An 8-week double-blind placebo-controlled study of 59 men already taking medication for high blood pressure found that 120 mg daily of coenzyme Q_{10} could significantly reduce blood pressure by about 9% as compared to placebo.[3]

Similar results were seen in other trials, but most of these were not double-blind.[4,5,6]

The usual dosage of CoQ_{10} is 30 to 100 mg 3 times daily. This supplement appears to be very safe. However, there are concerns that CoQ_{10}, like many other substances, might interact with the blood-thinning drug Coumadin (warfarin).[7] Individuals taking Coumadin should not take CoQ_{10} (or any other supplement) except under physician supervision. (See the chapter on **CoQ$_{10}$** for a more complete description of CoQ_{10}.)

Impotence

Visit Us at TNP.com

OTHER PROPOSED TREATMENTS

A number of other herbs and supplements may also be somewhat helpful for hypertension.

Fish Oil

Fish oil, a source of omega-3 fatty acids, is also commonly described as beneficial in the treatment of hypertension. However, the research record is mixed and at best shows a slight benefit.[8–14]

A typical dosage is 3 to 9 g daily. Fish oil frequently causes unpleasant burping. (See the chapter on **fish oil** for more information regarding safety issues.)

Minerals: May Be Effective in Case of Deficiency

Adequate intake of **calcium** (see page 234), **magnesium** (see page 351), and **potassium** (see page 390) is necessary for good blood pressure control. When your body lacks adequate amounts of these minerals, supplementation may improve blood pressure.[15–22]

A dosage of 750 to 1,000 mg daily of calcium and 350 mg daily of supplemental magnesium should suffice. Individuals with severe kidney disease should not take magnesium or calcium supplements (or any other supplement) except on the advice of a physician. Additionally, those with severe heart disease, cancer, hyperparathyroidism, sarcoidosis, or a history of kidney stones should not take calcium except on the advice of a physician. The best source of potassium is fruits and vegetables.

Hawthorn

The herb hawthorn is often said to reduce blood pressure, but there is no evidence that this is the case.[23] (See the chapter on **hawthorn** for more information on use and safety issues.)

Vitamin C: Possibly Effective

According to a 30-day double-blind study of 39 individuals taking medications for hypertension, treatment with 500 mg of **vitamin C** (see page 444) daily can reduce blood pressure by about 10%.[24] Smaller benefits were seen in studies of individuals with normal blood pressure or borderline hypertension.[25,26] However, in another study of 363 individuals given vitamin C (1,000 mg per day), vitamin E, beta-carotene, or placebo, no differences in blood pressure were seen among the groups.[27] Other studies have returned inconclusive results.[28,29]

The bottom line: Whether vitamin C truly affects blood pressure remains unclear.

Other Treatments

Several studies have found that **glucomannan** (see page 307), a dietary fiber derived from the tubers of *Amorphophallus konjac,* may improve high blood pressure.[30,31,32]

Weak evidence suggests that another type of fiber, **chitosan** (see page 247), may inhibit the expected rise in blood pressure after a high-salt meal.[33]

Highly preliminary evidence suggests that hibiscus tea may help reduce blood pressure.[34]

Animal studies suggest that **kelp** (see page 340) might help to lower blood pressure; however, we don't know if this effect would apply to humans.[35]

The herbs **astragalus** (see page 212), *Coleus forskohlii* (see page 259), and **maitake** (see page 354), and the supplements **beta-carotene** (see page 217), **flaxseed oil** (see page 285), and **taurine** (see page 420) are sometimes recommended for high blood pressure, but as yet there is no real evidence that they work.

Because **atherosclerosis** is the main harm caused by hypertension, treatments listed in the chapter on atherosclerosis should be considered as well.

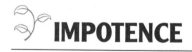

IMPOTENCE

Principal Proposed Treatments   There are no well-established natural treatments for impotence.

Other Proposed Treatments   DHEA (Dehydroepiandrosterone), L-Arginine, Ginkgo, Zinc, Ashwagandha, Damiana, Ginseng, Muira Puama, Pygeum, Suma

Not Recommended Treatments   Yohimbe, Licorice

Impotence, or erectile dysfunction, is the inability to achieve an erection. Impotence may occur for any of at least 15 possible causes, including diabetes, drug side effects, pituitary tumors, hardening of the arteries, hormonal imbalances, and psychological factors. A few of these conditions respond to specific treatment. For example, if a blood pressure drug is causing impotence, the best approach is to change drugs. If a pituitary tumor is secreting the hormone prolactin, treating that tumor may result in immediate improvement. However, in most cases, conventional treatment of impotence is nonspecific.

Generic treatment options include the drug Viagra, mechanical devices that utilize a vacuum to produce an erection, drugs for self-injection, and implantation of penile prostheses. Psychotherapy can also be helpful for treating all varieties of impotence, even when an organic cause can be identified.

PROPOSED TREATMENTS

The following natural treatments are widely recommended for impotence, but they have not been scientifically proven effective at this time.

DHEA

A double-blind, placebo-controlled study enrolled 40 men with difficulty achieving or maintaining an erection, who also had low measured levels of **DHEA** (see page 268).[1] The results showed that DHEA at a dose of 50 mg daily significantly improved sexual performance.

L-Arginine

In a double-blind trial, 50 men with problems developing an erection received either 5 g of **L-arginine** (see page 208) per day or placebo for 6 weeks.[2] More men in the treated group experienced improvement in sexual performance than in the placebo group.

Ginkgo

A slight amount of research suggests that ginkgo may be useful in impotence. One study of 60 men whose impotence was due to poor blood circulation demonstrated a 50% success rate after 6 months.[3] However, because this was not a double-blind study, the improvement noted may have been due to the power of suggestion.

Recent reports suggest that ginkgo may also be useful in reversing the impotence caused by drugs in the Prozac family as well as other types of antidepressant medications.[4-8] (For more information on use and safety issues, see the chapter on **ginkgo.**)

Zinc

Zinc (see page 463) deficiency is known to negatively affect sexual function. Because zinc is one of the most commonly deficient minerals in the diet, it is logical to assume that supplementation with zinc may be helpful for some men. A typical dosage for impotence is 15 to 30 mg daily, taken with 1 to 2 mg of **copper** (see page 262) as supplemental zinc interferes with copper absorption. Too much zinc can be toxic, so do not exceed this dose.

Other Treatments

Many other herbs are also reputed to improve sexual function, including **ashwagandha** (see page 212), **damiana** (see page 265), **ginseng** (see page 301), muira puama, **pygeum** (see page 395), and **suma** (see page 420). However, there is as yet no real evidence that they work.

Not Recommended Treatments

The herb **yohimbe** (see page 461) is the source of the drug yohimbine, which has been shown to be modestly better than placebo for impotence. However, this is a fairly dangerous treatment, and we do not recommend it.

The herb **licorice** (see page 344) may reduce testosterone levels in men.[9] For this reason, men with impotence, infertility, or decreased libido may want to avoid this herb.

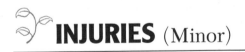

INJURIES (Minor)

Related Terms   Contusion, Sports Injuries, Strains, Bruises, Sprains

Principal Proposed Treatments   Proteolytic Enzymes

Other Proposed Treatments   OPCs, Horse Chestnut, Vitamin C, Citrus Bioflavonoids

Unless you never leave your couch, you are likely to injure yourself sometime. Although minor injuries such as bruises and sprains will heal without treatment, they can be quite unpleasant.

Conventional treatment for minor sprains and strains involves intensive icing for the first 72 hours. Bruises are generally not treated at all.

PRINCIPAL PROPOSED TREATMENTS

A supplement called proteolytic enzymes may be helpful for minor injuries. (For natural recommendations useful for treating related conditions, see the chapters on **easy bruising, minor burns, minor wounds,** and **surgery support.**)

Proteolytic Enzymes

Proteolytic enzymes (see page 393) help you digest the proteins in food. Your pancreas produces the proteolytic enzymes trypsin and chymotrypsin, and others, such as papain and **bromelain** (see page 229), are found in foods. Proteolytic enzymes are primarily used as a digestive aid for people who have trouble digesting proteins. However, for reasons that are not clear, these enzymes may also be helpful for minor injuries, reducing swelling, bruising, and pain, and shortening recovery time.

What Is the Scientific Evidence for Proteolytic Enzymes?

A double-blind placebo-controlled study of 44 individuals with sports-related ankle injuries found that treatment with a proteolytic enzyme combination (also containing bioflavonoids) resulted in faster healing and reduced the time away from training by about 50%.[1] Three other small, double-blind studies, involving a total of about 80 athletes, found that treatment with proteolytic enzymes significantly speeded healing of bruises and other mild athletic injuries as compared to placebo.[2,3,4]

A double-blind placebo-controlled trial involving 71 people with finger fractures found that treatment with a trypsin-chymotrypsin combination significantly improved recovery.[5]

In a controlled study, 74 boxers with bruises on their faces and upper bodies were given bromelain until all signs of bruising had disappeared;[6] another 72 boxers were given placebo. Fifty-eight of the group taking bromelain lost all signs of bruising within 4 days, compared to only 10 of the group taking placebo. Unfortunately, this study was apparently not double-blind, meaning that some of its results may have been due to the power of suggestion.

Additional evidence for the effectiveness of proteolytic enzymes in healing injuries comes from studies involving surgery. For more information, see the chapter on **surgery support**.

Dosage

The combination proteolytic enzymes used in the studies described above were special proprietary formulas; it is not clear what would be an equivalent dose of other proteolytic enzymes. Probably the best advice would be to follow the label instructions.

In studies, bromelain has been given at 120 to 400 mg daily beginning prior to surgery and continuing for a few days afterward.

Note: Bromelain "thins the blood" and could increase risk of bleeding during or after surgery. For this reason, physician supervision is essential.

Safety Issues

Proteolytic enzymes are believed to be quite safe, although there are some concerns that they might further damage the exposed tissue in an ulcer (by partly digesting it).

One proteolytic enzyme, pancreatin, may interfere with folate absorption (see the chapter on **folate** for more information). In addition, bromelain might increase the blood-thinning effects of warfarin (Coumadin) and possibly other anticoagulants.

OTHER PROPOSED TREATMENTS

Oligomeric Proanthocyanidins (OPCs)

OPCs (oligomeric proanthocyanidins; see page 373), substances found in grape seed and pine bark, may be helpful for injuries as well.

A 10-day double-blind placebo-controlled study enrolling 50 participants found that OPCs improved the rate at which edema disappeared following sports injuries.[7] In addition, a double-blind placebo-controlled study of 63 women with breast cancer found that 600 mg of OPCs daily for 6 months reduced postoperative edema and pain.[8] Also, in a double-blind placebo-controlled study of 32 people who had "face-lifts" and were followed for 10 days, swelling disappeared much faster in the treated group.[9]

A typical dose of OPCs is 150 to 300 mg daily, although 600 mg daily was used in one study described above. OPCs appear to be quite safe. However, if you are taking warfarin (Coumadin), heparin, aspirin, or other drugs that "thin" the blood, high doses of OPCs might lead to a risk of excessive bleeding.

Horse Chestnut

The herb **horse chestnut** (see page 325) has been traditionally used to treat **varicose veins** (see page 184) and other problems involving blood vessels and swelling. The active ingredient in horse chestnut is a substance called escin. One double-blind study of 70 people found that about 10 g of 2% escin gel, applied externally to bruises in a single dose 5 minutes after the bruises were induced, reduced their tenderness.[10]

Used externally, horse chestnut should be safe.

Vitamin C and Bioflavonoids

Vitamin C (see page 444) is known to play a role in wound healing. Citrus bioflavonoids and the related substances **oxerutins** (see page 377), appear to reduce leakage from capillaries.

Preliminary evidence from a somewhat poorly reported double-blind trial of 40 college football players suggests that a combination of vitamin C and citrus bioflavonoids taken before practice can reduce the severity of athletic injuries.[11]

Based on evidence from a double-blind study of individuals recovering from minor surgery or other minor injuries, oxerutins may be helpful as well.[12]

INSOMNIA

Principal Proposed Treatments   Valerian (Alone or Combined with Melissa), Melatonin

Other Proposed Treatments   Kava, St. John's Wort, 5-HTP (5-Hydroxytryptophan), Ashwagandha, Astragalus, Chamomile, He Shou Wu, Hops, Lady's Slipper Orchid, Passionflower, Skullcap, Vitamin C

According to recent reports, many people today have a serious problem getting a good night's sleep. Our lives are simply too busy for us to get the 8 hours we really need. To make matters worse, many of us suffer from insomnia. When we do get to bed, we may stay awake thinking for hours. Sleep itself may be restless instead of refreshing.

Most people who sleep substantially less than 8 hours a night experience a variety of unpleasant symptoms. The most common are headaches, mental confusion, irritability, malaise, immune deficiencies, depression, and fatigue. Complete sleep deprivation can lead to hallucinations and mental collapse.

The best ways to improve sleep are lifestyle changes: eliminating caffeine and sugar from your diet, avoiding stimulating activities before bed, adopting a regular sleeping time, and gradually turning down the lights.

Many drugs can also help with sleep. Such medications as Ambien, Restoril, Ativan, Valium, Xanax, and chloral hydrate are widely used for sleep problems. However, these medications tend to promote tolerance and dependency on the drug, and can even cause addiction.

Recently, physicians have come to regard some forms of insomnia as a variation of depression. This conclusion comes from a kind of reverse reasoning: We know that depression almost always disturbs sleep, and that antidepressants frequently help insomnia. Therefore, maybe some cases of insomnia really are depression in disguise.

Antidepressants can be used in two ways to correct sleep problems. Low doses of certain antidepressants immediately bring on sleep because their side effects include drowsiness. However, this effect tends to wear off with repeated use.

For chronic sleeping problems, full doses of antidepressants may be necessary. Antidepressants are believed to work by actually altering brain chemistry, which produces a beneficial effect on sleep. Desyrel (trazodone) and Serzone (nefazodone) are two of the most commonly prescribed antidepressants when improved sleep is desired, but most other antidepressants can be helpful as well.

PRINCIPAL PROPOSED TREATMENTS

Although the scientific evidence isn't yet definitive, the herb valerian and the hormone melatonin are widely accepted as treatments for certain forms of insomnia.

Valerian: Appears to Improve Sleep Gradually

Over 200 plant species belong to the genus *Valeriana*, but the species used for insomnia is *Valeriana officinalis*. This perennial grows abundantly in moist woodlands in Europe and North America and is under extensive cultivation to meet market demands. The root is used for medicinal purposes.

Valerian (see page 428) has a long traditional use for insomnia. Galen recommended valerian for insomnia in the second century A.D. The herb became popular in Europe from the sixteenth century onward as a sedative and was widely used in the United States as well until the 1950s. Rumors have it that Valium was named to imitate the sound of valerian, although there is no chemical similarity between the two.

Scientific studies of valerian in humans did not begin until the 1970s. The results ultimately led to its approval by Germany's Commission E in 1985. Presently, valerian is an accepted over-the-counter drug for insomnia in Germany, Belgium, France, Switzerland, and Italy.

Valerian is commonly recommended as an aid for occasional insomnia. However, the results of a recent study suggest that it may be more useful for long-term improvement of sleep.[1]

What Is the Scientific Evidence for Valerian?

Constituents of valerian as well as whole-valerian extracts have been shown to act as sedatives in laboratory animals.[2,3,4] Studies in humans have also found that valerian is an effective sleeping aid.

A recent 28-day double-blind placebo-controlled study followed 121 people with histories of significant sleep disturbance.[5] This study looked at the effectiveness of 600 mg of an alcohol-based valerian extract taken 1 hour before bedtime.

Valerian didn't work right away. For the first couple of weeks, valerian and placebo were running neck and neck. However, by day 28 valerian had pulled far ahead. Effectiveness was rated as good or very good by participant evaluation in 66% of the valerian group and in 61% by doctor evaluation, whereas in the placebo group, only 29% were so rated by participants and doctors.

This study provides good evidence that valerian is effective for insomnia. However, it has one confusing aspect: the 4-week delay before effects were seen. In another large study, valerian produced an immediately noticeable effect on sleep,[6] and that is what most practitioners believe to be typical. Why valerian took so long to work in this one study has not been explained.

Additional evidence for valerian's effectiveness comes from a double-blind placebo-controlled study of 78 elderly patients.[7] In this case, sleep improved by the end of the study, at 14 days.

The combination of valerian and **lemon balm** (see page 359), also known as melissa, has been tried for insomnia. A 30-day double-blind placebo-controlled study of 98 individuals without insomnia found that a valerian–lemon balm combination improved sleep quality as compared to placebo.[8] Similarly, a double-blind crossover study of 20 people with insomnia compared the benefits of the sleeping drug Halcion (0.125 mg) against placebo and a combination of valerian and lemon balm, and found them equally effective.[9]

We don't really know how valerian acts to induce sleep. Research suggests that the neurotransmitter GABA may be involved, although this has been disputed.[10–16] Conventional sleeping pills affect GABA as well.

Dosage

For insomnia, the standard dosage of valerian is 2 to 3 g of dried root, 270 to 450 mg of a water-based valerian extract (3–6:1), or 600 mg of an alcohol-based extract (4–7:1) taken 30 to 60 minutes before bedtime.[17] If the results of the most recent study are correct, 4 weeks of continuous treatment may be necessary to achieve full results.

Valerian is not recommended for children under 3 years old.[18]

Safety Issues

Valerian is on the FDA's GRAS (generally recognized as safe) list, and is approved for use as a food. In animals, it takes enormous doses of valerian to produce any serious adverse effects.[19]

In a suicide attempt, one young woman took approximately 20 g of valerian (20 to 40 times the recommended dose). Only mild symptoms developed, including stomach cramps, fatigue, chest tightness, tremors, and lightheadedness. All of these resolved within 24 hours, after two treatments with activated charcoal.[20] Her lab tests—including tests of her liver function—remained normal. Keep in mind that this does not mean that you can safely exceed the recommended dose!

One report did find toxic results from herbal remedies containing valerian mixed with several other herbal ingredients, including skullcap. Four individuals who took these remedies later developed liver problems.[21] However, skullcap products are sometimes contaminated with the liver-toxic herb germander, and this could have been the explanation.

There have also been about 50 reported cases of overdose with a combination preparation called Sleep-Qik, containing valerian as well as conventional medications.[22,23] Researchers specifically looked for liver injury, but found no evidence that it occurred.

There are some safety concerns about valepotriates, constituents of valerian, because they can affect DNA and cause other toxic effects. However, valepotriates are not present to a significant extent in any commercial preparations.[24,25]

Although no animal studies or controlled human trials have found evidence that valerian ever causes withdrawal symptoms when use is stopped, one case report is sometimes cited in support of the possibility that this might occur.[26] It concerns a 58-year-old man who developed delirium and rapid heartbeat after surgery. According to the patient's family, he had been taking high doses of valerian root extract (about 2.5 to 10 g per day) for many years. His physicians decided that he was suffering from valerian withdrawal. However, considering the many other factors involved (such as multiple medications and general anesthesia), it isn't really possible to conclude that valerian caused his symptoms.

Except for the unpleasant odor, valerian generally causes no side effects.[27,28] A few people experience mild gastrointestinal distress, and there have been rare reports of people developing a paradoxical mild stimulant effect from valerian.

Valerian does not appear to impair driving ability or produce morning drowsiness when it is taken at night.[29–32] However, there does appear to be some impairment of attention for a couple of hours after taking valerian.[33] For this reason, it isn't a good idea to drive immediately after taking it.

There have been no reported drug interactions with valerian. A 1995 study found no interaction between alcohol and valerian as measured by concentration, attentiveness, reaction time, and driving performance.[34] However, valerian extracts may prolong drug-induced sleeping time in mice, rats, and rabbits.[35,36] Thus, it is possible that valerian could compound the effects of other central-nervous-system depressants.

Safety in young children, pregnant or nursing women, or those with severe liver or kidney disease has not been established.

Melatonin: Rapid Effect on Sleep

The body uses **melatonin** (see page 357) as part of its normal control of the sleep-wake cycle. The pineal gland makes serotonin and then turns it into melatonin when exposure to light decreases. Strong light (such as sunlight) slows melatonin production more than weak light does, and a completely dark room increases the amount of melatonin made more than a partially darkened room does.[37]

Taking melatonin as a supplement seems to stimulate sleep when the natural cycle is disturbed. It has been most studied as a treatment for jet lag. In addition, it may be helpful for individuals who work the night shift and want to change sleeping time on the weekends, as well as for those with ordinary insomnia.

What Is the Scientific Evidence for Melatonin?

There is reasonably good evidence that melatonin can help you fall asleep when your bedtime rhythm has been disturbed,[38–42] although there have been negative studies as well.[43]

One double-blind placebo-controlled study enrolled 320 people and followed them for 4 days after plane travel. The participants were divided into four groups and given a daily dose of 5 mg of standard melatonin, 5 mg of slow-release melatonin, 0.5 mg of standard melatonin, or placebo.[44] The group that received 5 mg of standard melatonin slept better, took less time to fall asleep, and felt more energetic and awake during the day than the other three groups.

According to one review of the literature, melatonin treatment for jet lag is most effective for those who have crossed a significant number of time zones, perhaps eight.[45] One study on travelers found *no* benefit, but it may be that the change in time zones experienced by these travelers wasn't great enough to require melatonin.[46]

Good results were seen in a small double-blind trial of patients in a pulmonary intensive care unit.[47] It is famously difficult to sleep in an ICU, and the resulting sleep deprivation is not helpful for those recovering from disease or surgery. In this study of 8 hospitalized individuals, 3 mg of controlled-release melatonin "dramatically improved" sleep quality and duration.

A study of 19 individuals with schizophrenia who had disturbed sleep patterns found that 2 mg of controlled-release melatonin improved sleep.[48]

Mixed results have been seen in other studies involving swing-shift workers and people with ordinary insomnia.[49–60]

Melatonin might be particularly helpful for individuals who rely on benzodiazepine drugs to sleep.[61] In addition, people trying to quit using sleeping pills may find melatonin helpful. A double-blind placebo-controlled study of 34 individuals who regularly used such medications found that melatonin at a dose of 2 mg nightly (controlled-release formulation) could help them discontinue the use of the drugs.[62]

Note: There can be risks in discontinuing benzodiazepine drugs. Consult your physician for advice.

Dosage

Melatonin is typically taken about 30 minutes before bedtime on the first 4 days after traveling; however, the optimum dose is not clear.

Melatonin is available in two forms: quick-release and slow-release. There is some debate as to which one is better.

Safety Issues

Melatonin is probably safe for occasional use (as in plane travel), but its safety when used on a regular basis remains unknown. Keep in mind that melatonin is not really a food supplement: It is a hormone, just like estrogen, thyroid, or cortisone.

Based on theoretical ideas of how melatonin works, some authorities specifically recommend against its use in depression, schizophrenia, autoimmune diseases, and other serious illnesses and for pregnant or nursing women. Do not drive or operate machinery for several hours after taking melatonin. In addition, melatonin may impair balance.[63]

OTHER PROPOSED TREATMENTS

The following natural treatments are widely recommended for insomnia, but they have not been scientifically proven effective at this time.

Kava

The antianxiety herb kava is also said to be helpful for insomnia. A typical dose of standardized extract should provide about 210 mg of kavalactones and should be taken 1 hour before bedtime. (For more information on use and safety issues, see the chapter on **kava.**)

St. John's Wort

Because prescription antidepressants can help you sleep, it has been suggested that the herb St. John's wort may be useful in the same way.

St. John's wort does not cause immediate drowsiness like some pharmaceutical antidepressants. Rather, if it is effective, the results will develop gradually. (For more information on this herb's uses and safety issues, see the chapter on **St. John's wort.**)

Tryptophan and 5-Hydroxytryptophan

For many years, people used tryptophan as a sleeping aid. However, an accidental poisonous contaminant in one batch caused many cases of a terrible illness called eosinophilic myalgia. Tryptophan has since been taken off the shelves.

The substance 5-HTP (5-hydroxytryptophan) has recently become widely available as a substitute. Because it is made by a completely different manufacturing process (starting from a plant rather than bacteria), one would not expect the same contaminant to appear. Surprisingly, however, in September 1998 the FDA released a report stating that there was some evidence that commercial 5-HTP preparations might contain a similar contaminant.

We suggest you check with your physician for the most recent information.

A typical dosage is 100 to 300 mg at bedtime. (For more information on uses and safety issues, see the chapter on **5-HTP.**)

Other Herbs and Supplements

Many other herbs are reputed to offer sedative or relaxant benefits, including **ashwagandha** (see page 212), **astragalus** (see page 212), **chamomile** (see page 244), **He shou wu** (see page 322), **hops** (see page 324), lady's slipper, **passionflower** (see page 382), and **skullcap** (see page 410). **Vitamin C** (see page 444) is also sometimes recommended. However, there is as yet little scientific evidence that these treatments really work.

INTERMITTENT CLAUDICATION

Related Terms   Peripheral Vascular Disease

Principal Proposed Treatments   Ginkgo, L-Carnitine, Inositol Hexaniacinate, Arginine

Probably Ineffective Treatments   Vitamin E, Beta-Carotene

The arteries supplying the legs with blood may become seriously blocked in advanced stages of **atherosclerosis** (hardening of the arteries; see page 16). This can lead to severe, crampy pain when you walk more than a short distance, because the muscles are starved for oxygen. In fact, the intensity of intermittent claudication is often measured in the distance a person can walk without pain.

Conventional treatment for intermittent claudication consists of measures to combat atherosclerosis, the drug Trental (pentoxifylline), and other medications. In advanced cases, surgery to improve blood flow may be necessary.

PRINCIPAL PROPOSED TREATMENTS

A number of natural treatments may be helpful, but it isn't clear whether it is safe to combine them with the medications that may be prescribed at the same time. Medical supervision is definitely necessary for this serious disease.

Because they work so differently, it has been suggested that the two treatments described in this section, ginkgo and carnitine, might enhance each other's effectiveness when taken together.

Ginkgo

Germany's Commission E authorizes the use of **ginkgo** (see page 298) for the treatment of intermittent claudication. Several preliminary double-blind studies suggest that ginkgo can produce a significant increase in pain-free walking distance, probably by improving circulation.[1,2]

One study enrolled 111 patients and followed them for 24 weeks.[3] Participants were measured for pain-free walking distance by walking up a 12% slope on a treadmill at 2 miles an hour. At the beginning of treatment, both the placebo and ginkgo (120 mg) groups were able to walk about 350 feet without pain.

At the end of the trial, although both groups had improved (the power of placebo is amazing!), the ginkgo group had improved significantly more, showing about a 40% increase in pain-free walking distance as compared to only a 20% improvement in the placebo group.

Similar improvements were also seen in a double-blind placebo-controlled trial of 60 individuals who had achieved maximum benefit from physical therapy.[4]

Taking a higher dose of ginkgo may provide enhanced benefits in intermittent claudication. A 24-week, double-blind placebo-controlled study of 74 individuals found that ginkgo at a dose of 240 mg per day was more effective than 120 mg per day.[5]

Ginkgo generally does not cause side effects, but fears that it may interact with blood-thinning medications make its use in intermittent claudication difficult. To safely use ginkgo, you may have to decline conventional treatment, and this could be a very risky decision. For more details about other uses and safety issues, see the chapter on **ginkgo.**

L-Carnitine

The vitamin-like substance **L-carnitine** (see page 238) also appears to be of some benefit in intermittent claudication. Although it does not increase blood flow, carnitine appears to increase walking distance by improving energy utilization in the muscles.[6]

A recent double-blind study followed 245 people, half of whom were treated with a special form of L-carnitine called L-propionyl-carnitine; the other half took placebo.[7] A dosage of 2,000 mg daily produced an average 73% improvement in walking distance, compared to a 46% improvement in the placebo group. Reductions in pain levels were also reported.

The optimum dosage of L-propionyl-carnitine appears to be 1 to 3 g daily. This apparently safe supplement is not associated with any significant side effects, toxicities, or drug interactions. However, individuals on kidney dialysis should not use L-carnitine (or any other supplement) except on medical advice.

Inositol Hexaniacinate

The supplement inositol hexaniacinate, a special form of **vitamin B$_3$** (see page 437), appears to be helpful for intermittent claudication. Double-blind studies involving a total of about 400 individuals have found that it can improve walking distance for people with intermittent claudication.[8–11] For example, in one study, 100 individuals were given either placebo or 4 g of inositol hexaniacinate daily. Over a period of 3 months, walking distance improved significantly in the treated group.[12]

The usual dose of inositol hexaniacinate is about 1 to 4 g daily. However, due to the risk of liver inflammation, medical supervision is essential.

Arginine

The supplement **arginine** (see page 208) may be able to improve walking distance for people with intermittent claudication. In one study, after 2 weeks of treatment, participants could walk 66% farther than they could at the beginning of the study.[13]

A typical supplemental dosage of arginine is 2 to 3 g per day.

Antioxidants

A double-blind placebo-controlled trial of 1,484 individuals with intermittent claudication found no benefit from **vitamin E** (50 mg daily), **beta-carotene** (20 mg daily), or a combination of the two (see pages 451 and 217, respectively).[14]

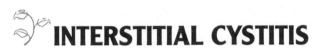

INTERSTITIAL CYSTITIS

Principal Proposed Treatments   Arginine

Other Proposed Treatments   Aortic Glycosaminoglycans, TENS, Dietary Changes

Interstitial cystitis (IC) is a severe, chronic inflammation of the bladder that's both disruptive and painful. Many more women than men suffer from the condition—of the 700,000 people with IC, 90% are female.

The symptoms of IC are notoriously variable and can differ from one person to another, or for one person from day to day. People with IC usually have an urgent and frequent need to urinate. They may experience recurring discomfort, tenderness, pressure, or intense pain in the bladder and surrounding pelvic area. This pain often intensifies as the bladder fills and may be exacerbated by sexual intercourse.

IC is generally diagnosed after other conditions with similar symptoms, such as **bladder infection** (see page 28), **herpes** (see page 86), and **vaginal infection** (see page 182), have been excluded.

The cause of IC is unknown. Although its symptoms resemble a bladder infection, IC does not appear to be caused by bacteria. One theory proposes that IC is caused by an infectious agent that simply hasn't been detected yet. A different theory holds that IC is an autoimmune reaction; still another, that it is related to allergies.

Because it varies so much in symptoms and severity, IC may be not one disease but several.

A variety of treatments are often tried alone or in combination before one is found that works. Oral antihistamines such as hydroxyzine (Atarax) and certirizine (Zyrtec) may provide relief, and the drowsiness they produce often wears off over time. Other medications used for IC include pentosan polysulfate sodium (Elmiron), pyridium, and anti-inflammatory drugs.

Distending the bladder by filling it to capacity with water for 2 to 8 minutes is frequently useful, but although the beneficial effects may persist for months, symptoms usually return eventually. In some cases, medications such as dimethyl sulfoxide and heparin may be introduced into the bladder with a catheter; actual surgical alteration of the bladder is rarely used to treat IC.

PRINCIPAL PROPOSED TREATMENTS

There is some evidence that the supplement arginine might be helpful for IC.

Arginine

Arginine (see page 208) is an amino acid found in many foods including dairy products, meat, poultry, and fish. It's important to many mechanisms in the body, including cell division, wound healing, ammonia removal, immune function, and hormone secretion.

The body also uses arginine to make nitric oxide, which helps to relax smooth muscles like those found in blood vessels and the bladder. Based on this known mechanism, arginine has been proposed as a treatment for various conditions that may be caused by limited blood flow. Similarly, some researchers theorize that arginine's effects on nitric oxide synthesis might help relax the bladder, making it a useful treatment for IC.[1,2]

What Is the Scientific Evidence for Arginine?

Preliminary evidence suggests that oral doses of arginine may reduce the pain and urinary symptoms of IC.

A 3-month double-blind trial of 53 people with IC found that individuals given 1,500 mg of arginine daily experienced greater improvement than those given placebo.[3] However, because a number of participants dropped out of the study, the results can't be taken as conclusive.

Another double-blind study found arginine had no benefit as compared to placebo, but again the study was too small to mean much.[4]

Other, very small, open studies of arginine for interstitial cystitis have found contradictory results.[5,6]

Dosage

A typical supplemental dosage of arginine is 2 to 3 g per day.

Safety Issues

At recommended doses, oral arginine appears to be safe and essentially side-effect free, although minor gastrointestinal upset can occur. However, there are some potential safety concerns with high-dose arginine, based on animal studies and in-hospital intravenous administration.

Arginine has been found to stimulate the body's production of gastrin, a hormone that increases stomach acid.[7] For this reason, there are concerns that arginine could be harmful for individuals with ulcers or for those taking drugs that are hard on the stomach.

Arginine might also alter potassium levels in the body, especially in people with severe liver disease.[8] This is a potential concern for individuals taking drugs that alter potassium balance (such as potassium-sparing diuretics and ACE inhibitors), as well as those with severe kidney disease. If you fall into any of these categories, do not use high-dose arginine except under physician supervision.

Maximum safe doses of arginine in pregnant or nursing women, young children, and people with severe liver or kidney disease have not been established.

OTHER PROPOSED TREATMENTS

Glycosaminoglycans

There is some evidence that in interstitial cystitis the surface layer of the bladder is deficient in protective natural substances called glycosaminoglycans.[9] This in turn might allow the bladder to become inflamed; it might also initiate autoimmune reactions.

Based on these highly preliminary findings, taking supplemental **glycosaminoglycans** (see page 207) have been suggested for interstitial cystitis. However, there is no evidence as yet that they would be helpful.

TENS

Transcutaneous electrical stimulation, or TENS, is primarily used (with mixed results) in the treatment of muscular pain. It has also been tried in interstitial cystitis, but thus far the evidence that it works is highly preliminary.[10]

Diet

Although there is no solid scientific evidence that dietary changes can relieve IC, many people find that certain foods increase their symptoms. The most frequently cited offenders are coffee, chocolate, ethanol, carbonated drinks, citrus fruits, and tomatoes.[11] Based on these reports, it may be worthwhile to experiment with your diet.

IRRITABLE BOWEL SYNDROME

Related Terms   Spastic Colon

Principal Proposed Treatments   Peppermint Oil, Friendly Bacteria, Flaxseed

Other Proposed Treatments   *Coleus forskohlii,* Slippery Elm, Glutamine, Avoidance of Allergenic Foods

Irritable Bowel Syndrome

Visit Us at TNP.com

The symptoms of irritable bowel syndrome (IBS) include one or more of the following: alternating diarrhea and constipation, intestinal gas, bloating and cramping, abdominal pain, painful bowel movements, mucous discharge, and undigested food in the stool. Despite all these distressing symptoms, in IBS the intestines appear to be perfectly healthy when they are examined. Thus the condition belongs to a category of diseases that physicians call *functional*. This term means that while the function of the bowel seems to have gone awry, no injury or disturbance of its structure can be discovered.

The cause of IBS remains unknown. Medical treatment for irritable bowel syndrome consists mainly of increased dietary fiber plus drugs that reduce bowel spasm. In addition, various forms of psychotherapy, including hypnosis, have been tried, with some success.[1–6]

PRINCIPAL PROPOSED TREATMENTS

Peppermint

Peppermint (see page 384) oil is widely used for IBS. However, the research evidence is a bit contradictory.[7–11] The proper dosage is 1 or 2 capsules (0.2 ml per capsule) 3 times daily between meals. Because dosage amounts of peppermint needed to relieve lower bowel cramping can cause heartburn, the best formulations are enteric coated to pass intact through the stomach (this is usually stated on the label).

When taken as directed, peppermint is believed to be reasonably safe in healthy adults.[12] However, peppermint can cause jaundice in newborn babies, so do not try to use it for colic. Excessive intake of peppermint oil can cause nausea, loss of appetite, heart problems, loss of balance, and other nervous system problems.

Safety in pregnant or nursing women or those with severe liver or kidney disease has not been established.

Friendly Bacteria (Probiotics)

Friendly bacteria (see page 200) may be helpful for IBS.

In a 4-week double-blind placebo-controlled trial of 60 individuals with IBS, probiotic treatment with *Lactobacillus plantarum* reduced intestinal gas significantly.[13] The benefits persisted for an additional year after treatment was stopped.

Benefits were also seen in a smaller double-blind trial using *L. acidophilus*.[14]

Flaxseeds

In a double-blind study, 55 people with chronic constipation caused by irritable bowel syndrome received either ground **flaxseed** (see page 286) or psyllium seed (a well-known treatment for constipation) daily for 3 months.[15] Those taking flaxseed had significantly fewer problems with constipation, abdominal pain, and bloating than those taking psyllium. The flaxseed group had even further improvements in constipation and bloating while continuing their treatment in the 3 months after the double-blind study ended. The researcher concluded that flaxseed relieved constipation more effectively than psyllium.

OTHER PROPOSED TREATMENTS

The herbs ***Coleus forskohlii*** (see page 259) and **slippery elm** (see page 411) as well as the supplement **glutamine** (see page 310) are also sometimes recommended for IBS, but there is little to no evidence as yet that they really work.

Food allergies (see page 82) may also play a role in IBS, and diets based on identifying and eliminating allergenic foods are reportedly successful at times.[16–22]

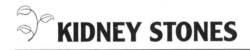

KIDNEY STONES

Related Terms   Renal Calculi, Nephrolithiasis, Urolithiasis, Calcium Oxalate Stones

Principal Proposed Treatments   Citrate

Other Proposed Treatments   Magnesium, Vitamin B$_6$, Goldenrod, Parsley, Fish Oil, GLA (Gamma-Linolenic Acid), Aortic GAGs, Vitamin A, Vitamin C, Calcium

If you've ever passed a kidney stone, you do not want to repeat the experience! The sharp and irregular stones travel down the slender tube (ureter) leading from the kidney to the urethra, following the path by which urine exits the body. While tiny stones may pass

unnoticed, a larger stone can induce some of the worst pain that humans experience.

Most kidney stones are composed of calcium and oxalic acid, substances present in the urine that can crystallize inside the kidneys. Although these chemicals occur in everyone's urine, our natural biochemistry is usually able to prevent them from crystallizing. However, sometimes these protective methods fail and a stone develops. This chapter focuses mainly on these "calcium oxalate stones."

Less commonly, kidney stones may be made from calcium and phosphate, from another substance called struvite (usually the result of an infection) or, rarely, from uric acid or cystine.

It isn't known why some people develop kidney stones and others do not. However, once you've had a stone, you are fairly likely to develop another.

Low fluid intake greatly increases the risk of developing virtually all types of stones.[1,2,3] For this reason, individuals at risk of developing stones are often advised to increase their fluid intake. However, while there is evidence that fluids in the form of coffee, tea, beer, and wine can decrease risk of kidney stone development, apple juice and grapefruit juice appear to have the opposite effect.[4,5]

High intakes of sodium[6,7] and protein (particularly animal protein) may also increase the risk of calcium oxalate stones,[8,9] although some studies have found that protein has no such effect.[10] Oxalate-rich foods such as spinach and cocoa may also increase the risk of developing calcium oxalate stones. Vitamin D affects calcium levels in the body, and prolonged use of extremely excessive doses of vitamin D has been known to cause kidney stones. Strangely, however, high-calcium foods don't seem to increase the risk of calcium oxalate stones (see Other Proposed Treatments).

Conventional treatment for kidney stones varies depending on symptoms as well as the location and chemical composition of the stones. For those who pass a stone spontaneously, the main treatments are painkillers and fluids. The chemical composition of passed stones can be analyzed to determine their cause. Other stones may be detected earlier, when they are still in the kidney. Treatment depends on their location and symptoms. Those causing problems may be treated with "extracorporeal shock-wave lithotripsy," a technique that can break up these stones from outside the body, allowing them to pass more easily. Occasionally, however, surgery may be necessary.

"Silent" stones, or those causing no symptoms, are often treated with preventive measures alone. These methods include increasing fluids, modifying the diet, and taking drugs or supplements to alter the chemistry of the urine.

PRINCIPAL PROPOSED TREATMENTS

Citrate

Citrate, or citric acid, is an ordinary component of our diet, present in high amounts in citrus fruits. Citrate binds with calcium in the urine, thereby reducing the amount of calcium available to form calcium oxalate stones. It also prevents tiny calcium oxalate crystals from growing and massing together into larger stones. Finally, it makes the urine less acidic, which inhibits the development of both calcium oxalate and uric acid stones.

One form of citrate supplement, potassium citrate, was approved by the FDA in 1985 for the prevention of two kinds of kidney stones: calcium stones (including calcium oxalate stones) and uric acid stones.

In a 3-year double-blind study of 57 people with a history of calcium stones and low urinary citrate levels, those given potassium citrate developed fewer kidney stones than they had previously. In comparison, the group given placebo had no change in their rate of stone formation.[11]

Potassium-magnesium citrate, a relatively new citrate source, was studied in a 3-year trial involving 64 participants with a history of calcium oxalate stones.[12] During the study, new stones formed in only 12.9% of those taking the potassium-magnesium citrate supplement, compared to a whopping 63.6% of those taking placebo.

Citrate is also available in the form of calcium citrate. Besides increasing citrate in the urine, this supplement has the advantage of being a readily absorbed form of calcium for those seeking to increase their calcium intake for other health reasons.[13] However, calcium citrate has not yet been studied as a preventive for kidney stones.

Some physicians have proposed drinking citrus juices as a means of increasing urinary citrate levels. Like potassium citrate, orange juice decreases urinary acidity and raises urinary citrate, but it also raises urinary oxalate, which might tend to work against its beneficial effects.[14] Lemon juice may be preferable, as it has almost five times the citrate of orange juice. A small study found that drinking 2 liters of lemonade a day doubled urinary citrate in people with decreased urinary citrate.[15] Avoid regular consumption of grapefruit juice, though: in one large-scale study, women drinking 8 ounces of grapefruit juice daily increased their risk of stones by 44%.[16]

It was first thought that citrate supplements were only helpful against kidney stones in individuals who didn't excrete the normal amount of citrate in their urine.[17] However, some researchers now suggest that citrate treatment may also be useful for those at risk for stones whose citrate excretion is normal.[18]

Dosage

The proper dosage of citrate depends on the chemical form and should be individualized under medical supervision.

Safety Issues

Potassium citrate can irritate the gastrointestinal tract, causing upset stomach or bloating in 9 to 17% of people.[19] Potassium-magnesium citrate may potentially cause the same problem, although one study found it to be no more irritating than placebo.[20]

Supplements containing potassium have the potential to raise blood levels of potassium too high, primarily in people with impaired kidneys or those taking a potassium-sparing diuretic such as triamterene. Taking too much citrate can also result in overly alkaline blood, again particularly in people with kidney disease.

Citrate-induced reduction of urinary acidity can lead to decreased blood levels and effectiveness of numerous drugs, including lithium, methotrexate, oral diabetes drugs, aspirin and other salicylates, and tetracycline antibiotics.[21] In addition, the urinary antiseptic methenamine is less effective in alkaline urine. Conversely, the blood levels of other drugs could increase, possibly increasing risk of toxicity. These drugs include stimulants such as ephedrine and methamphetamine, as well as the drugs flecainide and mecamylamine.

OTHER PROPOSED TREATMENTS

There is some evidence that magnesium and vitamin B_6 might help prevent kidney stones. Other herbs and supplements are often recommended as well, although there is little evidence that they work. Vitamin C and calcium are often said to raise the risk of kidney stones, but evidence suggests that in most (but not all) cases they might actually help prevent them.

Magnesium

Magnesium (see page 351), in the form of magnesium oxide or magnesium hydroxide, may help to prevent calcium oxalate stone development. Magnesium inhibits the growth of these stones in the test tube[22] and decreases stone formation in rats.[23]

However, human studies on magnesium have shown mixed results.[24–27] In one 2-year open study, 56 participants taking magnesium hydroxide had fewer recurrences of kidney stones than 34 participants not given magnesium.[28] In contrast, a double-blind (hence, more reliable) study with 124 participants found that magnesium hydroxide was essentially no more effective than placebo.[29]

Vitamin B_6

Vitamin B_6 (see page 439) might help prevent calcium oxalate stones in certain individuals. Deficiencies in this vitamin increase the amount of oxalate in the urine of animals and humans,[30] and a small uncontrolled study found that supplementation decreased oxalate excretion in people with a history of stones.[31] In addition, a 14-year study of more than 85,000 women with no history of kidney stones found that women with high intakes of B_6 developed fewer stones than those with the lowest in-

take.[32] On the other hand, a large-scale study of more than 45,000 men found no link between B_6 and stones.[33]

Miscellaneous Herbs and Supplements

In Europe, the herb **goldenrod** (see page 313) is sometimes used to help wash out kidney stones. It is believed to increase the flow of urine and therefore might help pass kidney stones and soothe inflamed tissues. However, there is as yet no evidence that it helps.

Germany's Commission E has also recommended the following herbs for kidney stones based primarily on their apparent ability to increase the flow of urine: asparagus, birch leaf, bishop's weed fruit, couch grass, **parsley** (see page 381), horsetail, java, lovage, petasites, shiny restharrow, and stinging nettle herb and root combination.[34] However, there is little to no evidence that they are really effective.

Several other supplements, including **fish oil** (see page 282), **GLA** (see page 304), **glycosaminoglycans** (GAGs; see page 207), and **vitamin A** (see page 432) are sometimes recommended for kidney stones, but there is little solid evidence that they work.[35–38]

Vitamin C and Calcium: Help or Harm?

One of the biggest controversies surrounding the causes of kidney stones has to do with **vitamin C** (see page 444). Early studies suggested that high vitamin C intake could increase oxalate in the urine and thereby potentially raise the risk of kidney stones. However, more recent research indicates that this conclusion was due to imperfect measurement techniques.[39] In large-scale observational studies, individuals who consume large amounts of vitamin C have shown either no change or a decreased risk of kidney stone formation.[40,41,42] Nonetheless, it seems that in some individuals high vitamin C intake can lead to a rapid increase in urinary oxalate, and in one case stones developed within a few days.[43] The bottom line: People with a history of kidney stones should probably limit vitamin C supplements to about 100 mg daily.[44]

There is also a controversy about **calcium** (see page 234). In the past, doctors frequently advised people with a history of calcium oxalate stones to reduce their calcium consumption. The reasoning was obvious: Since you need calcium to make such stones, reducing calcium intake might be expected to protect against them. Surprisingly, large observational studies have since suggested that higher calcium intake actually *lowers* the risk of developing these stones.[45] This effect, however, may be limited to calcium consumed as part of the diet. In a later study, the researchers explored how calcium supplements, compared to dietary calcium, affected the risk of kidney stones in more than 90,000 women. They found that dietary calcium decreased the risk of stones while supplemental calcium slightly increased the risk.[46]

Many of the women taking supplements took them on an empty stomach, and the researchers theorized that calcium supplements might be more effective at decreasing the risk of stones if taken with food. It is also possible that different types of calcium supplements have different effects on the development of kidney stones.

The bottom line: Restriction of calcium—whether supplemental or dietary—may still be appropriate for certain people.[47] Ask your physician for advice specific to you.

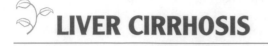

LIVER CIRRHOSIS

Related Terms   Cirrhosis of the Liver, Biliary Cirrhosis, Alcoholic Liver Cirrhosis

Principal Proposed Treatments   Milk Thistle

Other Proposed Treatments   SAMe, BCAAs, OPCs, Taurine, Phosphatidylcholine, Calcium and Vitamin D, Antioxidants

The liver is a marvelously sophisticated chemical laboratory, capable of carrying out thousands of chemical transformations on which the body depends. The liver produces important chemicals from scratch, modifies others to allow the body to use them better, and neutralizes an enormous range of toxins. Without a functioning liver, you can't live for very long.

Unfortunately, a number of influences can severely damage the liver. Alcohol is the most common. This powerful liver toxin harms the liver in three stages: these are called alcoholic fatty liver, alcoholic hepatitis, and alcoholic cirrhosis. Although the first two stages of injury are usually reversible, alcoholic cirrhosis is not. Generally, more than 10 years of heavy alcohol abuse is required to cause liver cirrhosis. Other causes include hepatitis C infection, primary biliary cirrhosis, and drug toxicity.

A cirrhotic liver is firm and nodular to the touch, and in advanced cases is shrunken in size. These changes reflect severe damage to its structure. A high percentage of liver cells have died, and fibrous scar-like tissue permeates the organ.

A cirrhotic liver cannot perform its chemical tasks, leading to wide-ranging impairment of bodily functions, such as the development of jaundice (yellowing of the skin due to unprocessed toxins), mental confusion, emaciation, and skin changes. In addition, the fibrous tissue impedes blood that is supposed to pass through the liver. This leads to abdominal swelling as fluid backs up (ascites), and to bleeding in the esophagus as veins expand to provide an alternative fluid path. Ultimately, coma develops, often triggered by internal bleeding or infection.

Treatments for liver cirrhosis begin with stopping the use of alcohol and all other liver-toxic substances. A number of treatments such as potassium-sparing diuretics can ameliorate symptoms to some extent, but they do not cure the disease.

The liver is too complex for a man-made machine to duplicate its functions, so there is no equivalent of kidney dialysis for liver cirrhosis. Only a liver transplant can help. Unfortunately, this is a very difficult operation, with a high failure rate. In addition, the supply of usable livers is inadequate to meet the need.

PRINCIPAL PROPOSED TREATMENTS
Milk Thistle

The herb **milk thistle** (see page 361) appears to offer numerous liver-protective benefits. In Europe, it is used to treat viral hepatitis, alcoholic fatty liver, alcoholic hepatitis, and drug- or chemical-induced liver toxicity. An intravenous preparation made from milk thistle is used as an antidote for poisoning by the liver-toxic deathcap mushroom, *Amanita phalloides*.

Milk thistle appears to be helpful for liver cirrhosis as well, significantly prolonging survival.

What Is the Scientific Evidence for Milk Thistle?

A double-blind placebo-controlled study followed 146 people with liver cirrhosis for 3 to 6 years. In the group treated with milk thistle, the 4-year survival rate was 58% as compared to only 38% in the placebo group.[1]

Another double-blind placebo-controlled trial followed 172 individuals with liver cirrhosis for 4 years, and also found a significant reduction in mortality with milk thistle.[2]

However, a 2-year double-blind placebo-controlled study that followed 125 individuals with alcoholic cirrhosis found no reduction in mortality.[3] It may be that the study was not long enough to reproduce the benefits seen in the other studies.

Dosage

The standard dosage of milk thistle for liver cirrhosis is 200 mg 3 times daily of an extract standardized to contain 70% silymarin (a chemical in the herb); alternatively, this can be stated as 420 mg of silymarin daily.

Some evidence supports the idea that silymarin bound to phosphatidylcholine is better absorbed.[4,5] This form should be taken at a dosage of 100 to 200 mg twice daily.

Safety Issues

Milk thistle appears to be essentially nontoxic. Animal studies have not shown any negative effects even when high doses were administered over a long period of time.[6,7] A study of 2,637 participants reported in 1992 showed a low incidence of side effects, limited mainly to mild gastrointestinal disturbance.[8] However, on rare occasions, severe abdominal discomfort may occur.[9]

On the basis of its extensive use as a food in England at the turn of the twentieth century, milk thistle is believed to be safe for pregnant and nursing mothers, and researchers have enrolled pregnant women in studies of the herb.[10] However, safety in young children, pregnant or nursing women, and individuals with severe renal disease has not been formally established. No harmful drug interactions are known.

One report has noted that silibinin (a constituent of silymarin) can inhibit a bacterial enzyme called beta-glucuronidase, which plays a role in the activity of certain drugs, such as oral contraceptives.[11] This could conceivably interfere with the action of these drugs.

OTHER PROPOSED TREATMENTS

SAMe: May Improve Survival in Liver Cirrhosis

Individuals with liver cirrhosis have difficulty synthesizing the substance **SAMe** (S-adenosylmethionine; see page 403) from the amino acid **methionine** (see page 360).[12,13] For this reason, supplemental SAMe (best known as a treatment for depression and arthritis) has been tried as a treatment for cirrhosis. However, as yet the evidence that it works is not strong.

A 2-year double-blind placebo-controlled trial followed 117 people with liver cirrhosis.[14] Overall, those given SAMe didn't do significantly better than those given placebo. However, when the results were reevaluated to eliminate individuals with severe liver cirrhosis, a significant reduction in mortality and liver transplantation was seen with SAMe.

A typical dose of SAMe is 400 mg 3 times daily. SAMe appears to be quite safe, according to both human and animal studies.[15–18] Its most common side effect is mild digestive distress. Like other substances with anti-depressant activity, SAMe might trigger a manic episode in individuals with **bipolar disorder** (manic-depressive illness; see page 27).[19–24]

SAMe might interfere with the action of the Parkinson's drug levodopa.[25] In addition, there may also be risks involved in combining SAMe with standard antidepressants.[26] For this reason, you shouldn't try either combination except under physician supervision.

BCAAs: Might Be Helpful for Hepatic Encephalopathy

In advanced liver cirrhosis, individuals experience severe mental confusion and may slip into a coma. This condition is called hepatic encephalopathy. One of the primary causes of hepatic encephalopathy is excessive ammonia levels in the body.

There is some reason to believe that special amino acids called BCAAs (branched-chain amino acids) might be helpful for individuals with hepatic encephalopathy, based on how they are metabolized in the body.[27] However, the evidence that BCAAs actually help is not yet conclusive.

For more information, see the chapter on **BCAAs**.

OPCs: Might Help Prevent Internal Bleeding

Individuals with cirrhosis are susceptible to internal bleeding. Highly preliminary evidence suggests that OPCs (oligomeric proanthocyanidins) might help prevent this problem.[28]

OPCs are best documented as a treatment for **varicose veins** (see page 184), where they are thought to work in part by stabilizing blood vessels. Individuals with cirrhosis have what amounts to internal varicose veins, caused by the shunting of fluid around the damaged liver. For more information, see the chapter on **OPCs**.

Other Natural Treatments That Might Help

The amino acid **taurine** (see page 420) might help reduce muscle cramps in individuals with cirrhosis.[29]

One study suggests that a diet high in protein from vegetable sources rather than animal sources might be helpful,[30] presumably due to differences in amino acid content.

Preliminary evidence from animal studies suggest that the supplement **phosphatidylcholine** (see page 248) might help protect against the development of alcoholic liver cirrhosis.[31]

The bones of individuals with biliary cirrhosis often become thin. Taking **calcium** (see page 234) and **vitamin D** (see page 449) supplements might help.[32,33] Antioxidants such as **beta-carotene** (see page 217), **vitamin C** (see page 444), **vitamin E** (see page 451), and **lipoic acid** (see page 347) have been tried for biliary cirrhosis, with promising results.[34]

LUPUS

Related Terms   Systemic Lupus Erythematosus, SLE

Principal Proposed Treatments   DHEA

Other Proposed Treatments   Flaxseed, Fish Oil, Beta-Carotene, Magnesium, Selenium, Vitamin B_3, Vitamin B_{12}, Vitamin E, Pantothenic Acid, Food Allergen Identification and Avoidance, Alfalfa (an Herb to Avoid)

Systemic lupus erythematosus (lupus or SLE for short) is an autoimmune disease that primarily affects women of childbearing age. Its cause is unknown, but is believed to involve both genetic inheritance and factors in the environment. Whatever the cause, individuals with SLE develop antibodies against substances in their own bodies, including DNA. These antibodies cause widespread damage and are believed to be primarily responsible for the many symptoms of this disease.

SLE may begin with such symptoms as fatigue, weight loss, fever, malaise, and loss of appetite. Other common early symptoms include muscle pain, joint pain, and facial rash. As SLE progresses, symptoms may develop in virtually every part of the body. Kidney damage is one of the most devastating effects of SLE, but many other serious problems may develop as well, including seizures, mental impairment, anemia, and inflammation of the heart, blood vessels, eyes, and digestive tract.

Conventional treatment for SLE revolves around anti-inflammatory drugs. In mild cases, taking nonsteroidal anti-inflammatory drugs (NSAIDs) may help; more severe forms of SLE require long-term use of corticosteroid anti-inflammatory drugs such as prednisone. The side effects of these medications can be quite serious themselves. So-called cytotoxic agents (azathioprine, cyclophosphamide, and chlorambucil) might also be helpful, but they have many side effects as well.

Close physician supervision is always required with lupus due to the risk of complications in so many organs.

PRINCIPAL PROPOSED TREATMENTS

Increasing evidence tells us that the hormone dehydroepiandrosterone (DHEA) may be helpful for the treatment of lupus, when used as a part of a comprehensive, physician-directed treatment approach.

DHEA

Dehydroepiandrosterone (DHEA) (see page 268), a hormone produced by the adrenal glands, is the most abundant steroid hormone found in the bloodstream. Your body uses DHEA as the starting material for making the sex hormones testosterone and estrogen. DHEA has been tried as a treatment for a variety of medical conditions, including **osteoporosis** (see page 136), but it is showing its greatest promise in the treatment of SLE.

What Is the Scientific Evidence for DHEA?

A 12-month double-blind placebo-controlled trial of 381 women with mild or moderate lupus evaluated the effects of DHEA at a dose of 200 mg daily.[1] Although many participants in both groups improved (the power of placebo is amazing!), DHEA was more effective than placebo, reducing many symptoms of the disease. Similarly positive results were seen in earlier small studies.[2,3]

Even if DHEA is not strong enough to completely control symptoms of SLE on its own, it might allow a reduction in dosage of the more dangerous standard medications. In addition, it might directly help offset some of the side effects of corticosteroid treatment, such as accelerated osteoporosis.[4,5] (**Calcium**, **vitamin D**, and **ipriflavone** might also help prevent corticosteroid-induced osteoporosis. See these chapters for more information.)

DHEA itself is relatively safe (especially in comparison to corticosteroids and cytotoxic drugs). One study found no significant side effects in 50 women who took up to 200 mg of DHEA daily for up to 1 year.[6] However, even at the low dose of 25 mg per day, DHEA may decrease levels of HDL ("good") cholesterol.[7,8] In addition, DHEA may cause **acne** (see page 2) and growth of facial hair.[9,10]

The safety of DHEA in young children, pregnant or nursing women, and individuals with severe liver or kidney disease has not been established. We also don't know whether DHEA interacts with other hormone treatments, such as estrogen, although it certainly stands to reason that it might. In particular, DHEA might raise the risk of various hormone-related cancers, such as breast cancer.

OTHER PROPOSED TREATMENTS

Flaxseed contains lignans and alpha-linolenic acid, substances with a wide variety of effects in the body. In particular, flaxseed may antagonize the activity of a substance called platelet-activating factor (PAF) that plays a role in SLE kidney disease (lupus nephritis). Preliminary evidence suggests that flaxseed might help prevent or treat lupus nephritis.[11,12]

Fish oil (see page 282) contains omega-3 fatty acids, which have some anti-inflammatory effects. Fish oil has been found useful in **rheumatoid arthritis** (see page 151), a disease related to SLE. The results of a small double-blind crossover trial suggest that fish oil might be useful for SLE as well, but more study is needed.[13] Current evidence suggests that fish oil is specifically *not* effective for lupus nephritis.[14,15]

Other treatments sometimes recommended for SLE include **beta-carotene** (see page 217), **magnesium** (see page 351), **selenium** (see page 407), **vitamin B₃** (see page 437), **vitamin B₁₂** (see page 442), **vitamin E** (see page 451), **pantothenic acid** (see page 380), and food allergen identification and avoidance. However, there is no real evidence as yet that these treatments work for lupus.

Alfalfa: An Herb to Avoid

The herb **alfalfa** (see page 202) contains a substance called L-canavanine, which can worsen SLE or bring it out of remission. Individuals with SLE should avoid alfalfa entirely.[16,17]

MACULAR DEGENERATION

Principal Proposed Treatments
   Antioxidants: Vitamin C, Vitamin E, Selenium, Beta-Carotene, Lutein, Zeaxanthin, Lycopene, Bilberry, Ginkgo, Grape Seed (as a Source of OPCs)
   Wine

Other Proposed Treatments   Zinc

The lens of the eye focuses an image of the world on a portion of the retina called the *macula*, the area of finest visual perception. After cataracts, damage to the macula is the second most common cause of visual impairment in those over 65. Smoking, high blood pressure, and atherosclerosis are associated with macular degeneration. Bright light also appears to play a role by creating damaging natural substances in the eye, called free radicals. Gradual deterioration of the macula is called macular degeneration.

In the most common form of macular degeneration, a substance known as lipofuscin accumulates in the lining of the retina. No conventional medical treatment is available for this disease, although mainstream researchers are seriously investigating the antioxidants described here.

A much less common form of macular degeneration involves the abnormal growth of blood vessels. This can be treated very successfully, if attended to soon enough, but may lead to irreversible blindness if left untreated. For this reason, medical consultation in all cases of macular degeneration (or any other type of vision loss) is essential.

PRINCIPAL PROPOSED TREATMENTS

Because research suggests that macular degeneration may be related to free radical damage, it's natural to reason that antioxidant nutrients may be able to protect against it. However, more research is necessary for firm conclusions.

An observational study of 2,152 subjects, aged 43 to 86, found that vitamin C supplementation was associated with a decreased incidence of early age-related macular degeneration.[1] Another observational study enrolling almost 2,000 people found that high intake of vitamin C or vitamin E was associated with less macular degeneration.[2]

It may be that combinations of many antioxidants, such as those found in foods, are most beneficial. One 18-month, double-blind study found that a daily supplement containing 750 mg of vitamin C, 200 IU of vitamin E, 50 mcg of selenium, and 20,000 IU of beta-carotene (along with other ingredients) stopped the progression of macular degeneration.[3] (See the chapters on **vitamin C, vitamin E,** and **selenium** for more information and safety issues.)

Various dietary carotenes may also be associated with a lower incidence of macular degeneration.[4,5] Carotenes (carotenoids) are a group of substances that are found in many fruits and vegetables, especially yellow-orange and dark-green ones. **Beta-carotene** (see page 217) is the most famous carotene. However, the less well-known carotenes **lutein** (see page 348) and zeaxanthin may be more closely correlated with protection from macular degeneration. These are principally found in dark-green leafy vegetables, such as spinach and collard greens. It has been suggested that lutein may protect the macula

Male Infertility

from light-induced damage by dyeing it yellow, thereby acting as a kind of natural sunglasses.[6,7] It also acts in the usual antioxidant fashion by neutralizing free radicals.[8] **Lycopene** (see page 349), a carotenoid found in tomatoes, may also be helpful.

Flavonoids are another group of naturally occurring chemicals, found in many plants, that may offer a variety of beneficial effects. Weak but interesting evidence suggests that the flavonoid-rich herbs **bilberry** (see page 220), **ginkgo** (see page 298), and **OPCs** (see page 373) may prevent or treat macular degeneration.[9,10,11]

Moderate wine consumption appears to help prevent macular degeneration.[12] Like these herbs, wine contains high levels of flavonoids.

OTHER PROPOSED TREATMENTS

The mineral **zinc** (see page 463) may also help prevent macular degeneration, although the study results are a bit contradictory.[13,14,15] A typical dosage is 15 to 30 mg daily, combined with 1 to 3 mg of **copper** (see page 262) to avoid zinc-induced copper deficiency. Too much zinc can be toxic, so do not exceed this dose.

MALE INFERTILITY

Principal Proposed Treatments   There are no well-established natural treatments for male infertility.

Other Proposed Treatments   Vitamin B$_{12}$, Zinc
 Antioxidants: Vitamin E, Vitamin C
 Ashwagandha, Pygeum, L-Arginine, Beta-Carotene, L-Carnitine, Coenzyme Q$_{10}$ (CoQ$_{10}$), PABA (Para-Aminobenzoic Acid), Selenium, Docosahexaenoic Acid (DHA)

Not Recommended Treatments   Licorice

Male infertility, the inability of a man to produce a pregnancy in a woman, can be caused by a great variety of problems, from anatomical defects to hormonal imbalances. In about half of all cases, however, the source of the problem is never discovered.

The good news is that without any treatment at all, about 25% of supposedly infertile men bring about a pregnancy within a year of the time they first visit a physician for treatment. In other words, infertility is often only low fertility in disguise.

PROPOSED TREATMENTS

The following natural treatments are widely recommended for male infertility, but they have not been scientifically proven effective at this time.

Vitamin B$_{12}$

Mild B$_{12}$ deficiencies are relatively common in people over 60.[1,2] Such deficiencies lead to reduced sperm counts and lowered sperm mobility. Thus **vitamin B$_{12}$** (see page 442) supplementation has been tried for improving fertility in men with abnormal sperm production.

In one double-blind study of 375 infertile men, supplementation with vitamin B$_{12}$ produced no benefits on average in the group as a whole.[3] However, in a particular subgroup of men with sufficiently low sperm count

and sperm motility, B$_{12}$ appeared to be helpful. Such "dredging" of the data is suspect from a scientific point of view, however, and this study cannot be taken as proof of effectiveness.

Vitamin B$_{12}$ is believed to be extremely safe.

Zinc

Zinc (see page 463) is also an essential nutrient for proper sperm production, and deficiency may result in lowered testosterone levels.[4] One small, uncontrolled study found not only an increase in sperm counts, but also an actual increase in pregnancy rate when men with low testosterone were given zinc supplements.[5] However, participants with normal testosterone levels did not benefit. The usual recommended dosage of zinc is about 15 to 30 mg daily, coupled with 1 mg of **copper** (see page 262) for balance. Too much zinc can be toxic, so do not exceed this dose.

Antioxidants

Free radicals, dangerous chemicals found naturally in the body, may damage sperm. For this reason, a number of studies have evaluated the benefits of antioxidants for male infertility.

In a double-blind placebo-controlled study of 110 men whose sperm showed subnormal activity, daily treatment with 100 IU of vitamin E resulted in improved sperm activity and increased rate of pregnancy in their

Visit Us at TNP.com

partners.[6] (For more information and safety issues, see the chapter on **vitamin E.**)

Preliminary studies suggest that vitamin C may improve sperm count and function.[7] However, a recent double-blind study of 31 individuals that tested both vitamin C and vitamin E found no benefit.[8] The dosages studied ranged from 200 to 1,000 mg daily. (For a discussion of safety issues, see the chapter on **vitamin C.**)

Other Herbs and Supplements

Many other substances have been suggested as treatments for infertility, including the herbs **ashwagandha** (see page 212) and **pygeum** (see page 395), as well as the supplements **L-arginine** (see page 208), **beta-carotene** (see page 217), **L-carnitine** (see page 238), **coenzyme Q$_{10}$** (see page 256), **PABA** (see page 379), and **selenium** (see page 407). However, the evidence that they really work is negligible, and studies on the last three supplements have shown more negative than positive results.

Docosahexaenoic acid (DHA), a component of **fish oil** (see page 282), has also been evaluated as a possible treatment for infertility, but a double-blind trial of 28 men with impaired sperm activity found no benefit.[9]

All the treatments listed in the chapter on **impotence** have also been proposed as treatments for male infertility.

Not Recommended Treatments

The herb **licorice** (see page 344) may reduce testosterone levels in men.[10] For this reason, men with impotence, infertility, or decreased libido may want to avoid this herb.

MENOPAUSAL SYMPTOMS (Other Than Osteoporosis)

Principal Proposed Treatments   Black Cohosh, Soy Isoflavones

Other Proposed Treatments   Progesterone Cream, Flaxseed, Vitamin C, Bioflavonoids, Essential Fatty Acids, Gamma Oryzanol, Licorice, Suma, Chasteberry, Vitamin E, Red Clover, Alfalfa, Dong Quai, Estriol

The hormonal changes of menopause can produce a wide variety of symptoms, ranging from hot flashes and vaginal dryness to anxiety, depression, and insomnia. Many of these symptoms are undoubtedly caused by the natural decrease in estrogen production that occurs at menopause; however, the human body is so complex that other hormonal factors also play a role.

Menopause is not a disease. It is clearly a natural process, but one that has fallen out of favor in modern society. We no longer consider it as an inevitable transition but instead regard it as a condition requiring treatment. No longer do women accept as merely part of life the decrease in libido, pain during intercourse, years of hot flashes, and other uncomfortable problems that may accompany menopause. This raises an important point: How close to nature do we want to live? One of the most valued ideals of alternative medicine is the desire to trust nature, but sometimes we may want to draw a line. For example, in a state of nature, infant and maternal mortality is high. This process of survival of the fittest helps humanity as a species to be stronger, but it is not something that a compassionate society can tolerate. Thus, no matter what our ideals, we frequently find ourselves tampering with nature. The treatment of menopause is simply one example among many.

Conventional medicine recommends the use of replacement estrogen to provide three benefits: eliminating the symptoms of menopause, protecting against osteoporosis, and maintaining the protection against cardiovascular disease that premenopausal women enjoy.

Estrogen-replacement therapy is quite effective at achieving these goals. However, like most medical treatments, it creates counterbalancing risks. The most frightening issue is the increased risk of breast cancer that appears to be associated with replacement estrogen. The decision whether to use estrogen-replacement therapy should involve a careful examination of the risks and benefits in consultation with a physician. Specially modified estrogens, such as Evista (raloxifene), appear to help osteoporosis and reduce the incidence of breast cancer, but they do not reduce symptoms of menopause.

PRINCIPAL PROPOSED TREATMENTS

Several natural treatments may reduce menopausal symptoms. However, we do not know for sure whether any of these reduce the risk of cardiovascular disease or osteoporosis. (See the chapters on **atherosclerosis** and

Menopausal Symptoms

osteoporosis for natural ways to reduce the risk of these conditions.)

Black Cohosh: Widely Used in Europe for Menopausal Symptoms

Black cohosh (see page 223) is a tall perennial herb that was originally found in the northeastern United States. Native Americans used it mainly for women's health problems but also as a treatment for arthritis, fatigue, and snakebite. European colonists rapidly adopted the herb for similar uses.

In the late nineteenth century, black cohosh was the main ingredient in the wildly popular Lydia E. Pinkham's Vegetable Compound for menstrual cramps. Migrating across the Atlantic, black cohosh became a popular European treatment for women's problems, arthritis, and high blood pressure. In the 1980s, black cohosh was approved by Germany's Commission E for use in menopause.

However, contrary to many reports, black cohosh does not work like estrogen. There is no evidence that it can prevent osteoporosis or heart disease, two of estrogen's most famous benefits.

What Is the Scientific Evidence for Black Cohosh?

The best evidence for black cohosh as a treatment for menopause comes from a double-blind study that followed 80 women for 12 weeks, comparing the benefits of black cohosh, conjugated estrogens (0.625 mg), and placebo.[1] According to the reported results, black cohosh was actually more effective than estrogen, both in relieving symptoms and in normalizing the appearance of vaginal cells under microscopic evaluation. Similar results were seen in open studies.[2,3]

Based on these and other results, black cohosh came to be described as a phytoestrogen—a plant that produces effects similar to estrogen. However, a recent double-blind study that evaluated two different dosages of black cohosh did not find any change in vaginal-cell appearance or indeed any other objective measurements that would indicate an estrogen-like effect.[4] An animal study has also found no evidence that black cohosh works like estrogen.[5]

If it doesn't act like estrogen, how does black cohosh work? The answer is that we really don't know.

Dosage

The standard dosage of black cohosh is 1 to 2 tablets twice daily of a standardized extract manufactured to contain 1 mg of 27-deoxyacteine per tablet.

Make sure not to confuse black cohosh with **blue cohosh** (*Caulophyllum thalictroides;* see page 225). Blue cohosh is potentially more dangerous because it contains chemicals that are toxic to the heart. One published case report documents profound heart failure in a child born to a mother who used blue cohosh to induce labor.[6]

Safety Issues

Black cohosh seldom produces any obvious side effects, other than occasional mild gastrointestinal distress. Studies in rats have shown no significant toxicity when black cohosh was given at 90 times the therapeutic dosage for a period of 6 months.[7] Because 6 months in a rat corresponds to decades in a human, this study appears to make a strong statement about the long-term safety of black cohosh.

Unlike estrogen, black cohosh does not stimulate breast cancer cells growing in a test tube.[8,9] However, this should not be taken as a guarantee that black cohosh does not increase the risk of breast cancer. Since we don't fully understand how black cohosh works, and because it has shown estrogen-like effects in some studies, women who have already had breast cancer should not take black cohosh except on the advice of a physician.

Black cohosh has been shown to slightly lower blood pressure and blood sugar in certain animals.[10,11] For this reason, it's possible that the herb could interact with drugs for high blood pressure or diabetes, although no such problems have been reported.

Black cohosh is generally not recommended for pregnant women or nursing mothers, and safety in young children and those with severe liver or kidney disease has not been established.

Soy Isoflavones: May Reduce Symptoms

Soy contains phytoestrogens called **isoflavones** (see page 335), which appear to produce far-reaching effects in the body. The most famous of these isoflavones are **genistein** (see page 294) and daidzein. These substances, perhaps along with other constituents of soy, appear to be effective in reducing menopausal hot flashes. In one double-blind study of 104 women, daily doses of 60 g of soy protein significantly reduced flushing associated with menopause.[12] Similarly positive results were seen in a 6-week double-blind placebo-controlled trial of 39 women.[13] However, soy does not appear to reduce vaginal dryness.

Some, but not all, studies suggest that soy isoflavones may be able to help one of the most feared complications of menopause: osteoporosis.[14–22] There is much stronger evidence that a semisynthetic isoflavone named ipriflavone (chemically similar to what is found in soy) definitely helps osteoporosis, although it does not reduce menopausal symptoms. (See the chapters on **osteoporosis**, **ipriflavone**, or **isoflavones** for more information.)

Visit Us at TNP.com

Soy appears to be protective against heart disease and breast and uterine cancer. However, there are indications that soy may not be safe for those who have already had breast cancer.

The best dosage of soy for menopausal symptoms is unclear. One or two cups of soy milk or slices of tofu daily appears to be helpful.[23] Various products containing concentrated isoflavones from soy or red clover have recently come on the market, but we know little about their effectiveness or optimum dosage.

There are some concerns that soy isoflavones may impair thyroid function or reduce absorption of thyroid medication, at least in children.[24,25,26] For this reason, individuals with impaired thyroid function should use soy with caution.

OTHER PROPOSED TREATMENTS

One double-blind placebo-controlled study suggests that cream containing the hormone progesterone (available over the counter) is effective against hot flashes.[27] However, contrary to widespread advertising, progesterone did not offer any benefits for osteoporosis. (See the chapter on **progesterone** for more information.)

Highly preliminary research suggests that **flaxseeds** (see page 286) may help decrease menopausal symptoms.[28]

Vitamin C (see page 444); bioflavonoids; essential fatty acids; an extract of rice bran called **gamma oryzanol** (see page 290); and the herbs **St. John's wort** (see page 414),[29] **licorice** (see page 344), **suma** (see page 420), and **chasteberry** (see page 245) are reportedly helpful for menopause. However, there is as yet little to no scientific evidence to turn to.

Although **vitamin E** (see page 451) is often recommended for menopausal hot flashes, there is no real evidence that it is effective. One 9-week double-blind placebo-controlled trial followed 104 women with hot flashes associated with breast cancer treatment, but it found marginal benefits at best.[30]

Isoflavone-rich extracts of the herb **red clover** (see page 397) have been suggested as a treatment for menopausal symptoms as well. However, a 28-week double-blind placebo-controlled crossover study of 51 postmenopausal women found no reduction in hot flashes among those given 40 mg of red clover isoflavones daily.[31] No benefits were seen in another double-blind placebo-controlled trial, which involved 37 women also given isoflavones from red clover at a dose of either 40 mg or 160 mg daily.[32]

Alfalfa (see page 202) has been investigated in the laboratory (but not yet evaluated in people) as a source of plant estrogens, which might make it helpful for menopause.[33,34,35]

The herb **dong quai** (see page 272) is also frequently recommended for menopausal symptoms, but a recent double-blind study found it to be entirely ineffective.[36]

ESTRIOL—A SAFER FORM OF ESTROGEN?

For over a decade, some alternative medicine practitioners have popularized the use of a special form of estrogen called **estriol** (see page 278), claiming that, unlike standard estrogen, it doesn't increase the risk of cancer. However, this claim is unfounded.

There is no real doubt that estriol is effective. Controlled and double-blind trials have found oral or vaginal estriol effective for reducing hot flashes, night sweats, insomnia, vaginal dryness, recurrent **urinary tract infections** (see page 28), and **osteoporosis** (see page 136).[37-45]

Estriol may cause less vaginal bleeding as a side effect than other forms of estrogen, although this has not been proven.[46,47]

However, like other forms of estrogen, oral estriol stimulates the growth of uterine tissue. This leads to risk of uterine cancer.

In a placebo-controlled study of 1,110 women, uterine tissue stimulation was seen among women given estriol orally (1 to 2 mg daily) as compared to those given placebo.[48] Another large study found that oral estriol increased the risk of uterine cancer.[49] In another study of 48 women given estriol 1 mg twice daily, uterine tissue stimulation was seen in the majority of cases.[50]

In contrast, a 12-month double-blind trial of oral estriol (2 mg daily) in 68 Japanese women found no effect on the uterus.[51] It may be that the high levels of soy in the Japanese diet altered the results.

Additionally, test tube studies suggest that estriol is just as likely to cause breast cancer as any other form of estrogen.[52]

The bottom line: If you use estriol, you should consider it like any other form of estrogen.

MIGRAINE HEADACHES

Principal Proposed Treatments   Feverfew, Magnesium

Other Proposed Treatments   5-HTP (5-Hydroxytryptophan), Fish Oil, Vitamin B_2 (Riboflavin), Butterbur, Calcium, Chromium, Folate, Ginger, Vitamin C, Allergen-Free Diet, Acupuncture

The term *migraine* refers to a class of headaches sharing certain characteristic symptoms. The two main subcategories of migraine are the common and the classic migraine.

In common migraines, headache pain usually occurs in the forehead or temples, often on one side only and typically accompanied by nausea and a preference for a darkened room. Headache attacks last from several hours up to a day or more. They are usually separated by completely pain-free intervals.

In the rarer form of migraine, called classic migraine, headache pain is accompanied by a visual disturbance known as an aura. Otherwise, symptoms are similar to those of the common migraine.

Migraines can be triggered by a variety of causes, including fatigue, stress, hormonal changes, and foods such as alcohol, chocolate, peanuts, and avocados. However, in many people, migraines occur with no obvious triggering factor.

The cause of migraine headaches has been a subject of continuing controversy for over a century. Opinion has swung back and forth between two primary beliefs: that migraines are related to epileptic seizures and originate in the nervous tissue of the brain; or that blood vessels in the skull cause headache pain when they dilate or contract (so-called vascular headaches). Most likely, several factors are involved, and more than one stimulus can light the fuse that leads to a full-blown migraine attack.

Conventional treatment of acute migraines has lately been revolutionized by the drug sumatriptan (Imitrex). This drug can completely abort a migraine headache in many individuals. It works by imitating the action of serotonin on blood vessels, causing them to contract. Drugs made from ergot mold are also effective.

People interested in prevention can choose from a bewildering variety of drugs, including ergot drugs, antidepressants, beta-blockers, calcium channel–blockers, and antiseizure medication. Picking the right one is mostly a matter of trial and error.

PRINCIPAL PROPOSED TREATMENTS

Scientific evidence suggests that the herb feverfew and the mineral magnesium can help prevent migraine headaches.

Keep in mind that serious diseases may occasionally first present themselves as migraine-type headaches. If you suddenly start having migraines without a previous history, or if the pattern of your migraines changes significantly, it is essential to seek medical evaluation.

Feverfew: Dried Leaf May Reduce Frequency and Severity of Headaches

Feverfew (see page 280) was widely used in ancient times as a treatment for headaches and other conditions. However, it fell out of favor for several centuries until an unexpected but fortunate event occurred in the late 1970s. At that time, the wife of the chief medical officer of the National Coal Board in England suffered from serious migraine headaches. When this fact became known to workers in the industry, a sympathetic miner suggested that she try a folk treatment he knew about. She followed his advice and chewed feverfew leaves. The results were dramatic: Her migraines almost completely disappeared.

Her husband was impressed, too, and used his high office to gain the ear of a physician who specialized in migraine headaches, Dr. E. Stewart Johnson of the London Migraine Clinic. Johnson subsequently tried feverfew on 10 of his patients. The results were so good that he subsequently gave the herb to 270 of his patients. A whopping 70% reported considerable relief.

Thoroughly excited now, Dr. Johnson enrolled 17 feverfew-using patients in an interesting type of double-blind study.[1] Half were continued on feverfew, and the other half transferred without their knowledge to placebo. Over a period of 6 months, the participants withdrawn from feverfew demonstrated a dramatic increase in headaches, nausea, and vomiting.

Unfortunately, this study had some serious flaws. It was too small, and because the participants were already feverfew users who felt it worked for them, it didn't say anything about the effectiveness of feverfew in the population at large. This type of error in a study is called *self-selection*. Nonetheless, the study brought a flood of response from the public and ultimately led to three preliminary but properly performed double-blind experiments.

Today, feverfew is used mainly for the prevention of chronic, recurrent migraine headaches, especially in the United Kingdom. Those who use it say that their headaches become less frequent and less severe, and may even stop altogether. However, feverfew must be taken religiously every day for best results.

Reportedly, feverfew taken at the onset of a migraine attack can provide some benefit, but no studies have yet been performed to confirm this. It is not at all effective for cluster or tension headaches.

What Is the Scientific Evidence for Feverfew?

Two double-blind studies suggest that regular use of feverfew leaf can help prevent migraine headaches and reduce their severity when they do come.

The so-called Nottingham trial followed 59 individuals for 8 months.[2] For 4 months, half received a daily capsule of feverfew leaf, and the other half received placebo. The groups were then switched and followed for an additional 4 months. Treatment with feverfew produced a 24% reduction in the number of migraines and a significant decrease in nausea and vomiting during the headaches.

A recent double-blind study of 57 people with migraines, who were given feverfew leaf daily, also showed distinct reductions in headache severity.[3] Unfortunately, the authors did not report whether the frequency of headaches improved.

However, the herb world was surprised when a Dutch study of 50 people showed no difference whatsoever between placebo and a special feverfew extract standardized to its parthenolide content.[4] This unexpected result reversed a widely held view about how feverfew works.

For many years it was assumed that the active ingredient in feverfew was a substance named parthenolide. Many articles were published explaining exactly how parthenolide prevented migraines.[5–8] On the basis of this premature explanation, indignant authors complained that samples of feverfew on the market vary as much as 10 to 1 in their parthenolide content. No less an authority than the herbal expert Varro Tyler said that "standardization of the herbal material on the basis of its parthenolide content is urgently required if this potentially valuable herb is to be used effectively."[9]

However, everyone was jumping the gun. The special feverfew extract used in the negative Dutch study was standardized to a high parthenolide content. Apparently, this extract lacked some essential substance or group of substances that is present in the whole leaf, which was used in the positive studies. Without these unknown constituents, it seems that feverfew does not work. What those substances may have been remains mysterious.

Dosage

Given the recent confusion surrounding parthenolide, previous dosage recommendations for feverfew based on parthenolide content have been cast in doubt. At the present time, the best recommendation is probably to take 80 to 100 mg of powdered whole feverfew leaf daily.

When taken at the onset of a migraine headache, higher amounts of feverfew are often used. However, the optimum dosage has not been determined.

Safety Issues

Among the many thousands of people who use feverfew as a folk medicine in England, no reports of serious toxicity have been published.

In the 8-month Nottingham clinical trial of 76 participants (59 completed the study), no significant differences in side effects were found between treated individuals and the placebo group, nor were any changes in measurements on blood tests and urinalysis noted.[10]

In a survey of 300 study participants, 11.3% reported mouth sores after chewing feverfew leaf, occasionally accompanied by general inflammation of tissues in the mouth.[11] A smaller percentage reported mild gastrointestinal distress.[12] However, mouth sores do not seem to occur in people who use encapsulated feverfew.

Animal studies confirm the safety of feverfew. No adverse effects were seen at doses 100 and 150 times the human daily dose in rats and guinea pigs respectively.[13]

However, because feverfew was an old folk remedy used to promote abortions, it should probably not be taken during pregnancy. Feverfew might slightly inhibit the activity of blood-clotting cells known as platelets,[14] so it should not be combined with strong anticoagulants, such as Coumadin (warfarin) or heparin, except on medical advice. Feverfew might also increase the risk of stomach problems if combined with anti-inflammatory drugs such as aspirin.[15,16,17] Safety in young children and those with severe liver or kidney disease has also not been established.

Magnesium: May Help Prevent Migraines

Magnesium (see page 351) is another natural treatment that appears to be effective for the prevention of migraine headaches. A recent 12-week double-blind study followed 81 people with recurrent migraines.[18] Half received 600 mg of magnesium daily (in the rather unusual form of trimagnesium dicitrate), and the other half received placebo.

By the last 3 weeks of the study, the frequency of migraine attacks was reduced by 41.6% in the treated group, compared to 15.8% in the placebo group. The only side effects observed were diarrhea (18.6%) and digestive irritation (4.7%).

Similar results have been seen in other double-blind studies.[19,20] There was one study that did not find a benefit,[21] but there were many problems with its design.[22]

Preliminary studies suggest that magnesium may also be helpful for menstrual migraines.

Since many people are deficient in magnesium anyway, it's hard to go wrong taking a magnesium supplement. The usual nutritional dose is in the neighborhood

Visit Us at TNP.com

of 350 to 450 mg daily, but 600 mg (as used in the study) should be safe, unless you suffer from severe heart or kidney disease.

OTHER PROPOSED TREATMENTS

Several other herbs and supplements are widely recommended for migraine headaches, but as yet there is little scientific proof that they are effective.

5-HTP

A number of drugs are used to prevent migraine headaches, including antidepressants in the Prozac family. Although we don't know for sure, many of them appear to work by either changing serotonin levels or producing serotonin-like effects in the body. Since the body uses **5-HTP** (see page 198) to make serotonin, supplemental 5-HTP might also affect serotonin levels and has been tested as a treatment for migraines.

In a 6-month trial of 124 people, 5-HTP proved equally effective as the standard drug methysergide.[23] The most dramatic benefits seen were a reduction in the intensity and duration of migraines. Since methysergide has been proven better than placebo for migraine headaches in earlier studies, the study results provide meaningful, although not airtight, evidence that 5-HTP is also effective.

Similarly good results were seen in another comparative study, using a different medication.[24]

However, in one study, 5-HTP was less effective than the drug propranolol.[25] Also, in a study involving children, 5-HTP failed to demonstrate benefit.[26] Other studies that are sometimes quoted as evidence that 5-HTP is effective for migraines actually enrolled adults or children with many different types of headaches (including migraines).[27,28,29]

Putting all this evidence together, it appears likely that 5-HTP can help people with frequent migraine headaches, but further research needs to be done. In particular, we need a large double-blind study that compares 5-HTP against placebo over a period of several months.

However, there are some safety concerns regarding 5-HTP. See the full chapter on 5-HTP for more information.

Fish Oil

Preliminary double-blind studies suggest that high doses of **fish oil** (see page 282) may be helpful for migraine headaches.[30,31]

Vitamin B_2 (Riboflavin)

According to a 3-month double-blind placebo-controlled study of 55 people with migraines, **vitamin B_2** (see page 436) can significantly reduce the frequency and duration of migraine attacks.[32]

Vitamin B_2 is an essential nutrient that is believed to be very safe. This study found that, when given at least 2 months to work, vitamin B_2, at a daily dose of 400 mg, can produce dramatic migraine relief. The majority of the participants experienced a greater than 50% decrease in the number of migraine attacks as well as the total days with headache pain. A larger and longer study is needed to follow up on these results.

Butterbur

The herb **butterbur** (see page 233) was tested as a migraine preventive in a double-blind placebo-controlled study involving 60 men and women who experienced at least 3 migraines per month.[33] After 4 weeks without any conventional medications, participants were randomly assigned to take either 50 mg of butterbur extract or placebo twice daily for 3 months.

The results were positive: both the number of migraine attacks and the total number of days of migraine pain were significantly reduced in the treatment group as compared to the placebo group. Three out of four individuals taking butterbur reported improvement, as compared to only one out of four in the placebo group. No significant side effects were noted.

The usual dosage of butterbur as a migraine preventive is 50 mg twice daily of an extract that has been processed to remove potentially dangerous chemicals called pyrrolizidine alkaloids. Pyrrolizidine alkaloids are liver-toxic and possibly carcinogenic.[34,35] **Warning**: Use of any butterbur product that still contains these alkaloids is definitely not recommended. Safety in young children, pregnant or nursing women, or people with severe kidney or liver disease has not been established.

Other Supplements

Calcium (see page 234), **chromium** (see page 251), **folate** (see page 288), **ginger** (see page 296), and **vitamin C** (see page 444) have also been reported to be helpful for migraines, but there is as yet not much scientific evidence for any of these treatments.

Other Treatments

Identifying and eliminating **allergenic foods** (see page 82) from your diet appears to be helpful in reducing the frequency of migraine attacks.[36]

At least one small double-blind study using real and "sham" treatments suggests that acupuncture can reduce the intensity and number of migraine attacks.[37] Furthermore, the improvements were found to continue for at least a year after the cessation of acupuncture treatment.

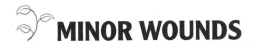

MINOR BURNS

Related Terms   Superficial Burn, First-Degree Burn, Scald

Principal Proposed Treatments   There are no well-established natural treatments for minor burns.

Other Proposed Treatments   Honey, Potato Peel, Gotu Kola, *Aloe vera*, Calendula, Chamomile, Goldenseal, Comfrey, Vitamin C, Vitamin E, Beta-Carotene, Ornithine Alpha-Ketoglutarate, Arginine, Zinc, Copper, Selenium, DHEA

Burns can be caused by heat, electricity, chemicals, and sun exposure. They vary in severity from causing minor pain to being life-threatening. First-degree burns are the mildest type, only damaging the top layer of skin. The skin gets red, painful, and tender. Though the skin may swell, no blisters form and the area turns white when touched.

Second-degree burns cause damage to deeper layers of the skin. The skin looks much like a first-degree burn except that blisters form at the surface. The blisters may be red or whitish and are filled with a clear fluid. Third-degree burns are the worst type of burn, extending through all layers of the skin and causing nerve damage. Because of this nerve damage, third-degree burns generally aren't painful and have no feeling when touched—an ominous sign. The skin may be white, blackened, or bright red. Blisters may also be present.

Only first-degree burns should be self-treated. More severe burns require a doctor's supervision to prevent infection and scarring. Third-degree burns and extensive second-degree burns can cause permanent injury or death.

The best treatment for minor burns is to cool the burn as quickly as possible by immersing the area in cold water. The burned area should be kept clean until it heals.

PROPOSED TREATMENTS

Although there are no well-established natural treatments for minor burns, several preliminary studies suggest a few options for reducing pain and speeding healing.

A series of studies done in India found that a combination of raw honey and gauze was significantly better than conventional types of bandages for superficial burns treated at a hospital.[1,2,3] The burns covered with honey healed faster and with less frequent infection than the burns covered with other types of bandages.

Potato peel has also been used successfully in developing countries as a replacement for more expensive conventional bandages.[4]

Highly preliminary studies suggest the herb **gotu kola** (see page 315) may speed healing of burns and reduce scarring.[5]

Aloe vera (see page 204) is often recommended as a treatment for minor burns; however, no evidence exists to support this claim.[6,7] Other popular topical burn treatments include **calendula** (see page 237), **chamomile** (see page 244), **goldenseal** (see page 314), and comfrey.

Oral or topical **vitamin C** (see page 444), **vitamin E** (see page 451), and **beta-carotene** (see page 217), alone or in combination, might be helpful for preventing sunburn.[8–21] However, the evidence at this time is preliminary and contradictory. (See the **sunburn** chapter for more information.)

Finally, there is some evidence that hospitalized individuals with severe burns may benefit from nutritional support with certain supplements, including **ornithine alpha-ketoglutarate** (OKG; see page 376), **arginine** (see page 208), **zinc** (see page 463), **copper** (see page 262), **selenium** (see page 407), and **DHEA** (dehydroepiandrosterone; see page 268).[22–25]

MINOR WOUNDS

Related Terms   Lacerations, Scrapes, Cuts

Principal Proposed Treatments   Careful Wound Cleaning

Other Proposed Treatments   Gotu Kola, Amino Acid Cream, Vitamin A, Vitamin C, Vitamin E, Zinc, Calendula, Cartilage, Chamomile, Chitosan, Goldenseal, Royal Jelly, St. John's Wort, Garlic, *Aloe vera*, Bee Propolis

Visit Us at TNP.com

Minor cuts are an ordinary fact of life, and nearly always heal on their own. There is no evidence that antibacterial gels and creams will help wounds heal faster, or prevent infection. In fact, by keeping the air away from a wound, these treatments might actually interfere with healing.

The best approach to minor wounds is also the simplest and most natural: clean the wound well, and keep it clean and exposed to the air. If signs of infection develop, such as redness, oozing, or swelling, a physician should be consulted.

PROPOSED TREATMENTS

Highly preliminary evidence suggests that the herb **gotu kola** (see page 315) might have general wound-healing properties, as well as help to prevent or treat keloid scars (a particular type of scar that is enlarged and bulging).[1,2,3]

A small double-blind trial found that the amino acids cysteine, **glycine** (see page 311), and threonine applied as a combination cream could help the healing of leg ulcers.[4] A variety of nutrients including **vitamins A** (see page 432), **C** (see page 444), and **E** (see page 451), and **zinc** (see page 463),[5] taken both orally and topically, have also been tried as a treatment for minor wounds, and creams containing A and E are common staples in the hospital. A number of topical herbs have been tried as well, including **calendula** (see page 237),[6] **cartilage** (see page 241),[7] **chamomile** (see page 244), **chitosan** (see page 247),[8] **goldenseal** (see page 314), royal jelly,[9] and **St. John's wort** (see page 414), but there is no real evidence as yet that any of these approaches work.

Numerous herbs have antibacterial properties, and for this reason might be helpful for preventing wound infection. However, one of the strongest antibacterial herbs, **garlic** (see page 291), can also burn the skin. In addition, if a wound is serious enough that infection is a real risk, physician supervision is essential.

The gel of the **Aloe vera** (see page 204) plant has a long folk history in the treatment of skin conditions. There is some evidence from human and animal studies that aloe might be helpful for wound healing,[10,11] but one study found that aloe gel actually slowed the healing of surgical wounds.[12]

Animal studies suggest that the honeybee product **propolis** (see page 216) applied topically may be of benefit in healing wounds.[13,14]

MULTIPLE SCLEROSIS

Principal Proposed Treatments   There are no well-established natural treatments for multiple sclerosis.

Other Proposed Treatments   Adenosine Monophosphate (AMP), Bee Venom, Biotin, Calcium, Evening Primrose Oil, Fish Oil, Ginkgo, Glycine, Linoleic Acid, Magnesium, Phenylalanine, Proteolytic Enzymes, Selenium, Threonine, Vitamin B_1, Vitamin B_{12}, Vitamin D, Vitamin E, Vitamin C

Multiple sclerosis (MS) is a disease affecting the fatty sheath that covers nerve fibers in the brain and spinal cord. This sheath, made of a substance called myelin, normally insulates the nerve fibers, allowing nerve impulses to move swiftly and efficiently between brain, spinal cord, and body. In MS, patchy areas of this insulating material are destroyed and replaced by scar tissue, which results in the slowing or blocking of nerve signals. People with MS may experience symptoms such as blurred vision, muscle weakness and spasticity, difficulty walking, poor coordination, bladder problems, numbness, and fatigue. In its most common form, the disease begins between the ages of 20 and 40 with an initial attack of symptoms followed by partial or complete remission. Further attacks usually follow and can eventually lead to progressive disability. Another form of the disease progresses more quickly.

Although the cause of MS isn't known for sure, scientists generally assume that MS is an autoimmune disease in which the immune system attacks the body's own myelin cells. Scientists theorize that something, perhaps a toxin or virus, triggers this autoimmune response in susceptible people. Not everyone appears to be equally susceptible. Gene studies suggest that genetics plays a role in who gets the disease, but other factors seem to be important as well. For example, MS tends to be more common the farther one goes from the equator.[1] The disease is also more prevalent in societies with greater dietary intake of meat and animal fat, lower intake of unsaturated fats compared to saturated fats, and lower intake of fish.[2,3,4] Not everyone agrees that all of these factors actually contribute to the disease. Some factors may simply be statistically associated with the actual cause.

There is no cure as yet for MS, but several new drugs—including two forms of the antiviral substance interferon and an unrelated drug, glatiramer acetate (Copaxone)—appear able to reduce the frequency of relapses in people with certain forms of MS. One of these drugs, interferon beta1a (Avonex), has been found to actually slow the rate of disability. Other medications reduce the severity of acute attacks or treat specific symptoms such as muscle spasticity.

PROPOSED TREATMENTS

While there are no well-documented natural treatments for multiple sclerosis, there are a few options that may provide some help.

There is some evidence that changing the type and amount of fat in the diet might alter the course of MS. Based on observations from population studies linking diets lower in fat or saturated fat to lower rates of MS, physician R.L. Swank developed a special low-fat diet for MS in which unsaturated fats replace most saturated fat. This approach, called the Swank diet, has been used by many people with MS. When he analyzed the long-term effects of the diet on his patients, Swank found that those adhering closely to the diet for 20 to 34 years developed significantly less disability than those who ate more saturated fat.[5,6] Because these were not controlled trials, they do not actually prove that the Swank diet works. Nonetheless, the possible connection between MS and fatty acids continues to arouse interest, and a variety of essential fatty acids have been proposed as possible treatments for MS (see below). Although a link between fat intake and MS is intriguing, research has not yet provided clear-cut evidence that any of these treatments help.

Linoleic Acid

One of the omega-6 essential fatty acids, a group of fats as necessary to the body as vitamins, linoleic acid is found in high concentration in sunflower and safflower oil as well as most other vegetable oils. Several researchers have investigated whether linoleic acid in the form of sunflower seed oil can help MS, but the results of their research were equivocal.

Three groups of investigators performed double-blind studies, using olive oil as a placebo, to see if linoleic acid supplements could affect the symptoms or course of MS.[7,8,9] Two of these studies (one involving 75 people, the other 116) found that those taking linoleic acid had shorter and less-severe attacks of MS compared to those taking placebo.[10,11] However, in the two years of the trials, the frequency of attacks and overall levels of disability were not significantly affected. The third study of 76 people found that linoleic acid had no effects on

either MS attacks or degrees of disability over 2½ years, as compared to olive oil.[12]

Another researcher suggests that these studies may have been too short—that it may take far longer than two years for linoleic acid to exert its effects on myelin.[13] Olive oil also contains important fatty acids; others have wondered if the olive oil could have been an effective treatment on its own, thereby obscuring the benefits of linoleic acid. Finally, yet another researcher carefully examining the study reports found that linoleic acid might have been effective in those individuals with less severe MS symptoms.[14,15]

Although interesting, this type of after-the-fact analysis must be interpreted with caution. More studies are needed to confirm whether linoleic acid, taken early in the course of MS or at other times, has the power to prevent, delay, or improve disability.

Dosage

In the three double-blind studies described above, participants received 17 to 20 g of linoleic acid per day, the equivalent of 1 ounce of sunflower seed oil.

Safety Issues

As a nutrient found in food, linoleic acid is considered to be safe. However, maximum safe dosages for young children, pregnant or nursing women, or people with severe liver or kidney disease have not been determined.

Other Essential Fatty Acids

There has been much excitement about other essential fatty acids as treatments for MS, including omega-3 fatty acids found in **fish oil** (see page 282) and **gamma-linolenic acid** (GLA; see page 304), an omega-6 fatty acid present in evening primrose oil. Evidence of their effectiveness, however, is still relatively weak.

Blood tests among people with MS have found lower levels of omega-3 fatty acids in their body fluids and tissues compared to those without MS.[16,17] Preliminary research also suggests that omega-3 supplements may decrease the production of certain inflammatory chemicals (including cytokines and interleukins) in people with and without MS.[18] One uncontrolled study noted fewer relapses among people with MS taking cod liver oil (a form of fish oil that also provides vitamins A and D), **calcium** (see page 234), and **magnesium** (see page 351).[19]

However, these findings by themselves do not prove that supplements will help treat the disease; for that, double-blind placebo-controlled studies are needed. Unfortunately, the only reported double-blind study of fish oil for MS had inconclusive results. In this 2-year study of 292 people with MS, comparing fish oil's omega-3 fatty acids with an olive oil placebo, there were no significant differences between the two groups.[20]

Visit Us at TNP.com

Some researchers have suggested that gamma-linolenic acid (GLA), might be beneficial in MS.[21] So far, however, little evidence suggests that it helps, and one uncontrolled study found it ineffective.[22,23,24]

Threonine

Early evidence suggests that threonine, a naturally occurring amino acid, might be able to decrease the muscle spasticity that often occurs with MS.

Two small double-blind studies found a modest but statistically significant improvement in muscle spasticity among people who took threonine compared to those who took placebo.[25,26] In one study of 26 people with MS, the improvement was so slight after 8 weeks of treatment that it was detectable by doctors but not by the participants themselves.[27] In the other, both researchers and a few of the 33 participants noticed improvement after 2 weeks of treatment, with some individuals reporting fewer spasms and milder pain.[28] Interestingly, this shorter trial that showed more improvement also used lower doses—6 g daily of L-threonine, as opposed to 7.5 g daily of threonine. No significant side effects were noted in either study.

Vitamin B$_{12}$

Because several studies have found MS to be occasionally associated with **vitamin B$_{12}$** (see page 442) deficiency,[29,30,31] some doctors recommend that people with MS be screened for this condition, and treated with B$_{12}$ if deficient.[32] (Vitamin B$_{12}$ deficiency can sometimes cause neurological problems on its own.) One highly preliminary study suggested that massive doses of B$_{12}$ could improve certain test results ("evoked potentials"), but not disability, in people with chronic progressive MS.[33] However, a double-blind study of 50 people with MS found that high doses of injected hydroxocobalamin, a form of B$_{12}$, did not affect the course of disease or number of relapses.[34]

Vitamin D

Our bodies normally obtain **vitamin D** (see page 449) in one of two ways: through our diet or through exposure of our skin to the sun. More than one group of researchers has noted that areas with less sunshine tend to have a higher incidence of MS, unless the residents eat more fish that is rich in vitamin D.[35–38] This has led to a theory that vitamin D might confer some protection against MS. So far, no human studies have adequately tested this hypothesis, although one open study (mentioned above) did investigate a combination of calcium, magnesium, and vitamin D given in the form of cod liver oil.[39]

Phenylalanine and TENS

Phenylalanine (see page 385) is an essential amino acid, meaning that we need it for life and our bodies can't manufacture it from other chemicals. We normally obtain all the phenylalanine we need for nutritional purposes from high-protein foods. Supplemental phenylalanine has been studied for MS only in combination with another treatment: transcutaneous nerve stimulation (TENS), a portable electrical device used to decrease pain and muscle spasticity.

Two small double-blind trials compared phenylalanine to placebo among a total of 16 people with MS being treated with TENS.[40] In both studies, those treated with phenylalanine and TENS experienced less muscle spasticity, fewer bladder symptoms, and less depression after 4 weeks of treatment than those treated with TENS and placebo. Following the double-blind studies, the same physician used phenylalanine and TENS on 50 people, 49 of whom were reported to improve.[41]

Other Treatments

Other treatments sometimes suggested for MS include adenosine monophosphate (AMP), bee venom, **biotin** (see page 221), **ginkgo** (see page 298), **glycine** (see page 311), **proteolytic enzymes** (see page 393), **selenium** (see page 407), **vitamin B$_1$** (see page 434), **vitamin C** (see page 444), and **vitamin E** (see page 451), but little to no evidence supports these recommendations. One double-blind study found that ginkgolide B, a chemical in ginkgo, was ineffective in treating MS attacks.[42] Bee venom has generated a great deal of interest over the years, despite the lack of reliable research supporting its use. Georgetown University researchers are currently conducting a study of its safety in people with MS.

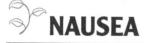

NAUSEA

Principal Proposed Treatments   Ginger, Vitamin B$_6$

Other Proposed Treatments   Vitamin K, Vitamin C, Acupressure/Acupuncture, Lowfat Diet

Nausea

Visit Us at TNP.com

Nausea can be caused by many factors, including stomach flu, viral infections of the inner ear (labyrinthitis), motion sickness, pregnancy, and chemotherapy. If you are continually nauseous, it can be more disabling than chronic pain. Successful treatment can make an enormous difference in your quality of life.

The sensation of nausea can originate in either the nervous system or the digestive tract itself. Most conventional treatments for nausea, such as Dramamine and Compazine, act on the nervous system, but products like Pepto-Bismol soothe the digestive tract directly.

PRINCIPAL PROPOSED TREATMENTS

The herb ginger has become a widely accepted treatment for nausea of various types. Vitamin B_6 may be helpful for the nausea of pregnancy.

Ginger: May Help Several Types of Nausea

Native to southern Asia, **ginger** (see page 296) is a 2- to 4-foot perennial that produces grass-like leaves up to a foot long and almost an inch wide. Ginger root, as it is named in the grocery store, actually consists of the underground stem of the plant with its bark-like outer covering scraped off.

Ginger has been used as food and medicine for millennia. Ginger's modern use dates back to the early 1980s, when a scientist named D. Mowrey noticed that ginger-filled capsules reduced his nausea during an episode of flu. Subsequent research ultimately led Germany's Commission E to approve ginger as a treatment for indigestion and motion sickness.

Ginger is typically not as effective as standard drugs for motion sickness, but it has the advantage of not causing drowsiness. Some physicians recommend ginger over other motion sickness drugs for older individuals who are unusually sensitive to drowsiness or loss of balance.

Ginger is also used for the nausea and vomiting of pregnancy, and some conventional medical textbooks mention it. However, physicians are hesitant to recommend any treatment during pregnancy until full safety studies have been performed, and although it is a food, these studies have not yet been completed for ginger (see Safety Issues).

European physicians sometimes give their patients ginger before and just after surgery to prevent the nausea that many people experience when they awaken from anesthesia. However, this treatment should be attempted only with a physician's approval.

What Is the Scientific Evidence for Ginger?

Scientific evidence suggests that ginger can be helpful for various forms of nausea.

Nausea and Vomiting of Pregnancy   A preliminary double-blind study performed in Denmark concluded that ginger can significantly reduce the nausea and vomiting that often accompany pregnancy.[1] Effects became apparent in 19 of 27 women after 4 days of treatment.

Motion Sickness   The first scientific study of ginger for motion sickness followed 36 college students with a known tendency toward motion sickness.[2] They were treated with either ginger or the standard antinausea drug dimenhydrinate and then placed in a rotating chair to see how much motion they could stand. Both treatments seemed about equally effective. Another study also found equivalent benefit between ginger and dimenhydrinate in a group of 60 passengers on a cruise through rough seas.[3] A study of 79 Swedish naval cadets found that ginger could decrease vomiting and cold sweating, but it didn't significantly decrease nausea and vertigo.[4]

However, a 1984 study funded by NASA found that ginger was not any more effective than placebo at reducing the symptoms of nausea caused by a vigorous nausea-provoking method.[5] Negative results were also seen in another study that used a strong nausea stimulus.[6]

Put all together, these studies paint a picture of a treatment that is somewhat effective for motion sickness but cannot overcome severe nausea.

Post-Surgical Nausea   A double-blind British study compared the effects of ginger, placebo, and the drug metoclopramide in the treatment of nausea following gynecological surgery.[7] The results in 60 women showed that both treatments produced similar benefits compared to placebo.

A similar British study followed 120 women receiving gynecological surgery.[8] Whereas nausea and vomiting developed in 41% of participants given placebo, in the groups treated with ginger or metoclopramide (Reglan), these symptoms developed in only 21% and 27%, respectively.

However, a double-blind study of 108 people undergoing similar surgery showed no benefit with ginger as compared to placebo.[9] Negative results were also seen in another study.[10]

Warning: Do not use ginger either before or immediately after surgery or labor and delivery without a physician's approval. Not only is it important to have an empty stomach before undergoing anesthesia, there are theoretical concerns that ginger may affect bleeding.

Dosage

For most purposes, the standard dosage of powdered ginger is 1 to 4 g daily taken in 2 to 4 divided doses.

To prevent motion sickness, it is probably best to begin treatment 1 or 2 days before the trip and continue it throughout the period of travel.

In the nausea and vomiting of pregnancy, the best form of ginger is probably freshly brewed tea made from boiled ginger root or powdered ginger and diluted to taste. If chilled, carbonated, and sweetened, this would become the original form of ginger ale, a famous anti-nausea beverage.

Safety Issues

Ginger is on the FDA's GRAS (generally recognized as safe) list and seldom causes any side effects.

Like onions and **garlic** (see page 291), extracts of ginger interfere with blood clotting in test tubes.[11,12,13] This has led to a theoretical concern that ginger should not be combined with drugs such as Coumadin (warfarin), Trental (pentoxifylline), or even aspirin. European studies with actual oral ginger in normal quantities have not found any effect on clotting,[14,15,16] but combination treatment might still cause problems.

Maximum safe dosages for young children, pregnant or nursing women, or those with severe liver or kidney disease have not been established.

Vitamin B$_6$

A large double-blind study suggests that 30 mg daily of **vitamin B$_6$** (see page 439) can reduce the sensation of nausea in morning sickness.[17] At this dose, vitamin B$_6$ should be entirely safe.

OTHER PROPOSED TREATMENTS

Although the following natural treatments are widely recommended to relieve nausea, there is as yet no convincing scientific evidence that they work.

Vitamin K and Vitamin C

On the basis of studies conducted in the 1950s, a combination of vitamin K (at the enormous dose of 5 mg) and vitamin C (25 mg) is sometimes recommended for morning sickness.[18] Please keep in mind that supplemental vitamin K can interfere with prescription blood-thinning drugs such as Coumadin (warfarin) and heparin. See the chapters on **vitamin K** and **vitamin C** for more information.

Acupressure/Acupuncture

An acupuncture point on the inside of the arm, about 1 to 2 inches below the wrist crease, is traditionally used to alleviate nausea. It is usually stimulated either with acupuncture needling or application of pressure.

A double-blind placebo-controlled study of 94 individuals undergoing cesarean section found that pressure on this point (acupressure) during and after surgery reduced nausea and vomiting.[19]

Acupressure or acupuncture have been evaluated for other forms of nausea, including morning sickness, general anesthesia, chemotherapy, and motion sickness, with generally positive results.[20–32]

Other Recommendations

Diets high in saturated fat (animal fat) can increase morning sickness in some people.[33]

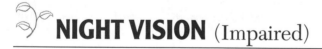

NIGHT VISION (Impaired)

Principal Proposed Treatments   Bilberry

Other Proposed Treatments   OPCs (Oligomeric Proanthocyanidins), Vitamin A, Zinc

The ability to see in poor light depends on the presence of a substance in the eye called rhodopsin, or visual purple. It is destroyed by bright light but rapidly regenerates in the dark. However, for some people, the adaptation to darkness or the recovery from glare takes an unusually long time. There is no medical treatment for this condition.

PRINCIPAL PROPOSED TREATMENTS

The herb bilberry is widely used as a treatment for impaired night vision. However, the scientific evidence is not yet as strong as it should be.

Bilberry: Widely Used in Europe for Impaired Night Vision

The herb **bilberry** (see page 220), a close relative of the American blueberry, is the most commonly mentioned natural treatment for impaired night vision. This use dates back to World War II, when pilots in Britain's Royal Air Force reported that a good dose of bilberry jam just before a mission improved their night vision, often dramatically. After the war, medical researchers investigated the constituents of bilberry and subsequently recommended it for a variety of eye disorders. However, the scientific evidence that it works is weak and contradictory.

A double-blind crossover trial of 15 individuals found no short- or long-term improvements in night vision attributable to bilberry.[1] Similarly negative results were seen in a double-blind placebo-controlled crossover trial of 18 subjects.[2]

In contrast, two much earlier placebo-controlled studies of bilberry found that the herb improved vision in semidarkness, shortened time necessary to adapt to darkness, and speeded recovery from glare.[3,4] However, the effect was not found to persist with continued use. A later double-blind placebo-controlled study on 40 healthy subjects found that a single dose of bilberry extract improved visual response for 2 hours.[5] Other small studies have also found benefits, but since they did not use a placebo group, they are not valid as evidence.[6,7,8]

The effects of bilberry are believed to be due to a group of chemicals called anthocyanosides. These naturally occurring antioxidants appear to have numerous important effects on the eye.[9,10]

The standard dosage of bilberry is 120 to 240 mg twice daily of an extract standardized to contain 25% bilberry anthocyanosides.

As one might expect of a food, bilberry is quite safe. Enormous quantities have been administered to rats without toxic effects.[11,12] One study involving 2,295 participants showed no serious side effects and only a 4% occurrence of mild reactions such as gastrointestinal distress, skin rashes, and drowsiness.[13] Although safety in pregnancy has not been proven, clinical trials have enrolled pregnant women.[14] However, safety in young children, nursing women, and those with severe liver or kidney disease has not been established.

Bilberry has no known drug interactions.

OTHER PROPOSED TREATMENTS

OPCs (see page 373) have also been recommended for improving night vision, although the evidence that they help is highly preliminary.[15,16]

There is no question that deficiencies of **vitamin A** (see page 432) and **zinc** (see page 463) can also negatively affect night vision. Since zinc is commonly lacking in many people's diets, taking 15 to 20 mg of zinc daily (along with 1 to 3 mg of **copper** [see page 262] for balance) may be advisable.

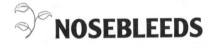

NOSEBLEEDS

Related Terms   Epistaxis

Principal Proposed Treatments   Citrus Bioflavonoids

Other Proposed Treatments   OPCs (Oligomeric Proanthocyanidins), Bilberry, Vitamin C, Proteolytic Enzymes, Shepherd's Purse

Who among us has never had a nosebleed? Whether a dab of blood on a tissue or a terrifying flood, a nosebleed can arise from many causes: dry winter air, colds, injuries, or the common if unsavory habit of picking one's nose. In many cases, no cause can be identified with certainty.

Sometimes nosebleeds arise more frequently because of faulty or weak *collagen*, a strengthening protein present in blood vessel walls and the surrounding connective tissue. Collagen problems may lead to nosebleeds in people who take corticosteroids and those with a condition called "fragile capillaries."

Corticosteroids, including nasal steroids used for allergies, can thin the collagen in the mucous membranes lining the nose. In fragile capillaries, weak or defective collagen in blood vessel walls may contribute to bleeding. People with collagen problems may have problems with bleeding gums, heavy menstrual periods, and **bruising** (blood collecting under the skin; see page 74) in addition to nosebleeds.

Rarely, the cause of nosebleeds and other bleeding lies in the blood itself. Anything that reduces blood clotting may lead to nosebleeds. Drugs such as warfarin (Coumadin) or heparin, or regular use of aspirin, can decrease the blood's tendency to clot. **Caution**: if you are taking such medications and begin to experience nosebleeds, talk to your doctor. Even natural substances such as **ginkgo** (see page 298), high-dose **vitamin E** (see page 451), and **garlic** (see page 291) may increase the tendency to bleed.

Conventional treatments for nosebleeds include various maneuvers for stopping acute bleeding, followed by the diagnosis and treatment of any underlying problems. Sometimes a physician can prevent future nosebleeds by cauterizing the blood vessel responsible.

PRINCIPAL PROPOSED TREATMENTS
Citrus Bioflavonoids

One supplement that may help prevent nosebleeds is **citrus bioflavonoids** (see page 254). Bioflavonoids (or flavonoids) are plant substances that bring color to many fruits and vegetables. Citrus fruits are a rich source of bioflavonoids, including diosmin, hesperidin, rutin, and naringen. One study has found that citrus bioflavonoids can help decrease symptoms of easy bleeding, such as nosebleeds, among people with fragile capillaries.

What Is the Scientific Evidence for Citrus Bioflavonoids?

A double-blind study of 96 people with fragile capillaries found that a combination of the bioflavonoids diosmin and hesperidin decreased symptoms of capillary fragility, such as nosebleeds and bruising.[1] In this 6-week trial, participants—41% of whom had problems with nosebleeds—took 2 tablets daily of the bioflavonoid combination or placebo. Those who received bioflavonoids had significantly greater improvements in both their symptoms and their capillary strength compared to those taking placebo. Unfortunately, the researchers didn't state how much the nosebleeds improved.

Dosage

A typical dosage of citrus bioflavonoids is 600 to 1,200 mg per day.

Safety Issues

Citrus bioflavonoids appear to be quite safe. In the study described above, the treatment caused no more side effects than placebo.[2] However, bioflavonoids may have some anticoagulant properties when taken in high doses, and therefore should be used only under medical supervision by individuals on blood-thinner drugs, such as warfarin (Coumadin) and heparin.

OTHER PROPOSED TREATMENTS

Although there are no other well-documented treatments for nosebleeds, numerous substances are used to treat other conditions that involve capillary fragility. It is possible, but certainly not proven, that some of these same treatments may be helpful for nosebleeds.

OPCs (Oligomeric Proanthocyanidins)

OPCs (see page 373) are bioflavonoid-like compounds found in large amounts in grape seed and grape extract products. Test tube studies have found that OPCs protect collagen, partly by inhibiting an enzyme that breaks

it down.[3] One rather poorly designed double-blind study of 37 people—most of whom had fragile capillaries—found that OPCs were more effective than placebo in decreasing capillary fragility[4]; however, the study authors left many questions unanswered in their report, making it hard to determine how seriously to take their results, and they did not address nosebleeds specifically.

The double-blind study of OPCs used a 100-mg dose daily for 15 days, although the authors felt some people would do better with 150 mg per day.[5] These compounds appear to be quite safe.

Anthocyanosides

Anthocyanosides are present in high concentrations in **bilberry** (see page 220), a food related to the blueberry. Like OPCs, anthocyanosides may strengthen capillaries through their effects on collagen. The normal dosage for bilberry is 120 to 240 mg twice daily of an extract standardized to contain 25% anthocyanosides. As one might expect of a food, bilberry appears to be quite safe.

Vitamin C

Vitamin C (see page 444) is vital for the development of normal collagen. People with scurvy (severe vitamin C deficiency) may bleed easily from the nose, as well as developing spontaneous bruises and other bleeding symptoms. True vitamin C deficiency is extremely rare in Western countries; marginal deficiencies are more likely to occur in people without access to much fresh food, such as some elderly people in institutions. However, there is no evidence as yet that vitamin C supplementation helps to decrease nosebleeds in the absence of true scurvy.

Other Treatments

The herb shepherd's purse (*Capsella bursae pastoris*) has been traditionally used as a topical application to control nosebleeds, although scientific evidence of its effectiveness is lacking. The herb should not be used during pregnancy because it can stimulate uterine contractions. Other proposed natural treatments for fragile capillaries include **proteolytic enzymes** (see page 393), such as **bromelain** (see page 229) and the digestive enzymes trypsin and chymotrypsin. Again, there is as yet no evidence showing that these substances can help prevent nosebleeds.

NUTRITION FOR CIGARETTE SMOKERS

Principal Proposed Treatments   Multivitamin and Mineral Supplements, Healthful Diet

Other Proposed Treatments   Vitamin E, Vitamin C

Herbs and Supplements to Avoid   High-Dose Beta-Carotene

Cigarette smoking is one of the biggest risk factors for cancer and heart disease. The more cigarettes a person smokes and the longer it's kept up, the greater the risk of dying from cancer, heart attack, or stroke. Probably less well known is that smokers are also much more likely to catch colds and other infections.

Of course, the best remedy for these risks and problems is quitting, but it's not easy. Because cigarette smoking poses such a public health risk, many studies have attempted to discern whether vitamin supplementation among smokers might help avert cancer and heart disease. However, the results have not been particularly promising, and one supplement, beta-carotene, may actually be dangerous for smokers.

PRINCIPAL PROPOSED TREATMENTS

People who smoke often have deficiencies in numerous nutrients, including **zinc** (see page 463), **calcium** (see page 234), **folate** (see page 288), **vitamins C** (see page 444) and **E** (see page 451), **beta-carotene** (see page 217), **lycopene** (see page 349), and essential fatty acids.[1–15] There are many possible causes for this depletion, including free radicals in cigarette smoke that destroy natural antioxidants; however, the most important single cause might be poor diet rather than smoking itself.[16]

Whatever the cause, there is little doubt that smokers would benefit from general nutritional support in the form of a multivitamin/mineral tablet. In addition, a diet high in fruits, vegetables, and fish will supply nutrients not found in multivitamins which help prevent cancer and heart disease.

OTHER PROPOSED TREATMENTS

As mentioned above, cigarette smoke contains free radicals, substances that can damage many parts of the body. Because of this, high dosages of antioxidants have been tried for the prevention of cigarette-related diseases. However, the results have not been promising. Vitamins E and C have not proven particularly helpful, and beta-carotene may be harmful.

Large double-blind trials found neither a beneficial nor a harmful effect of vitamin E in heart disease or lung cancer.[17–19] However, vitamin E consumption might significantly reduce risk of prostate cancer in smokers.[20]

A small double-blind placebo-controlled study including 20 smokers suggests that vitamin C supplements may improve arterial function, but the effects aren't long-lasting.[21]

Beta-Carotene: A Supplement to Avoid

Although nutritional doses of the antioxidant nutrient beta-carotene help to supply needed **vitamin A** (see page 432), there is evidence that smokers should avoid high doses of beta-carotene.

An enormous double-blind placebo-controlled study called the Alpha-Tocopherol, Beta-Carotene Cancer (ATBC) Prevention study enrolled 29,133 Finnish male smokers and examined the effects of vitamin E and beta-carotene supplements on lung cancer rates among them.[22] The results showed that 20 mg of beta-carotene daily for 5 to 8 years *increased* the risk of lung cancer by 18%.

In addition, a statistical analysis of the ATBC study including 1,862 smokers with heart problems found that individuals taking either beta-carotene or a beta-carotene/vitamin E combination had significantly increased risk of fatal heart attack compared to those taking placebo.[23] Another statistical review of the study analyzed the effects of beta-carotene on individuals with angina pectoris, one of the first symptoms of heart disease.[24] Results indicated that beta-carotene was associated with a slight increase in angina.

Another large double-blind placebo-controlled trial enrolling 18,314 smokers, former smokers, and workers exposed to asbestos studied the effects of a different combination, beta-carotene and vitamin A, on lung cancer and cardiovascular disease.[25] Evidence from the trial suggests that 30 mg of beta-carotene and 25,000 IU (international units) of vitamin A taken together daily have no beneficial effects and may be harmful. Individuals taking the supplements had a 28% higher incidence of lung cancer than the placebo group; a 17% higher death rate from lung cancer; and a 26% higher death rate from cardiovascular disease. The trial was stopped 21 months early based on these findings.

The bottom line: Although nutritional dosages of beta-carotene (in the neighborhood of 3 mg daily for adults) are probably healthful, smokers should avoid doses of beta-carotene greater than in the range of 20 to 30 mg daily.

Osteoarthritis

OSTEOARTHRITIS

Principal Proposed Treatments   Glucosamine, Chondroitin Sulfate, SAMe (S-Adenosylmethionine), Niacinamide

Other Proposed Treatments   Devil's Claw, White Willow, Healthy Diet, Boswellia, Ginger, Turmeric, Yucca, MSM (Methyl Sulfonyl Methane), Green-Lipped Mussel, Beta-Carotene, Boron, Bromelain, Cartilage, Cat's Claw, Chamomile, Copper, Dandelion, Feverfew, Molybdenum, D-Phenylalanine, Selenium, Vitamin C, Vitamin E, Zinc

In osteoarthritis, the cartilage in joints has become damaged, disrupting the smooth gliding motion of the joint surfaces. The result is pain, swelling, and deformity.

The pain of osteoarthritis typically increases with joint use and improves at rest. For reasons that aren't clear, although x rays can find evidence of arthritis, the level of pain and stiffness experienced by people does not match the extent of injury noticed on x rays.

Many theories exist about the causes of osteoarthritis, but we don't really know what causes the disease. Osteoarthritis is often described as "wear and tear" arthritis. However, evidence suggests that this simple explanation is not correct. For example, osteoarthritis frequently develops in many joints at the same time, often symmetrically on both sides of the body, even when there is no reason to believe that equal amounts of wear and tear are present. Another intriguing finding is that osteoarthritis of the knee is commonly (and mysteriously) associated with osteoarthritis of the hand. These factors, as well as others, have led to the suggestion that osteoarthritis may actually be a body-wide disease of the cartilage.

During one's lifetime, cartilage is constantly being turned over by a balance of forces that both break down and rebuild it. One prevailing theory suggests that osteoarthritis may represent a situation in which the degrading forces get out of hand. Some of the proposed natural treatments for osteoarthritis described later may inhibit enzymes that damage cartilage.

When the cartilage damage in osteoarthritis begins, the body responds by building new cartilage. For several years, this compensating effort can keep the joint functioning well. Some of the natural treatments described below appear to work by assisting the body in repairing cartilage. Eventually, however, building forces cannot keep up with destructive ones, and what is called end-stage osteoarthritis develops. This is the familiar picture of pain and impaired joint function.

The conventional medical treatment for osteoarthritis consists mainly of analgesic medications, such as Tylenol, and anti-inflammatory drugs, such as Aleve and Orudis. The main problem with anti-inflammatory drugs is that they can cause ulcers. Another possible problem is that they may actually speed the progression of osteoarthritis by interfering with cartilage repair and promoting cartilage destruction.[1-5] In contrast, some of the treatments described below appear to actually slow the course of the disease.

Recently, the use of extracts of cayenne pepper has found its way into conventional medicine. Briefly, it consists of the regular application of cayenne cream to the affected joint, ultimately resulting in a decreased sensation of pain. Unfortunately, this truly natural treatment seldom provides more than modest relief.

PRINCIPAL PROPOSED TREATMENTS

There are several very useful natural treatments for osteoarthritis. Not only do they reduce pain without causing any side effects, some may slow the progression of osteoarthritis.

Glucosamine: Safe Pain Relief That Lasts

One of the best-documented alternative approaches to the treatment of osteoarthritis is the supplement **glucosamine** (see page 308). Glucosamine is a small molecule formed of a sugar attached to a chemical structure called an amine. Taking glucosamine supplements provides a natural raw material for rebuilding cartilage. It seems to stimulate the activity of cartilage cells and perhaps also protect cartilage from damage.[6-13]

In Portugal, Spain, and Italy, glucosamine has been a primary treatment for osteoarthritis since the 1980s, and it is also widely used by veterinarians in the United States. Not only can it reduce symptoms, a major study tells us that it can also slow the course of arthritis. For this reason it is sometimes called a "chondroprotective" drug ("chondro" refers to cartilage).

In the long view, this is even more important than relieving symptoms. No conventional treatment for osteoarthritis protects the joints or hinders the progression of the disease. This effect may make glucosamine one of the most important treatments for arthritis.

What Is the Scientific Evidence for Glucosamine?

Reasonably solid studies have found that supplementation with glucosamine sulfate can relieve the pain of osteoarthritis. For example, one recent double-blind study compared the effectiveness of glucosamine sulfate and placebo in 252 people with osteoarthritis of the

Visit Us at TNP.com

knee.[14] The results showed that after 4 weeks the participants treated with glucosamine sulfate were in less pain and could move better than those given a placebo. No more side effects were noted in the participants who took glucosamine than in those who did not.

Another study found glucosamine equally effective to the standard arthritis drug Feldene.[15] A total of 329 participants were given 20 mg of Feldene, glucosamine, placebo, or glucosamine plus Feldene daily. Improvement was monitored through the Lequesne Index, a rating scale that evaluates the severity of osteoarthritis. Equivalent benefit was seen in all the treated groups. After 90 days, treatment was then stopped, and the participants were followed for an additional 8 weeks.

Interestingly, whereas the benefits of Feldene rapidly disappeared following the end of treatment, glucosamine was still producing a full effect at the end of the post-treatment period.

Other studies, enrolling a total of more than 350 participants, have found equivalent benefit between glucosamine and ibuprofen.[16,17]

However, not every study has been positive. A recent 2-month double-blind placebo-controlled trial of 98 individuals with osteoarthritis of the knee found no benefit.[18] The authors suggest that the relatively advanced osteoarthritis found in these participants was responsible for the negative outcome. Negative results were also seen in a double-blind placebo-controlled trial of glucosamine chloride.[19]

Nonetheless, overall, it certainly appears that glucosamine is effective for reducing symptoms of osteoarthritis. In addition, it appears to provide another important benefit: slowing the progression of the disease.

A 3-year double-blind placebo-controlled study of 212 individuals found that glucosamine can protect joints from further damage.[20] Over the course of the study, individuals given glucosamine showed some actual improvement in pain and mobility, while those given placebo worsened steadily. Even more importantly, x rays showed that glucosamine treatment prevented progressive damage to the knee joint.

Dosage

Glucosamine is usually taken as glucosamine sulfate, at a dosage of 500 mg 3 times daily. A 1,500-mg dose taken once daily may also work.[21] Keep in mind that it is not truly a cure because it must be taken forever for good results. It also does not produce complete relief. However, it often appears to help significantly. Pain ordinarily begins to improve in about a week and the benefit continues to increase for a month or more.

Safety Issues

Glucosamine is believed to be nontoxic and has not been associated with significant side effects.[22,23] This gives it a huge potential advantage over standard drug treatment, which can cause ulcers. However, recent animal studies and case reports have raised concerns that glucosamine might be harmful for individuals with diabetes. It may raise blood sugar levels[24–28] and also increase the risk of long-term diabetes side effects such as cataracts.[29]

Chondroitin Sulfate: Relieves Pain and May Slow Progression of Osteoarthritis

Reasonably good evidence supports the use of **chondroitin sulfate** (see page 250) for the pain of osteoarthritis as well. In addition, provocative evidence suggests that it may help prevent your arthritis from gradually getting worse.

Like glucosamine, chondroitin plays a natural role in the body's manufacture of cartilage. In Europe, chondroitin sulfate is usually injected directly into arthritic joints (under no circumstances should you try this yourself!). However, in the United States, oral chondroitin sulfate is the most popular form of this supplement.

For years it was questioned whether oral chondroitin sulfate could possibly work. Because of its large molecular size it is difficult to see how chondroitin sulfate could find its way through the lining of the digestive tract to be absorbed into the bloodstream. However, in 1995 researchers found evidence that up to 15% of chondroitin is actually absorbed.[30]

Scientists are unsure how chondroitin sulfate works, but one of three theories (or all of them) might explain its mode of action. Some evidence suggests that chondroitin may inhibit the enzymes that break down cartilage in the joints.[31] Another theory holds that chondroitin sulfate increases the amount of hyaluronic acid in the joints. (Hyaluronic acid is a protective fluid that keeps the joints lubricated.) Finally, as a building block of cartilage, available chondroitin might simply help the body rebuild damaged joints.

Perhaps the most exciting development is the recent evidence that suggests chondroitin sulfate can actually slow the progression of osteoarthritis. This would make it a true chondroprotective drug (see the previous discussion under the heading Glucosamine). However, more research is needed.

What Is the Scientific Evidence for Chondroitin Sulfate?

Much of the early research on chondroitin sulfate was published in French or Italian journals and has not been translated into English. However, the results of four double-blind placebo-controlled clinical trials were recently published in English. They provide substantial evidence that chondroitin sulfate is an effective treatment for osteoarthritis. Some show evidence that chondroitin sulfate can reduce the symptoms of osteoarthritis, while others suggest that, like glucosamine, it can slow or perhaps even stop the progression of the disease.

Reducing Symptoms   Studies involving a total of more than 250 people and lasting from 3 months to 1 year have found chondroitin effective for reducing the symptoms of arthritis.

A recent 6-month double-blind placebo-controlled study followed 85 individuals with osteoarthritis of the knee.[32] Participants received either 400 mg of chondroitin sulfate twice a day or placebo. Researchers evaluated improvement in arthritis symptoms by recording the level of pain as judged by the participant, the need for other medications, the time necessary to walk 20 meters on flat ground, and the overall effectiveness of the treatment as rated by physicians and participants.

After 1 month of treatment there was a 23% decrease in joint pain in the chondroitin sulfate group versus only a 12% decrease in the placebo group. By 6 months there was a 43% improvement in the chondroitin sulfate group versus only a 3% improvement in the placebo group (the placebo effect seems to have worn off after a while). While walking speed did not improve in the placebo group, there was a small but significant progressive improvement among individuals taking chondroitin. Physicians judged the improvement as good or very good in 69% of those taking chondroitin sulfate, but only in 32% of those taking placebo.

Another study enrolled more participants (127) and followed them for a period of 3 months.[33] The results were again positive. Finally, a third double-blind study involved only 42 participants, but followed them for a full year. Chondroitin sulfate took months to reach its full effect, but eventually relieved symptoms considerably better than placebo.[34] Positive results were also seen in earlier studies, including one that found chondroitin about as effective as the anti-inflammatory drug dicoflenac.[35–38]

Slowing the Disease   An important feature of this last study was that the individuals taking a placebo showed progressive joint damage over the year, but among those taking chondroitin sulfate no worsening of the joints was seen. In other words, chondroitin sulfate seemed to protect the joints of osteoarthritis sufferers from further damage.

A longer and larger double-blind placebo-controlled trial also found evidence that chondroitin sulfate can slow the progression of osteoarthritis.[39] One hundred and nineteen people were enrolled in this study, which lasted a full 3 years. Thirty-four of the participants received 1,200 mg of chondroitin sulfate per day; the rest received placebo. Over the course of the study researchers took x rays to determine how many joints had progressed to a severe stage.

During the 3 years of the study only 8.8% of those who took chondroitin sulfate developed severely damaged joints, whereas almost 30% of those who took placebo progressed to this extent. Unfortunately, the report did not state whether this difference was statistically significant.

Additional evidence comes from animal studies. Researchers measured the effects of chondroitin sulfate (administered both orally and via injection directly into the muscle) in rabbits, in which cartilage damage had been induced in one knee by the injection of an enzyme.[40] After 84 days of treatment, the damaged knees in the animals that had been given chondroitin sulfate had significantly more cartilage left than the knees of the untreated animals. Taking chondroitin sulfate by mouth was as effective as taking it through an injection.

Looking at the sum of the evidence, it does appear that chondroitin sulfate may actually protect joints from damage in osteoarthritis. However, at the present time, the evidence is better for glucosamine sulfate.

Dosage

The usual dosage of chondroitin sulfate is 400 mg taken 3 times daily. Chondroitin sulfate is often sold in combination with glucosamine. Preliminary information from one animal study suggests that this mixture may be superior to either treatment alone.[41]

There are large differences between chondroitin products based on their chemical structure. This can be expected to lead to significant differences in absorption and hence effectiveness.[42] It may be advisable to use the exact products that were tested in double-blind trials.

Safety Issues

Chondroitin sulfate has not been associated with any serious adverse effects. Participants in clinical trials have found mild digestive system distress to be the only real complaint.

SAMe: Helpful, but Very Expensive

SAMe (**S-adenosylmethionine**; see page 403) is a substance that occurs naturally in the body and plays a role in numerous biochemical functions. When used for osteoarthritis, it appears to reduce pain, decrease swelling, and improve mobility about as effectively as standard anti-inflammatory drugs, with significantly fewer side effects and risks. Indirect evidence suggests that SAMe may slow the progression of osteoarthritis, but, unlike glucosamine and chondroitin, we have no direct proof that SAMe offers this benefit. At present, this is an extremely expensive supplement.

What Is the Scientific Evidence for SAMe?

A substantial body of scientific evidence supports the use of SAMe in arthritis.[43] Numerous double-blind studies involving over a thousand participants in total suggest that it is approximately as effective as standard anti-inflammatory drugs.

One of the best double-blind studies enrolled 732 patients and followed them for 4 weeks.[44] Over this period, 235 of the participants received 1,200 mg of SAMe per day, while a similar number took either placebo or 750 mg daily of the standard drug naproxen. The majority of these patients had experienced moderate symptoms of osteoarthritis of either the knee or of the hip for an average of 6 years.

The results indicate that SAMe provided as much pain-relieving effect as naproxen and that both treatments were significantly better than placebo. However, differences did exist between the two treatments. Naproxen worked more quickly, producing readily apparent benefits at the 2-week follow-up, whereas the full effect of SAMe was not apparent until 4 weeks. By the end of the study, both treatments were producing the same level of benefit.

Animal evidence suggests that SAMe may help protect cartilage from damage.[45,46]

Dosage

SAMe is usually started at an initial dosage of 200 mg twice daily, which is then increased over 1 to 2 weeks up to 1,200 mg per day. The reason for this gradual approach is that if full doses are taken from the beginning many people develop stomach distress.

After symptoms improve, doses as low as 200 mg twice daily may suffice to keep pain under control.

Recently, SAMe has come on the U.S. market at a recommended dosage of 400 mg daily. This dosage labeling makes SAMe appear more affordable (if you're only taking 400 mg per day, you'll spend only about a third of what you'd pay for the full therapeutic dosage), but it is unlikely that SAMe will actually work when taken at such a low dosage.

Safety Issues

SAMe appears to be quite safe, according to both human and animal studies.[47–50] The most common side effect is mild digestive distress. However, SAMe does not actually damage the stomach.[51]

Like other substances with antidepressant activity, SAMe might trigger a manic episode in those with **bipolar disorder** (manic-depression; see page 27).[52,53,54]

Safety in young children, pregnant or nursing women, or those with severe liver or kidney disease has not been established.

SAMe might interfere with the action of the Parkinson's drug levodopa.[55] In addition, there may also be risks involved in combining SAMe with standard antidepressants.[56] For this reason, you shouldn't try either combination except under physician supervision.

Niacinamide

There is some evidence that **vitamin B$_3$** (see page 437) in the form of niacinamide may provide some benefits for those with osteoarthritis. In a double-blind study, 72 individuals with arthritis were given either 3,000 mg daily of niacinamide (in 5 equal doses) or placebo for 12 weeks.[57] The results showed that treated participants experienced a 29% improvement in symptoms, whereas those given placebo worsened by 10%. However, at this dose, liver inflammation is a concern that must be taken seriously.

OTHER PROPOSED TREATMENTS

The following natural treatments are widely recommended for osteoarthritis, but they have not yet been established as effective.

Devil's Claw: Reduces Arthritis Pain

Several preliminary double-blind studies involving a total of over 200 people suggest that the herb **devil's claw** (see page 267) can soothe the pain of various types of arthritis.[58]

A typical dosage of devil's claw is 750 mg 3 times daily of a preparation standardized to contain 3% iridoid glycosides. Devil's claw appears to be quite safe, with no evidence of toxicity at doses many times higher than recommended.[59] A 6-month open study of 630 people with arthritis who took devil's claw showed no side effects other than occasional mild gastrointestinal distress.[60] For the latter reason, it is recommended that those with ulcers not take devil's claw.

Safety in young children, pregnant or nursing women, or those with severe liver or kidney disease has not been established.

White Willow: Natural Aspirin

The herb **white willow** (see page 457) contains the aspirin-like substance salicin. Preliminary evidence suggests willow extracts can relieve osteoarthritis pain.[61]

Standardized willow bark extracts should provide 120 to 240 mg of salicin daily.

Aspirin and related anti-inflammatory drugs are notorious for irritating or damaging the stomach. However willow appears to be gentler in this regard.[62,63]

Nonetheless, willow could still cause the side effects associated with aspirin such as stomach irritation and even bleeding ulcers if used over the long term. All the other risks of aspirin therapy apply as well. For example, white willow should not be given to children, due to the risk of Reye's syndrome. It should also not be used by people with aspirin allergies, bleeding disorders, ulcers, kidney disease, liver disease, or diabetes, and it may interact adversely with alcohol, "blood thinners," other

Visit Us at TNP.com

Osteoporosis

anti-inflammatories, methotrexate, metoclopramide, phenytoin, probenecid, spironolactone, and valproate.

Safety in pregnant or nursing women, or those with severe liver or kidney disease has not been established.

Healthy Diet: Can Slow the Progression of Arthritis

There is considerable evidence that a diet high in **vitamin C** (see page 444), **vitamin E** (see page 451), and **beta-carotene** (see page 217) can slow the progression of osteoarthritis, by as much as 70%.[64] These nutrients are found in fruits, vegetables, whole grains, nuts, and seeds. However, we don't know whether taking supplements of these vitamins is just as effective. As described in detail in the chapter on beta-carotene, when you get vitamins from foods you also get numerous other healthful substances.

Miscellaneous Herbs and Supplements

One small double-blind study suggests that direct application of **stinging nettle leaf** (see page 369) to a painful joint may improve symptoms.[65]

Weak evidence suggests that the herbs **boswellia**, **ginger**, **turmeric**, **yucca**, and the supplement **MSM** might be useful for osteoarthritis. See the chapters on these topics for more information.

Evidence from animal studies suggests that green-lipped mussel may help alleviate osteoarthritis symptoms.[66,67,68] Other herbs and supplements sometimes recommended for osteoarthritis include **beta-carotene** (see page 217), **boron** (see page 227), **bromelain** (see page 229), **cartilage** (see page 241), **cat's claw** (see page 242), **chamomile** (see page 244), **copper** (see page 262), **dandelion** (see page 266), **feverfew** (see page 280), molybdenum, **D-phenylalanine** (see page 385), **selenium** (see page 407), vitamin C, vitamin E, and **zinc** (see page 463). However, there is little to no evidence as yet that these treatments are effective.

❧ OSTEOPOROSIS

Principal Proposed Treatments   Calcium, Vitamin D, Ipriflavone, Isoflavones, Genistein, Trace Minerals, Fish Oil, GLA (Gamma-Linolenic Acid)

Other Proposed Treatments   Vitamin K, DHEA (Dehydroepiandrosterone), Copper, Folate, Horsetail, Magnesium, Manganese, Pregnenolone, Strontium, Vanadium, Vitamin B_{12}, Boron, Progesterone, Estriol

In centuries past, the fragile bones and stooped stature of the aged were taken for granted. Today, however, prevention of osteoporosis is a real possibility.

Many factors are now known or suspected to accelerate the rate of bone loss. These include smoking, alcohol, low calcium intake, excessive phosphorus intake (such as found in soft drinks), lack of exercise, various medications, and several medical illnesses. Excessive consumption of **vitamin A** (see page 432) may also increase risk of osteoporosis,[1] and rapid weight loss may increase the risk in postmenopausal women.[2] Women are much more prone to osteoporosis than men and, for this reason, the following discussion focuses almost entirely on them.

Conventional medical treatment for osteoporosis in women centers mainly on hormone-replacement therapy. Although supplemental estrogen undoubtedly slows and perhaps even reverses osteoporosis, recent concern about the increased risk of breast cancer has caused many women and their physicians to rethink the use of this therapy. The so-called designer estrogen raloxifene (Evista) may offer benefits without this risk. Other drugs, such as Fosamax (a nonhormonal drug), can also help build bone.

Weight-bearing exercise is strongly recommended.

PRINCIPAL PROPOSED TREATMENTS

There is good evidence that calcium supplements may be able to slow the progression of osteoporosis. A combination of calcium and vitamin D may be able to produce even better effects, and it appears that the semisynthetic substance ipriflavone may actually reverse the disease to some extent. The combination of ipriflavone and calcium has also been tested and found more effective than calcium alone.

Calcium and Vitamin D

Calcium (see page 234) is necessary to build and maintain bone. You need **vitamin D** (see page 449), too, as the body cannot absorb calcium without it. (Although your body can manufacture vitamin D when exposed to the sun, in this age of sunblock, supplemental vitamin D may be necessary.) Numerous good studies indicate that

Visit Us at TNP.com

calcium supplements can help prevent and slow osteoporosis.[3] Calcium supplementation at the recommended doses appears to be able to reduce bone loss in postmenopausal women in every bone site except the spine.[4,5] Good evidence also tells us that when vitamin D is taken along with calcium the results are even better.[6] Combination treatment may be able to slow osteoporosis in the spine, and in some cases actually reverse osteoporosis to some extent. It may also protect against bone loss caused by corticosteroid drugs such as prednisone.[7]

While estrogen is more powerful than calcium alone, taking calcium along with estrogen may offer additional benefits.[8] Calcium supplements also help adolescent girls "put calcium in the bank,"[9] although regular exercise may be more important.[10]

Adding various trace minerals (**zinc** [see page 463], 15 mg; **copper** [see page 262], 2.5 mg; and **manganese** [see page 354], 5 mg) along with calcium and vitamin D seems to produce further improvement.[11,12] Essential fatty acids, such as **fish oil** (see page 282) and **GLA** (see page 304) from evening primrose oil, may also enhance the effectiveness of calcium.[13,14,15]

Dosage

Appropriate dietary intake of calcium is as follows: 210 to 270 mg daily for infants; 500 to 800 mg daily for children 1 to 8 years old; 1,300 mg daily for children and young adults 9 to 18 years old; 1,000 mg of calcium per day for adults 19 to 50 years old; and 1,200 mg per day for adults 51 years and over. Pregnant or nursing women should take 1,000 mg (unless they are under 19 years of age, in which case the dosage is 1,300 mg). Your body can absorb only about 500 mg of calcium at any one time, so you need to split up the daily dose into several parts.[16]

Some forms of calcium appear to be better absorbed and more effective than others.[17,18] Perhaps the best forms of calcium are calcium citrate and calcium citrate malate.

Because calcium competes with the absorption of other minerals, you should consider taking a multimineral supplement as well.

The usual recommendation for vitamin D ranges from 200 to 600 IU daily depending on age. However, some of the studies cited here used dosages greater than 800 IU daily. Such doses are probably safe,[19] but should be taken under medical supervision.

Safety Issues

In general, a daily intake of calcium up to 2,000 mg is safe.[20] Greatly excessive intake of calcium can cause numerous side effects, including dangerous or painful deposits of calcium within the body. If you have cancer, hyperparathyroidism, or sarcoidosis, you should take calcium only under the supervision of a physician.

People with **kidney stones** (see page 109) or a history of kidney stones are often cautioned not to take supplemental calcium. The reason for this warning is that kidney stones are commonly made of calcium oxalate crystals. However, studies have found that increased intake of calcium from food actually reduces the risk of kidney stones.[21,22] Calcium supplements, on the other hand, might increase kidney stone risk, especially if they are not taken with meals.[23] The bottom line: Restriction of calcium—whether supplemental or dietary—may still be appropriate for certain people.[24]

Vitamin D is safe when taken at a dosage of 400 to 800 IU daily. When used at doses considerably higher than this, vitamin D can build up in the body and cause toxic symptoms. However, the actual dosage at which intake becomes toxic is a matter of dispute.[25,26] Individuals with sarcoidosis or hyperparathyroidism should not take vitamin D, except on medical advice.

Ipriflavone

Ipriflavone (see page 332) is a semisynthetic variation of soy isoflavones (see following section). Ipriflavone appears to help prevent osteoporosis by interfering with bone breakdown. Estrogen works in much the same way, but ipriflavone does not appear to produce estrogenic effects anywhere else in the body other than in bone. For this reason, it probably doesn't increase the risk of breast or uterine cancer. However, it also doesn't reduce the hot flashes, night sweats, mood changes, or vaginal dryness of menopause.

Numerous double-blind placebo-controlled studies involving a total of over 1,000 participants have examined the effects of ipriflavone on osteoporosis.[27–32] Overall, it appears that ipriflavone can stop the progression of osteoporosis and perhaps reverse it to some extent.

For example, a 2-year double-blind study followed 198 postmenopausal women who had evidence of bone loss.[33] At the end of the study, there was a gain in bone density of 1% in the ipriflavone group compared to a loss of 0.7% in the placebo group.

Taking calcium plus ipriflavone may also be an excellent idea. In one study, 60 women, who had already been diagnosed with osteoporosis and had already suffered one spinal fracture, were given either 1,000 mg of calcium or 1,000 mg of calcium with ipriflavone.[34] After 6 months, the ipriflavone group had an increase of bone density in the spine of 3.5%, compared to a 2.1% net loss in the calcium-only group.

Ipriflavone may also be helpful for preventing osteoporosis in women who are taking Lupron or corticosteroids, medications that accelerate bone loss.[35,36]

There is some evidence that combining ipriflavone with estrogen may improve anti-osteoporosis benefits.[37,38] However, we do not know whether such combinations

Osteoporosis

increase or decrease the other benefits and adverse effects of estrogen-replacement therapy.

Finally, for reasons that are not at all clear, ipriflavone appears to be able to reduce pain in osteoporosis-related fractures that have already occurred.[39,40,41]

Dosage

The proper dosage of ipriflavone has been well established through studies: 200 mg 3 times daily or 300 mg 2 times daily. (A lower dose is necessary for those with kidney failure. Please consult your physician for details.)

Safety Issues

To date, 2,769 people have been treated with ipriflavone, for an average duration of more than 1 year. The incidence of side effects in those treated with ipriflavone was no more than what was observed in those taking placebo.[42]

However, because ipriflavone is eliminated by the kidneys, concerns have been raised about the use of ipriflavone by patients with kidney problems.[43]

Ipriflavone does not appear to affect the uterus, brain, breast, or vaginal tissue of postmenopausal women or the thyroid gland and uterus of experimental animals.[44] However, given the lack of large, long-term, cancer-risk studies for ipriflavone, women who have had breast cancer should use ipriflavone only on a physician's advice.

Also, although ipriflavone itself does not affect tissues outside of bone, some evidence suggests that if it is combined with estrogen, estrogen's effects on the uterus are increased.[45,46] This might mean that the risk of uterine cancer would be elevated over taking estrogen alone. It should be possible to overcome this risk by taking progesterone along with estrogen, which is standard medical practice in any case. However, this finding does make one wonder whether ipriflavone–estrogen combinations raise the risk of breast cancer too, an estrogen side effect that has no easy solution. At present, there is no available information on this important subject.

Additionally, ipriflavone may interfere with certain drugs by affecting the way they are processed in the liver. For example, it may raise blood levels of the older asthma drug theophylline.[47,48,49] It could also raise levels of caffeine, meaning that if you drink coffee while taking ipriflavone you might stay up longer than you expect! Additionally, ipriflavone could interact with tolbutamide (a drug for diabetes), phenytoin (used for epilepsy), and Coumadin (a blood thinner).[50] Such interactions are potentially dangerous, especially since phenytoin and Coumadin cause osteoporosis, and some people might be tempted to try taking ipriflavone at the same time.

Isoflavones

Isoflavones (see page 335) are water-soluble chemicals found in many plants. Some isoflavones are known as phytoestrogens, meaning they cause effects in the body somewhat similar to those of estrogen. The most investigated phytoestrogen isoflavones, genistein and daidzein, are found in **soy products** (see page 411) and the herb **red clover** (see page 397). Isoflavones may offer many benefits, including, it now appears, help against osteoporosis.

In one study that evaluated the benefits of soy isoflavones in osteoporosis, a total of 66 postmenopausal women took either placebo (soy protein with isoflavones removed) or soy protein containing 56 or 90 mg of soy isoflavones daily for 6 months.[51] The group that took the higher dosage of isoflavones showed significant gains in spinal bone density. There was little change in the placebo or low-dose isoflavone groups. This study suggests that soy isoflavones may be effective for osteoporosis.

Very nearly the same results were seen in a similar study as well. This 24-week double-blind study of 69 postmenopausal women found that isoflavone-rich soy products can significantly reduce bone loss from the spine.[52]

Similar benefits have been seen in animal studies.[53–59] However, a couple of animal studies and one human trial failed to find benefit.[60,61,62]

In animal studies, **genistein** (see page 294) alone has been found to help protect bone, perhaps by building new bone cells.[63,64,65] However, studies need to be done on humans before genistein can be definitively recommended for osteoporosis.

Estrogen and most other medications for osteoporosis work by fighting bone breakdown. Soy may work in the other way, by helping increase new bone formation.[66,67]

Dosage

The optimum dosage of isoflavones obtained from food is not known. We know that Japanese women eat up to 200 mg of isoflavones from soy daily, but we don't really know what amount of natural isoflavones is ideal. Most experts recommend 25 to 60 mg daily.

Roasted soybeans have the highest isoflavone content: about 167 mg for a 3.5-ounce serving. Tempeh is next, with 60 mg, followed by soy flour with 44 mg. Processed soy products such as soy protein and soy milk contain about 20 mg per serving. The same isoflavones found in soy are also contained in certain red clover products; check the label to determine the content.

Safety Issues

Studies in animals have found soy isoflavones essentially nontoxic.[68]

Nonetheless, because isoflavones work somewhat like estrogen, there are at least theoretical concerns that they may not be safe for women who have already had breast

Visit Us at TNP.com

cancer. Furthermore, evidence from one highly preliminary study in humans found changes suggestive of increased breast cancer risk after women took a commercial soy protein product.[69] Preliminary studies and reports have raised concerns that intensive use of soy products by pregnant women could exert a hormonal effect that impacts unborn fetuses.[70,71]

Red clover isoflavones probably present similar risks.

Finally, while fears have been expressed by some experts that soy isoflavones might interfere with the action of oral contraceptives, one study of 40 women suggests that such concerns are groundless.[72] Another trial found that soy does not interfere with the action of estrogen-replacement therapy in menopausal women.[73]

In addition, soy isoflavones may impair thyroid function or reduce absorption of thyroid medication, at least in children.[74,75,76] For this reason, individuals with impaired thyroid function should use soy with caution.

OTHER PROPOSED TREATMENTS

Evidence suggests (but doesn't prove) that vitamin K may help prevent osteoporosis.[77–86] The optimum dose is not known, although one study points to a daily intake of more than 100 mcg. See the chapter on **vitamin K** for more information about safety and other uses.

Increasing evidence suggests that the hormone **DHEA** (see page 268) may be helpful for fighting osteoporosis, especially in women over 70.[87–90]

Very preliminary evidence suggests that black tea, which is quite similar but not identical to **green tea** (see page 318), may help protect against osteoporosis.[91]

A wide variety of other food supplements have also been suggested as useful for the prevention or reversal of osteoporosis, including **copper** (see page 262), **folate** (see page 288), **horsetail** (see page 326), **magnesium** (see page 351), **manganese** (see page 354), **pregnenolone** (see page 391), strontium, **vanadium** (see page 430), and **vitamin B$_{12}$** (see page 442). However, there is as yet little direct evidence that they really work.

Boron (see page 227) is frequently mentioned as a treatment for osteoporosis as well.[92] However, there are some concerns that boron may raise levels of the body's own estrogen, especially in women on estrogen-replacement therapy, and therefore might present an increased risk of cancer.[93,94]

Although it has long been believed that eating a lot of animal-based protein increases the risk of osteoporosis, the results of a recent large study contradict this idea. This observational study of over 40,000 women suggests that the more animal protein you eat, the less likely you are to develop osteoporosis.[95] Protein was also found to protect bone in a double-blind study.[96]

The Progesterone Story

Many books promote the idea that natural **progesterone** (see page 392) prevents or even reduces osteoporosis. In this case, the term *natural* indicates that we are using the same progesterone found in the body. It is still made synthetically, but it is called "natural progesterone" to distinguish it from its chemical cousins known as progestins. Generally, prescription "progesterone" is actually a progestin.

The progesterone/osteoporosis story began with test tube and other preliminary studies suggesting that progesterone or progestins can stimulate the activity of cells that build bone.[97,98] Subsequently, a poorly designed and uncontrolled study (really, a series of case histories from one physician's practice) purportedly demonstrated that progesterone cream can slow or even reverse osteoporosis.[99,100,101]

However, a 1-year double-blind trial of 102 women given either progesterone cream (providing 20 mg progesterone daily) or placebo cream, along with calcium and multivitamins, found no evidence of any improvements in bone density attributable to progesterone.[102]

Furthermore, in a 3-year study of 875 women, combination treatment with estrogen and oral progesterone was no more effective for osteoporosis than estrogen alone.[103]

The Estriol Story

For over a decade, some alternative medicine practitioners have popularized the use of a special form of estrogen called **estriol** (see page 278), claiming that, unlike standard estrogen, it doesn't increase the risk of cancer. However, this claim is unfounded.

Controlled trials performed in Japan have found that estriol helps prevent bone loss in menopausal women,[104–108] although one small study found no benefit.[109]

However, like other forms of estrogen, oral estriol stimulates the growth of uterine tissue. This leads to risk of uterine cancer.

In a placebo-controlled study of 1,110 women, uterine tissue stimulation was seen among women given estriol orally (1 to 2 mg daily) as compared to those given placebo.[110] Another large study found that oral estriol increased the risk of uterine cancer.[111] In another study of 48 women given estriol 1 mg twice daily, uterine tissue stimulation was seen in the majority of cases.[112]

In contrast, a 12-month double-blind trial of oral estriol (2 mg daily) in 68 Japanese women found no effect on the uterus.[113] It may be that the high levels of soy in the Japanese diet altered the results. Additionally, test tube studies suggest that estriol is just as likely to cause breast cancer as any other form of estrogen.[114]

The bottom line: if you use estriol, you should consider it like any other form of estrogen.

Parkinson's Disease

PARKINSON'S DISEASE

Related Terms   Paralysis Agitans, Parkinsonism

Principal Proposed Treatments   CDP-Choline (Also Called Citicholine)

Other Proposed Treatments   Coenzyme Q_{10}, 5-HTP (5-Hydroxytryptophan), Glutathione, L-Methionine, N-Acetyl Cysteine, NADH, Octacosanol, D-Phenylalanine, Phosphatidylserine, SAMe, Vitamin B_6, Vitamin C, Vitamin E

Parkinson's disease is a chronic disorder typically affecting people over age 55. The condition is caused by the death of nerve cells in certain parts of the brain, leading to characteristic problems with movement. These include a "pill rolling" tremor in the hands (so called because it appears that the individual is rolling a small object between thumb and forefinger), difficulty initiating walking, a shuffling gait, decreased facial expressiveness, and trouble talking. Thinking ability may become impaired in later stages of the disease, and depression is common.

Although the underlying cause of Parkinson's disease is unknown, many researchers believe that free radicals may play a role in destroying at least some of the nerve cells. Large population studies provide some indications that people with higher intakes of antioxidants, which neutralize free radicals, may have lower rates of the disease. However, the results of these population studies are inconsistent: one study of 41,836 older women found that among the antioxidants studied, only **vitamin C** (see page 444) and **manganese** (see page 354) were linked to lower rates of Parkinson's disease—while intake of **vitamin E** (see page 451), for example, seemed unrelated.[1] In contrast, a smaller study of 5,342 older people found that individuals who consumed more vitamin E had a lower incidence of Parkinson's disease, but vitamin C and other antioxidants seemed unrelated.[2] Obviously, more research is needed.

The nerve cells that are affected in Parkinson's disease work by supplying dopamine, a neurotransmitter, to another part of the brain. Most treatments for Parkinson's disease work by artificially increasing the brain's dopamine levels. Simply taking dopamine pills won't work, however, because the substance cannot travel from the bloodstream into the brain. Instead, most people with Parkinson's disease take levodopa (L-dopa), which can pass into the brain and be converted there into dopamine. Many people take levodopa with carbidopa, a drug that increases the amount of levodopa available to make dopamine.

At first, levodopa produces dramatic improvement in symptoms; however, over time, levodopa becomes less effective and more likely to produce side effects. Other drugs may be tried, including bromocriptine, selegiline, and pergolide. There are also surgical treatments, such as pallidotomy, that can decrease symptoms.

PRINCIPAL PROPOSED TREATMENTS

Most research into natural treatments has focused on one of three goals: reducing the presence of free radicals in the brain in an effort to preserve dopamine-producing cells, enhancing the effects of levodopa or naturally-occurring dopamine, or treating the mental symptoms that sometimes accompany advanced Parkinson's disease. So far, the most useful natural treatment appears to be CDP-choline, a dietary supplement that may enhance levodopa's effectiveness.

CDP-Choline

Short for cytidinediphosphocholine, CDP-choline (sometimes called citicholine) is a substance that occurs naturally in the human body. It is closely related to choline, a nutrient commonly put in the B-vitamin family. Evidence suggests that CDP-choline may enhance the effects of levodopa and decrease some symptoms of Parkinson's disease.

For reasons that are not completely clear, CDP-choline seems to increase the amount of dopamine in the brain.[3,4] Most studies investigating this in people with Parkinson's disease have used intravenous or intramuscular injections of CDP-choline. However, in one study, CDP-choline was taken in oral form.

What Is the Scientific Evidence for CDP-Choline?

In a 4-week single-blind study of 74 people with Parkinson's disease, researchers tested whether oral CDP-choline might help levodopa be more effective.[5] Researchers divided participants into two groups: one group received their usual levodopa dose, the other received half their usual dose without knowing which dosage they were getting. All the participants took 1,200 mg a day of oral CDP-choline.

Even though 50% of the participants were taking only half their usual dose of levodopa, both groups scored equally well on standardized tests designed to evaluate the severity of Parkinson's disease symptoms.

Visit Us at TNP.com

A number of other single- and double-blind studies have found that intravenous or intramuscular injections of CDP-choline either reduced symptoms of Parkinson's disease or allowed decreased doses of levodopa without loss of effectiveness.[6–9]

Dosage

In the study of oral CDP-choline described previously, participants took 400 mg of CDP-choline 3 times a day.[10]

Safety Issues

In general, CDP-choline appears to be safe.[11] The study of oral CDP-choline for Parkinson's disease reported only a few brief, nonspecific side effects such as nausea, dizziness, and fatigue.[12] In a study of 2,817 elderly people who took oral CDP-choline for up to 60 days for problems other than Parkinson's disease, side effects were few and mild and reported in only about 5% of participants.[13] Two-thirds of these side effects were gastrointestinal (nausea, stomach pain, and diarrhea), and none required stopping the medication. The CDP-choline dose in this study was 550 to 650 mg per day, about half the dose used for Parkinson's disease.

The safety of CDP-choline in pregnant or nursing women, young children, or people with severe liver or kidney disease has not been established.

OTHER PROPOSED TREATMENTS

Three natural treatments have been studied for use in depression or dementia accompanying Parkinson's disease. In addition, several other treatments have been suggested for prevention or treatment of Parkinson's disease as a whole.

SAMe

Whether a symptom of the disease or a response to disability, depression affects many people with Parkinson's disease, and long-term use of levodopa may contribute to this problem. Research suggests that levodopa can deplete the brain of a substance called **S-adenosylmethionine** (see page 403), or SAMe for short.[14,15] As SAMe has been found in a number of small studies to have antidepressant effects,[16] it is possible that depleting it might trigger depression.

Researchers conducted a trial to determine if taking SAMe supplements could decrease depression in 21 individuals with Parkinson's disease who were taking levodopa.[17] In this double-blind study, each participant received either a combination of oral and injected SAMe or placebo daily for 30 days, followed by the alternate treatment for another 30 days. Although other symptoms of Parkinson's didn't change, 72% of people taking SAMe felt that their depression was improved after 2 weeks, while only 30% noted improvement with placebo. It is not yet known if oral SAMe alone would have similar effects.

Although SAMe might appear to be an excellent accompaniment to levodopa, there is another side to the issue. During treatment with levodopa, SAMe participates in breaking it down and gets used up in the process. It is possible that taking extra SAMe could lead to decreased effectiveness of levodopa.[18] In the short-term study described above, SAMe did not interfere with levodopa's effects, but longer-term use might do so.

The bottom line: If you have Parkinson's disease, it's safest to use SAMe—if at all—only under the supervision of a physician.

The dose in this study was 400 mg of oral SAMe twice a day along with a daily SAMe injection of 200 mg. When oral SAMe is used by itself for other conditions, it is typically taken in dosages of 400 mg 3 to 4 times per day. This regimen may easily exceed $200 a month. In order to reduce costs, some people take this dosage for a few weeks, then try decreasing it. As little as 200 mg twice daily may suffice to keep people feeling better once the full dosage has "broken through" the symptoms.

For a discussion of safety issues regarding SAMe, see the chapter.

5-HTP

Another natural substance, 5-HTP (5-hydroxytryptophan), is often used for depression and has also been tried for depression in Parkinson's disease. However, the evidence that it works is extremely preliminary.[19]

Note: Avoid 5-HTP if you take carbidopa. Using the two substances together might increase your chance of developing symptoms resembling those of the disease scleroderma.[20,21,22]

For more information on this supplement, see the **5-HTP** chapter.

Phosphatidylserine

Phosphatidylserine (see page 387), or PS for short, is a major component of cell membranes. Several studies have found PS supplementation effective for improving mental function in individuals with **Alzheimer's disease** (see page 5). One trial examined its use in 62 people, all of whom had both Parkinson's disease and Alzheimer's-type dementia. The results appeared to indicate some benefit, but due to the incompleteness of the report on this trial, it is difficult to draw conclusions.[23]

Vitamin E

Because of indications that free radicals play a role in causing Parkinson's disease, treatment with high doses of **vitamin E** (see page 451) have been tried to see if they

Periodontal Disease

can slow down the progression of Parkinson's disease. However, a large study yielded disappointing results. In this trial, 800 individuals newly diagnosed with Parkinson's disease took 2,000 IU of tocopherol (synthetic vitamin E) or placebo daily for an average of 14 months.[24,25,26] Vitamin E had no effects in delaying symptoms of the disease—nor did it reduce side effects of levodopa.

Vitamin C

One problem with levodopa treatment for Parkinson's disease is the so-called "on-off effect," in which a person taking levodopa will move more freely for some hours, followed by sudden "freezing up." **Vitamin C** (see page 444) has been tried as a remedy for "on-off effects" in a small double-blind study,[27] but the results were so minimal that the researchers didn't feel justified in recommending it.

Other Treatments

A few other treatments for Parkinson's disease, with minimal or conflicting evidence, include **NADH** (see page 368),[28,29,30] glutathione,[31] **octacosanol** (see page 372),[32] and the amino acids **D-phenylalanine**[33] (see page 385) and **L-methionine** (see page 360).[34,35] Caution is advised with the latter three, as they might interfere with the effectiveness of L-dopa.[36,37]

Treatments sometimes mentioned but essentially lacking any scientific data include **N-acetyl cysteine** (see page 366), **beta-carotene** (see page 217), **coenzyme Q$_{10}$** (see page 256), the hormone **pregnenolone** (see page 391), and **vitamin B$_6$** (see page 439). Be aware of the cautions regarding vitamin B$_6$, noted below.

Other Safety Issues

If you have Parkinson's disease, it is best to avoid taking the herb **kava** (see page 338). Preliminary reports suggest that kava may counter the effects of dopamine and possibly reduce the effectiveness of medications for Parkinson's.[38]

Other substances may also interact with Parkinson's drugs. **Iron** (see page 333) supplements can interfere with absorption of levodopa and carbidopa, and should not be taken within 2 hours of either medication.[39] Amino acid supplements such as **BCAAs** (branched-chain amino acids; see page 213) can temporarily decrease levodopa's effectiveness,[40] as may methionine and phenylalanine, two amino acids studied for treatment of Parkinson's disease.[41]

Vitamin B$_6$ in doses higher than 5 mg per day might also impair the effectiveness of levodopa, and should be avoided.[42] However, if you take levodopa/carbidopa combinations, this restriction may not necessarily apply. Talk with your physician about an appropriate dose of vitamin B$_6$.

As noted previously, SAMe, 5-HTP, and octacosanol may all interact with some Parkinson's drugs.

PERIODONTAL DISEASE

Related Term   Gum Disease

Principal Proposed Treatments   There are no well-established natural treatments for periodontal disease.

Other Proposed Treatments   Folate Mouthwash, Coenzyme Q$_{10}$ (CoQ$_{10}$), Zinc, Vitamin C, Calcium, Magnesium, Vitamin B$_{12}$, Bloodroot, Tea Tree Oil, Cranberry Juice

Periodontal disease begins with gum inflammation and progresses to pockets of infection, bone loss, and loosening of the teeth. It is present in 90% of individuals over the age of 65.

Conventional prevention and treatment include regular flossing, using mouthwash that contains extracts of the herb thyme (such as thymol, found in Listerine), and using special toothbrushing appliances. If the condition becomes advanced, special deep-cleaning techniques and even surgery may be necessary.

PROPOSED TREATMENTS

Folate

Preliminary studies suggest that **folate** (see page 288) mouthwash may help in periodontal disease. However, oral folate supplementation does not appear to be especially effective.[1–4]

Cranberry Juice

One test tube study suggests that **cranberry** (see page 263) juice might be useful for treating or preventing gum disease.[5] However, there is one kink to work out before cranberry could be practical for this purpose: the sweeteners added to cranberry juice aren't good for your teeth, but without them cranberry juice is very bitter.

Coenzyme Q$_{10}$ (CoQ$_{10}$)

The supplement **CoQ$_{10}$** (see page 256) is sometimes claimed to be an effective treatment for periodontal disease. However, the studies on which this idea is based are too flawed to be taken as meaningful.[6]

Other Herbs and Supplements

Other treatments proposed for periodontal disease include **zinc** (see page 463), **vitamin C** (see page 444), **calcium** (see page 234), **magnesium** (see page 351), **vitamin B$_{12}$** (see page 442), **bloodroot** (see page 224), and **tea tree** (see page 421) oil. However, as yet none of these suggestions can be regarded as proven.

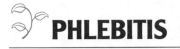

PHLEBITIS

Related Terms   Saphenous Thrombophlebitis, Thrombophlebitis, Superficial Phlebitis, Deep Vein Thrombosis

Principal Proposed Treatments   There are no well-established natural treatments for phlebitis.

Other Proposed Treatments   Bromelain, Aortic Glycosaminoglycans (GAGs), Horse Chestnut

The term *phlebitis* refers to an inflammation of a vein, usually in the leg, frequently accompanied by blood clots that adhere to the wall of the vein. When the affected vein is close to the surface, the condition is called superficial phlebitis. This condition usually resolves on its own without further complications. However, when phlebitis occurs in a deep vein, a condition called deep vein thrombosis (DVT), a clot could dislodge from the vein and lodge in the lungs. This is a life-threatening condition.

Symptoms of superficial phlebitis include pain, swelling, redness, and warmth around the affected vein. The vein feels hard to the touch because of the clotted blood.

Deep vein thrombosis is harder to diagnose. It can occur without any symptoms until the clot reaches the lungs. However, in about half of the cases, there are warning symptoms including swelling, pain, and warmth in the entire calf, ankle, foot, or thigh (depending on where the involved vein is located). Although these symptoms can also be caused by more benign conditions, deep vein thrombosis is such a life-threatening disorder that physician consultation is necessary.

Risk factors for any type of phlebitis include recent surgery or childbirth, varicose veins, inactivity, or sitting for long periods (such as on a long airplane ride). Prolonged placement of intravenous catheters can also cause phlebitis, possibly requiring antibiotic treatment.

Conventional treatments for superficial phlebitis include analgesics for pain, warm compresses, and compression bandages or stockings to increase blood flow. In more severe cases, anticoagulants or minor surgery may be required.

Deep vein thrombosis requires more aggressive treatment, including hospitalization, strong anticoagulants, and a variety of possible surgical procedures.

PROPOSED TREATMENTS

There are no well-established natural treatments for phlebitis at this time.

Note: Because phlebitis is a potentially life-threatening disorder, you should seek a doctor's advice before attempting any natural treatments.

Bromelain

Bromelain (see page 229) is an enzyme found in the stems of pineapple. Because it has anti-inflammatory properties and may be able to prevent blood platelet aggregation, it has been suggested as a treatment for phlebitis.[1,2,3] However, there is no good evidence supporting this use as of yet.

Aortic Glycosaminoglycans

Aortic glycosaminoglycans (GAGs; see page 207) are substances found in the tissues of the body, including blood vessels. They are closely related to the anticoagulant drug heparin. Preliminary evidence suggests that aortic GAGs might be helpful in treating phlebitis,[4] although not all studies agree.[5]

Other Natural Treatments

Horse chestnut (see page 325) is often used for chronic venous insufficiency and **varicose veins** (see page 184), conditions related to phlebitis. For this reason, horse chestnut is sometimes recommended for phlebitis as well, although there is as yet no real evidence that it works.

Phlebitis

Visit Us at TNP.com

PHOTOSENSITIVITY

Related Terms   Photodermatitis, Phototoxicity, Porphyria Cutanea Tarda, Photoallergy, Polymorphous Light Eruptions, Erythropoietic Protoporphyria

Principal Proposed Treatments   Avoiding Photosensitizing Plants, Beta-Carotene

Other Proposed Treatments   Vitamin C, Vitamin E, AMP, Vitamin B_6, Nicotinamide, EGCG

Nearly everyone will burn if exposed to enough ultra-violet radiation from the sun or other sources. However, some people burn particularly easily or develop exaggerated skin reactions to sunlight. Doctors call this condition photosensitivity. For some people, taking certain medications or plant products—or rubbing them on their skin—can cause photosensitivity. Similar reactions are seen in diseases such as some forms of porphyria (a group of usually hereditary metabolic disorders) or lupus. In another condition, called polymorphous light eruptions, dramatic rashes can develop after fairly limited sun exposure.

The most important step toward treating photosensitivity is to identify whether an external substance is causing the reaction, and then eliminate it if possible. Antibiotics are among the most common photosensitizing drugs. Many other natural substances can also cause this reaction. Another commonsense step is to use sunscreen and wear protective clothing, or simply to stay out of the sun.

Some types of photosensitivity may respond to specific treatments such as oral beta-carotene, steroids, or other medications.

PRINCIPAL PROPOSED TREATMENTS

As with conventional treatment, natural treatment begins with identifying any potential photosensitizing substances, including herbs. Beta-carotene may be helpful for treating polymorphous light eruptions or the photosensitivity of porphyria.

St. John's Wort and Other Plants: Can Cause Photosensitivity

A number of common herbs and plant products are known to provoke extreme reactions to sunlight in some individuals. One of the more well-known culprits is **St. John's wort** (see page 414), which has caused fatal photosensitivity reactions in cattle that grazed on it. In humans, no such problems have been reported at normal doses.[1] However, in one study of highly sun-sensitive people, double doses of the herb produced mild increases in reaction to ultraviolet radiation.[2] If you are particularly sun sensitive, exert extra sun precautions

when taking St. John's wort and don't exceed recommended doses.

Photosensitivity can also result from touching or eating other plants, including celery, dill, fennel, fig, lime, parsley, and parsnip, as well as arnica, artichoke, chrysanthemum, dandelion, lettuce, endive, marigold, and sunflower.[3,4] Lest you swear off gardening or salads altogether, be aware that most people do not react to these plants. Essential oils—of lime, for example—may be more problematic than the plant itself.

Beta-Carotene: May Help, but Evidence Is Conflicting

Beta-carotene (see page 217), a plant pigment giving color to carrots and yams, may be beneficial for at least two kinds of photosensitivity: polymorphous light eruptions (PLE)[5,6] and photosensitivity caused by certain types of porphyria.[7,8,9] It is the best-studied supplement for photosensitivity, although only four studies on it have been placebo-controlled and these had conflicting results.[10,11,12] According to one theory, beta-carotene prevents skin damage by neutralizing free radicals, harmful chemicals created in the skin by the action of radiation.[13]

One characteristic of beta-carotene is that it gives a deep yellow color to human skin when taken in high doses for several months. Since supplementation must go on for a while to see results, this side effect makes it difficult to conduct a truly double-blind study in which neither researchers nor the participants know who is taking the active compound and who is taking placebo. Once people begin to turn yellow, they are likely to figure out what they're taking, possibly affecting the study outcome. Therefore, even the results of placebo-controlled studies of beta-carotene are open to question.

What Is the Scientific Evidence for Beta-Carotene?

Three controlled trials of beta-carotene for polymorphous light eruptions found mixed results. A 10-week study in 50 people with PLE given beta-carotene plus canthaxanthin (another carotene) or placebo found evidence of significant benefit.[14] However, in two other controlled trials of beta-carotene alone, lasting 12 to 15 weeks (the number of participants was not reported), modest benefits were seen in one study and no benefits at all in the other.[15] None of these studies were truly double-blind (for the reason mentioned above).

Many uncontrolled studies have reported that beta-carotene extends the time that people with erythropoietic protoporphyria (EPP) can safely spend in the sun.[16,17,18] However, an 11-month controlled trial found no benefit.[19] A few case reports suggest beta-carotene may also be helpful in another kind of porphyria called porphyria cutanea tarda.[20] However, such studies cannot rule out the power of suggestion.

Several studies have found beta-carotene to be helpful in preventing ordinary sunburn,[21–24] but, again, other studies found no benefit.[25,26]

Dosage

In the research on beta-carotene for EPP, the adult dose used was 100 to 200 mg per day (sometimes up to 300).[27] Doses of 100 to 200 mg were used in studies on polymorphous light eruption.[28,29] In one of these, a combination of beta-carotene with canthaxanthin was given at a dose of 100 mg per day.[30] According to some researchers, full benefits may require 1 to 3 months of treatment to become apparent.[31] However, because of recent safety concerns with beta-carotene supplements, it is important to take high-dose supplements only under medical supervision (see Safety Issues below).

Safety Issues

Beta-carotene has long been considered a safe supplement. The only side effects reported from high-dosage beta-carotene are diarrhea and a yellowish tinge to the hands and feet. These symptoms disappear once use is discontinued or changed to lower doses. However, evidence has begun to accumulate that long-term use of beta-carotene might slightly increase risk of heart disease and cancer.[32–36] For this reason, high doses of beta-carotene supplements should only be taken on medical advice.

OTHER PROPOSED TREATMENTS

Other treatments sometimes recommended for preventing the photosensitivity of porphyria include **vitamins C** (see page 444) and **E** (see page 451), EGCG (a bioflavonoid found in **green tea;** see page 318), adenosine monophosphate (AMP), and **vitamin B$_6$** (see page 439). However, evidence for the effectiveness of these treatments is fairly minimal.

One gram daily of vitamin C was given to 12 people with EPP in a double-blind placebo-controlled trial.[37] Although 8 of the 12 reported improved sunlight tolerance, the study was too small for the results to be statistically significant.

In an uncontrolled study of AMP in 21 people with porphyria cutanea tarda, many showed decreased photosensitivity, much to the surprise of the investigator.[38] Two cases of EPP were also reportedly improved by vitamin B$_6$.[39] In addition, nicotinamide—another B vitamin—was found to help prevent polymorphous light eruptions in an uncontrolled study of 42 people.[40]

Evidence that vitamin C and vitamin E may help prevent **sunburn** (see page 171) in people without photosensitivity provides indirect evidence that these substances may be helpful for photosensitivity as well. However, a small double-blind placebo-controlled trial of individuals with polymorphous light eruption found no benefit with combined vitamin C (3 g per day) and vitamin E (1,500 IU per day).[41]

Studies on laboratory animals found that topical vitamin C and vitamin E, alone or together, helped prevent burning on exposure to ultraviolet light.[42–45] Two placebo-controlled human studies, one only partially blinded, found that a combination of oral vitamin C and E also modestly reduced skin redness from UV radiation.[46,47] However, placebo-controlled human studies of oral vitamin E or C taken alone found that they didn't help.[48,49]

Theoretically, EGCG may also reduce photosensitivity. Research suggests that spreading it on the skin may help prevent sunburn caused by ultraviolet rays in both animals and people.[50,51]

PMS (Premenstrual Syndrome)

Principal Proposed Treatments   Calcium, Chasteberry

Other Proposed Treatments   Ginkgo, Magnesium, Vitamin E, Multivitamin and Mineral Supplement, GLA (Gamma-Linolenic Acid), Progesterone Cream

Probably Ineffective Treatments   Vitamin B$_6$

Many women experience a variety of unpleasant symptoms in the week or two before menstruating. These include irritability, anger, headaches, anxiety, depression, fatigue, fluid retention, and breast tenderness. These symptoms undoubtedly result from hormonal changes of the menstrual cycle, but we don't know the cause of PMS or exactly how to treat it.

Conventional treatments include antidepressants, antianxiety drugs, beta-blockers, diuretics, oral contraceptives, and other hormonally active formulations. None of these treatments is entirely effective except for those that take the drastic step of inducing artificial menopause.

PRINCIPAL PROPOSED TREATMENTS

There is fairly good evidence that calcium supplements can significantly reduce all the major symptoms of PMS. There is also some evidence that the herbs chasteberry and ginkgo can lessen the symptoms of PMS. Vitamin B$_6$ is widely recommended as well, but its scientific record is mixed at best.

Calcium: May Improve All Symptoms of PMS

A recent study found surprisingly positive results using **calcium** (1,200 mg daily; see page 234) for the treatment of PMS symptoms. These results have made a big impact because the study was large (about 500 women) and was performed at a prestigious medical center, Columbia University.[1]

Participants took 300 mg of calcium (as calcium carbonate) 4 times daily. Compared to placebo, calcium significantly reduced mood swings, pain, bloating, depression, back pain, and food cravings. Similar findings were also seen in earlier preliminary studies.[2,3]

For healthy women, calcium is safe when taken at this dosage. However, if you have cancer, hyperparathyroidism, or sarcoidosis, you should take calcium only under the supervision of a physician.

Chasteberry: Especially Effective for Breast Tenderness

The herb **chasteberry** (see page 245) is widely used in Europe as a treatment for PMS symptoms. More than most herbs, chasteberry is frequently called by its Latin names: *vitex* or *Vitex agnus-castus*. A shrub in the verbena family, chasteberry is commonly found on riverbanks and nearby foothills in central Asia and around the Mediterranean Sea. After its violet flowers have bloomed, a dark brown, peppercorn-size fruit develops, with a pleasant odor reminiscent of peppermint. It is the fruit that is used medicinally.

The modern use of chasteberry dates back to the 1950s, when the German pharmaceutical firm Madaus Company first produced a standardized extract. It has become a standard European treatment for PMS, cyclical breast tenderness, and menstrual irregularities.

Reportedly, chasteberry can reduce many of the symptoms of PMS, but it is probably most dramatically effective for breast tenderness. This is probably because chasteberry suppresses the release of prolactin, a hormone that affects the breasts. Unlike other herbs used for women's health problems, research has shown that chasteberry does not contain any chemicals that act like estrogen or progesterone. Rather, it acts on the pituitary gland to suppress the release of prolactin.[4–7] Prolactin naturally rises during pregnancy to stimulate milk production and other physiological changes.

What Is the Scientific Evidence for Chasteberry?

Chasteberry is widely used in Germany as a general treatment for PMS. However, the scientific record for chasteberry lacks properly designed double-blind studies.

German gynecologists clearly believe that chasteberry is effective for PMS. In surveys involving about 3,000 women who had been prescribed chasteberry, physicians rated the overall effect of the treatment as good or very good about 90% of the time.[8,9] Based on the women's own reports, good results were seen in about 60% of participants, but only 30% reported complete relief. Chasteberry may be particularly effective in reducing the cyclic breast pain of PMS.[10]

However, these were not double-blind studies. Since there is a very high level of placebo response in PMS, often reaching 70%,[11] proper double-blind studies are necessary to determine the actual effectiveness of chasteberry.

A recently reported double-blind study followed 175 women with PMS for 3 months. Half of them received a standard chasteberry preparation, and the other half took 200 mg of pyridoxine (vitamin B$_6$) daily.[12] Over the 3-month study period, chasteberry was associated with "a considerably more marked alleviation of typical PMS complaints, such as breast tenderness, edema, inner tension, headache, constipation and depression." Overall, 77% of the participants treated with chasteberry showed improvement.

The main problem with this study is that pyridoxine itself is not a proven treatment for PMS; so the fact that chasteberry proved superior is not necessarily very meaningful (see the following discussion under the heading Vitamin B$_6$: May Not Be Effective).

Dosage

The typical dose of dry chasteberry extract is 20 to 40 mg given once a day. Chasteberry is sold often as a liquid extract to be taken at a dosage of 40 drops each morning. However, extracts that require higher or lower dosing are also available. We recommend following the label instructions.

Safety Issues

No detailed studies of the safety of chasteberry have been conducted. However, its widespread use in Germany has not led to any reports of significant adverse effects,[13] with the exception of a single case of excessive ovarian stimulation possibly caused by chasteberry.[14] In a study of over 1,500 women, mild side effects such as nausea, headache, and allergic skin reactions were reported by less than 2.5% of participants.[15]

Because it lowers prolactin levels, chasteberry is not an appropriate treatment for pregnant or nursing mothers. Its safety in adolescents or those with severe liver or kidney disease has not been established.

No known drug interactions are associated with chasteberry. However, it's quite conceivable that the herb could interfere with other hormonal medications, such as birth control pills, or drugs that affect the pituitary, such as bromocriptine.

Vitamin B$_6$: May Not Be Effective

Vitamin B$_6$ (see page 439) has been used for PMS for many decades, both by European and U.S. physicians. However, the results of scientific studies are mixed at best. A recent, properly designed, double-blind study found no benefit from vitamin B$_6$.[16] A dozen or more other double-blind studies have investigated the effectiveness of vitamin B$_6$ for PMS, but actually the negative studies cancel out the positive ones.[17] Some books on natural medicine report that the negative studies used too little B$_6$, but in reality there was no clear link between dosage and effectiveness.

The maximum safe dosage of vitamin B$_6$ for self-use is 50 mg twice daily. Higher doses should be used only under a physician's supervision because of the potential risk of nerve injury. Preliminary evidence suggests that the combination of B$_6$ and magnesium might be more effective than either treatment alone.[18]

OTHER PROPOSED TREATMENTS

Ginkgo: For Breast Tenderness and Other PMS Symptoms

One double-blind placebo-controlled study evaluated the benefits of *Ginkgo biloba* (see page 298) extract for women with PMS symptoms.[19] This trial enrolled 143 women, 18 to 45 years of age, and followed them for two menstrual cycles. Each woman received either the ginkgo extract (80 mg twice daily) or placebo on day 16 of the first cycle. Treatment was continued until day 5 of the next cycle, and resumed again on day 16 of that cycle.

The results were impressive. As compared to placebo, ginkgo significantly relieved major symptoms of PMS, especially breast pain and emotional disturbance.

Magnesium

Preliminary studies suggest that **magnesium** (see page 351) may also be helpful in PMS. A double-blind placebo-controlled study of 32 women found that magnesium taken from day 15 of the menstrual cycle to the onset of menstrual flow could significantly improve premenstrual mood changes.[20]

Another small, double-blind study (20 participants) found that magnesium supplementation might help prevent menstrual migraines.[21]

Magnesium is usually supplemented in the range of 200 to 600 mg daily, but for PMS it is sometimes given at a dosage of 500 to 1,000 mg daily starting on day 15 of the menstrual cycle and continuing through the beginning of menstruation. This dosage should be safe in healthy women, but if you suffer from any medical problems, you should check with a physician before trying it. As mentioned earlier, preliminary evidence suggests that combining vitamin B$_6$ with magnesium might improve the results.[22]

Vitamin E

Weak evidence suggests that **vitamin E** (see page 451) may be helpful for PMS.[23] A typical dosage of vitamin E is 400 IU daily.

Multivitamin and Mineral Supplements

Preliminary evidence suggests that combined treatment with a multivitamin and mineral supplement may be helpful in PMS.[24–27]

GLA: Primarily for Cyclic Breast Tenderness

Evening primrose oil, a source of GLA, is used for the breast pain that often occurs with premenstrual syndrome called **cyclic mastalgia** (see page 58). It may be helpful with other PMS symptoms as well, but the scientific evidence is weak.[28]

A typical dosage of evening primrose oil is 3 g daily. It must be taken for at least 4 to 6 weeks for noticeable effect, and maximum benefits may require 4 to 8 months to develop. Evening primrose oil appears to be safe. (See the chapter on **GLA** for more information about use and safety issues.)

Additional Treatments

Progesterone cream (see page 392) is another method widely recommended for PMS, but there is little evidence that it is effective.[29] Highly preliminary evidence suggests that **St. John's wort** (see page 414) might be helpful for PMS.[30]

PSORIASIS

Principal Proposed Treatments   There are no well-established natural treatments for psoriasis.

Other Proposed Treatments   Fish Oil, Oregon Grape, *Aloe vera* Cream, Cartilage, Beta-Carotene, Burdock, Chromium, *Coleus forskohlii*, Goldenseal, Topical Licorice Cream, Milk Thistle, Red Clover, Selenium, Taurine, Vitamin E, Zinc, Fumaric Acid, Vitamin A, Vitamin D

Up to 2% of Americans suffer from psoriasis, a skin condition that leads to an intensely itchy rash with clearly defined borders and scales that resemble silvery mica. The fingernails are also frequently involved, showing pitting or thickening.

Medical treatment for psoriasis includes applications of topical steroids and peeling agents that expose the underlying skin for the steroid to contact. Ultraviolet light can also be used, sometimes combined with coal tar applications or medications called psoralens. Synthetic versions of vitamin A can also be helpful. For especially problematic psoriasis, low doses of the anticancer drug methotrexate have proven quite effective.

PROPOSED TREATMENTS

The following natural treatments are widely recommended for psoriasis, but they have not been scientifically proven effective at this time.

Fish Oil

There is some evidence that eicosapentaenoic acid (EPA) from **fish oil** (see page 282) may be a bit helpful in psoriasis. One 8-week double-blind study followed 28 people with chronic psoriasis.[1] Half received 1.8 g of EPA daily (supplied by 10 capsules of fish oil), and the other half received placebo. By the end of the study, researchers saw significant improvement in itching, redness, and scaling, but not in the size of the psoriasis patches.

However, another double-blind study followed 145 people with moderate to severe psoriasis for 4 months and found no benefit as compared to placebo.[2]

Fish oil appears to be safe. The most common problem is fishy burps.

However, because fish oil has a mild "blood-thinning" effect, it should not be combined with powerful blood-thinning medications, such as Coumadin (warfarin) or heparin, except on a physician's advice. However, contrary to some reports, fish oil does not seem to cause bleeding problems when it is taken by itself.[3]

Also, fish oil does not appear to raise blood sugar levels in people with diabetes.[4] Nonetheless, if you have diabetes, you should not take any supplement except on the advice of a physician.

Fish oil may temporarily raise the level of LDL ("bad") cholesterol, but this effect seems to be short-lived and levels return to normal with continued use.[5,6]

If you decide to use cod liver oil as your fish oil supplement, make sure you do not exceed the safe maximum intake of **vitamin A** (see page 432) and **vitamin D** (see page 449). These vitamins are fat soluble, which means that excess amounts tend to build up in your body, possibly reaching toxic levels. Pregnant women should not take more than 2,667 IU of vitamin A daily because of the risk of birth defects; 5,000 IU per day is a reasonable upper limit for other individuals. Look at the bottle label to determine how much vitamin A you are receiving. (It is less likely that you will get enough vitamin D to produce toxic effects.)

Oregon Grape

Preliminary evidence suggests that the herb **Oregon grape** (*Mahonia;* see page 375) may help reduce symptoms of psoriasis, although it does not seem to be as effective as standard medications.[7,8,9]

A double-blind placebo-controlled study involving 82 people with psoriasis tested the effectiveness of topical application of *Mahonia*.[10] Participants used a placebo ointment on one side of their bodies and *Mahonia* on the other. According to the participants' assessments, the *Mahonia* ointment produced significantly better results. However, the physicians did not observe significant differences between the two. One possible design flaw was that the treatment salve was darker in color than the placebo, possibly allowing participants to guess which was which.

Another study found that dithranol, a conventional drug used to treat psoriasis symptoms, was more effective than *Mahonia*.[11] Regrettably, the authors fail to state whether this study was double-blind. Forty-nine participants applied one treatment to their left side and the other to their right for 4 weeks. Skin biopsies were then analyzed and compared with samples taken at the beginning of the study. The physicians evaluating changes in skin tissue were unaware which treatments had been used on the samples. Greater improvements were seen in the dithranol group.

A large open study in which 443 participants with psoriasis used *Mahonia* topically for 12 weeks found the herb to be helpful for 73.7% of the group.[12] Without a placebo group, it's not possible to know whether *Mahonia* was truly responsible for the improvement seen, but the trial does help to establish the herb's safety and tolerability (see the chapter on Oregon grape for more information about safety issues).

Laboratory research suggests *Mahonia* has some effects at the cellular level that might be helpful in psoriasis, such as slowing the rate of abnormal cell growth and reducing inflammation.[13,14]

Aloe

Aloe vera (see page 204) cream may be helpful for psoriasis, according to a double-blind study that enrolled 60 men and women with mild to moderate symptoms of psoriasis.[15] Participants were treated with either topical *Aloe vera* extract (0.5%) or a placebo cream, applied 3 times daily for 4 weeks. Aloe treatment produced significantly better results than placebo, and these results were said to endure for almost a year after treatment was stopped. The study authors also reported a high level of

complete "cure," but what exactly they meant by this was not reported clearly.

Other Herbs and Supplements

Based on very preliminary evidence, shark **cartilage** (see page 241) has been proposed as a treatment for psoriasis.[16]

Beta-carotene (see page 217), **burdock** (see page 232), **chromium** (see page 251), *Coleus forskohlii* (see page 259), **goldenseal** (see page 314), topical **licorice** (see page 344) cream, **milk thistle** (see page 361), **red clover** (see page 397), **selenium** (see page 407), **taurine** (see page 420), **vitamin E** (see page 451), and **zinc** (see page 463) are also sometimes mentioned as possible treatments for psoriasis. However, as yet there is no real evidence that they work.

A somewhat toxic natural substance called fumaric acid is sometimes recommended for psoriasis as well. **Vitamin A** (see page 432) or special forms of **vitamin D** (see page 449) taken at high levels may improve symptoms, but these are dangerous treatments that should be used only under the supervision of a physician.

RAYNAUD'S PHENOMENON

Principal Proposed Treatments   There are no well-established natural treatments for Raynaud's phenomenon.

Other Proposed Treatments   Inositol Hexaniacinate
    Essential Fatty Acids: Fish Oil, GLA (Gamma-Linolenic Acid)
    Ginkgo

Raynaud's phenomenon is a little understood condition in which the fingers and toes show an exaggerated sensitivity to cold. Classic cases show a characteristic white, blue, and red color sequence, as the digits lose blood supply and then rewarm. Some people develop only one or two of these signs.

The cause of Raynaud's phenomenon is unknown.

Conventional treatment consists mainly of reassurance and the recommendation to avoid exposure to cold and the use of tobacco (which can worsen Raynaud's). In severe cases, a variety of drugs can be tried.

PROPOSED TREATMENTS

The following natural treatments are widely recommended for Raynaud's phenomenon, but they have not yet been scientifically proven effective.

Inositol Hexaniacinate

According to one preliminary double-blind study, the special form of niacin (**vitamin B$_3$;** see page 437) called

inositol hexaniacinate may be helpful for Raynaud's phenomenon.[1] The dosage used in the study was 4 g daily. At this level of supplementation, regular blood tests to rule out liver inflammation are highly recommended. All forms of niacin may cause facial flushing.

Essential Fatty Acids

High doses of fish oil have also shown good results for Raynaud's phenomenon in preliminary double-blind studies.[2,3] However, a very high dosage must be used, perhaps 12 g daily. See the chapter on **fish oil** for specific safety information.

Another preliminary double-blind study suggests that high doses of GLA may be useful as well.[4,5] (For more information on use and safety issues, see the chapter on **GLA.**)

When taking essential fatty acids, it is a good idea to take vitamin E as well to prevent the fats from being damaged by free radicals. (For more information on use and safety issues, see the chapter on **vitamin E.**)

Visit Us at TNP.com

Ginkgo

Although no direct evidence shows that ginkgo is helpful for Raynaud's phenomenon, it has been shown to in-crease circulation in the fingertips[6] and thus may be useful. (For more information on use and safety issues, see the chapter on **ginkgo.**)

RESTLESS LEGS SYNDROME

Principal Proposed Treatments   There are no well-established natural treatments for restless legs syndrome.

Other Proposed Treatments   Magnesium, Folate, Iron, Vitamin E, Vitamin C, Vitamin B_{12}

People with restless legs syndrome (RLS) often feel an intense urge to move their legs, particularly when sitting still or trying to fall asleep. Unlike those with nighttime leg cramps—a different condition—people with RLS don't experience pain. Instead, they may describe an uncomfortable "creepy-crawly sensation" inside their legs. Walking relieves the symptoms, but as soon as people settle down again, the urge to move recurs. The feeling is sometimes described as "wanting to ride a bicycle under the covers."

RLS tends to run in families, often emerging or worsening with age. People with RLS frequently have another condition as well, called periodic leg movements in sleep (PLMS). People with PLMS kick their legs frequently during the night, disrupting their own sleep and that of their bed partner.

Since RLS is occasionally linked to other serious diseases, it's advisable to see a doctor if you have its symptoms.

Conventional medical treatment for RLS usually involves taking a levodopa/carbidopa combination, better known as a treatment for Parkinson's disease. The drug quinine has been used in the past, but one double-blind study found it to be ineffective.[1] Because of this and a risk of dangerous side effects, quinine is no longer used for this purpose.

PROPOSED TREATMENTS

Preliminary evidence suggests that symptoms of RLS may be relieved by supplementation with one of several minerals or vitamins, including magnesium, folate, iron and vitamin E. However, no double-blind studies have, as yet, found any of these treatments to be effective.

Magnesium

Preliminary studies suggest that supplemental **magnesium** (see page 351) may be helpful, even when magnesium levels are normal.[2,3] An open study of 10 people with insomnia related to RLS or periodic leg movements in sleep found that their sleep improved significantly when they took magnesium nightly for 4 to 6 weeks.[4]

Folate

Based on numerous case reports of improvement, **folate** (see page 288) is also sometimes recommended for RLS. Symptoms decreased in one study of 45 patients given 5 to 30 mg of folate daily.[5] However, because this was not a double-blind experiment, the value of the results is questionable. Keep in mind that such high doses of folate should be administered only under medical supervision. Folate may be of particular benefit to pregnant women with RLS who are deficient in this vitamin.[6]

Iron

A number of studies have linked RLS to low levels of **iron** (see page 333) in the blood.[7] In one analysis of the medical records of 27 people with RLS, those with the most severe symptoms had lower-than-average levels of serum ferritin, one measure of iron deficiency.[8] In another study in which 18 elderly people with RLS were compared with 18 elderly people without the condition, those with RLS also had reduced levels of serum ferritin.[9] When 15 of these people were given iron, all but one experienced a reduction in symptoms. Those with the lowest initial ferritin levels improved the most. However, because this was not a double-blind study, it isn't clear how much of the observed benefit was due to the placebo effect.

In contrast to these results, a recent double-blind study of 28 people found that iron didn't relieve RLS any better than placebo.[10] However, in this particular study, participants had normal levels of iron on average. The study didn't effectively measure whether iron might help RLS among people with iron deficiencies.

One theory holds that mild iron deficiency may cause RLS by decreasing the amount of a neurotransmitter called dopamine. This theory is supported by findings that conventional drugs that increase dopamine activity (such as the Parkinson's medication mentioned above) can also alleviate RLS.[11]

Restless Legs Syndrome

Visit Us at TNP.com

Tests for anemia won't necessarily pick up the low-grade iron deficiency that is linked to RLS. Be sure your doctor tests specifically for iron deficiency, not just anemia.

Vitamin E

Vitamin E (see page 451) may also help with this condition. Seven out of nine people with RLS given 400 to 800 IU daily of vitamin E experienced virtually complete control of symptoms, while the other two had partial relief.[12] Other anecdotal reports suggest that vitamin C may be useful, and that **vitamin B$_{12}$** (see page 442) may benefit people with RLS who are deficient in this nutrient.[13,14] However, until properly designed studies are performed, we cannot draw firm conclusions.

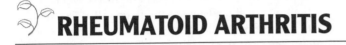

RHEUMATOID ARTHRITIS

Principal Proposed Treatments   Fish Oil

Other Proposed Treatments   Boswellia, Devil's Claw, Curcumin (Turmeric), Bromelain, *Tripterygium wilfordii*, Yucca, GLA (Gamma-Linolenic Acid), Zinc, Vitamin E, MSM (Methyl Sulfonyl Methane), Beta-Carotene, Betaine Hydrochloride, Boron, Burdock, Cat's Claw, Cayenne, Chamomile, Copper, Feverfew, Folate, Ginger, L-Histidine, Horsetail, Magnesium, Manganese, Molybdenum, Pantothenic Acid, D-Phenylalanine, Pregnenolone, Proteolytic Enzymes, Sea Cucumber, Vitamin C, White Willow, Chinese Herbs, Selenium, Dietary Changes, Flaxseed Oil

Rheumatoid arthritis is an autoimmune disease in the general family of **lupus** (see page 114). For reasons that are not understood, in rheumatoid arthritis the immune system goes awry and begins attacking innocent tissues, especially cartilage in the joints. Various joints become red, hot, and swollen under the onslaught. The pattern of inflammation is usually symmetrical, occurring on both sides of the body. Other symptoms include inflammation of the eyes, nodules or lumps under the skin, and a general feeling of malaise.

Rheumatoid arthritis is more common in women than in men and typically begins between the ages of 35 and 60. The diagnosis is made by matching the pattern of symptoms with certain characteristic laboratory results.

Medical treatment consists mainly of two categories of drugs: anti-inflammatory drugs in the ibuprofen family (nonsteroidal anti-inflammatory drugs, or NSAIDs) and drugs that may be able to put rheumatoid arthritis into full or partial remission, the so-called disease-modifying antirheumatic drugs (DMARDs).

Anti-inflammatory drugs relieve symptoms of rheumatoid arthritis but do not change the overall progression of the disease, whereas the DMARDs seem to affect the disease itself. A good analogy might be the various options available to "treat" a house "suffering" from a severe termite infestation. You could remove heavy furniture, tiptoe about instead of holding public dances, and put large beams under the joists. However, none of these methods would do anything to stop the gradual destruction of your house. These methods are like NSAIDs and other supportive techniques in that they treat only the symptoms.

A more definitive approach would be to hire an exterminator and kill the termites. In medical terms, this would be described as a disease-modifying treatment. Because medical treatments for chronic diseases are seldom as completely effective as this example, a closer analogy might be spraying a chemical that slows the spread of termites but does not stop them.

In rheumatoid arthritis, the drugs believed to alter the course of the disease (to slow it down or stop it) include gold compounds, D-penicillamine, antimalarials, sulfasalazine, and methotrexate. They are unrelated to one another but work somewhat similarly in practice.

Unfortunately, all the drugs in this category are quite toxic and reliably cause severe side effects. Because of this toxicity, for years a so-called pyramid approach was taken with people with rheumatoid arthritis. Physicians started with NSAIDs to help with the pain and inflammation, and progressed to successively stronger and more toxic medications only when the basic treatments failed. Natural treatments such as those described here might also be useful in early stages.

However, over the last few years, research has found that severe joint damage occurs very early in rheumatoid arthritis. This evidence has caused many authorities to suggest early, aggressive treatment with disease-modifying drugs to prevent joint damage. Nonetheless, this approach has not been universally adopted, and many physicians still prescribe NSAIDs for early stages of rheumatoid arthritis. The treatments described here may be reasonable alternative options.

Visit Us at TNP.com

Rheumatoid Arthritis

Visit Us at TNP.com

PRINCIPAL PROPOSED TREATMENTS

Rheumatoid arthritis is a difficult disease, and no alternative approach solves it easily. Even if you choose to use alternative methods, you should maintain regular visits to a rheumatologist to watch for serious complications. Finally, keep in mind that medical treatment may be able to slow the progression of rheumatoid arthritis. It is not likely that any of the alternative options have the same power.

Fish Oil

Fish oil (see page 282) is the only natural treatment for rheumatoid arthritis with significant documentation. According to the results of 12 double-blind placebo-controlled studies involving a total of over 500 participants, supplementation with omega-3 fatty acids can significantly reduce the symptoms of rheumatoid arthritis.[1] However, unlike some of the standard treatments, fish oil probably does not slow the progression of rheumatoid arthritis.

The most important omega-3 fatty acids found in fish oil are called EPA (eicosapentaenoic acid) and DHA (docosahexaenoic acid). Many forms of fish oil contain about 18% EPA and 12% DHA, for a total of about 30% by weight of omega-3 oils. In order to match the dosage used in several major studies, you should probably take enough fish oil to supply about 1.8 g of EPA (1,800 mg) and 0.9 g (900 mg) of DHA daily. Results may take 3 to 4 months to develop.

There are many forms of fish oil. If you decide to use cod liver oil as your fish oil supplement, make sure you do not exceed the safe maximum intake of **vitamin A** (see page 432) and **vitamin D** (see page 449). These vitamins are fat-soluble, which means that excess amounts tend to build up in your body, potentially reaching toxic levels. Otherwise, fish oil appears to be safe. The most common problem is fishy burps. It does have a mild "blood-thinning" effect, so it should not be combined with strong anticoagulant drugs such as Coumadin (warfarin) and heparin unless so instructed by a physician. However, contrary to some reports, fish oil does not seem to cause bleeding problems when it is taken by itself.[2] It also does not appear to raise blood sugar levels in people with diabetes.[3] However, if you have diabetes, you should not take any supplement except on the advice of a physician. Fish oil may temporarily raise the level of LDL ("bad") cholesterol, but this effect seems to be short-lived, and levels return to normal with continued use.[4,5]

Flaxseed oil (see page 285) has been offered as a more palatable substitute for fish oil, but it doesn't seem to work.[6]

Eating a lot of fish may be helpful.[7]

OTHER PROPOSED TREATMENTS

The following natural treatments are widely recommended for rheumatoid arthritis, but they have not yet been scientifically proven effective.

Boswellia

Boswellia serrata (see page 228) is a shrub-like tree that grows in the dry hills of the Indian subcontinent. It is the source of a resin called salai guggal, which has been used for thousands of years in Ayurvedic medicine, the traditional medicine of the region. It is very similar to a resin from a related tree, *Boswellia carteri*, which is also known as frankincense. Both substances have been used historically for arthritis.

Recent research has identified boswellic acids as the likely active ingredients in boswellia. In animal studies, boswellic acids have shown anti-inflammatory effects, but their mechanism of action seems to be quite different from that of standard anti-inflammatory medications.[8–11]

An issue of *Phytomedicine* that was devoted to boswellia briefly reviewed previously unpublished studies on the herb.[12] A pair of placebo-controlled trials involving a total of 81 people with rheumatoid arthritis found significant reductions in swelling and pain over the course of 3 months. Furthermore, a comparative study of 60 participants over 6 months found the boswellia extract relieved symptoms about as well as oral gold therapy. However, keep in mind that while gold shots can induce remission in rheumatoid arthritis, we have no evidence that boswellia can do the same.

Another double-blind study found no difference between boswellia and placebo.[13] The bottom line is that we need more research to know for sure whether boswellia is an effective treatment for rheumatoid arthritis.

The dosage of boswellia most often recommended is 400 mg 3 times a day of an extract that has been standardized to contain 37.5% boswellic acids. The full effect may take as long as 4 to 8 weeks to develop.

Few side effects have been reported with boswellia, other than an occasional allergic reaction or a mild upset stomach. However, due to the lack of formal safety studies, boswellia is not recommended for young children, pregnant or nursing women, or those with severe liver or kidney disease.

Devil's Claw

The herb **devil's claw** (see page 267) may be beneficial in rheumatoid arthritis. One double-blind study followed 89 people with rheumatoid arthritis for 2 months. The group given devil's claw showed a significant decrease in pain intensity and an improvement in mobility.[14]

Another double-blind study of 50 people with various types of arthritis showed that 10 days of treatment with devil's claw provided significant pain relief.[15]

A typical dosage of devil's claw is 750 mg 3 times daily of a preparation standardized to contain 3% iridoid glycosides.

Devil's claw appears to be quite safe, with no evidence of toxicity at doses many times higher than recommended.[16] A 6-month open study of 630 people with arthritis showed no side effects other than occasional mild gastrointestinal distress.[17] However, devil's claw is not advised for those with ulcers. Safety in young children, pregnant or nursing women, and individuals with severe liver or kidney disease has not been established.

Curcumin

Curcumin, an extract of the kitchen spice **turmeric** (see page 425), is often suggested as a treatment for rheumatoid arthritis because it appears to possess anti-inflammatory properties.[18] However, the one, small, double-blind study often cited as evidence for its effectiveness in this disease actually provides no such evidence at all.[19]

The typical dosage of curcumin is 400 to 600 mg 3 times daily. Curcumin is sometimes given in combination with an equal dose of an extract of the pineapple plant called **bromelain** (see page 229), which appears to possess anti-inflammatory properties of its own.[20]

Curcumin is thought to be quite safe.[21] Side effects are rare and are generally limited to occasional allergic reactions and mild stomach upset. However, safety in very young children, pregnant or nursing women, and those with severe liver or kidney disease has not been established. Because curcumin may stimulate contraction of the gallbladder,[22] individuals with gallbladder disease should take curcumin only under the supervision of a physician.

Additional Natural Treatments

The Chinese herb *Tripterygium wilfordii*, also called thunder god vine, has a long history of use for arthritis and skin diseases. A preliminary double-blind placebo-controlled crossover study of 70 individuals suggests that an extract of *Tripterygium wilfordii* may be beneficial in the treatment of rheumatoid arthritis.[23] However, more research is necessary before this can be considered a documented treatment for rheumatoid arthritis.

One preliminary and rather unimpressive double-blind study suggests that the herb **yucca** (see page 462) can help relieve the pain of rheumatoid arthritis.[24]

The essential fatty acid **gamma-linolenic acid** (GLA; see page 304), found in evening primrose oil and borage oil, may help relieve symptoms of rheumatoid arthritis.[25–28] **Zinc** (see page 463) has yielded mixed results in studies.[29,30,31] **Vitamin E** (see page 451) may reduce pain in rheumatoid arthritis, although it does not improve inflammation,[32] and may possibly help prevent rheumatoid arthritis.[33] Finally, very weak evidence suggests that the supplement **MSM** (see page 364) might be helpful as well.[34]

The following treatments are also sometimes proposed as effective for rheumatoid arthritis, but there is as yet little scientific evidence to turn to: **beta-carotene** (see page 217), **betaine hydrochloride** (see page 219), **boron** (see page 227), **burdock** (see page 232), **cat's claw** (see page 242), **cayenne** (see page 243), **chamomile** (see page 244), **copper** (see page 262), **feverfew** (see page 280), **folate** (see page 288), **ginger** (see page 296), **L-histidine** (see page 322), **horsetail** (see page 326), **magnesium** (see page 351), **manganese** (see page 354), molybdenum, **pantothenic acid** (see page 380), **D-phenylalanine** (see page 385), **pregnenolone** (see page 391), **proteolytic enzymes** (see page 393), sea cucumber, **vitamin C** (see page 444), **white willow** (see page 457), and Chinese herbal combinations. The antioxidant mineral **selenium** (see page 407) may help prevent rheumatoid arthritis;[35] studies are mixed on whether it is effective as a treatment.[36,37]

Identifying and avoiding **food allergens** (see page 82) may be helpful in some cases.[38] Adopting a vegetarian diet sometimes brings about improvement in mild rheumatoid arthritis.[39,40]

A 16-week double-blind placebo-controlled trial of 182 individuals with active rheumatoid arthritis evaluated the effectiveness of a combination herbal extract containing ashwagandha, boswellia, ginger, and turmeric.[41] The herbal extract showed no more effectiveness than placebo in nearly all measurements of disease severity; joint swelling alone showed improvement.

SEBORRHEIC DERMATITIS

Related Terms   Dandruff, Seborrhea

Principal Proposed Treatments   Aloe

Other Proposed Treatments   Vitamin B$_6$, Folate

Seborrheic dermatitis is an inflammation of the upper layers of the skin that causes scales on the scalp, face, and other parts of the body. When it affects newborns, it's called cradle cap.

Seborrheic dermatitis starts gradually. In adults, it often first appears as a condition similar to dandruff, but involving more inflammation of the scalp; itching, burning, or hair loss may occur. Seborrhea may also affect the skin behind the ears, on the eyebrows, on the bridge of the nose, around the nose, or on the trunk.

Besides inflammation of the scalp, newborns with cradle cap might get red bumps on their faces, scaling behind the ears, or a persistent diaper rash. Older children with seborrheic dermatitis may develop a thick, flaky rash.

Seborrhea tends to run in families and often worsens during cold weather. Researchers don't know what causes it and they haven't found a cure, but there are ways to control the condition. Special shampoos containing selenium sulfide, pyrithione zinc, salicylic acid, sulfur, or tar may be helpful for adult dandruff associated with seborrhea.

Corticosteroids may be used for intensely inflammatory lesions; but milder treatments, such as salicylic acid in mineral oil or medicated baby shampoo, are used to treat young children and infants who have scalp rashes.

PRINCIPAL PROPOSED TREATMENTS

There is some evidence that the herb aloe might offer some relief to people with seborrheic dermatitis.

Aloe

The gel inside the cactus-like leaves of the **aloe** (see page 204) plant (*Aloe vera*) has traditionally been used to treat burns and cuts. A recent study indicates it may also help relieve the symptoms of seborrheic dermatitis.

In this double-blind placebo-controlled study, 44 adults with seborrheic dermatitis applied either an aloe ointment or a placebo cream to affected areas 2 times daily for 4 to 6 weeks. Compared to the placebo group, those who used aloe reported that their symptoms improved significantly (62% versus 25%). Doctors who examined the participants also concluded that those using aloe had a significant decrease in scaliness, itching, and number of affected areas.[1]

Dosage

For seborrheic dermatitis, apply aloe gel 2 times daily on the affected areas.

Safety Issues

Other than occasional allergic reactions, no serious problems have been reported with topical aloe gel.

OTHER PROPOSED TREATMENTS

Highly preliminary studies in the 1950s and 60s suggest that **folate** (see page 288) taken orally, or **vitamin B$_6$** (see page 439) applied topically, may relieve some symptoms.[2,3]

Essential fatty acids, **zinc** (see page 463), **iron** (see page 333), and **vitamins A** (see page 432), **E** (see page 451), **D** (see page 449), **B$_1$** (see page 434), **B$_2$** (see page 436) and **C** (see page 444) have also been suggested as treatments for seborrheic dermatitis but there is no real evidence as yet that they work.[4]

SEXUAL DYSFUNCTION IN WOMEN

Related Terms   Female Sexual Arousal Disorder, Hypoactive Sexual Desire Disorder, Antidepressant-Induced Sexual Dysfunction

Principal Proposed Treatments   There are no well-established natural treatments for sexual dysfunction in women.

Other Proposed Treatments   DHEA (Dehydroepiandrosterone), *Ginkgo biloba,* Yohimbe Plus Arginine

Sexual impotence in men is a fairly well-known disorder, especially since former Senator Bob Dole has become a spokesman for the cause. However, sexual dysfunction in women is less often discussed. This is possibly because men who are impotent are unable to have sex, whereas women with sexual dysfunction are usually able to have sex but are not interested or don't fully enjoy it.

Though the common belief is that women have psychological rather than physical reasons for sexual dysfunction—and this may be true in some cases—women also have physical causes that may interfere with their ability to enjoy sex. Possible causes include side effects from drugs such as antidepressants or sedatives, hormonal insufficiency, painful intercourse, or adrenal insufficiency. Women experiencing sexual dysfunction should consult a physician to attempt to find its cause, as the problem may indicate a more serious disorder.

Conventional treatments for sexual dysfunction depend on its cause: counseling when the cause is psychological; switching or reducing dosage of drugs when they are at fault; hormone replacement therapy when there is a deficiency; treating the cause of painful intercourse; and correcting adrenal insufficiency. Drugs for these conditions are currently under active investigation. Some occasionally helpful options among those presently available include amantadine, cyproheptadine, buspirone, nefazodone, sildenafil, and bupropion.

PROPOSED TREATMENTS

Although there is no good evidence for natural treatments for sexual dysfunction, several substances have shown promising results in preliminary trials. These include DHEA, *Ginkgo biloba,* yohimbine, and arginine.

DHEA

The hormone **DHEA** (dehydroepiandrosterone; see page 268) may be helpful for sexual dysfunction in women over 70, and those women with adrenal failure. However, we strongly advise physician supervision when using this substance.

DHEA is produced by the adrenal glands. Levels of DHEA decline naturally with age, and fall precipitately in cases of adrenal failure. Because both elderly people and those with adrenal insufficiency report a drop in libido, several studies have examined whether supplemental DHEA can increase libido in these groups.

A 12-month double-blind placebo-controlled trial evaluated the effects of DHEA (50 mg daily) in 280 individuals between the ages of 60 and 79.[1] The results showed that women over 70 experienced an improvement in libido and sexual satisfaction. Other participants did not experience benefit. Effects were not seen until the sixth month, which may explain why similar trials that only lasted 3 months did not find any effect from DHEA.[2,3]

One 4-month double-blind placebo-controlled study of 24 women with adrenal failure found that 50 mg per day of DHEA (along with standard treatment for adrenal failure) improved libido and sexual satisfaction.[4] DHEA is not usually prescribed to individuals with adrenal failure, but this study suggests that it should be.

Keep in mind, however, that although it is sold as a "dietary supplement," DHEA is a potent synthetic hormone that has far-reaching effects throughout the body. Even at the low dose of 25 mg per day, it may decrease levels of HDL ("good") cholesterol.[5,6] In addition, DHEA may cause acne and male-pattern hair growth.[7,8]

There are also conflicting reports linking DHEA to some types of cancer.[9–12] Because DHEA is converted to other hormones in the body, it may also affect hormone-influenced diseases such as breast cancer.

The safety of DHEA in young children and pregnant or nursing women has not been established.

The bottom line: DHEA may be effective, but it should be used only under a doctor's supervision.

Ginkgo biloba

Numerous case reports and preliminary studies suggest that the herb ***Ginkgo biloba*** (see page 298) may be an effective treatment for antidepressant-induced sexual dysfunction.[13–17]

Investigation of ginkgo began after an elderly man with sexual dysfunction caused by an antidepressant decided to take *Ginkgo biloba* to improve his memory. His sexual function improved so dramatically (and unexpectedly) that it caught the attention of researchers.[18]

Subsequent open trials found benefits in men and even greater benefits in women.[19] However, double-blind placebo-controlled studies are needed to reliably evaluate the potential benefits of ginkgo in treating anti-depressant-induced sexual dysfunction. Keep in mind that ginkgo is a "blood thinner" that can increase risk of bleeding, especially if combined with blood-thinning drugs such as warfarin (Coumadin), heparin, and aspirin.

Yohimbine and Arginine

Yohimbine is a drug derived from the bark of the **yohimbe** (see page 461) tree. Studies have only used the standardized drug, not the actual herb. **Arginine** (see page 208) is an amino acid.

One small double-blind study of yohimbine combined with arginine found an increase in measured phys-

ical arousal among 23 women with female sexual arousal disorder.[20] However, the women themselves did not report any noticeable effects. Only the combination of yohimbine and arginine produced results; neither substance was effective when taken on its own.

An open trial of yohimbine alone to treat sexual dysfunction induced by the antidepressant fluoxetine (Prozac) found improvement in eight out of nine people, two of whom were women.[21] However, in the absence of a placebo group, these results can't be taken as reliable; in addition, there are concerns about the safety of combining yohimbe with antidepressants.

Note: Yohimbine (and the herb yohimbe) are relatively dangerous substances in general. They should only be used under physician supervision. Arginine may also present some risks (see these chapters for safety issues).

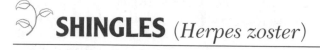

SHINGLES (*Herpes zoster*)

Related Terms   Post-Herpetic Neuralgia

Principal Proposed Treatments   Capsaicin, Proteolytic Enzymes

Other Proposed Treatments   Adenosine Monophosphate (AMP), Vitamin B_{12}, Vitamin E

Herpes zoster (shingles) is an acute, painful infection caused by the varicella-zoster virus, the organism that causes chickenpox. It develops many years after the original chickenpox infection, typically in the elderly or those with compromised immune systems. The first sign may be a tingling feeling, itchiness, or shooting pain on an area of skin. A rash may then appear, with raised dots or blisters forming. When the rash is at its peak, rash symptoms can range from mild itching to extreme pain. People with shingles on the upper half of the face should seek medical attention, as the virus may cause damage to the eyes.

Shingles usually resolves without complications within 3 to 5 weeks. However, in some people, especially the elderly, the pain persists for months or years. This condition, known as post-herpetic neuralgia (PHN), is thought to be due to continuing irritation of the nerves after the infection is over.

Conventional medical treatment for shingles includes antiviral drugs (acyclovir, famicyclovir, valacyclovir). When used properly, these lead to faster resolution of symptoms including lesions and acute neuralgia, and may reduce the incidence and severity of PHN. Steroids (prednisone) and tricyclic antidepressants (amitriptyline) are also prescribed to lessen shingles symptoms, and the former might help prevent PHN.

Individuals who do develop PHN may be treated with steroids, antidepressants, and topical creams (see Capsaicin, below). In severe cases, nerve blocks might be used.

PRINCIPAL PROPOSED TREATMENTS

For the initial attack of shingles, proteolytic enzymes may be helpful. Capsaicin cream is an FDA-approved treatment for PHN.

Proteolytic Enzymes

There is some evidence that **proteolytic enzymes** (see page 393) may be helpful for the initial attack of shingles.

Proteolytic enzymes are produced by the pancreas to aid in digestion of protein, and certain foods also contain these enzymes. Besides their use in digestion, these enzymes may have some effects in the body as a whole when taken orally. The most-studied proteolytic enzymes include papain (from papaya), **bromelain** (from pineapple; see page 229), and trypsin and chymotrypsin (extracted from the pancreas of various animals).

A double-blind study of 190 people with shingles compared proteolytic enzymes to the standard antiviral drug acyclovir.[1] Participants were treated for 14 days and their pain was assessed at intervals. Although both

Shingles

Visit Us at TNP.com

groups had similar pain relief, the enzyme-treated group experienced fewer side effects.

Similar results were seen in another double-blind study in which 90 individuals were given either an injection of acyclovir or enzymes, followed by a course of oral medication for 7 days.[2]

Proteolytic enzymes are thought to benefit cases of shingles by decreasing the body's inflammatory response and regulating immune response to the virus.

Dosage

When you purchase an enzyme, the amount is expressed not only in grams or milligrams but also in activity units or international units. These terms refer to the enzyme's potency (i.e., its digestive power).

Recommended dosages of proteolytic enzymes vary with the form used. Due to the wide variation, we suggest following label instructions. Proteolytic enzymes can be broken down by stomach acid. To prevent this from happening, supplemental enzymes are often coated with a substance that doesn't dissolve until it reaches the intestine. Such a preparation is called "enteric coated."

Safety Issues

Proteolytic enzymes are believed to be quite safe, although there are some concerns that they might further damage the exposed tissue in an ulcer (by partly digesting it). One proteolytic enzyme, pancreatin, may interfere with folate absorption (see the chapter on **folate**). In addition, the proteolytic enzyme papain might increase the blood-thinning effects of warfarin and possibly other anticoagulants.[3]

Capsaicin: Useful for Post-Herpetic Neuralgia

Capsaicin, the "hot" in hot peppers, has been found effective for treating the pain related to PHN, and has been approved by the FDA for that purpose. Capsaicin is thought to work by inhibiting chemicals in nerve cells that transmit pain (see also the chapter on **cayenne**).

Dosage

Topical capsaicin cream is available in 2 strengths, 0.025 and 0.075%. Both preparations are indicated for use in neuralgia. The cream should be applied sparingly to the affected area 3 to 4 times daily. Treatment should continue for several weeks as the benefit may be delayed. Capsaicin creams are approved over-the-counter drugs and should be used as directed.

Safety Issues

Over-the-counter creams containing concentrated capsaicin are recognized as safe, but caution should be used near the eyes and mucous membranes. Mild to moderate burning may occur at first, but it decreases over time.

OTHER PROPOSED TREATMENTS

Adenosine Monophosphate (AMP)

Adenosine monophosphate (AMP), a natural by-product of cell metabolism, has been studied as a possible treatment for initial shingles symptoms as well as PHN prevention.

In a double-blind placebo-controlled study of 32 people with shingles, AMP was injected 3 times a week for 4 weeks.[4] At the end of the 4-week treatment period, 88% of those treated with AMP were pain-free versus only 43% in the placebo group; all participants still in pain were then given AMP, and no recurrence of pain was reported in 3 to 18 months of follow-up. However, this was a highly preliminary study, and more evidence is needed before AMP can be considered a proven treatment for shingles.

Oral AMP has not been tried for this condition. **Note**: Do not self-inject AMP products meant for oral consumption.

Vitamins

Vitamin E (see page 451) and **B$_{12}$** (see page 442) have also been suggested as possible treatments for PHN, but the evidence that they work is extremely weak.[5,6,7]

Shingles

Visit Us at TNP.com

SPORTS PERFORMANCE

Principal Proposed Treatments
Repetitive, High-Intensity, Short-Burst Exercise: Creatine (Creatine Monophosphate)
Strength and Power: (Hydroxymethyl Butyrate) HMB
Post-Race Infection, Muscle Soreness: Vitamin C

Other Proposed Treatments   Alpha-Ketoglutarate (OKG), Amino Acids, Arginine, Beta-Carotene, Branched Chain Amino Acids (BCAAs), Bromelain, Caffeine, Calcium, Carnitine, Chromium, Ciwujia, Coenzyme Q_{10}, Conjugated Linoleic Acid (CLA), Cordyceps, Dihydroxyacetone Pyruvate (DHAP), Gamma Oryzanol, Ginseng, Guarana, Glucosamine, Glutamine, Horse Chestnut, Inosine, Ipriflavone, Iron, Lipoic Acid, Magnesium, Ma Huang (Ephedra), Manganese, Medium-Chain Triglycerides, Nicotinamide Adenine Dinucleotide (NADH), Octacosanol, Oligomeric Proanthocyanidins (OPCs), Ornithine, Pantothenic Acid/Pantethine, Phosphate, Phosphatidylserine (PS), Protein Hydrosylates, Protein Supplements (Soy or Whey Powder), Ribose, Selenium, Suma, Thymus Extract, *Tribulus terrestris*, Trimethylglycine (TMG), Vitamin B_1 (Thiamin), Vitamin B_2 (Riboflavin), Vitamin B_3 (Niacin), Vitamin B_6 (Pyridoxine), Vitamin E

Not Recommended Treatments   Androstenedione, Dehydroepiandrosterone (DHEA), Vanadium, Boron

In the competitive world of sports, the smallest advantage can make an enormous difference in the outcome of a contest. A supplement that could improve an athlete's strength, speed, or endurance could make the difference between tenth and first place in a race. Supplements that could enhance the training process or shorten the time to heal from an injury would be enormously valuable to serious athletes. Because of this, sports supplements are a big business, and many athletes try to enhance their abilities by using them.

A supplement that can improve an athlete's performance is called an "ergogenic aid"—but the big question is, "Are there *really* any ergogenic aids?" Proper training, good nutrition, and a healthy lifestyle definitely increase performance, but the case for supplements is much weaker. The best evidence is for creatine as an aid in repetitive, short-burst, high-intensity exercise. There is also a bit of evidence for hydroxymethyl butyrate (HMB) as an aid for bodybuilders and strength athletes. In addition, vitamin C may help prevent post-marathon colds.

However, many, many other sports supplements are available for sale with no more than highly preliminary evidence behind them. In addition, a few are probably dangerous.

For treatment of minor sports injuries, see the chapter on **injuries**.

PRINCIPAL PROPOSED TREATMENTS

In this section, we discuss sports supplements with some real evidence behind them: creatine, HMB, vitamin C, and sports beverages. Each has its own recommended use for athletes. We also address nutrition and training, the best-established ergogenic aids of all.

Creatine: For Repetitive, High-Intensity, Short-Burst Exercise

Creatine (see page 264) is one of the best-selling and best-documented supplements for enhancing athletic performance, although the scientific evidence that it works is still far from complete. The evidence that does exist points to benefits in forms of exercise that require repeated short-term bursts of high-intensity exercise, such as soccer and basketball.[1–4] Creatine has also been proposed to promote weight loss and reduce the proportion of fat to muscle in the body, but there is little evidence that it is effective for these purposes.[5]

Creatine is a naturally occurring substance that plays an important role in the production of energy in the body: the body converts it to phosphocreatine, a form of stored energy used by muscles. In theory, taking supplemental creatine will build up a reserve of phosphocreatine in the muscles, to help them perform on demand. Supplemental creatine may also help the body make new phosphocreatine faster when it has been used up by intense activity.

Creatine is not an essential nutrient because your body can make it from the amino acids L-arginine, glycine, and L-methionine. Provided that you eat enough protein (the source of these amino acids), your body will make all the creatine you need for good health. However, because meat is the most important dietary source of creatine and its amino acid building blocks, vegetarian athletes may potentially have difficulty producing enough creatine themselves.

What Is the Scientific Evidence for Creatine?

Several small double-blind studies suggest that creatine can improve performance in exercises that involve repeated short bursts of high-intensity activity.[6] The evidence is better for men than for women.

A double-blind study investigated creatine and swimming performance in 18 men and 14 women.[7] Men taking the supplement had significant increases in speed when doing 6 bouts of 50-meter swims started at 3-minute intervals, as compared with men taking placebo. However, their speed did not improve when swimming 10 sets of 25-yard lengths started at 1-minute intervals. It may be that the shorter rest time between laps was not enough for the swimmers' bodies to resynthesize phosphocreatine.

Interestingly, none of the women enrolled in the study showed any improvement with the creatine supplement. The authors of this study noted that women normally have more creatine in their muscle tissue than men do, so perhaps creatine supplementation (at least at this level) is not of benefit to women, as it appears to be for men. Further research is needed to fully understand this gender difference in response to creatine.

In an earlier double-blind study, 16 physical education students exercised 10 times for 6 seconds on a stationary cycle, alternating repetitions with a 30-second rest period.[8] The results showed that individuals who took 20 g of creatine for 6 days were better able to maintain cycle speed throughout the repetitions. Many other studies showed similar improvements in performance capacity involving repeated bursts of action.[9,10,11]

In contrast, studies of endurance or nonrepetitive exercise have not shown benefits from creatine supplementation.[12–16] Therefore, creatine probably won't help you with marathon running or single sprints.

Isometric exercise capacity (pushing against a fixed resistance), however, may improve with creatine. In addition, two double-blind placebo-controlled studies, each lasting 28 days, provide some evidence that creatine and creatine plus HMB can increase lean muscle and bone mass.[17] The first enrolled 52 college football players during off-season training, and the other followed 40 athletes engaged in weight training.

Dosage

For bodybuilding and exercise enhancement, a typical dosage schedule starts with a "loading dose" of 15 to 30 g daily (divided into 2 or 3 separate doses) for 3 to 4 days, followed by 2 to 5 g daily. Some authorities recommend skipping the loading dose. By comparison, we typically get only about 1 g of creatine in a normal daily diet.

Creatine's ability to enter muscle cells can be increased by combining it with glucose, fructose, or other simple carbohydrates. However, caffeine may block creatine's effects.[18]

Safety Issues

Creatine appears to be safe, at least in healthy athletes. No significant side effects have been found with the regimen of several days of a high dosage (15 to 30 g daily)

followed by 6 weeks of a lower dosage (2 to 3 g daily). A placebo-controlled study of 100 football players found no adverse consequences during 10 months to 5 years of creatine supplementation.[19] Three deaths have been reported in individuals taking creatine, but other causes were most likely responsible.[20]

However, there are some potential concerns with creatine. Because it is metabolized by the kidneys, fears have been expressed that creatine supplements could cause kidney injury, and there are two worrisome case reports.[21,22] While evidence suggests that creatine is safe for people whose kidneys are healthy to begin with, and who don't take excessive doses,[23,24] individuals with kidney disease, especially those on dialysis, should avoid creatine.

Another concern revolves around the fact that creatine is metabolized in the body to the toxic substance formaldehyde.[25] However, it is not clear whether the amount of formaldehyde produced in this way will cause any harm.

As with all supplements taken in very high doses, it is important to purchase a high-quality form of creatine, as contaminants present even in very low concentrations could conceivably build up and cause problems.

HMB: For Strength and Power Athletes

Technically "beta-hydroxy beta-methylbutyric acid," **HMB** (see page 323) is a chemical that occurs naturally in the body when the amino acid leucine breaks down.

Leucine is found in particularly high concentrations in muscles. During athletic training, damage to the muscles leads to the breakdown of leucine as well as increased HMB levels. Evidence suggests that taking HMB supplements might signal the body to slow down the destruction of muscle tissue.[26] However, while promising, the research record at present is contradictory and marked by an absence of large studies.

HMB is not an essential nutrient, so there is no established requirement. HMB is found in small amounts in citrus fruit and catfish. To get a therapeutic dosage, however, you need to take a supplement in powder or pill form.

What Is the Scientific Evidence for HMB?

According to most but not all of the small double-blind trials performed thus far, HMB may improve response to weight training.[27–33] HMB might help prevent muscle damage during prolonged exercise.[34]

Muscle Building   Studies on chick and rat muscles suggest that HMB reduces the amount of muscle protein that breaks down during exercise.[35]

In a controlled study, 41 male volunteers aged 19 to 29 were given either 0, 1.5, or 3 g of HMB daily for 3 weeks.[36] The participants also lifted weights 3 days a week for 90 minutes. The results suggested that HMB can enhance strength and muscle mass in direct proportion to intake.

In another controlled study reported in the same article, 32 male volunteers took either 3 g of HMB daily or placebo, and then lifted weights for 2 or 3 hours daily, 6 days a week for 7 weeks. The HMB group saw a significantly greater increase in its bench-press strength than the placebo group. However, there was no significant difference in body weight or fat mass by the end of the study.

Another double-blind placebo-controlled trial of 39 men and 36 women found that over 4 weeks HMB supplementation improved response to weight training.[37]

Two placebo-controlled studies in women found that 3 g of HMB had no effect on lean body mass and strength in sedentary women, but it did provide an additional benefit when combined with weight training.[38]

However, two double-blind placebo-controlled studies, each lasting 28 days, failed to detect any effect on body composition or strength.[39] The first enrolled 52 college football players during off-season training, and the other followed 40 athletes engaged in weight training. Although HMB at a dose of 3 or 6 g daily produced no effect different from placebo, creatine plus HMB did produce some improvements. Marginal results were seen in another double-blind trial.[40]

All of these studies were small, and therefore, their results are not reliable. Larger studies will be necessary to truly establish whether HMB is helpful for power athletes working to enhance strength and muscle mass.

Dosage

A typical therapeutic dosage of HMB is 3 g daily.

Be careful not to confuse HMB with gamma hydroxybutyrate (GHB), a similar supplement. GHB can cause severe sedation, especially when combined with other sedating substances, such as alcohol or antianxiety drugs.

Safety Issues

HMB seems to be safe when taken at standard doses.[41,42] However, full safety studies have not been performed, so HMB should not be used by young children, pregnant or nursing women, or those with severe liver or kidney disease, except on the advice of a physician.

As with all supplements taken in very large doses, it is important to purchase a quality product, as an impurity present even in very small percentages could add up to a real problem.

Vitamin C: Preventing the "Post-Marathon Sniffle"

While being active in sports can improve your physical (and mental) well-being, it also places higher stresses on your body, and can end up damaging your system. Pre-

ventative maintenance to the rescue! In addition to eating right and getting enough sleep, taking **vitamin C** (see page 444) may help as well.

Apart from providing some of our basic nutritional needs, this vitamin's greatest benefit to athletes is its potential for preventing colds.[43,44,45] Extremely intense exercise, such as training for and running in a marathon, is known to lower immunity, and endurance athletes frequently get sick after maximal exertion. When we exercise at a highly competitive level or train intensely for a competitive athletic event, we stress our bodies as we push them to perform, and sickness may be the result. Vitamin C might help prevent this, although not all studies agree. (See also Supplements for Recovery.)

As an additional bonus, vitamin C may also help reduce muscle soreness due to exertion.[46]

What Is the Scientific Evidence for Vitamin C?

Cold Prevention   According to a double-blind placebo-controlled study involving 92 runners, taking 600 mg of vitamin C for 21 days prior to a race made a significant difference in the incidence of sickness afterwards.[47] Within 2 weeks after the race, 68% of the runners taking placebo developed cold symptoms, versus only 33% of those taking the vitamin C supplement. As part of the same study, non-runners of similar age and gender to those running were also given vitamin C or placebo. Interestingly, for this group, the supplement had no apparent effect on the incidence of upper respiratory infections. Vitamin C seemed to be specifically effective in this capacity for those who exercised intensively!

Two other studies found that vitamin C could reduce the number of colds experienced by groups of people involved in rigorous exercise in extremely cold environments.[48] One study involved 139 children attending a skiing camp in the Swiss Alps, while the other enrolled 56 military men engaged in a training exercise in Northern Canada during the winter months. In both cases, the participants took either 1 g of vitamin C or placebo daily at the time their training program began. Cold symptoms were monitored for 1 to 2 weeks following training, and significant differences in favor of vitamin C were found.

However, one very large study of 674 marine recruits in basic training found no such benefit.[49] The results showed no difference in the number of colds between the treatment and placebo groups.

What's the explanation for this discrepancy? There are many possibilities. Perhaps basic training in the marines is significantly different from the other forms of exercise studied. Another point to consider is that the marines didn't start taking vitamin C right at the beginning of training, but waited 3 weeks. The study also lasted a bit longer than the positive studies mentioned above, continuing for 2 months; maybe vitamin C is more effective at preventing colds in the short term. Of course, another possibility is that it doesn't really work. More research is needed to know for sure.

Muscle Soreness   Recent studies on using vitamin C for muscle soreness have been based on the theory that muscle pain may stem in part from damage by free radicals—naturally occurring but dangerous substances that increase with exertion. Vitamin C acts as an antioxidant, neutralizing these free radicals. (Vitamin E, selenium, beta-carotene, coenzyme Q_{10}, and OPCs are also antioxidants; see Supplements for Recovery.)

One double-blind trial compared vitamin C, vitamin E, and placebo for muscle soreness in 24 male volunteers.[50] Vitamin C was found to relieve muscle soreness, while vitamin E did not. However, larger trials are needed to resolve whether or not vitamin C is effective in preventing muscle soreness.

Why Does Vitamin C Seem to Work Only Under Certain Conditions?   Several theories address vitamin C's successes at illness prevention in conjunction with exercise.[51] As mentioned above, heavy exercise is known to generate free radicals, which may cause damage to parts of the immune system. Vitamin C may protect the immune system from some of that damage, enabling it to better fight off colds. Heavy exercise may also slow the rate at which certain immune cells are made in our bodies. Perhaps not coincidentally, laboratory studies have found that vitamin C increases the rate at which these same cells are made. A hand-in-hand observation is that certain hormones produced during physical stress may depress the immune system, but vitamin C may be able to protect immune cells from damage done by these same hormones. In summary, vitamin C may combat some of the negative effects that exercise can have on our immune system, and thereby prevent infection.

Dosage

The doses used in the studies mentioned above ranged from 600 to 2,000 mg of vitamin C daily. We don't know for certain that such large doses are necessary to obtain a protective effect.

Safety Issues

Vitamin C is indisputably safe at dosages up to 500 mg daily in adults, and is probably safe for most individuals at significantly higher doses. In recognition of this, the U.S. government has issued recommendations regarding "tolerable upper intake levels" (ULs) for vitamin C. The UL can be thought of as the highest daily intake over a prolonged time known to pose no risks to most members of a healthy population. The ULs for vitamin C are as follows:

- Children 1–3 years, 400 mg
      4–8 years, 650 mg
      9–13 years, 1,200 mg
- Males and females 14–18 years, 1,800 mg
      19 years and older, 2,000 mg
- Pregnant women 2,000 mg (1,800 mg if under 19 years old)
- Nursing women 2,000 mg (1,800 mg if under 19 years old)

However, the maximum safe dosages of vitamin C for those with severe liver or kidney disease have not been determined.

Possible side effects from taking very high doses may include diarrhea, **copper** (see page 262) deficiency, and excessive **iron** (see page 333) absorption.

People with a history of kidney stones are advised against taking more than 100 mg of vitamin C daily,[52] and those with glucose-6-phosphate dehydrogenase deficiency (a genetic defect resulting in anemia), iron overload, kidney failure, or a history of intestinal surgery should use vitamin C only under medical supervision. Vitamin C may also reduce the blood-thinning effects of Coumadin (warfarin) and heparin.[53,54]

Nutrition and Training: Good for All Athletes

We may be stating the obvious, but supplements alone will not improve your strength or endurance in the absence of a good training program and a healthy diet. Increased muscle mass or stamina is the result of an appropriate exercise program supported by adequate intake of calories and essential nutrients, including fuel for energy, protein, fluids, vitamins, and minerals.

Just like your car requires more gasoline if you drive farther, your body requires more fuel if you exercise more. In addition to carbohydrates and fats which provide fuel during a workout, you need adequate protein to prevent the muscles that you're working so hard to build up from breaking down. One researcher's recommendation for protein intake is 1.2 to 1.4 g of protein per kg of body weight (1 kg equals about 2.2 pounds) if you pursue endurance-type sports, such as marathon running.[55] If you are involved in strength-building sports such as weight lifting, 1.4 to 1.8 g per kg body weight is suggested. These amounts are higher than the current recommended daily intakes for protein, which may be more appropriate for people with a less active lifestyle. Protein supplements such as **soy** (see page 411) or whey powders, or protein hydrosylates, are sometimes used to boost protein intake. However, taking protein in the form of separate amino acids does not appear to offer any additional benefit (see Amino Acids in Ergonomic Aids).

Whether adding vitamins and minerals over and above the amount suggested by the recommended daily

Sports Performance

Visit Us at TNP.com

intake is necessary or beneficial to athletes is an unresolved issue. Several vitamins and minerals are used as sports supplements, and we'll discuss them in the sections below.

Sports Beverages

Sports beverages may also be beneficial. Most obviously, they provide fluids, helping to avoid exercise-induced dehydration. In addition, they contain varying amounts of carbohydrates and electrolytes. These carbohydrates can be important because once your body has burned up all the fuel that was available in your bloodstream, it will begin to use the glycogen stored in your muscles, which can cause muscle wasting. Consuming carbohydrates has been found to prevent loss of muscle tissue during intense exercise, to delay fatigue, and even to improve performance times in some cases.[56]

The electrolytes in most sports drinks help to prevent dehydration and other potential problems related to electrolyte imbalances. Major electrolytes in your body include **potassium** (see page 390), sodium, and chloride, with potassium and sodium working together like a molecular seesaw: when the level of one goes up, the other goes down. All together, these three dissolved minerals play an essential chemical role in every function of your body. Making sure you have enough of them will enhance your performance and improve your recovery.

OTHER PROPOSED TREATMENTS

Numerous other supplements are commonly recommended for athletes. Unfortunately, the evidence that they work is marginal at best.

Some supplements are marketed as ergogenic aids, said to improve speed, strength, or endurance. These include medium-chain triglycerides (MCTs), ginseng, branched-chain amino acids (BCAAs), stimulants (ephedrine and caffeine), pyruvate (DHAP), nicotinamide adenine dinucleotide (NADH), B vitamins, coenzyme Q_{10}, carnitine, inosine, ribose, trimethylglycine (TMG), suma, phosphate, octacosanol, certain minerals (copper, magnesium, iron, and zinc), and a Chinese medicine called cordyceps. Certain commercial preparations that combine herbs and supplements are also marketed as ergogenic aids.

Supplements reputed to increase muscle mass or improve muscle/fat ratio include phosphatidylserine (PS), pyruvate, BCAAs, conjugated linoleic acid, lipoic acid, ipriflavone, gamma oryzanol, the herb *Tribulus terrestris*, and chromium.

Some sports supplements aren't aimed at improving performance directly but are instead intended to speed recovery time, whether by helping **injuries** (see page 101) to heal more quickly or restoring the body's natural balance after the stress of exertion. Like vitamin C, glut-

amine may help prevent colds following intense exercise. Various antioxidants may reduce muscle soreness. Other supplements are said to help prevent or treat athletic injuries, including glucosamine, oligomeric proanthocyanidins (OPCs), bromelain, other proteolytic enzymes, and horse chestnut.

In the following sections, we'll discuss these substances briefly, describing the level of evidence behind them.

Ergogenic Aids

Medium-Chain Triglycerides (MCTs)

Medium-chain triglycerides (MCTs; see page 356) are fats with an unusual chemical structure that allows the body to digest them easily. Most fats are broken down in the intestine and remade into a special form that can be transported in the blood. But MCTs are absorbed intact and taken to the liver, where they are used directly for energy. In this sense, they are processed very similarly to carbohydrates. For that reason, MCTs have been proposed as an alternative to "carbo-loading" for providing a concentrated source of easily utilized energy, although there is little evidence as yet that they really improve performance.[57,58,59] In one study, researchers felt that there was actually some impairment of performance due to a sensation of bloating.[60]

Phosphatidylserine

Phosphatidylserine (PS; see page 387) is a phospholipid and a major component of cell membranes. Good evidence suggests that PS can improve mental function, especially in the elderly.[61–73]

Recently, PS has also been marketed as a sports supplement, said to help bodybuilders and power athletes develop larger and stronger muscles. This is based on modest evidence that PS slows the release of cortisol following heavy exercise.[74,75,76] Cortisol is a hormone that causes muscle tissue to break down. For reasons that are unclear, the body produces increased levels of cortisol after heavy exercise. Strength athletes who believe natural cortisol release works against their efforts to rapidly build muscle mass hope that PS will help them advance more quickly. However, there is no direct evidence yet to support claims that PS actually helps to build muscles more quickly and with less training effort.

Ginseng

There are actually three different herbs commonly called **ginseng** (see page 301): Asian or Korean ginseng (*Panax ginseng*), American ginseng (*Panax quinquefolius*), and Siberian "ginseng" (*Eleutherococcus senticosus*). The latter is actually not ginseng at all, but the Russian scientists responsible for promoting it believe that it functions identically. According to some experts, another herb, ciwujia, is actually *Eleutherococcus,* while others claim it is a related but different species.

The evidence for *Panax ginseng* as a sports supplement is mixed. An 8-week double-blind placebo-controlled trial evaluated the effects of *Panax ginseng* with and without exercise in 41 individuals.[77] The participants were given either ginseng or placebo, and then underwent exercise training or remained untrained throughout the study. The results showed that ginseng improved aerobic capacity in individuals who did not exercise, but offered no benefit in those who did exercise. In a 9-week double-blind placebo-controlled trial of 30 highly trained athletes, treatment with *Panax ginseng* or *Panax ginseng* plus vitamin E produced significant improvements in aerobic capacity.[78] Another double-blind placebo-controlled trial of 37 individuals also found some benefit.[79]

However, negative results were seen with *Panax ginseng* in an 8-week double-blind trial that followed 31 healthy men in their twenties.[80] Negative results have been seen in other small trials of *Panax ginseng* as well.[81–86]

A double-blind study of 20 athletes over an 8-week period found that a standard *Eleutherococcus* formulation produced no improvement in physical performance.[87]

Branched-Chain Amino Acids (BCAAs): Leucine, Isoleucine, and Valine

Amino acids are molecules that form proteins when joined together. Three of them—leucine, isoleucine, and valine—are called **branched-chain amino acids** (BCAAs; see page 213), describing the shape of the molecules. Muscles have a particularly high BCAA content.

Both strength training and endurance exercise use up greater amounts of BCAAs than normal daily activities,[88] perhaps increasing an athlete's need for dietary intake of these amino acids. Sports such as mountaineering and skiing may cause even greater depletion of BCAAs because of metabolic changes that occur at higher altitudes. Athletes have tried BCAA supplements to build muscle, improve performance, postpone fatigue, and cure "overtraining syndrome" (see Supplements for Recovery); however, most of the evidence suggests that they do not work.[89–96]

Conjugated Linoleic Acid (CLA)

Conjugated linoleic acid (CLA; see page 261) is a mixture of different isomers, or chemical forms, of linoleic acid. Although linoleic acid itself is an essential fatty acid—a type of fat that your body needs as much as it needs vitamins—there is no evidence that you need CLA in your diet. If you choose to include it, supplements are the only practical source.

The evidence that CLA can help you lose fat while retaining muscle is highly preliminary at best.[97–100]

Amino Acids

Athletes use a number of amino acids as supplements for a variety of purposes, sometimes individually and sometimes in combination. Amino acids are sometimes taken as protein supplements, as they are the components from which proteins are formed. Some individual amino acids are also biochemically active, and taking them alone might alter your metabolism or change your hormone balance. However, evidence supporting the use of amino acids as ergogenic aids is sparse to nonexistent. The few clinical trials performed generally don't show positive results,[101,102] and there is no evidence that amino acids are better than whole protein.

Those amino acids believed by some to be ergogenic include **arginine** (see page 208), **glutamine** (see page 310), and ornithine (ornithine and glutamine combined form **ornithine alpha-ketoglutarate;** see page 376), as well as the branched-chain amino acids leucine, isoleucine, and valine, discussed above. Glutamine is also used for overtraining syndrome (see Supplements for Recovery).

Stimulants: Ma Huang (Ephedra), Caffeine (Coffee, Tea, Guarana, Cola, etc.)

A number of plant-derived stimulants are used by some athletes to improve their performance, including ephedrine from the Chinese herb **ma huang** (also called ephedra) and caffeine from coffee, tea, cola, or guarana (a plant native to South America). Both ephedrine and caffeine are central nervous system stimulants. Caffeine also appears to change the way your body burns calories, possibly allowing it to burn fats first and preserve muscle glycogen for later on in the competition—sort of like "saving the best for last."[103]

Ephedrine's value in enhancing sports performance has not been established; at the same time, there are serious safety issues associated with its use (see Safety Issues in the chapter on **ephedra**). Some sports federations have determined that specific amounts of ephedrine in an athlete's system are grounds for disqualification.

Caffeine does appear to improve performance during endurance-type exercises.[104] **Note**: The International Olympic Committee has set a tolerance limit for caffeine in the urine at 12 mcg/ml. If you're competing in a sport that follows similar regulations, you may want to have a cup of coffee or tea, but don't drink the whole pot.

Pyruvate (Dihydroxyacetone Pyruvate, DHAP)

Pyruvate (see page 395) supplies the body with pyruvic acid, a natural compound that plays important roles in the manufacture and use of energy. Pyruvate supplements

Sports Performance

have become popular with bodybuilders and other athletes based on slim evidence that pyruvate can reduce body fat and enhance the ability to use energy efficiently.[105–108] However, at the present time, there is only preliminary evidence that it really works in these ways. Other preliminary evidence suggests that pyruvate may slightly increase an athlete's capacity for endurance exercise.[109,110] Unfortunately, these studies were too small for the results to mean very much.

Nicotinamide Adenine Dinucleotide (NADH)

Short for nicotinamide adenine dinucleotide, **NADH** (see page 368) is an important cofactor ("assistant") that helps enzymes in their work throughout the body. NADH particularly plays a role in producing energy (ATP or adenosine triphosphate, your body's preferred fuel). It's possible that taking supplemental NADH could help speed up ATP synthesis. However, NADH has to undergo some chemical changes to participate in ATP formation, and we don't really know if supplemental NADH gets processed in a way that allows it to be effective. NADH is one of those supplements that appeared on the market before it was sufficiently evaluated. Its use is completely speculative at present.

B-Complex Vitamins

The recommended daily intakes for B vitamins are based on caloric intake. Because people who are exercising rigorously on a regular basis are likely to consume more calories than the average person, supplementation with B vitamins may thus be appropriate. **Vitamin B_2** (also called riboflavin; see page 436) and vitamin B_5 (**pantothenic acid;** see page 380) have also been proposed as performance enhancers for athletes, but there is no real evidence that either is effective for this.

Lipoic Acid

Lipoic acid (see page 347) is now being used by some athletes as an "insulin mimicker" because it appears to increase the body's utilization of blood sugar,[111,112] which in turn might help build muscle glycogen. However, no studies have yet been done to determine whether or not lipoic acid supplementation actually increases muscle glycogen, so this use is purely theoretical at present.

Coenzyme Q_{10} (CoQ$_{10}$ or Ubiquinone)

Coenzyme Q_{10} (CoQ$_{10}$; see page 256), also known as ubiquinone, is an antioxidant discovered by researchers at the University of Wisconsin in 1957. Its name comes from the word *ubiquitous,* meaning "found everywhere." Indeed, CoQ$_{10}$ is found in every cell in the body, where it plays a fundamental role in the mitochondria, the parts of the cell that produce energy from food. Its best-established use is for **congestive heart failure** (see page 54). CoQ$_{10}$ has also been used as a performance enhancer for athletes, but most clinical trials have found no significant improvement with CoQ$_{10}$, and one group reported significant worsening of performance with the supplement compared to placebo.[113–119]

Coenzyme Q_{10} might be of some value as a recovery supplement because of its antioxidant properties (see Supplements for Recovery).

Carnitine

Carnitine (see page 238) is a compound the body uses to turn fat into energy. It is not considered an essential nutrient, because the body can manufacture all it needs. However, supplemental carnitine may improve the ability of certain tissues to produce energy. Principal dietary sources of carnitine are meat and dairy products, but a supplement is necessary to obtain therapeutic dosages. Carnitine is widely touted as a physical performance enhancer, but there is no real evidence that it is effective, and some research indicates that it does not work in this capacity.[120]

Inosine

Inosine (see page 329) is an important chemical found throughout the body. It plays many roles, one of which is helping to make ATP, the body's main form of usable energy. Based primarily on this fact, inosine supplements have been proposed as an energy booster for athletes. However, most of the available evidence suggests that it doesn't work for this purpose.[121–125]

Ipriflavone

Ipriflavone (see page 332) is a semisynthetic version of an **isoflavone** (water-soluble chemicals found in many plants; see page 335) from **soy** (see page 411). Ipriflavone is also touted as a bodybuilding aid, but no real evidence supports this use.

Ribose

Ribose (see page 401) is a carbohydrate also vital for the manufacture of ATP. Ribose has been tried for improving exercise capacity in individuals with certain enzyme deficiencies and other rare conditions that cause muscle pain during exertion. There is weak evidence that it may help people with some of these conditions—but not others—to exercise without pain.[126,127]

Ribose has recently been touted as an important new athletic performance enhancer; however, there is as yet no evidence at all that it works. Although at least one animal study seems to show that skeletal muscle replenishes ATP ("ready to go" chemical energy for your cells) more quickly when ribose is added to the blood,[128] no research so far indicates improvement in sports performance with ribose supplements.

Visit Us at TNP.com

Gamma Oryzanol

Very preliminary evidence suggests that **gamma oryzanol** (see page 290), which is derived from rice bran oil, may increase endorphin release and aid muscle development.[129,130] These findings have created interest in using gamma oryzanol as a sports supplement. However, a 9-week double-blind placebo-controlled trial of 22 weight-trained males found no difference between placebo or 500 mg daily of gamma oryzanol in terms of performance, body composition, or hormone levels.[131]

Trimethylglycine (TMG)

Trimethylglycine (TMG; see page 423) is a naturally occurring compound that may help to prevent **atherosclerosis** (see page 16) and is therefore sometimes taken as a supplement. In the course of doing its work to keep your blood vessels clear, TMG is turned into another substance, dimethylglycine (DMG).

In Russia, DMG is used extensively as an athletic performance enhancer and has recently become popular among American athletes. TMG is cheaper, and may have the same effects as DMG, as it changes into DMG in the body. However, one small study suggests that DMG does not work,[132] making the use of TMG as a sports supplement seem rather pointless.

Suma

Suma (see page 420) is a large ground vine native to Central and South America. Sometimes called "Brazilian ginseng," native people have long used suma to promote robust health as well as to treat practically all illnesses. They called it *Para Toda*, which means "for all things."[133]

Russian Olympic athletes have used suma, along with other adaptogens, in the belief that it will enhance sports performance. In the United States, suma is sometimes recommended as a general body strengthener. However, there has been little formal scientific investigation of suma at this time.

Tribulus terrestris

Tribulus terrestris (see page 424) is a tropical plant with a long history of medicinal use. It has been tried for low libido in both men and women, **female infertility** (see page 79), and **impotence** (see page 100). In addition, it has been studied as a treatment for heart disease.[134]

One theory regarding how *T. terrestris* might help with sexual problems is that a component from the plant called protodioscine is converted to the hormone **DHEA** (see page 268) in our bodies.[135] DHEA is used by the body as a building block for both testosterone and estrogen (as well as other hormones).

This finding has led bodybuilders and strength athletes to try *T. terrestris* for increasing muscular development. So far, however, the scientific evidence seems to be against it; this is not surprising, as DHEA itself has not been found effective as a sports supplement.

One study involving 15 men compared the effects of *T. terrestris* (3.21 mg per kilogram of body weight—292 mg daily for a 200 lb man) against placebo on body composition and endurance among men engaged in resistance training.[136] At the end of the 8-week study, the only significant difference between the treatment and placebo groups was that the placebo group showed greater gains in endurance.

Nonetheless, *Tribulus terrestris* continues to be used by athletes. It is usually taken in dosages ranging from 250 to 750 mg a day, taken in divided doses with meals. *T. terrestris* is also available in 250 mg capsules standardized to provide 40% furostanol saponins.

No significant adverse effects have been noted in any of the clinical trials or human research studies of *T. terrestris*. In animal studies, toxicity was found to be extremely low in both the short and the long term. However, *T. terrestris* is known to have a toxic effect on sheep.[137,138,139]

Note: Women who are pregnant or nursing should not use this product, as it has the potential to alter hormonal chemistry significantly. Likewise, men with enlarged prostates, and anyone with a medical condition should not take *Tribulus terrestris* without first consulting a physician.

Phosphate

Phosphate has been studied as an ergogenic aid to improve aerobic capacity and endurance with greatly mixed results.[140,141] One unanswered question is whether the findings in some studies resulted from the ingestion of phosphate, or from the other compounds the phosphate was mixed with, such as sodium or calcium. Because the trials performed so far have used inconsistent methods and measurements, it isn't possible to know yet whether or not phosphate has any potential benefit as a sports supplement.

Octacosanol

Octacosanol (see page 372) is a naturally occurring waxy substance extracted from wheat germ oil; policosanol is a mixture of related substances that includes octacosanol, manufactured from sugar cane. Both are marketed as performance-enhancing dietary supplements. They are said to increase muscle strength and endurance and improve reaction time and stamina, but there is no reliable scientific evidence as yet to support these claims.

The only evidence for octacosanol as a performance enhancer comes from one small double-blind trial with marginal results.[142]

Sports Performance

Mineral Supplements

Magnesium (see page 351), **zinc** (see page 463), **iron** (see page 333), **copper** (see page 262), and **chromium** (see page 251) have all been bandied about as having potential to aid athletes in achieving their goals. However, all are believed by nutritionists to be helpful as supplements only if you are deficient in these minerals.[143,144] Although the majority of athletes are probably not deficient in most of these, use of a multivitamin supplementation with minerals will ensure that you're getting adequate amounts. Supplementation with individual minerals is not recommended except under a doctor's supervision, as it can cause imbalances rather than improve performance.

Chromium has been sold as a "fat burner" and is also said to help build muscle tissue. While studies evaluating its effects on weight loss are contradictory, the largest study did find some benefit.[145–149] However, studies evaluating its benefits as a performance enhancer or aid to bodybuilding have yielded almost entirely negative results.[150–157]

It's been suggested that athletes—and in fact most people—may not get enough chromium. The best solution for this is to make sure your multivitamin includes chromium at a dosage of 50 to 200 mcg daily. Animal studies on the safety and toxicity of chromium revealed it to be generally quite safe.[158] However, there is one report of kidney damage in a person who took 1,200 to 2,400 mcg of chromium for several months; in another report, as little as 600 mcg for 6 weeks was enough to cause damage.[159,160] There has also been one report of a severe skin reaction caused by chromium picolinate.[161] While these may be relatively rare reactions, physician supervision is recommended when using more than the recommended nutritional intake.[161]

Concerns have also been raised over the use of the picolinate form of chromium in individuals suffering from affective or psychotic disorders because picolinic acids can change the levels of neurotransmitters.[162] See Safety Issues in the chapter on chromium for more information.

Cordyceps

Cordyceps is a traditional Chinese medicinal substance, part fungus, part caterpillar. Its use as a sports supplement is based entirely on the belief that it combats the effects of aging, but there is no scientific evidence to support this idea.

Commercial Preparations

We don't have scientific evidence on every formula touted for improving sports performance. However, one small double-blind study of a mixture of various herbs and supplements marketed as SPORT® found it to be ineffective for improving sports performance in trained athletes.[163]

Supplements for Recovery

The stresses of sports competitions can sometimes weaken you, and injuries can keep an athlete out of training and impede performance. The less "downtime," the better. The substances discussed in this section have been proposed for sustaining health or speeding recovery, but none have been proven effective at this time.

Preventing Infections

Earlier in this chapter, we discussed the evidence that vitamin C might help prevent the infections that can follow intense exercise. The amino acid glutamine may be helpful for this purpose as well. This idea is based on findings that the amount of glutamine in the blood system of an athlete who has trained very hard is lower than the norm.[164] Glutamine is an important fuel source for some of our immune system cells, and it is possible that the drop in glutamine is associated with the high incidence of infections that occur in athletes who have overtrained.[165,166]

Indeed, one double-blind clinical trial involving 151 athletes found that supplementation with 5 g of glutamine immediately after heavy exercise, followed by another 5 g 2 hours later, reduced the incidence of infections quite significantly.[167] Only 19% of those taking glutamine reported infections, while 51% of the placebo group succumbed to illness. (For more information on dosage and safety, see the chapter on **glutamine**.)

Thymus extract (see page 422) is a supplement derived from the thymus gland of cows and is thought to enhance immune function. However, a double-blind placebo-controlled study failed to find any significant evidence of benefit with thymus extract.[168] In addition, there are significant safety issues with thymus extract (see the chapter for details).

Traumatic Injuries

Bruises and sprains are common among athletes. There is some evidence that various supplements may enhance recovery from these injuries. The most popular are **bromelain**, other **proteolytic enzymes**,[169–172] **oligomeric proanthocyanidin complexes (OPCs)**, and/or **horse chestnut**, although the evidence isn't strong. See the chapters on each of these topics for more information.

Some athletes also use **glucosamine** (see page 308), best known for its use in treating osteoarthritis, in the unproven belief that it can help prevent muscle injuries, relieve tendinitis, and repair damaged cartilage. However, there is no scientific evidence to support these ideas yet.

Visit Us at TNP.com

Muscle Soreness

Muscle soreness is a common problem among hard-training athletes. A treatment that could reduce such soreness might help an athlete train harder.

As mentioned previously, exercising increases the presence of free radicals, naturally occurring substances that can damage tissue. Some researchers have theorized that such damage may in part cause the muscle soreness, and perhaps muscle deterioration, that can accompany a strenuous workout.[173,174] Based on this theory, various antioxidants have been proposed to help prevent athletic muscle soreness, including selenium, beta-carotene, vitamin E, OPCs, and coenzyme Q_{10}, in addition to vitamin C, which is discussed above. As yet, there is little direct evidence that they work for this purpose.

Similarly, while vitamin E has been suggested as a treatment to prevent symptoms that can occur after endurance running, such as gastrointestinal bleeding, stomach cramps, nausea, or muscle injury, one double-blind trial found no significant benefit for any of these symptoms.[175]

The supplement phosphatidylserine (PS) might also help treat muscle soreness due to its effects on cortisol. (See Phosphatidylserine in Ergogenic Aids for details.)

NOT RECOMMENDED TREATMENTS

At least four commonly recommended supplements fall in the "not recommended" category.

Hormones

Although they are often sold as supplements, **androstenedione** (see page 206) and **dehydroepiandrosterone** (DHEA; see page 268) are really hormones. The long-term consequences of using these "supplements" are unknown. They alter your body's hormone balance, which may cause unpredictable side effects. For this reason, we do not recommend the use of these substances. In addition, there is no real evidence that they work.

Androstenedione is sometimes used by athletes based on the belief that it will increase the amount of testosterone in the system. The truth of this is still a bit uncertain. In a 7-day open study of 42 healthy men, 300 mg daily of androstenedione significantly increased testosterone levels.[176] However, in an 8-week double-blind placebo-controlled study of 20 healthy men undergoing weight training, 300 mg of androstenedione daily did not affect testosterone levels.[177] A third trial of men given 200 mg daily also found no change in testosterone.[178] On balance, it does not appear that androstenedione increases testosterone. However, there was one consistent fact in all of these trials: androstenedione increases estrogen levels significantly. This change would not be expected to improve sports performance. Indeed, in the 8-week trial mentioned above, no improvement in sports performance was seen.

Athletes have used DHEA on the belief that (like phosphatidylserine) it might limit the body's response to cortisol and thereby cause an increase in muscle tissue growth. However, study results have been mixed, so it's uncertain whether DHEA really interferes with cortisol or not.[179,180] In any case, most (but not all), studies have found no performance benefits from taking DHEA.[181,182,183]

Minerals

The mineral vanadium has been suggested for use by bodybuilders based on its effects on insulin, but there is no evidence that it works. A double-blind placebo-controlled study involving 31 weight-trained athletes found no benefit of supplementation at more than 1,000 times the nutritional dose.[184] Furthermore, there are serious safety concerns about taking vanadium at such high doses (see the chapter on **vanadium**). We do not recommend exceeding the nutritional dose of 10 to 30 mcg daily.

The mineral **boron** (see page 227) has also been proposed as a sports supplement based on its potential to alter the body's hormone balance. However, clinical studies suggest that boron supplementation is more likely to increase your estrogen levels than help you produce more testosterone.[185,186,187] Elevated estrogen levels have been associated with increased rates of some types of cancer, so we don't recommend taking supplemental boron. Far more research needs to be done on boron before it should be considered either safe or effective.

STRESS

Principal Proposed Treatments   Ginseng (*Panax* Species)

Other Proposed Treatments   *Eleutherococcus senticosus*, Ashwagandha, Astragalus, Suma, Rhodiola, Schisandra, Maitake, Shiitake, Kava, Valerian, Phosphatidylserine

The effects of stress on your health can be far-reaching. Some of the conditions often associated with stress include **insomnia** (see page 103), **high blood pressure** (see page 98), **ulcers** (see page 180), head-

Stress

aches, **anxiety** (see page 11), **depression** (see page 59), decreased memory, and drug or alcohol abuse. Stress is known to cause changes in the body's chemistry, altering the balance of hormones in our systems in ways that can lower our resistance to disease. As a result, we can become more susceptible to **flus** (see page 47), **colds** (see page 47), and other types of illness. Too much stress sometimes brings on outbreaks of **cold sores** (see page 86) or genital **herpes** (see page 86) for people who carry these viruses in their systems. Other chronic diseases such as **irritable bowel syndrome** (see page 108), **asthma** (see page 14), **Crohn's disease** (see page 57), and **rheumatoid arthritis** (see page 151) may also flare up during times of stress.

If it's possible to avoid situations that cause you to feel tense, unhappy, or worn down, that's obviously to your benefit. However, it isn't always possible to live a stress-free existence. Work deadlines, family demands, relationship problems, traffic jams, missed appointments, forgotten birthdays, personality conflicts, college exams—all of these things, and many more, can be sources of stress. Furthermore, though most of us associate stress with unpleasant events, even wonderful events in our lives, like weddings, vacations, and holidays, can be genuinely stressful.

Not everyone responds to these situations by getting "stressed out." There are those apparently unflappable folks whose pulse rate wouldn't even go up during an earthquake, and then there are those for whom being five minutes late constitutes reason for a state of total panic. How you manage the stress in your life can determine the impact it will have on you.

There are many different methods of dealing with stress. The basics for good health that we all know (but often forget) help in coping with stress: Eating a balanced diet and getting adequate rest help your body adapt and respond to the events in your life. Ironically, stress can interfere with your ability to take care of yourself in this way. When you're worrying so much you can't sleep, getting adequate rest becomes impossible. Stress can affect your eating habits too. So what else can you do? Exercise, meditation, and biofeedback are all widely accepted stress management tools that might help you break out of a stress-induced downward spiral.

For some people, stressful circumstances can trigger symptoms severe enough to warrant seeking medical attention. Conditions that are often associated with stress, such as **insomnia** (see page 103), **anxiety** (see page 11), **depression** (see page 59), and **panic attacks** (see page 11), are sometimes treated with sedatives, antipsychotic drugs, or antidepressants.

PRINCIPAL PROPOSED TREATMENTS

The primary natural approach to treating stress focuses on the use of so-called *adaptogens*. The term *adaptogen* refers to a hypothetical treatment described as follows: An adaptogen should help the body adapt to stresses of various kinds, whether heat, cold, exertion, trauma, sleep deprivation, toxic exposure, radiation, infection, or psychological stress. Furthermore, an adaptogen should cause no side effects, be effective in treating a wide variety of illnesses, and help return an organism toward balance no matter what may have gone wrong.

Although there is no solid evidence that there really are any such things as adaptogens, there is quite a bit of suggestive evidence that the herb *Panax ginseng* functions in this way.

Other plants that have been called adaptogens by some herbalists include *Eleutherococcus senticosus*, **ashwagandha** (see page 212), **astragalus** (see page 212), **suma** (see page 420), rhodiola, schisandra, and the Oriental mushrooms **maitake** (see page 354), shiitake, and **reishi** (see page 400). These are discussed in the section on Other Proposed Treatments.

Ginseng (*Panax* Species): The Most Famous Potential Adaptogen

If any herb is an adaptogen, **ginseng** is (see page 301). However, a number of herbs are referred to as ginseng. The original medicinal species of the herb is Asian or Korean ginseng (*Panax ginseng*). American ginseng (*Panax quinquefolius*) contains many of the same chemical compounds, although in slightly different proportions.

Siberian "ginseng" (*Eleutherococcus senticosus*) is actually not ginseng at all, and it's discussed in a separate section (see Other Proposed Treatments).

What Is the Scientific Evidence for Ginseng?

Most of the evidence regarding ginseng as an adaptogen comes from animal studies. However, studies in humans have found effects that are consistent with the possibility of benefits in stressful situations.

Adaptogenic Effects In animals, ginseng injections have been found to increase stamina; improve mental function; protect against radiation, infections, toxins, exhaustion, and stress; and activate white blood cells.[1] If you put these studies together, injected ginseng truly does appear to be an adaptogen, as reputed.

However, when ginseng is injected into the abdomen or bloodstream, it enters the body directly without going through the digestive tract. This mode of administration is strikingly different from taking ginseng by mouth.

Other studies have administered ginseng orally. The majority of studies examining the effects of ginseng on animals under conditions of extreme stress indicate that ginseng increases physical endurance and causes physiological changes that may help the body adapt to adverse conditions.[2–8] In addition, studies in mice found that consuming ginseng before exposure to a virus significantly increased the survival rate and number of antibodies produced.[9,10]

Immune System Stimulation   A double-blind placebo-controlled study suggests that *Panax ginseng* can improve immune system response to flu virus.[11] This trial enrolled 227 participants at three medical offices in Milan, Italy. Half were given ginseng at a dosage of 100 mg daily, and the other half received placebo. Four weeks into the study, all participants received influenza vaccine.

The results showed a significant decline in the frequency of colds and flus in the treated group compared to the placebo group (15 versus 42 cases). Also, antibody levels in response to the vaccination rose higher in the treated group than in the placebo group.

Two other studies found evidence that ginseng increases the number of immune cells in the blood,[12,13] although a third did not.[14]

Mental Function   Some of the possible effects of stress, as we've mentioned, include impairment of mental functions. Whether or not a given herb is an adaptogen, if that herb might improve your ability to remember things and stay focused, it could be of benefit. Therefore, we're including all of the information on the research about ginseng's effects on mental function here. In some cases, mental function was tested while the participants were under stress, making the studies even more relevant to our topic.

Two human studies suggest that *Panax ginseng* might improve some aspects of mental function. In the more recent investigation, 112 healthy middle-aged adults were given either ginseng or placebo for a 2-month period.[15] The results showed that ginseng improved abstract thinking ability. However, there was no significant difference in reaction time, memory, concentration, or overall subjective experience between the two groups.

An earlier, smaller trial enrolled 16 healthy men who also took either ginseng or placebo for 12 weeks.[16] For most of the tasks measured, there was no statistically significant difference between the men taking ginseng and those taking placebo. The one area in which the ginseng group performed significantly better was in mental arithmetic.

A double-blind study of the effects of ginseng on the work performance and well-being of nurses on night duty did not find significant differences between the treatment and placebo groups.[17]

Sense of Well-Being   Among stress' potential symptoms is a general decline in overall sense of well-being.

A double-blind study compared the effects of a nutritional supplement with and without ginseng extract on feeling of well-being in 625 people.[18] Quality of life was measured by a set of 11 questions. People taking the ginseng-containing supplement reported significant improvement compared to those taking the non-ginseng supplement. Similar findings were reported in a double-blind placebo-controlled study of 36 people newly diagnosed with **diabetes** (see page 65).[19] After 8 weeks, participants who had been taking 200 mg of ginseng daily reported improvements in mood, well-being, vigor, and psychophysical performance that were significant compared to the reports of control participants.

Sports Performance   The evidence for *Panax ginseng* as a sports supplement is mixed. An 8-week double-blind placebo-controlled trial evaluated the effects of *Panax ginseng* with and without exercise in 41 individuals.[20] The participants were given either ginseng or placebo, and then underwent exercise training or remained untrained throughout the study. The results showed that ginseng improved aerobic capacity in individuals treated with ginseng who did not exercise, but offered no benefit in those who did exercise. In a 9-week double blind placebo controlled trial of 30 highly trained athletes, treatment with *Panax ginseng* or *Panax ginseng* plus vitamin E produced significant improvements in aerobic capacity.[21] Another double-blind placebo-controlled trial of 37 individuals also found some benefit.[22]

However, negative results were seen with *Panax ginseng* in an 8-week double-blind trial that followed 31 healthy men in their twenties.[23] Negative results have been seen in other small trials of *Panax ginseng* as well.[24,25,26]

Dosage

The typical recommended daily dosage of *Panax ginseng* is 1 to 2 g of raw herb, or 200 mg daily of an extract standardized to contain 4 to 7% ginsenosides. In one study of American ginseng (*Panax quinquefolius*) for diabetes, the dose used was 3 g.[27]

Note: Because *Panax ginseng* is so expensive, some ginseng products actually contain very little of it. Adulteration of ginseng supplements with other herbs and even caffeine is not unusual.[28,29]

Safety Issues

The various forms of ginseng appear to be nontoxic in both short- and long-term use, according to the results of studies in mice, rats, chickens, and dwarf pigs.[30–33] Ginseng also does not seem to be carcinogenic, and side effects of ginseng are rare.

Safety in young children, pregnant or nursing women, or individuals with severe liver or kidney disease has not been established. Interestingly, Chinese tradition suggests that ginseng should not be used by pregnant or nursing women. However, contrary to some reports, ginseng does not appear to have estrogenic effects.[34]

For complete information on safety and drug interactions with ginseng, please see the section on Safety Issues in the chapter about **ginseng**.

OTHER PROPOSED TREATMENTS

Eleutherococcus (Eleutherococcus senticosus): Another Possible Adaptogen

In the 1940s, Dr. Brekhman, the same scientist who first dubbed ginseng an adaptogen, decided that a much less expensive herb, *Eleutherococcus senticosus*, is just as good as ginseng. A thorny bush that grows much more rapidly than true ginseng, this plant later received the misleading name of "Siberian" or "Russian ginseng." Its chemical makeup, however, is completely unrelated to that of *Panax ginseng*. As yet, there is little evidence that oral *Eleutherococcus* is an adaptogen.

What Is the Scientific Evidence for Eleutherococcus?

Although many scientific trials of *Eleutherococcus* have involved people (and in some trials, enormous numbers of participants), most were not double-blind and many were not controlled, making the results nearly meaningless. Animal studies of *Eleutherococcus* have also been reported, but the use of injections rather than oral doses makes their relevance limited as well.

A suggestion of adaptogenic effects comes from a double-blind placebo-controlled study of *Eleutherococcus*'s effects on the immune systems of healthy volunteers.[35] Participants took either 10 ml of extract of *Eleutherococcus* or placebo 3 times daily for a 4-week period. Blood samples were analyzed to determine changes in immune cells. A very large, statistically significant increase in numbers of cells important to immune functions was observed in the treatment group as compared to the placebo group. This finding supports, but definitely does not prove, that *Eleutherococcus* may increase resistance to disease.

More practical data was obtained in another double-blind placebo-controlled study involving 93 people in-

fected with herpes virus.[36] Use of *Eleutherococcus* significantly reduced the severity, frequency, and duration of herpes outbreaks relative to placebo during the 6-month trial.

On the negative side, a double-blind study of 20 athletes over an 8-week period found that a standard *Eleutherococcus* formulation produced no improvement in physical performance.[37]

Dosage

Eleutherococcus is taken at a daily dosage of 2 to 3 g of whole herb or 300 to 400 mg of extract.

Safety Issues

One case report suggests that taking *Eleutherococcus* simultaneously with the drug digoxin caused an erroneous reading on tests for digoxin levels.[38] If you are taking digoxin, use of *Eleutherococcus* is not advised, because it may make monitoring of digoxin levels inaccurate.

Other Possible Adaptogens

Preliminary evidence from one poorly reported double-blind placebo-controlled human trial of the herb rhodiola (*Rhodiola rosea*) suggests that it may improve physical and mental performance and sense of well-being.[39] Numerous other herbs are said to be adaptogens as well. These include ashwagandha, astragalus, maitake, reishi, shiitake, suma, and schisandra. However, there is little to no real evidence as yet that they work in this capacity.

Other Options

Insomnia (see page 103) and **anxiety** (see page 11) are both common complaints related to stressful circumstances. These symptoms themselves can often make stress worse. It works like this: You feel stressed and worried, so you can't fall asleep; then, because you're starting the next day already fatigued, the stressors you encounter are harder to deal with, making it even harder to sleep the next night. Whether your complaint is anxiety or insomnia, you can easily see how being able to calm down or get some sleep could help in the long run.

There are natural treatments that may help insomnia and anxiety. For more information, see the chapters on **kava** and **valerian**.

In stressful situations, levels of the hormone cortisol rise, setting off a chain-reaction of changes in the body. It is believed that lowered immunity, difficulty sleeping, and several other symptoms of stress are directly related to this increase in cortisol. Highly preliminary evidence suggests that the supplement phosphatidylserine might help reduce this effect.[40,41,42]

SUNBURN

Principal Proposed Treatments   Vitamin E, Vitamin C, EGCG

Other Proposed Treatments   Beta-Carotene, Mixed Carotenoids, Jojoba, *Aloe vera*, Poplar Bud

We're all familiar with sunburn—the short-term skin inflammation caused by overexposure to the sun. Besides the familiar redness, pain, blistering, and flaking, overexposure to sunlight can lead to long-term skin damage, including premature aging and an increased risk of skin cancer.

The chief culprit in sunburn is not the sun's heat but its ultraviolet radiation, which occurs in the forms UVA and UVB. This radiation acts on substances in our skin to form chemicals called free radicals. These free radicals appear to be partly responsible for the short-term damage of sunburn, and perhaps for long-term damage from the sun as well.

Conventional approaches to sunburn focus on prevention: staying out of the sun (especially when the sun is strongest), wearing protective clothing, and using sunscreen. Sunscreen blocks much of the radiation from our skin and helps prevent inflammation. A recent study of 1,383 Australians suggests that regular sunscreen use may also diminish the number of tumors caused by one form of skin cancer, squamous-cell carcinoma.[1]

Many drugs and herbs may increase your sensitivity to the sun. Some of the drugs that increase sun sensitivity are sulfa drugs, tetracycline, phenothiazines, and piroxicam. Herbs which might increase sensitivity to the sun include **St. John's wort** (see page 414) and **dong quai** (see page 272). Particular care should be taken when combining any of these substances, as they could amplify each other's effects.

PRINCIPAL PROPOSED TREATMENTS

Several studies have found that **vitamins C** (see page 444) and **E** (see page 451), and EGCG, a bioflavonoid present in **green tea** (see page 318), may help to prevent sunburn. Many manufacturers already add vitamin E to sunscreens. Taking these substances by mouth also appears to help.

Vitamins C and E

Antioxidants such as vitamins C and E neutralize free radicals in the blood and in other parts of our bodies. Test-tube and animal studies suggest that they perform the same job in the skin. Levels of these antioxidants in skin cells decrease after exposure to ultraviolet radiation, suggesting they may be temporarily depleted.[2,3]

What Is the Scientific Evidence for Vitamins C and E?

In several animal studies, vitamins C and E applied to the skin helped to protect against ultraviolet damage.[4–7] One study found that topical vitamin E seemed to work best against UVB, topical C protected more against UVA, and the two vitamins together worked better than either one by itself.[8] Vitamin E was effective even when applied to mouse skin 8 hours after ultraviolet exposure had occurred.[9] Combining the vitamins with sunscreen yielded the best result, adding to the UV-protection offered by sunscreen alone.[10]

In addition, preliminary evidence from a small double-blind placebo-controlled trial suggests that a face cream containing vitamin C could improve the appearance of sun-damaged skin.[11]

Oral use of combined C and E may be beneficial as well, although more research is needed. So far the benefits appear to be milder than those of sunscreen. One double-blind study of 10 people found that 2 g of vitamin C and 1,000 IU of E taken for 8 days resulted in a modest decrease in "sunburn" induced by ultraviolet light.[12] A 50-day placebo-controlled study of 40 people found that higher doses of these vitamins provided a sun-protection factor of about 2.[13] (Compare this to the sun protection factor of 15 or higher in many sunscreens.) However, so far research hasn't found that these vitamins, taken separately, are any more helpful than placebo.[14,15]

Dosage

It is unclear whether the doses of vitamin C and E so far investigated in humans are optimum. Mild positive results were found with a combination of 3 g of vitamin C and 2 g of vitamin E (d-alpha-tocopherol) per day in one study, and with 2 g of C and 1,000 IU of E in another. However, good evidence suggests that the body doesn't benefit from more than about 200 mg of vitamin C daily, and that any excess is excreted in the urine.[16] Vitamin E is typically supplemented at a dose of 400 to 800 IU daily. Doses above 800 IU should be taken only on the advice of a physician (see Safety Issues).

Topically, a 5% solution of tocopherol acetate helped prevent skin damage in mice when applied immediately or up to 8 hours after ultraviolet exposure.[17]

Safety Issues

Oral vitamin C is thought to be safe at up to 2000 mg per day in adults. However, high doses of vitamin C can lead to **copper** (see page 262) deficiency and excessive **iron** (see page 333) absorption.

There have been warnings that long-term vitamin C treatment can cause **kidney stones** (see page 109), but three large-scale observational studies found either a reduced rate of stone formation or no impact at all with higher vitamin C intake.[18,19,20] Still, people with a history of kidney stones should consider restricting their vitamin C intake to about 100 mg daily.[21]

Vitamin E is generally regarded as safe when taken at the recommended therapeutic dosage of 400 to 800 IU daily. However, vitamin E does have a "blood-thinning" effect that could lead to problems in certain situations. In one study of 28,519 men, vitamin E supplementation at the low dose of about 50 IU synthetic vitamin E per day caused an increase in fatal hemorrhagic strokes, the kind of stroke caused by bleeding. (However, it reduced the risk of a more common type of stroke, and the two effects essentially canceled out.)[22] Based on its blood-thinning effects, there are concerns that vitamin E could cause problems if it is combined with medications that also thin the blood, such as Coumadin (warfarin), heparin, Trental (pentoxifylline), and aspirin. Theoretically, the net result could be to thin the blood *too* much, causing bleeding problems. A study that evaluated vitamin E plus aspirin did in fact find an additive effect.[23] In contrast, the results of a study on vitamin E and Coumadin found no evidence of interaction, but it would still not be advisable to combine these treatments except under a physician's supervision.[24]

There is also at least a remote possibility that vitamin E could also interact with herbs that possess a mild blood-thinning effect, such as **garlic** (see page 291) and **ginkgo** (see page 298). Individuals with bleeding disorders such as hemophilia, and those about to undergo surgery or labor and delivery should also approach vitamin E with caution.

EGCG

Green tea contains a potent antioxidant known as epigallocatechin gallate, or EGCG. Applied to the skin, EGCG may help to minimize sunburn damage.

What Is the Scientific Evidence for EGCG?

According to several studies, mice given green tea to drink or receiving topical applications of green tea were protected against skin inflammation and carcinogenesis caused by exposure to UVB.[25,26] In one controlled human study, topical EGCG decreased skin inflammation as well as sources of free radicals in the skin after participants were exposed to UVB radiation.[27] The researchers concluded that EGCG added to sunscreen might help protect against inflammation, skin cancer, and premature aging of skin caused by sunlight. Unfortunately, the report did not state how many people were tested or whether the study was double-blind, making it difficult to determine the value of the results.

Dosage

In the human study noted above, 3 mg of EGCG was applied per square inch of skin.

Safety Issues

Green tea is widely consumed in many Asian countries and as a beverage or flavoring is presumably safe. No formal toxicology studies have been published on oral or topical EGCG.

OTHER PROPOSED TREATMENTS

Beta-Carotene and Mixed Carotenoids

Beta-carotene belongs to a large family of natural chemicals known as carotenoids or carotenes. Widely found in plants, carotenoids (along with another group of chemicals, the bioflavonoids) give color to fruits, vegetables, and other plants. **Beta-carotene** (see page 217) is important nutritionally because the body uses it to produce **vitamin A** (see page 432).

Beta-carotene, alone or in combination with other carotenoids, may be able to reduce the effects of sunburn, but study results are mixed.

What Is the Scientific Evidence for Carotenoids?

In a double-blind study, 20 young women took 30 mg daily of beta-carotene or placebo for 10 weeks before a 13-day stretch of controlled sun exposure at a sea-level vacation spot.[28] Those who'd taken the beta-carotene before and during the sun exposure experienced less skin redness than those taking placebo, even when both groups used sunscreen.

Two open studies of mixed carotenoids found similar results. These trials, one of 20 and one of 22 people, found that after taking mixed carotenoids for 12 to 24 weeks, participants could tolerate more ultraviolet radiation before developing skin redness.[29,30] Vitamin E (500 IU/day) taken along with beta-carotene in one of the studies didn't significantly affect the results.[31] However, since these two studies didn't include control groups, the results are less reliable.

However, not every study has found beta-carotene or mixed carotenoids to be helpful. In a double blind trial of 16 older women, high doses of beta-carotene taken for 23 days didn't provide any more protection than placebo against simulated sun exposure[32] nor did high doses of mixed carotenoids protect against UVA- and UVB-induced redness in a 4-week, uncontrolled study of 23 people.[33]

Surgery Support

Some carotenoid advocates explain these negative results by pointing at the short length of these negative trials. Carotene might simply need to be taken for longer than a month to make an impact on sunburn. However, an earlier 10-week study found that high doses of beta-carotene produced only very minor (though statistically significant) protection against sunburn among 30 men exposed to natural sunshine, compared to placebo.[34] The study authors didn't feel this small improvement was enough to warrant using beta-carotene to prevent sunburn.

Dosage

The proper dosage of beta carotene for protecting against sunburn is unclear.

In most of the studies where carotene supplements seemed to make a difference, participants took at least 25 mg of mixed carotenoids or 30 mg of beta-carotene per day for at least 10 weeks.[35,36]

Another trial with positive results used a more complex dosing schedule.[37] In this trial, 30 mg of carotenoids for 8 weeks didn't seem to make a difference, but improvement was noted when the dose was increased to 60 mg for the following 8 weeks, and 90 mg for the final 8

weeks. It is unclear if it was the dose increase or the duration of treatment that made a difference

However, in other studies, higher doses taken for a short time had no effect.[38,39]

Note: We are not sure at the present time whether it is advisable to take dosages of beta-carotene in this range (see Safety Issues below). Doses to maintain adequate nutrition are much lower, around 2 mg per day.

Safety Issues

While nutritional dose beta-carotene is safe, there are concerns that high-dose use of the supplement may increase the risk of cancer and heart disease.[40–45]

Excessive use of beta-carotene may also cause diarrhea and a yellowish tinge to the hands and feet. These symptoms disappear once you stop taking beta-carotene or move to lower doses.

Other Natural Treatments

Although research information is lacking, topical jojoba, poplar bud (*Populi gemma*), and **Aloe vera** (see page 204) are sometimes recommended for soothing sunburn pain and itch. However, one small study found that applying *Aloe vera* gel after UVB exposure had no effect on skin redness.[46]

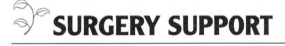

SURGERY SUPPORT

Related Terms   Anesthesia, Lymphedema, Operations, Postoperative Recovery

Principal Proposed Treatments   Proteolytic Enzymes, Oxerutins, Citrus Bioflavonoids, OPCs, Ginger, Acupuncture/Acupressure

Other Proposed Treatments   Bee Propolis, Magnet Therapy, Horse Chestnut, Multivitamin and Mineral Supplements

Herbs and Supplements to Avoid   Garlic, Ginkgo, Vitamin E, Others

Surgery, even relatively minor surgery, is a significant trauma to the body. The surgical incision itself can cause swelling (edema), pain, and bruising; anesthesia frequently causes nausea and bloating. Certain surgeries that damage the body's lymphatic system, such as radical mastectomy, can cause a specific form of long-lasting swelling called lymphedema.

Modern surgery involves numerous sophisticated nondrug techniques to help wounds heal rapidly and completely. Various medications can be used to help offset the side effects of anesthesia.

PRINCIPAL PROPOSED TREATMENTS

A variety of herbs, supplements, and other alternative therapies have been tried for problems encountered following surgery. However, keep in mind that many such

substances can interact with anesthetic drugs, and in some cases might increase risk of bleeding. For this reason, herbs and supplements should only be used for surgical support under the supervision of a physician.

Proteolytic Enzymes: May Be Helpful for Recovery from Surgery

Proteolytic enzymes (see page 393) may help reduce pain, bruising, and swelling after surgery.

Proteolytic enzymes help you digest the proteins in food. Your pancreas produces the proteolytic enzymes trypsin and chymotrypsin. Others, such as papain and **bromelain** (see page 229), are found in foods. The primary use of proteolytic enzymes is as a digestive aid for people who have trouble digesting proteins. However, for reasons that are not clear, these enzymes also appear to help recovery from injuries such as surgery.

Visit Us at TNP.com

What Is the Scientific Evidence for Proteolytic Enzymes?

Various proteolytic enzymes have been found helpful for aiding recovery from surgery.

A double-blind placebo-controlled trial of 80 individuals found that treatment with a proteolytic enzyme combination after knee surgery significantly improved the rate of recovery, as measured by mobility and swelling.[1]

Another double-blind placebo-controlled trial evaluated the effects of a proteolytic enzyme combination in 80 individuals undergoing oral surgery.[2] The results showed reduced pain, inflammation, and swelling in the treated group as compared to the placebo group.

In a controlled study of 53 individuals undergoing nasal surgery, bromelain was found to decrease bruising and swelling.[3]

A double-blind placebo-controlled study evaluated 160 women who received episiotomies (surgical cuts in the perineum) during childbirth.[4] Participants given 40 mg of bromelain 4 times daily for 3 days, beginning 4 hours after delivery, showed a statistically significant decrease in edema, inflammation, and pain. Ninety percent of patients taking bromelain demonstrated excellent or good responses compared to 44% in the placebo group. However, for reasons that aren't clear, another double-blind study of 158 women who received episiotomies failed to find significant benefit.[5]

In a double-blind controlled trial, 95 patients undergoing treatment for cataracts were given 40 mg of bromelain or placebo (along with other treatments) 4 times daily for 2 days prior to surgery and 5 days post-operatively.[6] Overall, less inflammation was noted in the bromelain-treated group compared to the placebo group.

Benefits were also seen in a small double-blind placebo-controlled crossover study of people undergoing dental surgery.[7]

However, no significant benefits were seen in a double-blind placebo-controlled trial of 154 individuals undergoing plastic surgery of the face.[8]

Dosage

The combination proteolytic enzymes used in the studies described above were special proprietary formulas; it is not clear what would be an equivalent dose of other proteolytic enzymes. Probably the best advice would be to follow the label instructions.

In studies, bromelain has been given at 120 to 400 mg daily beginning prior to surgery and continuing for a few days afterward.

Note: Bromelain "thins the blood" and could increase risk of bleeding during or after surgery. For this reason, physician supervision is essential.

Safety Issues

Proteolytic enzymes are believed to be quite safe, although there are some concerns that they might further damage the exposed tissue in an ulcer (by partly digesting it).

One proteolytic enzyme, pancreatin, may interfere with folate absorption (see the chapter on **folate** for more information). In addition, bromelain might increase the blood-thinning effects of warfarin (Coumadin) and possibly other anticoagulants.

Oxerutins and Other Bioflavonoids: May Be Helpful for Lymphedema and Ordinary Post-Surgical Swelling

Oxerutins (see page 377) have been widely used in Europe since the mid-1960s, primarily as a treatment for **varicose veins** (see page 184). Derived from a naturally occurring bioflavonoid called rutin, oxerutins were specifically developed to treat varicose veins and related venous problems. However, they may also be helpful for treating lymphedema and ordinary post-surgical edema. Oxerutins appear to work by strengthening the capillaries.

Bioflavonoids from citrus fruit may be helpful as well.

What Is the Scientific Evidence for Oxerutins?

Women who have undergone surgery for breast cancer may experience a lasting and troublesome side effect: swelling in the arm caused by damage to the lymph system. Along with the veins, the lymphatic system is responsible for returning fluid to the heart. When this system is damaged by breast cancer surgery, fluid accumulates in the arm. Three double-blind placebo-controlled studies enrolling a total of over 100 people have examined the effectiveness of oxerutins in lymphedema following breast cancer surgery.[9,10,11]

In a 6-month double-blind placebo-controlled study, oxerutins worked significantly better than placebo in reducing swelling, aiding comfort and mobility, and in other measures of lymphedema.[12]

Two smaller studies also found oxerutins to be more effective than placebo,[13,14] but the researchers were not sure that the improvement was large enough to make a real difference. Other researchers who have investigated oxerutins for lymphedema say that this treatment "convert[s] a slowly worsening condition into a slowly improving one."[15]

The **citrus bioflavonoids** (see page 254) diosmin and hesperidin might also be helpful for lymphedema following breast cancer surgery.[16] **Note**: Do not use bioflavonoid combinations containing tangeretin if you are taking tamoxifen for breast cancer.

Oxerutins might also be helpful for the ordinary swelling that occurs after any type of surgery. In one double-blind trial, researchers gave oxerutins or placebo for 5 days to 40 people recovering from minor surgery or other minor injuries, and found it significantly helpful in reducing swelling and discomfort.[17]

Dosage

A typical dosage of oxerutins for post-surgical edema is 3 g daily. Citrus bioflavonoids are usually taken at a dose of 500 mg twice daily.

Safety Issues

Oxerutins appear to be safe. In most studies, oxerutins have produced no more side effects than placebo.[18,19] Citrus bioflavonoids appear to be safe as well.[20,21]

Oxerutins and citrus bioflavonoids have been given to pregnant women in some studies, with no apparent harmful effects. However, their safety in pregnant or nursing women cannot be regarded as absolutely proven. In addition, the safety of oxerutins has not been established for individuals with severe liver or kidney disease.

OPCs: May Also Be Helpful for Lymphedema and Ordinary Post-Surgical Edema

OPCs (oligomeric proanthocyanidins; see page 373), substances found in grape seed and pine bark, may be helpful for recovery from surgery as well. Like oxerutins, to which they are chemically related, OPCs are thought to work by reducing leakage from capillaries.

A double-blind placebo-controlled study of 63 women with breast cancer found that 600 mg of OPCs daily for 6 months reduced postoperative symptoms of lymphedema.[22] Additionally, in a double-blind placebo-controlled study of 32 people who were followed for 10 days after a "face-lift," swelling disappeared much faster in the treated group.[23]

A typical dose of OPCs is 150 to 300 mg daily, although 600 mg daily was used in one study described above.

OPCs appear to be quite safe. However, if you are taking warfarin (Coumadin), heparin, aspirin, or other drugs that "thin" the blood, high doses of OPCs might cause a risk of excessive bleeding.

Ginger: May Be Helpful for Post-Surgical Nausea

European physicians sometimes give their patients **ginger** (see page 296) before and just after surgery to prevent the nausea that many people experience when they awaken from anesthesia. However, this treatment should be attempted only with a physician's approval.

What Is the Scientific Evidence for Ginger?

Studies evaluating ginger as a treatment for post-surgical nausea have returned conflicting results.

A double-blind British study compared the effects of ginger, placebo, and the drug metoclopramide in the treatment of nausea following gynecological surgery.[24] The results in 60 women showed that both treatments produced similar benefits compared to placebo.

A similar British study followed 120 women receiving gynecological surgery.[25] Whereas nausea and vomiting developed in 41% of participants given placebo, these symptoms developed in only 21% of the group treated with ginger and 27% of the group treated with metoclopramide (Reglan).

However, a double-blind study of 108 people undergoing similar surgery showed no benefit with ginger as compared to placebo.[26] Negative results were also seen in another study.[27]

Warning: Do not use ginger either before or immediately after surgery, or labor and delivery, without a physician's approval. Not only is it important to have an empty stomach before undergoing anesthesia, there are theoretical concerns that ginger may affect bleeding.

Dosage

The usual dosage of powdered ginger is 1 to 4 g daily taken in 2 to 4 divided doses.

Safety Issues

Ginger is on the FDA's GRAS (generally recognized as safe) list and seldom causes any side effects. However, ginger might "thin" the blood to some extent,[28,29,30] although this has been disputed.[31,32,33] For this reason, ginger should not be combined with drugs such as warfarin (Coumadin), pentoxifylline (Trental), or even aspirin. Ginger might also present a risk of increased bleeding during or after surgery, although this has not been observed in studies.

Maximum safe dosages for young children, pregnant or nursing women, or individuals with severe liver or kidney disease have not been established.

Acupuncture/Acupressure: May Also Be Helpful for Nausea

An acupuncture point on the inside of the arm, about 1 to 2 inches below the wrist crease, is traditionally used to alleviate nausea. It is usually stimulated either with acupuncture needling or application of pressure.

Most studies, but not all, have found that acupressure or acupuncture on this point can reduce post-surgical nausea.[34–41]

For example, a double-blind placebo-controlled study of 94 individuals undergoing cesarean section found that pressure on this point (acupressure) during and after surgery reduced nausea and vomiting.[42]

OTHER PROPOSED TREATMENTS

A preliminary controlled study found that the honeybee product **propolis** (see page 216) mouthwash following oral surgery significantly speeded healing time as compared to placebo.[43]

One small double-blind placebo-controlled study suggests that magnet therapy patches of the "unipolar" variety can help reduce pain and swelling after surgery.[44]

Just like OPCs, extracts of **horse chestnut** (see page 325) are sometimes recommended to help reduce swelling after sprains, other athletic injuries, and surgery. This use is based on the known effects of horse chestnut on blood vessels, and there is some evidence that it may be effective.[45] However, horse chestnut may also increase bleeding and should only be used under a doctor's supervision.

Good nutrition is essential to recovery from any physical trauma. For this reason, use of a multivitamin and mineral supplement in the weeks leading up to surgery, and for some time afterwards, might be advisable.

In addition, numerous herbs and supplements might help wounds heal better. (For more information, see the chapter on **minor wounds**.) However, these treatments should not be used for surgical wounds except on the advice of a physician.

Herbs and Supplements to Avoid

The herb **garlic** (see page 291) "thins" the blood. Case reports suggest that garlic can increase bleeding during or after surgery.[46,47,48] For this reason, it is probably advisable to avoid garlic supplements for a week prior to surgery, and not to restart it after surgery until all risk of bleeding is past.

Many of the herbs suggested for surgery support in this chapter also carry a risk of increasing bleeding.

Many other herbs and supplements might increase risk of bleeding as well, including **ginkgo** (see page 298), high-dose **vitamin E** (see page 451), **white willow** (see page 457), **devil's claw** (see page 267), **chamomile** (see page 244), papaya, **red clover** (see page 397), **reishi** (see page 400), **fish oil** (see page 282), and **phosphatidylserine** (see page 387).

Before undergoing any surgical procedure, you should inform your physician of all herbs or supplements you might be taking.

TARDIVE DYSKINESIA

Related Terms   Tardive Dyskinesis

Principal Proposed Treatments   Vitamin E

Other Proposed Treatments   Choline, CDP-Choline, Lecithin, DMAE, BCAAs, Niacin, Manganese, Vitamin B$_6$, Essential Fatty Acids, Vitamin C

Tardive dyskinesia (TD) is a potentially permanent side effect of drugs used to control schizophrenia and other psychoses. This late-developing (tardy, or tardive) complication consists of annoying, mostly uncontrollable movements (dyskinesias). Typical symptoms include repetitive sucking or blinking, slow twisting of the hands, or other movements of the face and limbs. TD can cause tremendous social embarrassment to particularly vulnerable individuals.

Several different theories have been proposed for the development of TD.[1] According to one, long-term treatment with antipsychotic drugs causes the brain to become overly sensitive to the neurotransmitter dopamine, resulting in abnormal movements. According to another, imbalances among different neurotransmitters can cause or aggravate symptoms. In a third theory, TD may arise in part from damage to the brain caused by free radicals generated by schizophrenia treatments. All of these theories may contain some truth.

Unfortunately, discontinuing medication that caused TD usually doesn't help, and may even worsen the dyskinesia as well as the underlying schizophrenia.[2] Drugs such as L-dopa and oxypertine may improve TD but present their own significant risk of side effects. Fortunately, newer medications for schizophrenia that are less likely to cause TD have been developed in recent years.

PRINCIPAL PROPOSED TREATMENTS
Vitamin E

Vitamin E (see page 451), an antioxidant, works to neutralize free radicals in the body. If the free-radical theory of TD is accurate, it makes sense that vitamin E might help prevent or treat the condition. In the early 1990s,

Tardive Dyskinesia

scientific evidence began to gather suggesting that vitamin E might, indeed, be a safe and effective TD treatment. Studies were persuasive enough that many conventional physicians began prescribing vitamin E for TD. However, the latest, largest, and longest-term study of vitamin E casts doubt on the effectiveness of this remedy.

What Is the Scientific Evidence for Vitamin E?

Between 1987 and 1998, at least five double-blind studies were published which indicated that vitamin E was beneficial in treating TD.[3,4] Although most of these studies were small and lasted only 4 to 12 weeks, one 36-week study enrolled 40 individuals.[5] Three small double-blind studies reported that vitamin E was not helpful.[6,7] Nonetheless, a statistical analysis of the double-blind studies done before 1999 found good evidence that vitamin E was more effective than placebo.[8] Most studies found that vitamin E worked best for TD of more recent onset.[9]

However, in 1999, the picture on vitamin E changed with the publication of one more study—the largest and longest to date.[10] This double-blind study included 107 participants from nine different research sites who took 1,600 IU of vitamin E or placebo daily for at least 1 year. In contrast to most of the previous studies, this trial found that vitamin E was not effective in decreasing TD symptoms.

Why the discrepancy between this study and the earlier ones? The researchers, some of whom had worked on the earlier, positive studies of vitamin E, were at pains to develop an answer.[11,12] They proposed a number of possible explanations. One was that the earlier studies were too small or too short to be accurate, and that vitamin E really didn't help at all. Another was the most complicated: that vitamin E might help only a subgroup of people who had TD—those with milder TD symptoms of more recent onset—and that fewer of these people had participated in the latest study. They also pointed to changes in schizophrenia treatment since the last study was done, including the growing use of antipsychotic medications that do not cause TD.

The bottom line: The effectiveness of vitamin E for a given individual is simply not known. Given the lack of other good treatments for TD, and the general safety of the vitamin, it may be worth discussing with your physician.

Dosage

Most of the vitamin E studies used daily doses of 1,200 to 1,600 IU, evenly divided into 2 or 3 doses each day.

Note: Medical supervision is necessary when using doses this high.

Safety Issues

Vitamin E is generally regarded as safe when taken at the recommended therapeutic dosage of 400 to 800 IU daily. However, vitamin E does have a "blood-thinning" effect that could lead to problems in certain situations. In one study of 28,519 men, vitamin E supplementation at the low dose of about 50 IU synthetic vitamin E per day caused an increase in fatal hemorrhagic strokes, the kind of stroke caused by bleeding. (However, it reduced the risk of a more common type of stroke, and the two effects essentially canceled out.)[13] Based on its blood-thinning effects, there are concerns that vitamin E could cause problems if it is combined with medications that also thin the blood, such as Coumadin (warfarin), heparin, Trental (pentoxifylline), and aspirin. Theoretically, the net result could be to thin the blood *too* much, causing bleeding problems. A study that evaluated vitamin E plus aspirin did in fact find an additive effect.[14] In contrast, the results of a study on vitamin E and Coumadin found no evidence of interaction, but it would still not be advisable to combine these treatments except under a physician's supervision.[15]

There is also at least a remote possibility that vitamin E could also interact with herbs that possess a mild blood-thinning effect, such as garlic and ginkgo. Individuals with bleeding disorders such as hemophilia, and those about to undergo surgery or labor and delivery should also approach vitamin E with caution.

In addition, vitamin E might enhance the body's sensitivity to its own insulin in individuals with adult-onset diabetes.[16,17] This could lead to risk of blood sugar levels falling too low. If you are taking oral hypoglycemic medications, do not take high-dose vitamin E without first consulting your physician.

OTHER PROPOSED TREATMENTS
Choline and Related Substances

According to one theory, TD symptoms may be caused or aggravated by an imbalance between two neurotransmitters, dopamine and acetylcholine. The nutrient **choline** (see page 248) and several related substances—**lecithin** (see page 343), CDP-choline, and **DMAE** (see page 270)—have been suggested as possible treatments, with the goal of increasing the amount of acetylcholine the body produces. Lecithin and CDP-choline are broken down by the body to produce choline, and choline provides one of the building blocks for acetylcholine. DMAE (2-dimethylaminoethanol, sometimes called deanol) may also increase production of acetylcholine, although this has been questioned.

Although a variety of small studies have been conducted on these substances, evidence for their effectiveness is mixed at best. Three small double-blind studies of lecithin had conflicting results: one found lecithin more helpful than placebo,[18] one found it to be barely superior,[19] and one found it no better than placebo.[20] In

Visit Us at TNP.com

two small double-blind trials of choline itself, some people experienced decreased TD symptoms on choline compared to placebo but other people did not, and several people grew worse.[21,22]

CDP-choline, a natural substance closely related to choline, has also been the subject of a couple of small studies with mixed results. An open study of 10 people found it helpful for TD,[23] but a tiny double-blind study found it ineffective.[24]

Of the various so-called *cholinergic* treatments for TD, the best studied is DMAE—but the preponderance of evidence suggests it is not effective. Although some case reports and open studies seemed to suggest that DMAE might decrease TD symptoms,[25,26] properly designed studies using double-blind methods and placebo-control groups have not borne this out. Of 12 double-blind studies reviewed, only one found DMAE to be significantly effective when compared with placebo.[27] A meta-analysis of proposed treatments for TD found DMAE to be no more effective than placebo.[28] It seems likely, though not entirely certain, that the benefits seen in open studies and individual cases resulted from the placebo effect. However, it is also possible that particular individuals respond well to DMAE—or to other cholinergic treatments—even if most don't.

Other Natural Treatments

Preliminary evidence suggests that **BCAAs** (branched-chain amino acids; see page 213) might decrease TD symptoms.[29] Other proposed treatments include **niacin** (see page 437),[30] **manganese** (see page 354),[31] **vitamin B6** (see page 439),[32,33,34] and essential fatty acids,[35,36] but so far evidence for their effectiveness is contradictory or weak. Two double-blind trials of evening primrose oil, which contains large amounts of the essential fatty acid **GLA** (gamma-linolenic acid; see page 304), found that it was not significantly more effective than placebo at reducing TD.[37]

Prevention: High-Dose Vitamins?

An informal 20-year study of more than 60,000 people treated with antipsychotic drugs plus high doses of vitamins found that only 34 of them (0.5%) developed TD.[38] This is far fewer than might be expected: the estimated rate of TD among people treated with traditional antipsychotic medications is 20 to 25%.[39] These results were based on reports from 80 psychiatrists who routinely used high-dose vitamins along with drugs to treat people with schizophrenia. Vitamins typically included **vitamin C** (see page 444), niacin, B6, and E in varying dosages. However, because the study design was very informal, it is not possible to draw firm conclusions from its results.

Phenylalanine: A Supplement to Avoid

There is some concern that the amino acid **phenylalanine** (see page 385), present in many protein-rich foods, may worsen TD.[40,41,42] In a double-blind study of 18 people with schizophrenia, those who took phenylalanine supplements had more TD symptoms than those who took placebo.[43]

TINNITUS

Principal Proposed Treatments   There are no well-established natural treatments for tinnitus.

Other Proposed Treatments   Ginkgo biloba, Vitamin A Combined with Vitamin E, Vitamin B12, Zinc, Glutamic Acid, Ipriflavone, Oxerutins, Melatonin, Periwinkle, Biofeedback, Massage, Acupuncture, Hypnosis

Tinnitus is the technical term for ringing in the ear, although it may actually involve sounds better described as buzzing, roaring, or hissing. The noise can be intermittent or continuous and can vary in pitch and loudness. Most people have experienced tinnitus occasionally for a minute or two. However, some people have tinnitus continuously, over long periods of time. It can range from a minor annoyance to a serious and nearly intolerable condition.

Exposure to loud noise can lead to tinnitus, as can ear obstructions, **ear infections** (see page 73), otosclerosis (abnormal bone growth in the ear), head injuries, or heart and blood vessel disorders. In some cases, treating the underlying disorder will relieve the tinnitus; however, in many cases the cause either can't be found or can't be treated.

One approach involves covering up the noise to make it more tolerable; this includes hearing aids, tinnitus maskers (devices worn in the ear that emit pleasant sounds), or simply playing music to cover the noise. Avoiding loud noises, nicotine, aspirin, caffeine, and alcohol may help, since these often aggravate tinnitus. Biofeedback, massage, acupuncture, and hypnosis have also been tried, but the results have been mixed.[1]

Drugs such as carbamazepine, benzodiazepines, and tricyclic antidepressants may be tried, although none of these have been proven effective for tinnitus.

PROPOSED TREATMENTS

Although there are no well-documented natural treatments for tinnitus, a number of studies have found promising results with several potential treatments.

Ginkgo biloba

There have been numerous studies of **Ginkgo biloba** (see page 298) extract for treating tinnitus.[2–6] However, only five used a placebo control, and only four were double-blind. Of the controlled studies, only one did not find any benefit of ginkgo over placebo, and that trial was small and used an unusual form of ginkgo extract.[7]

One of the best-designed of the positive studies was a controlled, randomized, double-blind study of 99 people.[8] Half of the group received placebo, and the other half took 40 mg of ginkgo extract 3 times a day for 12 weeks. The ginkgo group had a significant reduction in loudness of tinnitus as compared to the placebo group.

Other Natural Treatments

Vitamins A (see page 432) and **E** (see page 451) in combination, **vitamin B$_{12}$** (see page 442), **zinc** (see page 463), glutamic acid, **ipriflavone** (see page 332), oxerutins, and periwinkle have also been suggested for the treatment of tinnitus.[9–15] However, there is no real evidence as yet that they work for this condition.

Melatonin (see page 357) is sometimes used to help people with tinnitus sleep; however, it doesn't appear to have any effect on the tinnitus itself.[16,17]

ULCERATIVE COLITIS

Related Terms   Inflammatory Bowel Disease (Ulcerative Colitis, Crohn's Disease)

Principal Proposed Treatments   Nutritional Support

Other Proposed Treatments   Essential Fatty Acids, Probiotics, Glutamine, Boswellia, Bromelain, Glycosaminoglycans, Food Allergies

U lcerative colitis is a disease of the colon that is closely related to **Crohn's disease** (see page 57). The two are grouped in a category called inflammatory bowel disease (IBD), because they both involve inflammation of the digestive tract.

The major symptoms of ulcerative colitis include abdominal pain and bloody diarrhea. When the disease becomes severe, fever, weight loss, dehydration, and anemia may develop. Sometimes, constipation develops instead of diarrhea. Arthritis, skin sores, and liver inflammation may occur as well.

One of the most feared consequences of ulcerative colitis is dramatic dilation of the colon, which can lead to fatal perforation of the colon. Ulcerative colitis also leads to a greatly increased risk of colon cancer.

Ulcerative colitis tends to wax and wane, with periods of remission punctuated by severe flare-ups. Medical treatment aims at reducing symptoms and inducing and maintaining remission.

Sulfasalazine is one of the most common medications for ulcerative colitis. Given either orally or as an enema, it can both decrease symptoms and prevent recurrences. Corticosteroids such as prednisone are used similarly in more severe cases, sometimes combined with immunosuppressive drugs such as azathioprine. Partial removal of the colon may be necessary in severe cases.

PRINCIPAL PROPOSED TREATMENTS

Individuals with ulcerative colitis can easily develop deficiencies in numerous nutrients. Chronic bleeding leads to iron deficiency. Malabsorption, decreased appetite, drug side effects, and increased nutrient loss through the stool may lead to mild or profound deficiencies of protein, **vitamins A** (see page 432), **B$_{12}$** (see page 442), **C** (see page 444), **D** (see page 449), **E** (see page 451), and **K** (see page 456), **folate** (see page 288), **calcium** (see page 234), **copper** (see page 262), **magnesium** (see page 351), **selenium** (see page 407), and **zinc** (see page 463).[1–10] If you have ulcerative colitis, supplementation to restore adequate body stores of these nutrients is highly advisable and may improve specific symptoms as well as overall health. We recommend working closely with your physician to identify any nutrient deficiencies and evaluate the success of supplementation in correcting them.

OTHER PROPOSED TREATMENTS
Essential Fatty Acids

Small double-blind trials suggest that essential fatty acids such as those in **fish oil** (see page 282) might be helpful for reducing symptoms of ulcerative colitis.[11–14] However, another small double-blind placebo-controlled trial found no such benefit.[15] Larger studies will be necessary to discover for certain whether fish oil helps or not. Regular use of fish oil does not appear to help prevent disease flare-ups.[16,17]

A small double-blind placebo-controlled trial found some benefit in ulcerative colitis with evening primrose oil, a source of **GLA** (see page 304).[18]

Probiotics

Friendly bacteria, or **probiotics** (see page 200), might be helpful in ulcerative colitis. One 12-week double-blind study of 120 individuals found that a friendly strain of *Escherichia coli* helped prevent flare-ups as well as the standard drug mesalazine.[19] However, because the rate of flare-up was so low in both groups, larger, placebo-controlled studies will be necessary to fully establish the effectiveness of probiotics in ulcerative colitis.

Probiotics might be useful for individuals with ulcerative colitis who have had part or all of the colon removed. Such individuals frequently develop a complication called "pouchitis," inflammation of part of the remaining intestine. A 9-month double-blind trial of 40 individuals found that a combination of three probiotic bacteria could significantly reduce the risk of a pouchitis flare-up.[20] Participants were given either placebo or a mixture of various probiotics, including four strains of lactobacilli, three strains of bifidobacteria, and one strain of *Streptococcus salivarius*. The results showed that treated individuals were far less likely to have relapses of pouchitis.

Other Natural Treatments

Glutamine (see page 310),[21–24] **boswellia** (see page 228),[25] **bromelain** (see page 229),[26] and **glycosaminoglycans** (GAGs; see page 207) have been suggested for the treatment of ulcerative colitis, but the evidence that they work is highly preliminary at best.

There are indications that **allergies** (see page 82) to foods such as milk may play a role in ulcerative colitis,[27–32] although the evidence is not yet solid.

ULCERS

Principal Proposed Treatments   Deglycyrrhizinated Licorice (DGL)

Other Proposed Treatments   Rhubarb, Aloe, Bioflavonoids, Colostrum, Butterbur, Betaine Hydrochloride, Cat's Claw, Glutamine, Marshmallow, MSM (Methyl Sulfonyl Methane), Reishi, Selenium, Suma, Vitamin A, Vitamin C, Zinc

The highly concentrated acid produced by the stomach is quite capable of burning a hole through the tissue of the stomach and duodenum (part of the small intestine). That it usually does not do so is a tribute to the effectiveness of the methods that the body uses to protect itself. However, sometimes these protective mechanisms fail, and the ever-present acid begins to produce an ulcer.

Ulcer pain is caused by stomach acid coming into contact with unprotected tissue. Eating generally decreases ulcer pain temporarily because food neutralizes the acid. As soon as the food begins to be digested, the pain returns.

Conventional medical treatment for ulcers has gone through a slow revolution. A few decades ago, the prescribed response to ulcers was a bland diet—one low in spices and high in dairy products, which were believed to coat the stomach. However, eventually it was discovered that spicy foods are innocent and that milk itself is somewhat ulcer forming! The only other option at that time was surgery.

Next came antacids containing magnesium and aluminum (such as Maalox). However, these were seldom strong enough to allow the ulcer to heal fully. Ulcer treatment took a big step forward with the development of Tagamet (cimetidine), followed by Zantac (ranitidine), Pepcid (famotidine), and others. These drugs dramatically lower the stomach's production of acid. Later, a new class of even more potent acid suppressors appeared, led by Prilosec (omeprazole).

When stomach acid is suppressed, ulcer pain rapidly diminishes, and the ulcer heals. For a time, these drugs were regarded as the definitive answer to ulcers. This early enthusiasm began to fade when it became clear that ulcers frequently returned after the drugs were stopped. In the late 1980s, a new explanation for this problem began to surface. First regarded as a wacky theory, it has now become the accepted explanation.

We now believe that ulcers are caused by the bacteria *Helicobacter pylori*. Apparently, this previously ignored organism has the capacity to infect the stomach and, by so doing, to weaken the stomach lining. Only when antibiotics to kill *Helicobacter pylori* are combined with stomach acid suppressants do ulcers go away and stay away.

PRINCIPAL PROPOSED TREATMENTS

The most famous supplement used for ulcer disease is a special form of **licorice** (see page 344) known as deglycyrrhizinated licorice (DGL). This form of licorice eliminates the portion of the herb that can cause serious side effects.

Head-to-head comparison studies involving as many as 100 participants and lasting for up to 2 years suggest that DGL is more effective than the drug Tagamet at healing ulcers and keeping them from recurring.[1,2,3]

However, DGL has not been shown to kill *Helicobacter pylori*. For this reason, it probably must be taken continuously to prevent ulcers.

Preliminary evidence suggests that DGL might also help protect the stomach from damage due to non-steroidal anti-inflammatory drugs.[4]

The proper dosage of DGL is two to four 380-mg tablets chewed 20 minutes before meals. DGL tastes bad but is believed to be very safe, although extensive safety studies have not been performed. Side effects are rare. Safety in young children, pregnant or nursing women, and those with severe liver or kidney disease has not been established.

According to one report, whole licorice possesses significant estrogenic activity and, as such, shouldn't be taken by women who have had breast cancer.[5] Licorice may also reduce testosterone levels in men.[6] For this reason, men with impotence, infertility, or decreased libido may want to avoid this herb. It is not clear whether the same potential exists with DGL, but it is less likely.

Warning: Because ulcers can be dangerous, medical supervision of treatment is essential.

OTHER PROPOSED TREATMENTS

The following natural treatments are widely recommended, but they have not been scientifically proven effective at this time.

Rhubarb and **aloe** (see page 204) have been suggested as treatments for bleeding ulcers.[7] However, this condition is sufficiently dangerous that conventional medical treatment is far more appropriate.

Highly preliminary studies suggest that various bioflavonoids can inhibit the growth of *Helicobacter pylori*.[8] All fruits and vegetables provide bioflavonoids, but these substances can also be taken as supplements. The dosage depends on the type of bioflavonoid used. A typical dosage for **citrus bioflavonoids** (see page 254) is 500 mg 3 times daily.

Colostrum (see page 260) might help protect the stomach from damage caused by anti-inflammatory drugs, at least according to one study in rats and a small human trial.[9,10]

Very weak evidence also suggests that **butterbur** (see page 233) might help protect the stomach lining from ulcers.[11,12]

Betaine hydrochloride (see page 219), **cat's claw** (see page 242), **glutamine** (see page 310), **marshmallow** (see page 355), **MSM** (see page 364), **reishi** (see page 400), **selenium** (see page 407), **suma** (see page 420), **vitamin A** (see page 432), **vitamin C** (see page 444), and **zinc** (see page 463) have also been suggested as aids to ulcer healing, but there is as yet little to no scientific evidence that they are effective.

Contrary to some reports, the herb **turmeric** (see page 425) does not appear to be effective for treating ulcers,[13,14] and it might increase the risk of developing ulcers if taken at excessive doses.[15] Neither **garlic** (see page 291) nor **cayenne** (see page 243) appear to be helpful against *Helicobacter pylori,* the stomach bacteria implicated as a major cause of ulcers.[16,17] However, some evidence suggests that cayenne can protect the stomach against damage caused by anti-inflammatory drugs.[18,19,20]

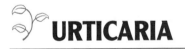

URTICARIA

Related Terms   Hives, Dermographism, Angioedema, Prickly Heat

Principal Proposed Treatments   There are no well-established natural treatments for urticaria.

Other Proposed Treatments   Elimination Diet, Acupuncture, Vitamin C, Vitamin B$_{12}$, Quercetin

Urticaria, commonly called hives, is an inflammation of the surface layers of the skin, and is characterized by small, itchy red or white welts (called wheals). Urticaria is usually caused by an allergic reaction; however, the allergenic trigger is often unknown. When a cause can be identified, it is frequently something taken by mouth, such as shellfish or other fish, dairy products, peanuts or other legumes, chocolate, fresh fruit, or medications.

Sometimes other allergens such as pollens, molds, or animal dander can produce hives. Hives can also be caused by heat (cholinergic urticaria or "prickly heat"), cold (cold urticaria), pressure (dermographism and pressure urticaria), light (solar urticaria), exercise, and certain infections such as **hepatitis B** (see page 189).

In most acute cases, urticaria disappears within hours or days without any treatment. Sometimes,

Vaginal Infection

however, it may continue for a prolonged period, or recur frequently. Such chronic cases are often very difficult to treat.

Urticaria is closely related to another condition called angioedema, which involves swelling in the deeper layers of the skin. When swelling occurs in the throat or tongue, angioedema can be life-threatening.

Urticaria and angioedema are also closely related to anaphylaxis, an extremely dangerous condition that can lead to death within minutes or hours. Anaphylaxis is an overwhelming allergic reaction that may lead to swelling of internal organs, collapse of blood circulation, shock, or suffocation. It may be caused by all the same factors that trigger hives; one of the most well-known causes is bee sting allergy. (See the chapter on **food allergies**.)

Conventional treatments for urticaria and angioedema include avoidance of triggering factors, antihistamines, and, occasionally, corticosteroids. When breathing is threatened, epinephrine shots and possibly hospitalization may be needed.

PROPOSED TREATMENTS

Because urticaria is frequently caused by allergens in food, the so-called *elimination diet* has been tried as a treatment for chronic symptoms.

There are many forms of the elimination diet. One of the most common involves starting with a highly restricted diet consisting only of foods that are seldom allergenic, such as rice, yams, and turkey. Other proponents of the elimination diet allow a greater range of foods at the outset. If dietary restriction leads to resolution or improvement of symptoms, foods are then reintroduced one by one to see which, if any, will trigger urticaria. (For more information see the chapter on **food allergies**.)

The results of preliminary studies suggest that the elimination diet can be effective in some cases of chronic or recurrent urticaria.[1,2,3] However, it is an arduous approach that is not for the faint of heart. Various forms of allergy testing have been advocated to make matters easier; the idea is to identify specific offending foods only, rather than eliminating practically everything. Unfortunately, food allergy testing appears to be somewhat unreliable.[4]

Acupuncture

In China, urticaria is often treated with acupuncture; however, the evidence that acupuncture works for this condition is very weak.[5]

Other Natural Treatments

Vitamins C (see page 444) and **B$_{12}$** (see page 442), and the flavonoid **quercetin** (see page 396), have also been suggested, but there is no evidence as yet that they really work for treating urticaria.

VAGINAL INFECTION

Related Terms   Vaginal Yeast Infection, Candida, Trichomonas, Bacterial Vaginosis, Gardnerella, Vaginitis

Principal Proposed Treatments   There are no well-established natural treatments for vaginal infection.

Other Proposed Treatments   Acidophilus, Tea Tree Oil, Boric Acid, Bee Propolis

There are three main causes of vaginal infections: the fungus (yeast) *Candida albicans* (see page 38), the parasite *Trichomonas vaginalis*, and the bacterial organism *Gardnerella vaginalis*.

Factors that can contribute to vaginal infections include the use of antibiotics (which kill friendly bacteria, allowing yeast to grow), corticosteroids and HIV (which suppress the immune system), oral contraceptives and pregnancy (which alter the vaginal environment by changing hormone levels), and **diabetes** (increased sugar levels provide a friendly environment for yeast; see page 65).

Conventional medical treatment for vaginal infections caused by *Candida* include vaginal suppositories containing antifungal medications, or in some cases, oral antifungal medications. Women with diabetes often find that yeast infections are less common when their blood sugar levels are well controlled.

Trichomonas infections are treated with oral metronidazole and *Gardnerella* infections with oral or vaginal metronidazole or vaginal clindamycin.

PROPOSED TREATMENTS

There are some promising natural treatments for vaginal infections caused by *Candida* and other organisms, but the scientific evidence for them is not yet strong.

Acidophilus

Friendly bacteria such as **acidophilus** (see page 200) are normally found in the vagina. When colonies of these organisms are present, it is difficult for unfriendly organisms such as *Candida* to become established. For this reason, women have been advised to use yogurt or other products containing acidophilus, both orally and in vaginal suppositories, to prevent or treat yeast infections. Although this practice seems to make good sense, there is surprisingly little evidence to support it.[1,2]

An unblinded crossover trial of 33 women with recurrent vaginitis found that those who ate yogurt containing *Lactobacillus acidophilus* for 6 months had a decreased incidence of vaginal infections during the year of the study.[3] However, many of the women refused to participate in the non-yogurt portion of the study after obtaining good results, and only 13 completed the study to the end. This, along with the lack of blinding, makes the results of the study unreliable.

In an uncontrolled trial of 38 women who had not responded to conventional treatments, a vaginal douche of *L. acidophilus* twice daily along with a vitamin B supplement produced normal vaginal flora in 76% of the women 1 week after treatment.[4] In another uncontrolled study of 28 women with recurrent vaginitis, participants were given vaginal suppositories containing *Lactobacillus* to be inserted twice daily for 7 days.[5] All of the women reported subjective improvement, which was confirmed with pelvic exam. However, because these studies were not controlled, the results are less than reliable.

Nonetheless, there are good reasons to believe that increasing the population of friendly bacteria in the vagina will tend to prevent infections. Both oral and topical use of acidophilus should have this effect.

Although many available products purport to contain acidophilus, a study of a variety of health food products found that many contained few or no active organisms.[6] For this reason, it may be preferable to use live-culture yogurt.

Tea Tree Oil

Tea tree oil (see page 421), an essential oil from the plant *Melaleuca alternifolia*, possesses antibacterial and antifungal properties,[7] and appears to spare friendly bacteria in the *Lactobacillus* family.[8]

Tea tree oil has been tried for various forms of vaginal infection, but there is little scientific evidence as yet that it works. In an uncontrolled trial, 96 women with trichomonal vaginitis were treated with tampons saturated in tea tree oil and left in the vagina for 24 hours, followed by daily vaginal douches with a tea tree oil solution.[9] The researcher reported good results with this regimen in 3 to 4 weeks. However, the study was poorly designed and has not been replicated.

If you wish to try tea tree oil, keep in mind that it can cause irritation to the skin and mucous membranes.[10]

Boric Acid

Boric acid is a chemical substance with antiseptic properties. A double-blind comparison study of 108 women with yeast infections found that 92% of those who used boric acid suppositories nightly for 2 weeks experienced full recovery, as compared to 64% of those given suppositories of the standard antifungal drug nystatin.[11]

Another small uncontrolled study of boric acid suppositories in women with chronic vaginal yeast infections also found benefit.[12]

However, there are safety concerns with boric acid. If taken internally, it is quite toxic. For this reason, it should not be applied to open wounds. In addition, it should not be used by pregnant women, nor applied to the skin of infants.[13]

Other Herbs and Supplements

Various tropical plants appear to possess antifungal properties, and have been tested as possible treatments for candidal yeast infections. The plant *Solanum nigrescens* has been tested in a single-blind comparison trial against the standard drug nystatin.[14] In this study, 100 women with *Candida* vaginitis treated twice daily for 2 weeks with *Solanum* suppositories showed results equivalent to those given nystatin suppositories. However, this plant can be toxic and should not be used except under physician supervision.

One preliminary study suggests **bee propolis** (see page 216) may be helpful for treating vaginal infections.[15]

Test tube studies have found antifungal properties from numerous other herbs, including the tropical tree *Tabeuia avellanedae*,[16] garlic extracts,[17,18,19] the plant alkaloid berberine sulfate,[20] and essential oils of various plants, including **cinnamon** (see page 254), eucalyptus, lemongrass, palmarosa, and **peppermint** (see page 384).[21,22,23] However, it is a long way from such studies to proof of safety and effectiveness in people.

Varicose Veins

Visit Us at TNP.com

VARICOSE VEINS

Principal Proposed Treatments   Horse Chestnut, Oxerutins and Other Bioflavonoids, OPCs (Oligomeric Proanthocyanidins), Gotu Kola, Bilberry, Red Vine Leaf (Grape Leaf)

Other Proposed Treatments   Butcher's Broom, Aortic Glycosaminoglycans, Bromelain, Collinsonia, Calendula

Walking upright has given our leg veins a difficult task. Although they lack the strong muscular lining of arteries, they must constantly return a large volume of blood to the heart. The movements of the legs act as a pump to push the blood upward while flimsy valves stop gravity from pulling it back down.

However, over time these valves often begin to fail. The blood then begins to pool in the deep veins of the leg, stretching the vein wall and injuring its lining. This situation is called *venous insufficiency*. Typically, the legs begin to feel heavy, swollen, achy, and tired. *Varicose veins*, a condition closely related to venous insufficiency, occur when veins near the surface of the skin are damaged. They visibly dilate and become distorted, resulting in a cosmetically unpleasant appearance.

Varicose veins affect women about two to three times as often as men. Occupations involving prolonged standing also increase the incidence of venous insufficiency. Pregnancy and obesity do so as well because the increase of pressure in the abdomen makes it more difficult for the blood to flow upward.

Conventional medical treatment of venous insufficiency consists mainly of reducing weight, elevating the legs, and wearing elastic support hose. Unsightly damaged veins can be destroyed by injection therapy or be surgically removed.

PRINCIPAL PROPOSED TREATMENTS

Why are some illnesses luckier than others? Next to prostate enlargement, varicose veins have the most extensive repertoire of scientifically researched herbal treatments: at least six herbal and nutritional treatments widely used in Europe for venous insufficiency.

These treatments have much in common. All of them appear to work by strengthening the walls of veins and other vessels. They primarily relieve symptoms of aching, heaviness, and swelling in the legs and ankles. These therapies are probably not able to significantly improve the appearance of the legs, but it is thought (though not proven) that the regular use of these treatments might help prevent more visible varicose veins from developing.

Warning: Symptoms similar to those caused by varicose veins can actually be due to more dangerous conditions such as **phlebitis** (see page 143) or thrombosis.

Medical evaluation is necessary prior to self-treating with the natural supplements described here.

Horse Chestnut: The Leading Herbal Treatment for Varicose Veins/ Venous Insufficiency

The most popular German herbal treatment for venous insufficiency is **horse chestnut** (see page 325). Closely related to the Ohio buckeye, this tree produces large seeds known as horse chestnuts. Medical use of horse chestnut dates back to nineteenth-century France, where extracts were used to treat hemorrhoids (which are really a form of varicose veins).

German scientific research into horse chestnut began in the 1960s and ultimately led to Germany's Commission E approving the herb for vein diseases of the legs. In 1995, this herb was the third most common prescription herb in Germany, after **ginkgo** (see page 298) and **St. John's wort** (see page 414).

What Is the Scientific Evidence for Horse Chestnut?

More than 800 individuals have been involved in double-blind placebo-controlled studies of horse chestnut for treating venous insufficiency.[1–9] One of the largest of these trials followed 212 people over a period of 40 days using a crossover design.[10] Participants initially received either horse chestnut or placebo and then were crossed over to the other treatment (without their knowledge) after 20 days. Horse chestnut treatment significantly reduced leg edema, pain, and sensation of heaviness when compared to placebo.

However, the design of this study was not quite up to modern standards. A better-designed double-blind study of 74 individuals also found benefit.[11]

Good results were also seen in a partially double-blinded placebo-controlled study that compared the effectiveness of horse chestnut versus compression stockings in 240 people over a course of 12 weeks.[12] Compression stockings worked faster to lessen swelling, but by 12 weeks the results were equivalent between the two treatments, and both were better than placebo.

Unlike many herbs, the active ingredients in horse chestnut have been identified to a reasonable degree of certainty. They appear to be a complex of related chemicals known collectively as escin. Escin reduces the rate of fluid leakage from stressed and irritated vessel walls. We don't really know how it does this, but the most prominent theory proposes that escin plugs leaking capillaries, prevents the release of enzymes that break down collagen and open holes in capillary walls, and forestalls other forms of vein damage.[13,14]

Dosage

The most common dosage of horse chestnut is 300 mg twice daily, standardized to contain 50 mg escin per dose, for a total daily dose of 100 mg escin. After good results have been achieved, the dosage can be reduced by about half for maintenance.

Horse chestnut preparations should certify that a toxic constituent called esculin has been removed (see Safety Issues). Also, a delayed-release formulation must be used to prevent gastrointestinal upset.

Safety Issues

Whole horse chestnut is classified as an unsafe herb by the FDA. Eating the nuts or drinking a tea made from the leaves can cause horse chestnut poisoning, the symptoms of which include nausea, vomiting, diarrhea, salivation, headache, breakdown of red blood cells, convulsions, and circulatory and respiratory failure possibly leading to death.[15] However, manufacturers of the typical European standardized extract formulations remove the most toxic constituent (esculin) and standardize the quantity of escin. To prevent stomach irritation caused by another ingredient of horse chestnut, the extract is supplied in a controlled-release product, which reduces the incidence of irritation to below 1%, even at higher doses.[16]

Properly prepared horse chestnut products appear to be quite safe.[17] After decades of wide usage in Germany, there have been no reports of serious harmful effects, and even mild reported reactions have been few in number.

In animal studies, horse chestnut and its principal ingredient escin have been found to be very safe, producing no measurable effects when taken at dosages seven times higher than normal. Dogs and rats have been treated for 34 weeks with this herb without harmful effects.[18] Studies in pregnant rats and rabbits found no injury to embryos at doses up to 10 times the human dose, and only questionable effects at 30 times the dose.

However, individuals with severe kidney problems should avoid horse chestnut.[19,20,21] In addition, injectable forms of horse chestnut can be toxic to the liver.[22]

Horse chestnut should not be combined with anticoagulant or "blood-thinning" drugs, as it may amplify their effect.[23,24] The safety of horse chestnut in young children and pregnant or nursing women has not been established. However, 13 pregnant women were given horse chestnut in a controlled study without noticeable harm.[25]

Oxerutins and Other Bioflavonoids: Widely Used in Europe

Oxerutins (see page 377) have been widely used in Europe since the mid-1960s but this supplement remains hard to find in North America. Derived from a naturally occurring bioflavonoid called rutin, oxerutins were specifically developed to treat varicose veins and related venous problems. It is not clear whether this particular derivative of rutin is more effective than other bioflavonoids used for these conditions, but oxerutins are by far the best studied. Numerous studies have found them effective for improving symptoms such as aching, swelling, and fatigue in the legs.

What Is the Scientific Evidence for Oxerutins and Other Bioflavonoids?

At least 17 double-blind placebo-controlled studies enrolling a total of more than 2,000 participants have examined oxerutins' effectiveness for treating varicose veins and venous insufficiency. All but one found oxerutins significantly more effective than placebo, giving substantial relief from swelling, aching, leg pains, and other uncomfortable symptoms, while causing no significant side effects. Together, these studies make a strong case for the use of oxerutins in these conditions.

For example, a 12-week double-blind placebo-controlled study enrolled 133 women with moderate, chronic venous insufficiency.[26] Half received 1,000 mg oxerutins daily, and the rest took placebo. All participants were also fitted with standard compression stockings, and wore them for the duration of the trial. The researchers measured subjective symptoms, such as aches and pains, as well as objective measures of edema in the leg.

Those who took oxerutins experienced significantly less lower-leg edema than the placebo group. Furthermore, these better results lasted through a 6-week follow-up period, even though participants were no longer taking oxerutins. The stockings, on the other hand, produced no lasting benefit after participants stopped wearing them. They gave symptomatic relief while they were worn, but they didn't improve capillary circulation in a lasting way, as oxerutins apparently did.

Several other double-blind placebo-controlled studies have also found benefits with oxerutins.[27–36] Additionally, there is some evidence that troxerutin—one of the compounds in the standardized mixture sold as oxerutins—may be effective when taken alone,[37] though perhaps not as effective as the standard mixture of oxerutins.[38]

Varicose Veins

Visit Us at TNP.com

Oxerutins are closely related to the natural flavonoid rutin, which is found primarily in citrus fruits and buckwheat. One study suggests that buckwheat tea might also be effective against varicose veins, presumably because of its rutin content.[39] Other **citrus-derived bioflavonoids** (see page 254) such as diosmin, hesperidin, and hidrosmin also appear to be effective, although the evidence is not as strong as for oxerutin.[40–45]

Dosage

For varicose veins, oxerutins are usually taken in dosages ranging from 900 mg to 1,200 mg daily. A typical dosage is 1,000 mg daily, taken in two separate daily doses of 500 mg. The bioflavonoids diosmin and hesperidin are taken at the same dosage.

Safety Issues

Oxerutins appear to be safe and well tolerated. In most studies, oxerutins have produced no more side effects than placebo. For example, in a study of 104 elderly people with venous insufficiency, 26 participants taking oxerutins reported adverse events, compared with 25 in the placebo group.[46] The most commonly observed side effects were gastrointestinal symptoms, headaches, and dizziness.[47]

Oxerutins have been given to pregnant women in some studies, with no apparent harmful effects. However, their safety in pregnant or nursing women cannot be regarded as absolutely proven. In addition, the safety of oxerutins has not been established for people with severe liver or kidney disease.

Extensive investigation of diosmin and hesperidin combination therapy has found it essentially nontoxic and free of drug interactions.[48] The combination was given to 50 pregnant women in a research study, without apparent harm to mothers or children.[49]

OPCs: Reasonably Good Evidence That Can They Help

Grape seed and pine bark contain high levels of special bioflavonoids called **OPCs** (oligomeric proanthocyanidin complexes; see page 373). Similar substances are found in cranberry, bilberry, blueberry, hawthorn, and other plants.

OPCs are interesting antioxidant chemicals that appear to have the ability to improve collagen (a type of strengthening tissue found in many parts of the body), reduce capillary leakage, and control inflammation.[50–53] In Europe, OPCs are widely used to treat venous insufficiency, varicose veins, **easy bruising** (see page 74), and **hemorrhoids** (see page 85).

What Is the Scientific Evidence for OPCs?

Placebo-controlled studies involving a total of about 400 participants suggest that OPCs provide significant bene-

fit for varicose veins.[54–58] For example, a double-blind study comparing grape seed OPCs against placebo in 71 individuals showed improvement in 75% of the treated group, as compared to 41% in the control group.[59] Similarly, a 2-month double-blind placebo-controlled trial of 40 individuals with chronic venous insufficiency found that 100 mg 3 times daily of OPCs from pine bark significantly reduced edema, pain, and the sensation of leg heaviness.[60]

Another placebo-controlled trial enrolled 364 individuals and found benefits, but it was poorly reported and somewhat difficult to interpret.[61]

Dosage

OPCs are generally taken at a dosage of 150 to 300 mg daily when used for varicose veins. Lower doses are sometimes recommended as a daily antioxidant supplement.

Safety Issues

Extensive studies have shown OPCs to be nontoxic.[62] Side effects are rare and are limited to mild gastrointestinal distress. However, safety in young children, pregnant or nursing women, and people with severe liver or kidney disease has not been established. OPCs may have some anticoagulant properties when taken in high doses, and should be used only under medical supervision by individuals on blood-thinning drugs such as Coumadin (warfarin), Trental (pentoxifylline), and heparin.

Gotu Kola: Also Effective

Another reasonably well documented treatment for venous insufficiency is the tropical creeper **gotu kola** (see page 315), which should not be confused with the caffeine-containing **kola nut** (used in original recipes for Coca-Cola; see page 258).

In India and Indonesia, gotu kola has a long history of use in promoting wound healing, treating skin diseases, and slowing the progress of leprosy. It was also reputed to prolong life, increase energy, and promote sexual potency.[63] In the 1970s, Italian and other European researchers discovered that gotu kola can significantly improve symptoms of venous insufficiency, and it subsequently became a popular European treatment for this condition.

In practice, 4 weeks of treatment with gotu kola frequently produces welcome benefits in the discomfort of chronic venous insufficiency. The active ingredients in gotu kola are believed to be asiaticoside, asiatic acid, madecassic acid, and madecassoside.[64]

What Is the Scientific Evidence for Gotu Kola?

There is significant scientific evidence for the effectiveness of gotu kola in varicose veins/venous insufficiency.

A vacuum suction chamber has been used in some gotu kola studies to evaluate the rate of fluid leakage in venous insufficiency. It produces swelling when applied to the skin of the ankle. When leg veins are leaking a lot of fluid, this swelling takes longer to disappear.

In one study of people with venous insufficiency, 2 weeks of treatment with gotu kola extracts was shown to reduce the time necessary for the swelling to disappear.[65]

A placebo-controlled study (whether it was double-blind was not stated) of 52 patients with venous insufficiency compared the effects of gotu kola extract at 180 mg daily and 90 mg daily against placebo.[66] After 4 weeks of treatment, researchers observed improvement in various measurements of vein function in all treated patients, but not in the placebo group. They also found that the higher dose was more effective than the lower dose. This kind of dose responsiveness is generally taken as good evidence that a treatment is actually effective.

Another study of double-blind design followed 87 people with varicose veins and compared the benefits of gotu kola at 60 mg and 30 mg daily against placebo.[67] Again, the results showed improvements in both treated groups, but greater improvement at the higher dose.

A double-blind study of 94 individuals with venous insufficiency of the lower limb compared the benefits of gotu kola extract at 120 mg daily and 60 mg daily against placebo.[68] The results also showed a significant dose-related improvement in the treated groups in symptoms such as subjective heaviness, discomfort, and edema.

A 1992 review of all the gotu kola studies available concluded that gotu kola extract provides a dose-related improvement in venous insufficiency symptoms, reducing foot swelling, ankle edema, and fluid leakage from the veins.[69]

Dosage

The usual dosage of gotu kola is 20 to 60 mg 3 times daily of an extract standardized to contain 40% asiaticoside, 29 to 30% asiatic acid, 29 to 30% madecassic acid, and 1 to 2% madecassoside.

Safety Issues

Studies suggest that oral asiaticoside at a dosage of 1 g per kilogram body weight is safe.[70] This leaves a wide margin of safety, since standard daily doses of gotu kola provide about 2,000 times less asiaticoside for an average adult. Studies have also found that doses of 16 g per kilogram body weight of fresh gotu kola leaves are nontoxic,[71] and studies in rabbits suggest that gotu kola extracts are not harmful to fetal development.[72]

The only reported side effect with gotu kola is rare allergic skin rash. Safety in pregnancy has not been established. However, Italian physicians have given it to pregnant women.[73] Safety in young children, nursing mothers, and individuals with severe liver or kidney disease has not been established.

Bilberry: May Be Useful

Although much more famous as a treatment for eye problems such as **impaired night vision** (see page 128), there is some evidence that **bilberry** (see page 220), a relative of the American blueberry, may be useful in varicose veins as well.

In a placebo-controlled study that followed 60 people with varicose veins for 30 days, bilberry extract significantly decreased pain and swelling.[74] Similar results were seen in another 30-day double-blind trial involving 47 participants.[75] Bilberry contains substances known as anthocyanosides that are closely related to grape seed OPCs. Like OPCs, they appear to strengthen connective tissue such as the walls of veins.[76,77,78] The standard dosage of bilberry is 120 to 240 mg twice daily of an extract standardized to contain 25% anthocyanosides.

Bilberry is a commonly eaten food and as such is believed to be safe. Enormous quantities have been administered to rats without toxic effects.[79] One study of 2,295 people given bilberry extract showed a 4% incidence of side effects such as mild digestive distress, skin rashes, and drowsiness.[80] Safety in young children, pregnant or nursing women, and people with severe kidney or liver disease has not been established. However, there are no known or suspected problems with these conditions, and pregnant women have been given bilberry in clinical trials.[81]

Red Vine Leaf (Grape Leaf)

Extracts of red vine leaf (*Folia vitis viniferae,* or grape leaf) have also been tried as a treatment for chronic venous insufficiency. A recent 12-week double-blind placebo-controlled study followed 219 individuals with chronic venous insufficiency.[82] In this study, daily doses of 360 mg and 720 mg red vine leaf extract both proved significantly more effective than placebo in reducing edema as well as improving pain and other symptoms. The researchers concluded that the higher dosage resulted in a slightly greater, more sustained improvement.

The usual dose of red vine leaf is 360 mg or 720 mg taken once daily.

In the double-blind study just described, side effects were largely limited to mild gastrointestinal distress and occasional reports of headaches. Blood tests and physical examination did not reveal any harmful effects. However, comprehensive safety studies have not yet been performed, and red vine leaf is not at present recommended for pregnant or nursing women, or individuals with severe liver or kidney disease.

OTHER PROPOSED TREATMENTS

The following natural treatments are widely recommended for varicose veins, but they have not yet been scientifically proven effective.

Butcher's Broom

Butcher's broom (see page 232) is so named because its branches were a traditional source of broom straw used by butchers. This Mediterranean evergreen bush has a long history of traditional use in the treatment of urinary conditions. Recent European interest has focused on the possible value of butcher's broom in the treatment of hemorrhoids and varicose veins, although there is as yet no more than preliminary evidence that it is effective.[83]

Butcher's broom is standardized to its ruscogenin content. A typical oral dose should supply 50 to 100 mg of ruscogenins daily.

Butcher's broom is believed to be safe when used as directed, although detailed studies have not been performed. Noticeable side effects are rare. However, safety in young children, pregnant or nursing women, and people with severe liver or kidney disease has not been established.

Aortic Glycosaminoglycans

A preparation made from the blood vessels of cows, known as **aortic glycosaminoglycans** (GAGs; see page 207), has been used in Italy as a remedy for varicose veins. Although it is said to be highly effective, the scientific evidence is not yet strong.[84,85,86]

The typical dosage is 100 mg daily. Aortic GAGs are believed to be safe because they are widely found in foods. Since aortic GAGs are essentially ground-up blood vessels from cows, they are probably safe to take, even in large quantities. The only concern that has been raised regards their ability to slightly decrease blood clotting. However, safety in young children, pregnant or nursing women, and individuals with severe liver or kidney disease has not been established.

Bromelain

Bromelain (see page 229) is not actually a single substance, but rather a collection of protein-digesting enzymes found in pineapple juice and in the stems of pineapple plants. Although there is no direct evidence on its use for varicose veins, bromelain has anti-edema effects similar to treatments used for varicose veins, suggesting that it might be helpful.

Collinsonia

The herb collinsonia, or stone root, has a long traditional history of use as a treatment for varicose veins and hemorrhoids, but it has not been scientifically evaluated to any meaningful extent. The dosage varies with the preparation.

Calendula

A cream made from the herb **calendula** (see page 237) is said to be somewhat cosmetically helpful in varicose veins, although there is little evidence that this is true.

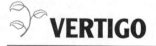

VERTIGO

Related Terms   Dizziness, Benign Positional Vertigo, Meniere's Disease, Benign Paroxysmal Positional Vertigo, Vertiginous Syndrome

Principal Proposed Treatments   There are no well-established natural treatments for vertigo.

Other Proposed Treatments   Ginkgo, Ginger, Oxerutins, Vitamin B$_6$, Hypnosis

Vertigo is closely related to dizziness, but involves the perception of actually seeing the room spin about you, similar to what happens when you spin around rapidly and then stop. Often, vertigo is accompanied by nausea and a loss of balance. Vertigo may pass quickly, or it may last for hours or even days.

There are many possible causes of vertigo including motion sickness, infection in the inner ear, vision problems, head injury, insufficient blood supply to the brain, and brain tumors. A condition called benign paroxysmal positional vertigo leads to attacks of vertigo triggered by certain head positions; its cause is believed to be de-posits of calcium in the inner ear. Another condition, Meniere's disease, is characterized by sudden, intense attacks of vertigo often accompanied by nausea and vomiting, along with ringing in the ears and progressive deafness. Its cause is unknown.

Conventional treatments for vertigo depend upon the cause and severity of the condition. Drugs for motion sickness and mild vertigo of any cause include meclizine, dimenhydrinate, and perphenazine. Scopolamine is prescribed for severe motion sickness. Benign paroxysmal positional vertigo is often treated through a series of exercises which help to alleviate symptoms.[1,2] For Meniere's disease, changes in diet are often recommended (including limiting sodium, sugar, and alcohol intake), sometimes in combination with diuretic drugs.

PROPOSED TREATMENTS

Several natural treatments have been tried for vertigo; however, the scientific evidence for these treatments is very preliminary at this time.

Ginkgo biloba

A double-blind placebo-controlled study of 67 people with vertigo found that 160 mg of *Ginkgo biloba* (see page 298) extract per day significantly reduced symptoms compared to placebo.[3] At the end of the 3-month study, 47% of the ginkgo group had completely recovered, as compared to only 18% of the placebo group.

Keep in mind that ginkgo is a "blood thinner": it can increase risk of bleeding, especially if combined with blood-thinning drugs such as warfarin (Coumadin), heparin, and aspirin.

Ginger

Evidence suggests that the herb **ginger** (see page 296) can be helpful for motion sickness.

One study enrolled 36 college students with a known tendency toward motion sickness.[4] They were given either ginger or the standard antinausea drug dimenhydrinate, and then placed in a rotating chair to see how much they could tolerate. Both treatments seemed about equally effective.

Another study also found equivalent benefit between ginger and dimenhydrinate in a group of 60 passengers on a cruise through rough seas.[5] A later study of 79 Swedish naval cadets found that ginger could decrease vomiting and cold sweating, but didn't significantly decrease nausea and vertigo.[6] In addition, a small double-blind study evaluated whether ginger could help with experimentally induced vertigo.[7] Ginger root powder significantly reduced vertigo compared to the placebo.

However, a 1984 study funded by NASA found that ginger was not any more effective than placebo.[8] Two other small studies have also failed to find any benefit.[9,10] The reason for this discrepancy in results may lie in the type of ginger used or the severity of the stimulus used to bring on motion sickness.

Other Natural Treatments

The supplements **oxerutins** (see page 377) and **vitamin B$_6$** (see page 439) are sometimes recommended for vertigo; however, the evidence supporting these treatments is very preliminary.[11,12]

Hypnosis has been tried for vertigo resulting from head trauma, with some apparent success.[13]

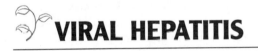

VIRAL HEPATITIS

Principal Proposed Treatments   Milk Thistle

Other Proposed Treatments   Licorice, Chinese and Japanese Herb Combinations, Green Tea, Thymus Extract, *Phyllanthus amarus,* Vitamin C, Liver Extracts, Taurine, Lecithin, Astragalus, Reishi

Hepatitis is an infection of the liver caused by one of several viruses, the most common of which are named hepatitis A, B, and C. Hepatitis A is spread mainly through contaminated food and water, whereas hepatitis B is transmitted by sexual contact and use of contaminated needles. The route of transmission of hepatitis C is not completely clear but is believed to be similar to that of hepatitis B.

When you first develop hepatitis, it is called acute hepatitis. Hepatitis can also become a long-term disease known as chronic hepatitis. All forms of hepatitis cause jaundice, liver tenderness, and severe fatigue. Hepatitis A is the mildest form and seldom causes symptoms continuing longer than a couple of months. Hepatitis B and C produce more severe symptoms, last two or three times longer, and can go on to become chronic.

Chronic hepatitis consists of persistent liver infection and inflammation that lingers long after the primary symptoms of the disease have disappeared. It can produce subtle symptoms of liver tenderness and continued fatigue and over time can gradually destroy the liver. Chronic hepatitis also appears to increase the risk of liver cancer.

The best treatment for hepatitis is prevention. You can avoid hepatitis A by practicing good hygiene and using the conventional treatment, known as immune globulins, while traveling in areas where the disease is common. Hepatitis B can be prevented by immunization and the same precautions taken against AIDS. AIDS precautions almost certainly decrease the transmission of hepatitis C as well.

Conventional medicine has little in the way of treatment for the initial hepatitis infection once it has started.

Visit Us at TNP.com

Treatment for chronic hepatitis is developing but is still quite imperfect. The most effective methods involve varieties of interferon.

PRINCIPAL PROPOSED TREATMENTS

In Europe, the herb milk thistle is commonly used along with other treatments for hepatitis. Keep in mind, though, that this is a very serious disease. Medical supervision is essential.

Milk Thistle: May Be Helpful for Chronic Hepatitis

Milk thistle (see page 361) may be useful as a supportive treatment for chronic hepatitis. Native to Europe, milk thistle has a long history of use as both a food and a medicine. At the turn of the twentieth century, English gardeners grew milk thistle to use its leaves like lettuce (after cutting off the spines), the stalks like asparagus, the roasted seeds like coffee, and the roots (soaked overnight) like oyster plant. The seeds and leaves of milk thistle were used for medicinal purposes as well.

German researchers in the 1960s were sufficiently impressed with the history and clinical effectiveness of milk thistle to begin examining it for active constituents. The most important ingredient appears to be silymarin (actually a set of four related substances), which appears to possess a wide variety of liver-protective benefits. It is one of the few herbs that have no real equivalent among standard medications.

In 1986, Germany's Commission E approved an oral extract of milk thistle standardized to 70% crude silymarin content as a treatment for "toxic liver damage; also the supportive treatment of chronic inflammatory liver diseases and hepatic cirrhosis." The herb is widely used in chronic viral hepatitis as well as alcoholic fatty liver, liver cirrhosis, alcoholic hepatitis, chemical-induced liver toxicity, and abnormal liver enzymes of unknown cause. In addition, milk thistle is often added as a protective agent when drugs that are known to be toxic to the liver are used. An intravenous preparation made from milk thistle is used as an antidote for poisoning by the death-cap mushroom, *Amanita phalloides.*

What Is the Scientific Evidence for Milk Thistle?

Preliminary double-blind studies of people with chronic hepatitis have shown significant improvement in symptoms such as fatigue, reduced appetite, and abdominal discomfort.[1,2,3] Laboratory signs of liver injury also showed improvement in these trials. However, larger research trials need to be performed before milk thistle can be called a proven treatment for chronic hepatitis. Milk thistle is probably not helpful during the initial acute hepatitis infection.[4]

As for most herbs, the mechanism of action of milk thistle remains in doubt. In mushroom poisoning and other liver-toxic exposure, silymarin is believed to get in the way of toxins trying to bind to liver cell membrane receptors by binding to the receptors itself.[5] This is called *competitive inhibition.* Incidentally, glutathione, a compound that our body normally produces to protect the liver and kidney from reactive chemicals, works in a similar fashion. Many other suggestions of how milk thistle may function have been made, but which one is correct remains unclear.[6–10]

Dosage

The standard dosage of milk thistle is 200 mg 2 or 3 times daily of an extract standardized to contain 70% silymarin.

Some evidence supports the idea that silymarin bound to phosphatidylcholine is better absorbed.[11,12] This form should be taken at a dosage of 100 to 200 mg twice daily.

Safety Issues

Milk thistle is believed to possess very little toxicity. Animal studies have not shown any negative effects even when high doses were administered over a long period of time.[13]

A study of 2,637 participants reported in 1992 showed a low incidence of side effects, limited mainly to mild gastrointestinal disturbance.[14] However, on rare occasions severe abdominal discomfort may occur.[15]

On the basis of its extensive use as a food, milk thistle is believed to be safe in pregnancy and lactation (milk production), and researchers have enrolled pregnant women in studies.[16] However, safety in young children, pregnant or nursing women, and individuals with severe renal disease has not been formally established. No drug interactions are known.

One report has noted that silibinin (a constituent of silymarin) can inhibit a bacterial enzyme called beta-glucuronidase, which plays a role in the activity of certain drugs, such as oral contraceptives.[17] This could interfere with their action.

OTHER PROPOSED TREATMENTS

The following natural treatments are widely recommended for hepatitis, but they have not been scientifically proven effective at this time.

Licorice

In Japan, an injectable combination of **licorice** (the herb, not the candy; see page 344) and certain amino acids is used for chronic hepatitis.[18] However, it is not clear whether oral licorice is equally useful, and the high dosages used for treatment of chronic hepatitis may cause an elevation of blood pressure.

Warning: According to one report, whole licorice possesses significant estrogenic activity and, as such, shouldn't be taken by women who have had breast cancer.[19] Licorice may also reduce testosterone levels in men.[20] For this reason, men with impotence, infertility, or decreased libido may want to avoid this herb.

Warning: Do not inject preparations of licorice designed for oral use.

Herb Combinations

Chinese and Japanese herbal medicines typically use combinations of herbs rather than just one. A multicenter, randomized, controlled clinical study looked at the effectiveness of a combination containing the herb *Radix bupleuri* in chronic hepatitis and found good results.[21] However, this combination has not been formally tested to verify its safety.

Other Herbs and Supplements

Some but not all observational studies suggest that **green tea** (see page 318) might help prevent various types of liver disease.[22]

Thymus extract (see page 422) has been tried as a treatment for hepatitis B and C. However, the results of small double-blind trials have not been positive.[23–26]

The herb ***Phyllanthus amarus*** (see page 389) has been extensively studied as a treatment for chronic hepatitis, but it does not appear to be effective.[27–36]

Other common natural medicine recommendations for hepatitis include high doses of **vitamin C** (see page 444), liver extracts, **taurine** (see page 420), lecithin, and the herbs **astragalus** (see page 212), and **reishi** (see page 400). However, there is as yet no solid scientific evidence that these approaches really work.

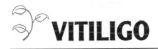

VITILIGO

Principal Proposed Treatments   Khellin, L-Phenylalanine

Other Proposed Treatments   Vitamin B$_{12}$, Folate, *Picrorhiza kurroa*, PABA, Hydrochloric Acid (HCl)

Vitiligo is a skin disease in which pigment-making cells, called melanocytes, are destroyed, leaving white irregular patches of skin where pigment used to be. The patches usually appear on the hands, feet, arms, face, and lips, but can also occur on the skin around the mouth, nose, eyes, and genitals. Hair growing from areas affected by vitiligo may also turn white. Although vitiligo in itself isn't painful, it can cause emotional distress.

Science hasn't identified the cause of vitiligo, but some researchers theorize that an autoimmune process plays a role. In an autoimmune disease, the body's immune system starts attacking innocent tissues. In vitiligo, antibodies may develop against melanocytes, ultimately destroying some of them. Vitiligo seems to be more common in people who have other autoimmune diseases; however, most people with vitiligo have no other autoimmune disease.

Most conventional vitiligo treatments combine ultraviolet light (UVA) exposure with oral or topical drugs that selectively sensitize the skin to UVA—such drugs are called "psoralens" because they are most commonly used to treat psoriasis. The results of this treatment are generally reasonably good. Another option is topical corticosteroids, which may be best for localized vitiligo.[1] In severe cases, surgical procedures including skin grafting and melanocyte transplantation may be considered, although these approaches are still experimental.

PRINCIPAL PROPOSED TREATMENTS

Most natural therapies for vitiligo also employ exposure to UVA or natural sunlight in conjunction with an oral or topical treatment.

Khellin

Khellin, an extract of the fruit of the Mediterranean plant khella (*Ammi visnaga*), is closely related to the standard psoralen drug methoxsalen. Both are used in conjunction with UVA to repigment vitiligo patches.

A double-blind placebo-controlled study of 60 people indicated that the combination of oral khellin and natural sun exposure caused repigmentation in 76.6% of the treatment group; in comparison, no improvement was seen in the control group receiving sunlight plus placebo.[2] A subsequent placebo-controlled study of 36 people found that a topical khellin gel plus UVA caused repigmentation in 86.1% of the treated cases, as opposed to 66.6% in the placebo group.[3]

Visit Us at TNP.com

Weight Loss

Dosage

A typical oral dosage of khellin is 100 mg daily.

Safety Issues

Khellin has no reported side effects when used topically. Oral doses, however, have caused various side effects ranging from nausea and vomiting to liver inflammation.

L-Phenylalanine

A handful of preliminary studies suggest that oral **L-phenylalanine** (see page 385), a natural amino acid, might also be helpful for vitiligo. It too is combined with either sunlight or controlled ultraviolet light.

Of four studies on the subject, only one was double-blind.[4] It found positive results; however, because only 24 individuals were enrolled, further research will be necessary to confirm its conclusions. The other studies were open, uncontrolled trials, and as such prove little.[5,6,7]

Dosage

The dosage in the studies ranged from 50 to 100 mg per kilogram of body weight.

Safety Issues

None of the four studies reported side effects. However, daily doses near or above 1,500 mg of L-phenylalanine can reportedly cause anxiety, headache, and even mildly elevated blood pressure.[8]

The safety of high dosages of L-phenylalanine has not been established for young children, pregnant or nursing women, or those with severe liver or kidney disease.

In addition, phenylalanine should not be combined with antipsychotic drugs or medications used for **Parkinson's disease** (see page 140).[9–12]

OTHER PROPOSED TREATMENTS

Vitamin B$_{12}$ and Folate

There is some evidence that people with vitiligo have lower than average levels of both **vitamin B$_{12}$** (see page 442) and **folate** (see page 288).[13] In addition, there is a particularly high incidence of vitiligo among individuals with pernicious anemia, a condition in which vitamin B$_{12}$ is poorly absorbed. However, this information does not prove that taking extra B$_{12}$ and folate will help. Furthermore, a much larger study of 100 people found no significant association between vitiligo and low levels of either vitamin.[14]

One uncontrolled study does suggest that vitamin B$_{12}$ and folate supplements might improve pigmentation in vitiligo, but because of its poor design the results prove little.[15]

Picrorhiza kurroa

The herb *Picrorhiza kurroa* is used by Ayurvedic physicians to treat fever, dyspepsia, asthma, bronchitis, and liver disease. One poorly designed single-blind study suggests the herb might increase effectiveness of the standard drug methoxsalen.[16]

PABA

PABA (para-aminobenzoic acid; see page 379) is best known as the active ingredient in sunblock. Based on a 1942 study, oral PABA has been suggested as a vitiligo treatment. The study, however, lacked a control group, so the results aren't meaningful.[17] Ironically, another study suggests that high oral doses of PABA can actually cause vitiligo.[18]

Hydrochloric Acid (HCl)

As noted above, vitiligo is sometimes associated with pernicious anemia. Pernicious anemia in turn is often linked to low levels of stomach gastric acid, a condition called achlorhydria.[19] For this reason, some physicians specializing in natural medicine recommend supplemental hydrochloric acid (HCl) to augment low gastric acid, but there is no evidence as yet that it helps.

WEIGHT LOSS

Related Terms   Obesity

Principal Proposed Treatments   Chromium, Fiber

Other Proposed Treatments   Pyruvate, 5-HTP (5-Hydroxytryptophan), HCA, Caffeine-Ephedra, Vitamin C, CLA, Evening Primrose Oil, Spirulina, Diacylglycerol, High-Protein/Low-Carbohydrate Diets

Losing weight can be a lifelong challenge. Researchers who study obesity consider it a chronic health condition that must be managed much like high blood pressure or high cholesterol. That means there's no easy cure.

Being overweight puts you at higher risk for heart disease, strokes, diabetes, osteoarthritis, and possibly several types of cancer.[1,2] The good news is that even modest weight loss diminishes such risks. Losing just 5 to 10% of your total weight can lower blood pressure, raise "good" cholesterol (high-density lipoprotein, or HDL), and improve blood sugar control.[3,4] The upshot may be a significantly increased life span.

In most cases, obesity is due to lifestyle factors such as diet and exercise. However, studies show that diet alone only sometimes reduces weight, and exercise alone seldom offers more than modest benefits. But the combination of improved diet and regular exercise is the best way to lose weight and keep it off.

Weight-loss drugs have had a patchy safety record. Prescription amphetamines for reducing appetite proved dangerously addictive, and other diet drug combinations such as fenfluramine-phentermine (Fen-Phen) have had dangerous side effects. New drugs may be safer and more effective.

PRINCIPAL PROPOSED TREATMENTS

Chromium: May Help in Fat Loss

Chromium (see page 251) is a mineral the body needs in only small amounts, but it's important to human nutrition.

Although it has principally been studied for improving blood-sugar control in people with diabetes, recent evidence suggests that chromium may also help reduce body fat, probably through its effects on insulin.[5,6,7]

A 3-month double-blind study of 122 moderately overweight people found that 400 mcg of chromium daily resulted in an average loss of 6.2 pounds of body fat, as opposed to 3.4 pounds in the placebo group. There was no loss of lean body mass.[8] These results suggest that chromium can help you lose fat without losing muscle.

However, six smaller double-blind placebo-controlled studies found chromium picolinate supplements produced no weight loss or change in lean body mass.[9–14] These conflicting results may be due to differences in study size, the dosage of chromium, and the individuals enrolled. Overall, chromium does appear to be promising.

Dosage

The U.S. government recommendations for chromium are as follows:

- Infants 0 to 6 months, 10 to 40 mcg
- Infants 7 to 12 months, 20 to 60 mcg
- Children 1 to 3 years, 20 to 80 mcg
- Children 4 to 6 years, 30 to 120 mcg
- Adults (and children 7 years and older), 50 to 200 mcg

The dosage of chromium used in weight-loss studies ranged somewhat higher than these guidelines, up to 200 to 400 mcg daily. There may be risks in taking excessive doses of chromium (see Safety Issues).

Safety Issues

At recommended doses, chromium is safe. However, chromium is a heavy metal that might conceivably build up and cause problems if taken to excess. There is one report of kidney damage in a person who took 1,200 to 2,400 mcg of chromium for several months; in another report, as little as 600 mcg for 6 weeks was enough to cause damage.[15,16] While these may be relatively rare reactions, physician supervision is recommended when using more than the recommended nutritional intake.

There has been one report of a severe skin reaction caused by a form of chromium called chromium picolinate.[17]

Concerns have also been raised over the use of this substance in individuals suffering from depression, bipolar disease, or psychosis, because picolinic acids can change neurotransmitter levels.[18] There are additional concerns, still fairly theoretical, that chromium picolinate could have adverse effects on DNA.[19]

If you have diabetes, you should consult a physician before trying chromium; you may need to have your diabetes medication adjusted.[20]

The maximum safe dosages of chromium for nursing women or people with severe liver or kidney disease have not been established.

Fiber: May Decrease Appetite

Dietary fiber is important to many intestinal tract functions including digestion and waste excretion. It also removes bile acids from the gut, and thus has a mild cholesterol-lowering effect. An increasing number of studies suggest that fiber may also help people lose weight. It's thought to work by decreasing appetite—it bulks up in the stomach and causes a full feeling.

Dietary fiber is primarily derived from the cell walls of plants. Whole, unprocessed grains, legumes, fruits, and vegetables all contain considerable proportions of fiber.

There are two kinds: soluble fiber, which swells up and holds water, and insoluble fiber, which does not. Soluble fiber is found in psyllium, apples, and oat bran. Most other plant-based foods contain insoluble fiber.

Weight Loss

Fiber supplements may contain a variety of soluble or insoluble fibers from grain, citrus, vegetable, and even shellfish sources.

What Is the Scientific Evidence for Fiber Supplements?

Several small studies have evaluated fiber supplements for helping overweight people lose weight.

For example, a double-blind placebo-controlled study found that among 97 mildly overweight women on a strict low-calorie diet, those who took 7 g of an insoluble fiber daily for 11 weeks lost 10.8 pounds compared to 7.3 pounds in the placebo group.[21]

However, a double-blind placebo-controlled study of 60 overweight children who were eating a normal, well-balanced diet found that 2 g each day of a fiber supplement had no effect on weight loss.[22]

One small study found that **chitosan** (see page 247), an insoluble fiber derived from crustaceans, didn't reduce body weight.[23] Preliminary evidence indicates that soluble guar fiber probably doesn't decrease appetite, whereas pectin fiber (from apples) may.[24,25]

Glucomannan (see page 307), a source of dietary fiber from the tubers of *Amorphophallus konjac,* has also been tried for weight loss, but with mixed results.[26–29]

Dosage

The typical dose of fiber used in such studies is 5 to 7 g per day.

Safety Issues

Fiber is essentially a food, and aside from a few reports of gastrointestinal discomfort, there are rarely any side effects associated with taking fiber supplements.

OTHER PROPOSED TREATMENTS

Pyruvate: Preliminary Evidence Is Encouraging

Pyruvate is a natural compound that plays important roles in the body's manufacture and use of energy. It's not an essential nutrient, since your body makes all it needs.

Evidence from several small double-blind studies suggests that **pyruvate** (see page 395) supplements may enhance weight loss.[30–35] Unfortunately, these studies were all too small for the results to be taken as fully reliable.

Although most products on the market contain only (or almost only) pyruvate, some also contain small amounts of a related compound, dihydroxyacetone, which the body converts to pyruvate. The combination of the two products is known as **DHAP** (see page 395).

Both pyruvate and dihydroxyacetone appear to be quite safe, aside from mild side effects such as occasional stomach upset and diarrhea. However, maximum safe dosages for children, women who are pregnant or nursing, or people with liver or kidney disease have not been established.

A typical therapeutic dosage of pyruvate is 30 g daily. Keep in mind that even a small percentage of contaminant in such an enormous dose could be harmful, so be sure to use a quality product.

5-HTP: A Promising Option

5-Hydroxytryptophan (5-HTP; see page 198) is a naturally occurring substance that your body manufactures on its way to making the brain chemical serotonin. Although it's primarily been studied as a possible antidepressant, preliminary evidence from three small double-blind placebo-controlled clinical trials suggests that 5-HTP may also help people lose weight.[36,37,38] It's thought to work by raising levels of serotonin, which in turn may influence eating behavior.

A typical therapeutic dosage of 5-HTP is 100 to 300 mg 3 times daily. No significant adverse effects have been reported in clinical trials of 5-HTP. Side effects appear to be limited to occasional mild digestive distress and possible allergic reactions.

However, an alarming report raised safety concerns about 5-HTP in 1998, when the U.S. Food and Drug Administration reported detecting a chemical compound known as "peak X" in some 5-HTP products. Peak X has a frightening history involving tryptophan, which is an amino acid related to 5-HTP. Until about 10 years ago, tryptophan was widely used as a sleep aid, but it was taken off the market when thousands of people using it developed a disabling and sometimes fatal blood disorder; the same contaminant, peak X, was found to be associated with that disaster.

Because the body turns tryptophan into 5-HTP, 5-HTP has been marketed as a safe replacement for the banned amino acid. It was assumed that 5-HTP could not possibly present the same contaminant risk as tryptophan because it is manufactured completely differently. However, the recent discovery that peak X exists in batches of 5-HTP is worrisome.

Another safety issue with 5-HTP involves its interaction with carbidopa, a medication used for Parkinson's disease. Several reports suggest that the combination can create skin changes similar to those that occur in the disease scleroderma.[39,40,41]

In addition, 5-HTP should not be combined with drugs that raise serotonin levels, such as SSRIs (e.g., Prozac), other antidepressants, or the pain medication tramadol. There is a chance you might raise serotonin levels too high, causing a dangerous condition called serotonin syndrome.

Safety in young children, pregnant or nursing women, and people with liver or kidney disease has not been established (although, in some studies children have been given 5-HTP without any apparent harmful effects).

Calcium and Vitamin D Supplements

Rapid weight loss in overweight postmenopausal women appears to accelerate osteoporosis slightly.[42] For this reason, taking **calcium** (see page 234) and **vitamin D** (see page 449) supplements—always a good idea—may be especially appropriate here.

Garcinia cambogia: No Evidence That It Works

Hydroxycitric acid (HCA; see page 328), a derivative of citric acid, is found primarily in a small, sweet, purple fruit called *Garcinia cambogia,* the Malabar tamarind. In animal studies, HCA suppressed appetite and thereby encouraged weight loss.[43–47]

It has also been suggested that HCA interferes with the body's ability to produce and store fat.[48–51]

However, the largest and best-designed human trial found no benefit with HCA,[52] and another small placebo-controlled human study found HCA had no effect on metabolism.[53]

Caffeine and Ephedra: May Be Effective, but Not Recommended

Caffeine and **ephedra** (also known as ma huang; see page 277) are central nervous system stimulants that, when combined, may help people lose weight.

Several well-designed studies examining the effect of a caffeine-ephedra combination indicate that it does promote weight loss.[54–57] However, these stimulants affect the heart, and should be used only under physician supervision.

Vitamin C: For Weight Loss, Too?

Vitamin C (see page 444), the single most popular vitamin supplement in the United States, has been tested in hundreds of clinical studies for dozens of illnesses from cancer to colds, and even for weight loss.

Results of two small double-blind placebo-controlled studies suggest that extremely overweight people who take vitamin C supplements may lose some weight,[58,59] but larger studies will have to be conducted before these results can be taken as recommendations.

Conjugated Linoleic Acid (CLA)

Conjugated linoleic acid (CLA; see page 261) is a mixture of different isomers, or chemical forms, of linoleic acid. This is an essential fatty acid—a type of fat that your body needs as much as it needs vitamins.

CLA has been proposed as a fat-burning substance, but the evidence that it works is mixed.[60–63]

Evening Primrose Oil: Questionable Benefit

Evening primrose is a native American wildflower, named for the late afternoon opening of its delicate flowers. Its seeds are one of the best natural sources of **cis-gamma-linolenic acid** (GLA; see page 304), an important member of the essential omega-6 family of fatty acids.

One double-blind study of 74 women found that evening primrose oil failed to produce any weight loss as compared to placebo; however, another investigation that restricted treatment to 47 people with a family history of obesity found it produced a small but significant weight loss.[64,65]

Other Treatments

Preliminary evidence suggests that a special type of fat known as diacylglycerol may help individuals lose fat, especially fat around the abdomen.[66] One double-blind placebo-controlled trial investigated the possible weight loss effects of **spirulina** (see page 413).[67] However, while individuals taking 8.4 g of spirulina daily lost weight, the difference between the spirulina group and the placebo group was not statistically significant. Larger and longer studies are needed to establish whether spirulina is indeed an effective treatment for obesity. Other treatments often recommended for weight loss, but with little scientific backing, include **pantothenic acid** (see page 380), **zinc** (see page 463), and **coenzyme Q_{10}** (see page 256).

What About High-Protein Diets?

High-protein, low-carbohydrate diets have some interesting scientific evidence behind them, but they have not yet been proven to work as claimed. However, contrary to some reports, they haven't been proven dangerous either.

According to advocates, a high-protein, low-carb diet can help you achieve your ideal weight, prevent heart disease, control diabetes, and prolong life. However, conventional medical authorities are skeptical, pointing to studies that show a diet centered around whole grains reduces the risk of heart disease and will probably help you live longer.

Because the high-protein, low-carb diet is the opposite of that, doctors are concerned that it isn't healthy for you. However, advocates of high-protein diets claim that their approach is even healthier than the whole-grain centered diet. Intriguing evidence suggests that there could be some truth to this idea.

What Is the Scientific Evidence for High-Protein Diets?

The rationale for the high-protein diet involves insulin. When you eat carbohydrates, the body releases insulin to process the sugars they contain. There is some reason to believe that the less insulin your body produces, the healthier you will be (within limits), and the easier it will be to lose weight.

Insulin release helps fat cells create fat. In addition, elevated insulin levels tend to lead to an increased risk of heart disease. One large study found that increased insulin levels were twice as strong a predictor of future heart disease as elevated cholesterol.[68]

A high-protein, low-carb diet tends to reduce insulin levels, and could therefore help prevent heart disease.

A large study lends support to this concept. It examined the relationship between protein intake and heart disease in 80,082 women during a 14-year period.[69] The results suggest that a diet replacing carbohydrates with protein does not increase heart disease risk and might even reduce it. In addition, high intake of refined carbohydrates (such as sugar and white flour) has been found to be a significant risk factor for heart disease.[70]

But does the high-protein diet help you lose weight? The answer is, "Maybe." The research reported so far is intriguing, but not definitive. Studies currently in progress should settle the issue in the next several years.

Safety Issues

If you have kidney problems, eating a high-protein diet could be dangerous. High-protein intake also reduces the effectiveness of medication for Parkinson's disease. Also, don't get too extreme and eliminate your entire carbohydrate intake: this will alter your metabolism in an unhealthy way. Finally, choose healthy protein sources such as fish, legumes, and lean meat.

P A R T

TWO

Herbs and Supplements

5-HTP (5-HYDROXYTRYPTOPHAN)

Principal Proposed Uses   Depression, Migraine Headaches, Other Types of Headaches

Other Proposed Uses   Obesity (Weight Loss), Fibromyalgia, Anxiety, Insomnia

Many antidepressant drugs work, at least in part, by raising serotonin levels. The supplement 5-hydroxytryptophan (5-HTP) has been tried in cases of depression for a similar reason: the body uses 5-HTP to make serotonin, so providing the body with 5-HTP might therefore raise serotonin levels.

As a supplement, 5-HTP has also been proposed for all the same uses as other antidepressants, including aiding weight loss, preventing migraine headaches, decreasing the discomfort of fibromyalgia, improving sleep quality, and reducing anxiety.

SOURCES

5-HTP is not found in foods to any appreciable extent. For use as a supplement, it is manufactured from the seeds of an African plant (*Griffonia simplicifolia*).

THERAPEUTIC DOSAGES

A typical dosage of 5-HTP is 100 to 200 mg 3 times daily. Once 5-HTP starts to work, it may be possible to reduce the dosage significantly and still maintain good results.

THERAPEUTIC USES

The primary use of 5-HTP is for **depression** (see page 59). Several small short-term studies have found that it may be as effective as standard antidepressant drugs.[1,2] Since standard antidepressants are also used for **insomnia** (see page 103) and **anxiety** (see page 11), 5-HTP has also been suggested as a treatment for those conditions, but there is only very preliminary evidence as yet that it works.[3]

Some, but not all, studies suggest that regular use of 5-HTP may help reduce the frequency and severity of **migraine headaches** (see page 120), as well as help other types of headaches.[4–10] Additionally, preliminary evidence suggests that 5-HTP can reduce symptoms of **fibromyalgia**[11] (see page 80) and perhaps help you lose weight.[12–15]

WHAT IS THE SCIENTIFIC EVIDENCE FOR 5-HTP (5-HYDROXYTRYPTOPHAN)?

Depression

Several small studies have compared 5-HTP to standard antidepressants.[16] The best one was a recent 6-week study of 63 people given either 5-HTP (100 mg 3 times daily) or an antidepressant in the Prozac family (fluvoxamine, 50 mg 3 times daily).[17] Researchers found equal benefit between the supplement and the drug. Actually, 5-HTP worked a little better at reducing depressed mood, anxiety, physical symptoms, and insomnia, but the differences were not statistically significant. There was no question that 5-HTP caused fewer and less severe side effects. The only real complaint with 5-HTP was occasional mild digestive distress, which is found with virtually all medications.

Migraine and Other Headaches

A number of drugs are used to prevent migraine headaches, including antidepressants in the Prozac family. Although we don't know for sure, many of them appear to work by either changing serotonin levels or producing serotonin-like effects in the body. There is some evidence that 5-HTP may help prevent migraines too.

In a 6-month trial of 124 people, 5-HTP proved equally effective as the standard drug methysergide.[18] The most dramatic benefits observed were reductions in the intensity and duration of migraines. Since methysergide has been proven better than placebo for migraine headaches in earlier studies, the study results provide meaningful, although not airtight, evidence that 5-HTP is also effective.

Similarly good results were seen in another comparative study, using a different medication.[19]

However, in one study, 5-HTP was less effective than the drug propranolol.[20] Also, in a study involving children, 5-HTP failed to demonstrate benefit.[21] Other studies that are sometimes quoted as evidence that 5-HTP is effective for migraines actually enrolled adults or children with many different types of headaches (including migraines).[22,23,24]

Putting all this evidence together, it appears likely that 5-HTP can help people with frequent migraine headaches, but further research needs to be done. In particular, we need a large double-blind study that compares 5-HTP against placebo over a period of several months.

Finally, an 8-week double-blind placebo-controlled trial of 65 individuals (mostly women) with tension headaches found that 5-HTP at a dose of 100 mg 3 times daily did not significantly reduce the number of headaches experienced; however it did reduce participants' need to use other pain-relieving medications.[25]

5-HTP

Visit Us at TNP.com

Obesity (Weight Loss)

The drug fenfluramine was one member of the now infamous phen-fen treatment for **weight loss** (see page 192). Although very successful, fenfluramine was later associated with damage to the valves of the heart, and was removed from the market. Because fenfluramine raises serotonin levels, it seems reasonable to believe that other substances that affect serotonin might also be useful for weight reduction.

Three small double-blind placebo-controlled clinical trials have examined whether 5-HTP can help you lose weight. The first study found that 5-HTP (80 mg daily) could reduce caloric intake despite the fact that the 19 participants made no conscious effort to eat less.[26] The second study, which used a much higher dosage (900 mg daily) in 20 overweight women, found that treatment helped the participants stick to their diets.[27] The result was improved weight loss.

The third trial, which enrolled 20 obese women, confirmed the results of the second with even slightly better results: After 12 weeks the average weight loss in the 5-HTP group was 10.3 pounds versus just 2.28 pounds in the placebo group.[28] These impressive results deserve more study.

A related double-blind placebo-controlled study suggests that 5-HTP may facilitate weight loss in overweight individuals with adult-onset diabetes.[29]

(For another approach to weight loss, specifically reducing fat, see the chapter on **chromium**.)

Fibromyalgia

Antidepressants are the primary conventional treatment for fibromyalgia, a little-understood disease characterized by aching, tender muscles, fatigue, and disturbed sleep. One study suggests that 5-HTP may be helpful as well. In this double-blind trial, 50 subjects with fibromyalgia were given either 100 mg of 5-HTP or placebo 3 times daily for a month.[30] Those receiving 5-HTP experienced significant improvements in all symptom categories, including pain, stiffness, sleep patterns, anxiety, and fatigue.

(For another approach to fibromyalgia, see the chapter on **SAMe**.)

SAFETY ISSUES

No significant adverse effects have been reported in clinical trials of 5-HTP. Side effects appear to be limited to occasional mild digestive distress and possible allergic reactions.

However, an alarming report has raised concerns about the safety of 5-HTP. In 1998, the U.S. Food and Drug Administration reported detecting a chemical compound known as "peak X" in some 5-HTP products. Peak X has a frightening history involving a supplement related to 5-HTP: tryptophan. Until about 10 years ago, tryptophan was widely used as a sleep aid. However, it was taken off the market when thousands of people using the supplement developed a disabling and sometimes fatal blood disorder. This same contaminant, peak X, was found to be associated with that disaster.

Since the body turns tryptophan into 5-HTP, the latter has been marketed as a safe replacement for the banned amino acid. Until recently, it was assumed that 5-HTP could not possibly present the same risk as tryptophan because it is manufactured completely differently. However, the recent discovery that the same substance exists in batches of 5-HTP is worrisome. At this time, there is no other information from the FDA regarding specific cautions on using 5-HTP, but you should pay close attention to reports that may follow up on this finding.

Another safety issue with 5-HTP involves an interaction with a medication used for Parkinson's disease: carbidopa. Several reports suggest that the combination can create skin changes similar to those that occur in the disease scleroderma.[31,32,33]

5-HTP should not be combined with drugs that raise serotonin levels, such as SSRIs (e.g., Prozac), other antidepressants, or the pain medication tramadol. There is a chance you might raise serotonin levels too high, causing a dangerous condition called serotonin syndrome.

According to one report, 5-HTP may cause seizures in children with Down's syndrome.[34]

Although safety in children has not been proven, children have been given 5-HTP in studies without any apparent harmful effects.[35,36,37] Safety in pregnant or nursing women and those with liver or kidney disease has not been established.

⚠ INTERACTIONS YOU SHOULD KNOW ABOUT

If you are taking

Prescription antidepressants (including **SSRIs, MAO inhibitors,** or **tricyclics**) or the pain drug **tramadol:** Do not take 5-HTP in addition except on a physician's advice.

The Parkinson's disease medication **carbidopa:** Taking 5-HTP at the same time might cause skin changes similar to those that develop in the disease scleroderma.

5-HTP

Visit Us at TNP.com

ACIDOPHILUS AND OTHER PROBIOTICS

Supplement Forms/Alternate Names   Lactobacillus, Bifidobacterium, B. bifidus, L. acidophilus, L. bulgaricus, L. casei, L. plantarum, L. reuteri, S. salivarius, S. thermophilus, Saccharomyces boulardii, Probiotics

Principal Proposed Uses   "Traveler's Diarrhea," Viral Diarrhea (in Children), Antibiotic-Associated Diarrhea, Irritable Bowel Syndrome, Vaginal Infection

Other Proposed Uses   Strengthening Immunity, High Cholesterol, Ulcerative Colitis, Canker Sores, Crohn's Disease, Colon Cancer Prevention, Milk Allergies, Yeast Hypersensitivity Syndrome

Lactobacillus acidophilus is a "friendly" strain of bacteria used to make yogurt and cheese. Although we are born without it, acidophilus soon establishes itself in our intestines and helps prevent intestinal infections. Acidophilus also flourishes in the vagina, where it protects women against yeast infections.

Acidophilus is one of several microbes known collectively as *probiotics* (literally, "pro life," indicating that they are bacteria and yeasts that help rather than harm). Others include the bacteria *L. bulgaricus, L. reuteri, L. plantarum, L. casei, B. bifidus, S. salivarius,* and *S. thermophilus* and the yeast *Saccharomyces boulardii.* Your digestive tract is like a rain forest ecosystem, with billions of bacteria and yeasts rather than trees, frogs, and leopards. Some of these internal inhabitants are more helpful to your body than others. Acidophilus and related probiotics not only help the digestive tract function, they also reduce the presence of less healthful organisms by competing with them for the limited space available.

Antibiotics can disturb the balance of your "inner rain forest" by killing friendly bacteria. When this happens, harmful bacteria and yeasts can move in and flourish. This is why women taking antibiotics sometimes develop vaginal infections.

Conversely, it appears that the regular use of probiotics can help prevent vaginal infections and generally improve the health of the gastrointestinal system. Whenever you take antibiotics, you should probably take probiotics as well, and continue them for some time after you are done with the course of treatment. There is reason to believe that regular use of probiotics can reduce your risk of developing infectious diarrhea while traveling through foreign countries. Probiotics may also help prevent diarrhea caused by antibiotics, as well as help prevent and treat childhood diarrhea.

SOURCES

Although we believe that they are helpful and perhaps even necessary for human health, we don't have a daily requirement for probiotic bacteria. They are living creatures, not chemicals, so they can sustain themselves in your body unless something comes along to damage them, such as antibiotics.

Cultured dairy products such as yogurt and kefir are good sources of acidophilus and other probiotic bacteria. Supplements are widely available in powder, liquid, capsule, or tablet form. Grocery stores and natural food stores both carry milk that contains live acidophilus.

THERAPEUTIC DOSAGES

Dosages of acidophilus are expressed not in grams or milligrams, but in billions of organisms. A typical daily dose should supply about 3 to 5 billion live organisms. Other probiotic bacteria are used similarly.

The typical dose of *S. boulardii* yeast is 500 mg twice daily (standardized to provide 3×10^{10} colony-forming units per gram), to be taken while traveling, or at the start of using antibiotics and continuing for a few days after antibiotics are stopped.

Because probiotics are not drugs, but rather living organisms that you are trying to transplant to your digestive tract, it is necessary to take the treatment regularly. Each time you do, you reinforce the beneficial bacterial colonies in your body, which may gradually push out harmful bacteria and yeasts growing there.

The downside of using a living organism is that probiotics may die on the shelf. In fact, a study reported in 1990 found that most acidophilus capsules on the market contained no living acidophilus.[1] The container label should guarantee living acidophilus (or bulgaricus, and so on) at the time of purchase, not just at the time of manufacture. Another approach is to eat acidophilus-rich foods such as yogurt, where the bacteria are most likely still alive.

To treat or prevent vaginal infections, mix 2 tablespoons of yogurt or the contents of a couple of capsules of acidophilus with warm water and use as a douche.

Finally, in addition to increasing your intake of probiotics, you can take fructo-oligosaccharides, supplements that can promote thriving colonies of helpful bacteria in the digestive tract. (Fructo-oligosaccharides are carbohydrates found in fruit. *Fructo* means "fruit," and an *oligosaccharide* is a type of carbohydrate.) Taking this supplement is like putting manure in a garden; it is thought to foster a healthy environment for the bacteria you want to have inside you. The typical daily dose of fructo-oligosaccharides is between 2 and 8 g.

THERAPEUTIC USES

Evidence suggests that acidophilus and other probiotics may be helpful for preventing traveler's diarrhea and diarrhea caused by antibiotics, as well as preventing and treating viral diarrhea in children; it may also help **irritable bowel syndrome** (see page 108).[2–21]

A few preliminary studies suggest that probiotics might be helpful for preventing **vaginal yeast infections** (see page 182).[22–27]

Preliminary evidence suggests that regular use of probiotics may improve immunity.[28,29]

Preliminary double-blind trials suggest that probiotics might help prevent heart disease by reducing **cholesterol** (see page 88) levels.[30,31]

Probiotics might be helpful in **ulcerative colitis** (see page 179).[32,33]

Probiotic treatment has also been proposed as a treatment for **canker sores** (see page 40) and **Crohn's disease** (see page 57), and as a preventative measure against colon **cancer** (see page 32), but there is no solid evidence that it is effective.[34]

There is some evidence that probiotics can help reduce symptoms of milk allergies when added to milk.[35]

Finally, probiotics may be helpful in a condition known as *yeast hypersensitivity syndrome* (also known as chronic candidiasis, chronic candida, systemic candidiasis, or just **candida;** see page 38). Although this syndrome is not recognized by conventional medicine, some practitioners of alternative medicine believe that it is a common problem that leads to numerous symptoms, including fatigue, digestive problems, frequent sinus infections, muscle pain, and mental confusion. Yeast hypersensitivity syndrome is said to consist of a population explosion of the normally benign candida yeast that live in the vagina and elsewhere in the body, coupled with a type of allergic sensitivity to it. Probiotic supplements are widely recommended for this condition because they establish large, healthy populations of friendly bacteria that compete with the candida that is trying to take up residence.

WHAT IS THE SCIENTIFIC EVIDENCE FOR ACIDOPHILUS AND OTHER PROBIOTICS?

Diarrhea

According to several studies, it appears that regular use of acidophilus and other probiotics can help prevent "traveler's diarrhea" (an illness caused by eating contaminated food, usually in developing countries).[36,37] One double-blind placebo-controlled study followed 820 individuals traveling to southern Turkey, and found that use of a probiotic called *Lactobacillus GG* significantly protected against intestinal infection.[38]

Other studies using *S. boulardii* have found similar benefits,[39,40,41] including a double-blind placebo-controlled trial enrolling 3,000 Austrian travelers.[42] The greatest benefits were seen in travelers who visited North Africa and Turkey. The researchers noted the benefit depended on consistent use of the product, and a dosage of 1,000 mg daily was more effective than 250 mg daily.

Probiotics may also help prevent or treat diarrhea in children. A double-blind study evaluated the possible benefits of the probiotic *L. reuteri* in 66 children with rotavirus diarrhea (rotavirus is a virus that can cause severe diarrhea in children).[43] The study found that treatment shortened the duration of symptoms, and the higher the dose, the better the effect.

Another double-blind placebo-controlled study found that *B. bifidum* and *Streptococcus thermophilus* can help protect against rotavirus infection in hospitalized infants.[44] The probiotics *L. casei* and *S. boulardii* may also help prevent diarrhea in infants and children.[45,46,47]

Keep in mind that diarrhea in young children can be serious. If it persists for more than a day, you should take your child to a physician.

Several double-blind and open trials suggest that probiotics, including *S. boulardii,* may also help reduce antibiotic-related diarrhea.[48–52] One study evaluated 180 individuals, who received either placebo or 1,000 mg of saccharomyces daily along with their antibiotic treatment, and found that the treated group developed diarrhea significantly less often.[53] A similar study of 193 individuals also found benefit.[54] However, a smaller study of saccharomyces did not find benefit.[55]

Small double-blind studies suggest *S. boulardii* might be helpful for treating chronic diarrhea in people with HIV, hospitalized patients being tube-fed, and individuals with Crohn's disease.[56–59]

Irritable Bowel Syndrome

People with irritable bowel syndrome (IBS) experience crampy digestive pain as well as alternating diarrhea and constipation and other symptoms. Although the cause of irritable bowel syndrome is not known, one possibility is a disturbance in healthy intestinal bacteria. Based on this theory, probiotics have been tried as a treatment for IBS.

In a 4-week double-blind placebo-controlled trial of 60 individuals with IBS, treatment with *L. plantarum* reduced intestinal gas significantly.[60] The benefits persisted for an additional year after treatment was stopped.

In another double-blind trial, 18 individuals with irritable bowel syndrome were given either placebo or a capsule containing 5 billion *L. acidophilus* organisms daily for 6 weeks.[61] Greater improvement was seen in the treated group than in the placebo group, but so many people dropped out of the study the results are difficult to evaluate.

Vaginal Yeast Infections

A review of the many studies on the use of oral and topical acidophilus to prevent vaginal yeast infections concluded that it may be effective, but more study is needed.[62,63]

Immunity

A number of studies suggest that various probiotics can enhance immune function,[64] but there is only one double-blind placebo-controlled study on the subject. This 12-week trial evaluated 25 healthy elderly individuals, half of whom were given milk containing a particular strain of *Bifidobacterium lactis*, the others milk alone.[65] The results showed various changes in immune parameters which the researchers took as possibly indicating improved immune function.

Cholesterol

An 8-week double-blind placebo-controlled trial of 70 overweight individuals found that a probiotic treatment containing *S. thermophilus* and *Enterococcus faecium* could reduce LDL ("bad") cholesterol by about 8%.[66] Similarly positive results were seen in other trials of the same or other probiotics.[67,68,69] However, a 6-month double-blind placebo-controlled trial found no long-term benefit.[70] Researchers speculate that participants stopped using the product regularly toward the later parts of the study.

Ulcerative Colitis

A 12-week double-blind study of 120 individuals with ulcerative colitis found that a friendly strain of *Escherichia coli* helped prevent flare-ups of the disease as effectively as the standard drug mesalazine.[71]

Individuals with severe ulcerative colitis who have had part or all of the colon removed frequently develop a complication called "pouchitis," inflammation of part of the remaining intestine. A 9-month double-blind trial of 40 individuals found that a combination of three probiotic bacteria could significantly reduce the risk of a pouchitis flare-up.[72] Participants were given either placebo or a mixture of various probiotics, including four strains of lactobacilli, three strains of bifidobacteria and one strain of *S. salivarius*. The results showed that treated individuals were far less likely to have relapses of pouchitis during the study period.

SAFETY ISSUES

There are no known safety problems with the use of acidophilus or other probiotics. Occasionally, some people notice a temporary increase in digestive gas.

⚠ INTERACTIONS YOU SHOULD KNOW ABOUT

If you are taking **antibiotics,** it may be beneficial to take probiotic supplements at the same time, and to continue them for a couple of weeks after you have finished the course of drug treatment. This will help restore the balance of natural bacteria in your digestive tract.

ALFALFA (*Medicago sativa*)

Alternate or Related Names   Lucerne, Purple Medick, Purple Medicle, Buffalo Herb, Purple Medic

Principal Proposed Uses   Nutritional Support

Other Proposed Uses   Lowering Cholesterol, Diabetes, Menopausal Symptoms, Antifungal, Allergies

Alfalfa is one of the earliest cultivated plants, used for centuries for feeding livestock. This probably is true in part because it is easy to grow, thrives in many varied climates throughout the world, and provides an excellent protein-rich food source for cattle, horses, sheep, and other animals. The name alfalfa comes from the Arabian *al-fac-facah*, for "father of all foods."[1] Its high protein content and abundant stores of vitamins make it a good nutritional source for humans, too. Historic (but undocumented) medicinal uses of alfalfa include treatment of

stomach upset, arthritis, bladder and kidney problems, boils, and irregular menstruation.

REQUIREMENTS/SOURCES

Alfalfa sprouts appear on many salad bars and in the grocery's produce section. Bulk powdered herb or capsules and tablets containing alfalfa leaves or seeds are available in pharmacies and health food stores.

Alfalfa

Visit Us at TNP.com

THERAPEUTIC DOSAGES

Since there is no documented therapeutic effect for alfalfa, there is no established dose. Bulk alfalfa can be used like a tea (1 to 2 teaspoons per cup, steeped in boiling water for 10 to 20 minutes). Tablets and capsules may be taken according to the manufacturer's recommendations.

THERAPEUTIC USES

Alfalfa is high in vitamin content, providing **beta-carotene** (see page 217), vitamin B-complex, vitamins **C** (see page 444), **E** (see page 451), and **K** (see page 456), and can be used as a nutritional supplement.[2] However, keep in mind that high doses of alfalfa may present some health risks (see Safety Issues below).

Numerous animal studies[3-14] and two very small, open studies using human volunteers[15,16] indicate that chemicals from alfalfa seeds, leaves, and roots might be helpful for lowering **cholesterol** (see page 88) levels in the blood, thereby reducing atherosclerotic plaque.

Studies using mice to investigate alfalfa's traditional use for **diabetes** (see page 65) found that it improved some symptoms.[17,18] Unfortunately, there have not been any clinical trials involving humans with diabetes.

Alfalfa has also been investigated in the laboratory (but not yet evaluated in people) as a source of plant estrogens, which might make it helpful for **menopause** (see page 117).[19,20,21] Alfalfa may also have some use in fighting fungi.[22,23,24] Rats fed a disease-causing fungus were able to eliminate more of the fungus from their systems when fed a diet high in alfalfa. It is has been suggested that one of the saponins from alfalfa causes damage to the cell membranes of fungi.

Finally, Alfalfa's proposed use to reduce hay fever symptoms has no scientific validation.

SAFETY ISSUES

Alfalfa in its various forms may present some health risks. Powdered alfalfa herb, alfalfa sprouts, and alfalfa seeds all contain L-cavanine, a substance that may cause abnormal blood cell counts, spleen enlargement, or recurrence of **lupus** (see page 114) in patients with controlled disease. However, heating alfalfa may correct this problem.

Researchers investigating alfalfa seeds' ability to lower cholesterol levels discovered that it had another effect on the lab animals used for testing. In some of the monkeys, it caused a disease very similar to lupus.[25] Further research on this effect revealed that monkeys that had abnormal blood cell counts when eating either alfalfa seeds or sprouts, and then recovered when alfalfa was no longer part of their diet, developed the symptoms again when given an isolated component of alfalfa called L-canavanine.[26] Alfalfa seeds and sprouts have a higher concentration of L-canavanine than the leaves or roots.

In a clinical trial of alfalfa seeds for lowering cholesterol involving only three human volunteers, one man who participated developed pancytopenia (an abnormally low number of all of the various types of blood cells) and enlargement of the spleen.[27] Additionally, there are two published case reports of patients who had lupus which was controlled with drug therapy, suffering relapses after consuming alfalfa tablets. Again, L-canavanine is thought responsible for these effects.

When alfalfa seeds were autoclaved (heated to extremely high temperatures) and fed to monkeys for a year, no ill effects were seen, and the monkeys' cholesterol levels decreased.[28] It may be that the L-canavanine can be destroyed by extreme heat, while the saponins that seem to be responsible for the beneficial effects of alfalfa remain intact. If so a heat-treated product might prove safe; however, much research remains to be done before we can know this for certain.

At present, it seems prudent that people who have been diagnosed with lupus, or those who suspect a predisposition to it based on family history, should probably avoid alfalfa. This includes the tablets used for supplements and the sprouts on the salad bar (go for the lettuce or the spinach instead).

Because of the estrogenic effects of some of alfalfa's components, alfalfa is not recommended for pregnant or nursing women or young children. In addition, the high **vitamin K** (see page 456) content in alfalfa could, in theory, make the drug warfarin (Coumadin) less effective.

Finally, a number of cases of food poisoning have been documented from fresh sprouts infected with bacteria that was present on the seeds prior to germination.[29,30,31] Unfortunately, sprouts can appear fresh and yet host enough bacteria to cause illness in people who eat them. Some health care workers recommend that those at higher risk for such infections—young children, those with chronic diseases, and the elderly—avoid eating sprouts altogether.

⚠ INTERACTIONS YOU SHOULD KNOW ABOUT

If you are taking warfarin (Coumadin), the high vitamin K content of alfalfa might make it less effective.

ALOE (*Aloe vera*)

Principal Proposed Uses
 Topical Uses: Wound Healing, Burn Healing, Psoriasis, Seborrhea.
 Oral Uses: Diabetes

Other Proposed Uses
 Oral Uses: AIDS, Asthma, Ulcers, Immune Weakness

The succulent aloe plant has been valued since prehistoric times for the treatment of burns, wound infections, and other skin problems. Medicinal aloe is pictured in an ancient cave painting in South Africa, and Alexander the Great is said to have captured an island off Somalia for the sole purpose of possessing the luxurious crop of aloe found there.

Most uses of aloe refer to the gel inside its cactus-like leaves. However, the skin of the leaves themselves can be condensed to form a sticky substance known as "drug aloe" or "aloes." It is a powerful laxative, and an unpleasant one. The uses described below refer only to aloe gel.

WHAT IS ALOE USED FOR TODAY?

We suspect millions of people would swear by their own experience that applying aloe to the skin can drastically reduce the time it takes for **burns** (see page 123) (including **sunburn;** see page 171) to heal. However, aloe has been found ineffective for treating sunburn and has never been properly evaluated for other types of burns.[1,2,3]

A study in animals suggests that topical aloe gel may improve **wound healing** (see page 123).[4,5] However, one report suggests that aloe can actually impair healing in severe wounds.[6]

There is actually better evidence (although still imperfect) for two lesser-known uses of topical aloe: **psoriasis** (see page 148) and **seborrhea** (see page 154).

Intriguing evidence suggests that aloe gel taken orally might be helpful for type 2 **diabetes** (see page 65).[7,8]

Oral *Aloe vera* is also sometimes recommended to treat AIDS, **asthma** (see page 14), **stomach ulcers** (see page 180), and general immune weakness. While the evidence for benefit in these conditions is slight to nonexistent, one of the constituents of aloe, acemannan, does seem to possess numerous interesting effects. Test-tube and animal studies suggest that it may stimulate immunity and inhibit the growth of viruses.[9,10,11] However, it remains to be discovered whether this preliminary research will translate into actual benefits in human beings. *Aloe vera* is definitely not a proven treatment for any of these conditions.

WHAT IS THE SCIENTIFIC EVIDENCE FOR ALOE?

Psoriasis

According to a double-blind study that enrolled 60 men and women with mild to moderate symptoms of psoriasis, *Aloe vera* cream may be helpful for this chronic skin condition.[12] Participants were treated with either topical *Aloe vera* extract (0.5%) or a placebo cream, applied 3 times daily for 4 weeks. Aloe treatment produced significantly better results than placebo, and these results were said to endure for almost a year after treatment was stopped. The study authors also reported a high level of complete "cure," but what exactly they meant by this was not reported clearly.

Seborrhea

Seborrhea is a fairly common skin condition, leading to oily, red, and scaly eruptions in such areas as the eyebrows, eyelids, nose, ear, upper lip, chest, groin, and chin. A double-blind placebo-controlled study of 44 individuals found that 4 to 6 weeks of treatment with aloe ointment could significantly reduce symptoms of seborrhea.[13]

Diabetes

Evidence from some but not all studies suggests that aloe gel can improve blood sugar control in individuals with type 2 diabetes.[14–19]

For example, a single-blind placebo-controlled trial evaluated the potential benefits of aloe in either 72 or 40 individuals with diabetes (the study report appears to contradict itself).[20] The results showed significantly greater improvements in blood sugar levels among those given aloe over the 2-week treatment period.

Another single-blind placebo-controlled trial evaluated the benefits of aloe in individuals who had failed to respond to the oral diabetes drug glibenclamide.[21] Of the 36 individuals who completed the study, those taking glibenclamide and aloe showed definite improvements in blood sugar levels over 42 days as compared to those taking glibenclamide and placebo.

Although these are promising results, large studies that are double- rather than single-blind will be needed to establish aloe as an effective treatment for hypoglycemia.

DOSAGE

For the treatment of diabetes, a dosage of 1 tablespoon of *Aloe vera* juice twice daily has been used in studies.

For internal use in treating AIDS and other conditions, some authorities recommend a dose of aloe standardized to provide 800 to 1,600 mg of the substance acemannan daily.

SAFETY ISSUES

Other than occasional allergic reactions, no serious problems have been reported with aloe gel, whether used internally or externally. However, comprehensive safety studies are lacking. Safety in young children, pregnant or nursing women, or those with severe liver or kidney disease has not been established.

In addition, keep in mind that if aloe is successful as a treatment for diabetes, blood sugar levels could fall too low, necessitating a reduction in medication dosage.

⚠ INTERACTIONS YOU SHOULD KNOW ABOUT

If you are using:

- Hydrocortisone cream: Aloe gel might help it work better.[22]
- Medications for diabetes: Oral use of aloe vera might cause your blood sugar levels to fall too low.

ANDROGRAPHIS (*Andrographis paniculata*)

Principal Proposed Uses   Colds (Prevention and Reducing Symptoms)

Other Proposed Uses   Heart Disease Prevention, Liver Protection, Stimulating Gallbladder Contraction

Andrographis is a shrub found throughout India and other Asian countries that is sometimes called "Indian echinacea." Historically, it has been used in epidemics, including the Indian flu epidemic in 1919, during which andrographis was credited with stopping the spread of the disease.[1]

WHAT IS ANDROGRAPHIS USED FOR TODAY?

Over the last decade, andrographis has become popular in Scandinavia as a treatment for **colds** (see page 47). It is beginning to become available in the United States as well. Reasonably good evidence tells us that it can reduce the severity of cold symptoms. It may also help prevent colds.

Although we don't know how andrographis might work for colds, some evidence suggests that it might stimulate immunity.[2] Interestingly, the ingredient of andrographis used for standardization purposes, andrographolide, does not appear to affect the immune system as much as the whole plant extract.

Preliminary studies in animals also suggest that andrographis may offer benefits for preventing **heart disease** (see page 16).[3,4,5] In addition, highly preliminary studies suggest that andrographis may help protect the liver from toxic injury, perhaps more successfully than the more famous liver-protective herb **milk thistle** (see page 361).[6,7,8] It also appears to stimulate gallbladder contraction.[9] Andrographis does not appear to have any antibacterial effects.[10]

WHAT IS THE SCIENTIFIC EVIDENCE FOR ANDROGRAPHIS?

Reducing Cold Symptoms

A few well-designed double-blind studies have found that andrographis can reduce the severity of symptoms.

A 4-day, double-blind placebo-controlled trial of 158 adults with colds found that treatment with andrographis significantly reduced cold symptoms.[11] Participants were given either placebo or 1,200 mg daily of an andrographis extract standardized to contain 5% andrographolide. The results showed that by day 2 of treatment, and even more by day 4, individuals who were given the actual treatment experienced significant improvements in symptoms as compared to participants in the placebo group. The greatest response was seen in earache, sleeplessness, nasal drainage, and sore throat, but other cold symptoms improved as well.

Good results were seen in two other double-blind placebo-controlled studies, involving a total of over 100 participants.[12,13]

Another double-blind study, which involved 152 adults, compared the effectiveness of andrographis (in doses of 3 g per day or 6 g per day, for 7 days) to acetaminophen for the treatment of sore throat and fever. The higher dose of andrographis (6 g) decreased symptoms of

Andrographis

Visit Us at TNP.com

fever and throat pain, as did acetaminophen, while the lower dose of andrographis (3 g) did not.

There were no significant side effects in either group.[14]

Preventing Colds

According to one double-blind placebo-controlled study, andrographis may increase resistance to colds.[15] A total of 107 students, all 18 years old, participated in this 3-month-long trial that used a dried extract of andrographis. Fifty-four of the participants took two 100-mg tablets standardized to 5.6% andrographolide daily—considerably less than the 1,200 to 6,000 mg per day that has been used in studies on treatment of colds. The other 53 students were given placebo tablets with a coating identical to the treatment. Then, once a week throughout the study, a clinician evaluated all the participants for cold symptoms.

By the end of the trial, only 16 people in the group using andrographis had experienced colds, compared to 33 of the placebo-group participants. This difference was statistically significant, indicating that andrographis reduces the risk of catching a cold by a factor of two as compared to placebo.

DOSAGE

A typical dosage of andrographis is 400 mg 3 times a day. Doses as high as 1,000 to 2,000 mg 3 times daily have been used in some studies. Andrographis is usually standardized to its content of andrographolide, typically 4 to 6%.

SAFETY ISSUES

Andrographis has not been associated with any side effects in human studies. In one study, participants were monitored for changes in liver function, blood counts, kidney function, and other laboratory measures of toxicity.[16] No problems were found.

However, some animal studies have raised concerns that andrographis may impair fertility. One study found that male rats became infertile when fed 20 mg of andrographis powder daily.[17] In this case, the rats stopped producing sperm and showed physical changes in some of the testicular cells involved in sperm production. Researchers also detected evidence of degeneration of other anatomical structures in the testicles. However, another study showed no evidence of testicular toxicity in male rats that were given up to 1 g per kilogram body weight daily for 60 days, so this issue remains unclear.[18]

One group of female mice also did not fare well on high dosages of andrographis.[19] When fed 2 g per kilogram body weight daily for 6 weeks (thousands of times higher than the usual human dose), all female mice failed to get pregnant when mated with males of proven fertility. Meanwhile, of the control females, 95.2% got pregnant when mated with a similar group of male mice.

While andrographis is probably not a useful form of birth control, these results are worrisome and suggest the need for more research. Safety in young children, pregnant or nursing women, or those with severe liver or kidney disease has not been established.

Also, because andrographis may stimulate gallbladder contraction, it should not be used by individuals with gallbladder disease except under physician supervision.

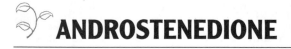

ANDROSTENEDIONE

Principal Proposed Uses   Performance Enhancement

Androstenedione is a hormone produced naturally in the body by the adrenal glands, the ovaries (in women), and the testicles (in men). The body first manufactures **DHEA** (see page 268), then turns DHEA into androstenedione, and finally transforms androstenedione into testosterone, the principal male sex hormone. Androstenedione is also transformed into estrogen.

Androstenedione is widely used by athletes who believe that it can build muscle and increase strength. However, there is no evidence that it works. U.S. baseball fans know that the all-time single-season home run champion, Mark McGwire, used androstenedione during his record-setting season. Whether it helped is anyone's guess. Hitting home runs is not only a matter of strength, but of timing and concentration as well. Nonetheless, if McGwire were playing in any other professional sport, or in the Olympics, he would have been suspended for using androstenedione.

SOURCES

Androstenedione is not an essential nutrient—your body manufactures it from scratch. It is found in meat and in some plants, but to get a therapeutic dosage, you will need to take supplements.

THERAPEUTIC DOSAGES

The typical recommended dose of androstenedione is 100 mg 2 times daily with food.

THERAPEUTIC USES

Androstenedione is said to enhance **athletic performance** (see page 158) and strength by increasing testosterone production, thereby building muscle. However, the balance of evidence suggests that the supplement increases estrogen levels more than it increases testosterone levels, and that it doesn't enhance athletic performance. [1–4]

WHAT IS THE SCIENTIFIC EVIDENCE FOR ANDROSTENEDIONE?

In a 7-day open study of 42 healthy men, 300 mg daily of androstenedione significantly increased testosterone levels.[5]

However, in an 8-week double-blind placebo-controlled study of 20 healthy men undergoing weight training, 300 mg of androstenedione daily did not affect testosterone levels.[6]

A third trial also failed to find any change in testosterone levels among men given 200 mg of androstenedione daily.[7]

On balance, it does not appear that androstenedione increases testosterone. However, one fact was consistent in all these trials: androstenedione increased estrogen levels significantly. This change would not be expected to improve sports performance. Indeed, in the 8-week trial mentioned above, no improvement in sports performance was seen.[8]

A 12-week double-blind study of 40 trained male athletes given either DHEA or androstenedione at 100 mg daily also found no improvement in lean body mass or strength, or change in testosterone levels.[9]

SAFETY ISSUES

Androstenedione can cause hair loss on the head and growth of body hair.[10] There are also concerns that androstenedione, like related hormones, might increase the risk of liver cancer and heart disease. In addition, because it raises estrogen levels, androstenedione might increase cancer risk in women.

One case report suggests another potential complication with the use of androstenedione.[11] An individual who was using androstenedione to improve his physique experienced priapism (painful continuous erection) for over 30 hours, requiring a visit to the emergency room. Previously he had experienced an episode lasting 2 to 3 hours that spontaneously resolved itself. While it isn't certain that androstenedione was the cause, it appears to be the most likely possibility.

⚠ INTERACTIONS YOU SHOULD KNOW ABOUT

If you are taking any **estrogen,** it is possible that androstenedione might raise cancer risk.

AORTIC GLYCOSAMINOGLYCANS

Supplement Forms/Alternate Names   Aortic GAGs, Mesoglycan, CSA, Chondroitin Polysulphate, Mucopolysaccharide, Chondroitin Sulfate A, GAGs

Principal Proposed Uses   Atherosclerosis, High Cholesterol, Varicose Veins, Hemorrhoids, Phlebitis, Kidney Stones, Interstitial Cystitis

Aortic glycosaminoglycans (GAGs) are important substances found in many tissues in the body, including the joints and the lining of blood vessels. Chemically, aortic GAGs are related to the blood-thinning drug heparin and the supplement chondroitin (for more information, see the chapter on **chondroitin).** Unlike chondroitin, aortic GAGs are primarily used to treat diseases of blood vessels. Preliminary evidence suggests that aortic GAGs may be helpful for atherosclerosis, varicose veins, phlebitis, and hemorrhoids.

SOURCES

Aortic GAGs are not essential nutrients because the body usually manufactures them from scratch. For supplement purposes, aortic GAGs are commercially extracted from the aorta (the largest artery) of cows—hence the name. Substances very similar to aortic GAGs can be produced from **cartilage** (see page 241), bone, or **chondroitin sulfate** (see page 250), and are often used interchangeably.

Aortic Glycosaminoglycans

Visit Us at TNP.com

THERAPEUTIC DOSAGES

The usual dosage of aortic GAGs is 100 mg daily.

THERAPEUTIC USES

Hardening of the arteries due to **atherosclerosis** (see page 16) is the major cause of heart disease and strokes. High **cholesterol** (see page 88), **hypertension** (see page 98), cigarette smoking, and other factors damage the inner lining of blood vessels, causing a series of dangerous changes.

There is some evidence that aortic GAGs may slow the development of atherosclerosis, by lowering cholesterol levels, "thinning" the blood, or through other effects.[1,2,3]

They may also be useful for various other diseases of blood vessels, including **varicose veins** (see page 184), **hemorrhoids** (see page 85), and **phlebitis** (see page 143).[4–8]

Warning: Do not self-treat phlebitis. It is a potentially deadly disease.

Preliminary evidence suggests aortic GAGs may be useful in treating **kidney stones** (see page 109).[9]

GAGs have also been proposed as a treatment for **interstitial cystitis** (see page 107), but there is as yet no real evidence for this potential use.

WHAT IS THE SCIENTIFIC EVIDENCE FOR AORTIC GLYCOSAMINOGLYCANS?

Atherosclerosis

In a recent study, one group of men with early hardening of the coronary (heart) arteries was given 200 mg daily of aortic GAGs, while the other group received no treatment.[10] After 18 months, the layering of the vessel lining was 7.5 times greater in the untreated group than in the aortic GAG group, a significant difference. Additional preliminary evidence that aortic GAGs might help atherosclerosis comes from other studies in animals and people.[11,12] However, in the absence of properly designed double-blind trials, the results can't be taken as truly reliable.

We don't know how aortic GAGs might help atherosclerosis. There is some evidence that they can reduce cholesterol levels and also "thin" the blood.[13]

Vein Diseases

Several Italian studies suggest that aortic GAGs may be helpful in varicose veins, phlebitis, and hemorrhoids.[14–18]

SAFETY ISSUES

Aortic GAGs are essentially ground-up blood vessels from cows, so they are probably safe to take even in large quantities. The only concern that has been raised regards their ability to slightly decrease blood clotting (see Interactions You Should Know About). Maximum safe dosages for young children, pregnant or nursing women, or those with severe liver or kidney disease have not been determined.

⚠ INTERACTIONS YOU SHOULD KNOW ABOUT

If you are taking drugs that powerfully decrease blood clotting, such as **Coumadin (warfarin), heparin, Trental (pentoxifylline),** or even **aspirin,** do not use aortic GAGs except under physician supervision. Because aortic GAGs interfere slightly with blood clotting, there is a chance that the combination could cause bleeding problems.

ARGININE

Supplement Forms/Alternate Names   Arginine Hydrochloride, L-Arginine

Principal Proposed Uses   Congestive Heart Failure, Intermittent Claudication, Impotence, Sexual Dysfunction in Women, Nutritional Support

Other Proposed Uses   Interstitial Cystitis, Colds (Prevention), Infertility

Arginine is an amino acid found in many foods, including dairy products, meat, poultry, and fish. It plays a role in several important mechanisms in the body, including cell division, wound healing, removal of ammonia from the body, immunity to illness, and the secretion of important hormones.

The body also uses arginine to make nitric oxide, a substance that relaxes the blood vessels. Based on this, arginine has been proposed as a treatment for various cardiovascular diseases, including congestive heart failure and intermittent claudication, as well as impotence, female sexual dysfunction, and an unpleasant urinary condition called interstitial cystitis. Arginine's effects on immunity have made it useful as part of an "immune cocktail" given to severely ill hospitalized patients and also, possibly, for preventing colds.

REQUIREMENTS/SOURCES

Normally, the body either gets enough arginine from food, or manufactures all it needs from other widely available nutrients. Certain stresses, such as severe burns, infections, and injuries, can deplete your body's supply of arginine. For this reason, arginine (combined with other nutrients) is used in a hospital setting to help enhance recovery from severe injury or illness.

Arginine is found in dairy products, meat, poultry, fish, nuts, and chocolate.

THERAPEUTIC DOSAGES

A typical supplemental dosage of arginine is 2 to 3 g per day. For congestive heart failure, higher dosages ranging from 5 to 15 g have been used in trials.

Warning: Do not try to self-treat congestive heart failure. If you have this condition, be sure to consult your physician before taking any supplements.

THERAPEUTIC USES

Small double-blind studies suggest that arginine may be helpful for the treatment of several seemingly unrelated conditions that are, in fact, all linked by arginine's effects on nitric oxide: **congestive heart failure** (see page 54), **impotence** (see page 100), **sexual dysfunction** (see page 155) in women, interstitial cystitis, and **intermittent claudication** (see page 106).[1–8]

In addition, one preliminary double-blind study suggests that arginine supplementation might help prevent **colds** (see page 47).[9]

Some reports suggest that arginine may be helpful in the treatment of infertility. However, studies in men have found no benefit.[10–15] The results of one controlled (but not blinded) study in women suggest that arginine might help standard fertility therapy (in vitro fertilization) work better.[16]

Preliminary studies failed to find arginine helpful for kidney failure or **asthma** (see page 14).[17]

There is some evidence that nutritional mixtures containing arginine may enhance recovery from major surgery, injury, or illness.[18]

WHAT IS THE SCIENTIFIC EVIDENCE FOR ARGININE?

Congestive Heart Failure

Three small double-blind studies enrolling a total of about 70 individuals with congestive heart failure found that oral arginine at a dose of 5 to 15 g daily could significantly improve symptoms as well as objective measurements of heart function.[19,20,21]

Intermittent Claudication

People with advanced hardening of the arteries, or atherosclerosis, often have difficulty walking due to lack of blood flow to the legs, a condition known as intermittent claudication. Pain may develop after walking less than half a block.

In a double-blind placebo-controlled study of 41 individuals, arginine at a dose of 8 g daily provided by a food bar improved pain-free walking distance by 66%.[22]

Good results were also seen in another study, although its convoluted design makes interpreting the results somewhat difficult.[23]

Impotence

In a double-blind trial, 50 men with problems developing an erection received either 5 g of arginine per day or placebo for 6 weeks.[24] More men in the treated group experienced improvement in sexual performance than in the placebo group.

Sexual Dysfunction in Women

Some postmenopausal women have difficulty feeling sexually aroused. A double-blind trial of 23 postmenopausal women found that a combination of arginine (6 g daily) and the drug yohimbine (used for impotence in men) increased sexual response.[25]

Interstitial Cystitis

Interstitial cystitis is a condition in which an individual feels like he or she has symptoms of a bladder infection, but no infection is present. Medical treatment for this condition is less than satisfactory. Some preliminary evidence suggests that arginine might help.

A 3-month double-blind trial of 53 individuals with interstitial cystitis found that participants given 1,500 mg of arginine daily experienced greater improvement than participants given placebo.[26] However, due to the number of people who dropped out of the study, the results can't be taken as conclusive.

Another double-blind trial found no evidence of benefit, but it was too small to prove anything.[27]

Artichoke

Colds

A 2-month double-blind study involving 40 children with a history of frequent colds concluded that arginine seemed to provide some protection against respiratory infections.[28] Of the children who were given arginine, 15 stayed well during the 60 days of the study. By contrast, only 5 of the children who took placebo stayed well, a significant difference.

Nutritional Support in Hospitalized Patients

Several nutritional products that contain arginine as well as other substances have been tried in hospital settings to enhance recovery following major surgery, illness, or injury. These mixtures are delivered "enterally," which means through a tube into the stomach. A review of 15 studies, about half of them double-blind and involving a total of 1,557 individuals, found that such products can reduce episodes of infection, time on ventilator machines, and length of stay in the hospital.[29]

However, because of the many nutrients contained in these so-called "immunonutrient" mixtures, it is not clear whether arginine deserves the credit.

SAFETY ISSUES

At moderate doses (2 to 3 g per day), oral arginine appears to be safe and essentially side-effect free, although minor gastrointestinal upset can occur. However, there are some potential safety issues regarding high-dose arginine. These cautions are based on findings from animal studies and hospital experiences of intravenous administration.

Arginine has been found to stimulate the body's production of gastrin, a hormone that increases stomach acid.[30] For this reason, there are concerns that arginine could be harmful for individuals with ulcers and people taking drugs that are hard on the stomach.

Arginine might also alter potassium levels in the body, especially in people with severe liver disease.[31] This is a potential concern for individuals who take drugs that also alter potassium balance (such as potassium-sparing diuretics and ACE inhibitors), as well as those with severe kidney disease. If you fall into any of these categories, do not use high-dose arginine except under physician supervision.

Maximum safe doses in pregnant or nursing women, young children, and those with severe liver or kidney disease have not been established.

⚠ INTERACTIONS YOU SHOULD KNOW ABOUT

If you are taking

- **Lysine** to treat herpes: Arginine might counteract the potential benefit.[32]
- **Drugs that are hard on the stomach** (such as **nonsteroidal anti-inflammatory medications**): Taking high doses of arginine might stress your stomach further.
- **Medications that can alter the balance of potassium** in your body (such as **potassium-sparing diuretics** or **ACE inhibitors**): High doses of arginine should be used only under physician supervision.

ARTICHOKE (*Cynara scolymus*)

Alternate or Related Names   Garden Artichoke, Globe Artichoke

Principal Proposed Uses   Dyspepsia (Indigestion)

Other Proposed Uses   High Cholesterol, Liver Protection

The artichoke is one of the oldest cultivated plants.[1] It was first grown in Ethiopia and then made its way to southern Europe via Egypt. Its image is found on ancient Egyptian tablets and sacrificial altars. The ancient Greeks and Romans considered it a valuable digestive aid and reserved what was then a rare plant for consumption in elite circles. In sixteenth-century Europe, the artichoke was also considered a "noble" vegetable meant for consumption by the royal and the rich.

In traditional European medicine, the leaves of the artichoke (not the flower buds, which are the parts commonly cooked and eaten as a vegetable) were used as a diuretic to stimulate the kidneys and as a "choleretic" to stimulate the flow of bile from the liver and gallbladder. (Bile is a yellowish-brown fluid manufactured in the liver and stored in the gallbladder; it consists of numerous substances, including several that play a significant role in digestion.)

Visit Us at TNP.com

In the first half of the twentieth century, French scientists began modern research into these traditional medicinal uses of the artichoke plant.[2] Their work suggested that the plant does indeed stimulate the kidney and gallbladder. Mid-century, Italian scientists isolated a compound from artichoke leaf called cynarin, which appeared to duplicate many of the effects of whole artichoke. Synthetic cynarin preparations were used as a drug to stimulate the liver and gallbladder and to treat elevated cholesterol from the 1950s to the 1980s; competition from newer pharmaceuticals has since eclipsed the use of cynarin.

WHAT IS ARTICHOKE USED FOR TODAY?

Artichoke leaf (as opposed to cynarin) continues to be used in many countries.

Germany's Commission E has authorized its use for "dyspeptic problems."[3] **Dyspepsia** (see page 71) is a rather vague term that corresponds to the common word "indigestion," indicating a variety of digestive problems including discomfort in the stomach, bloating, lack of appetite, nausea, and mild diarrhea or constipation.

In Europe, dyspepsia is commonly attributed to inadequate flow of bile from the gallbladder, which is why artichoke leaf is used as a treatment for this condition. Evidence tells us that artichoke leaf does indeed stimulate the gallbladder.[4,5,6] However, there is little real proof that gallbladder dysfunction is actually the cause of dyspepsia, and individuals whose gallbladder has been removed are not particularly likely to suffer from digestive distress. There is no solid evidence that artichoke leaf taken by itself improves dyspepsia. The only evidence we do have comes from open studies and a trial of a combination herbal treatment containing artichoke leaf.[7]

Better evidence suggests that artichoke leaf may help lower cholesterol.[8]

A number of animal studies suggest that artichoke protects the liver from damage by chemical toxins.[9] Artichoke's liver-protective effects have never, however, been proven in controlled clinical trials.

WHAT IS THE SCIENTIFIC EVIDENCE FOR ARTICHOKE?

High Cholesterol

According to a double-blind placebo-controlled study of 143 individuals with elevated cholesterol, artichoke leaf extract significantly improved cholesterol readings.[10] Total cholesterol fell by 18.5% as compared to 8.6% in the placebo group; LDL cholesterol by 23% versus 6; and LDL to HDL ratio decreased by 20% versus 7%.

An earlier double-blind placebo-controlled study of 44 healthy individuals failed to find any improvement in cholesterol levels attributable to artichoke leaf.[11] The researchers note, however, that study participants, on average, started the trial with lower than normal cholesterol levels (due to a statistical accident); improvement, therefore, couldn't be expected!

Artichoke leaf may work by interfering with cholesterol synthesis.[12] Besides cynarin, a compound in artichoke called luteolin may play a role in reducing cholesterol.[13]

DOSAGE

Germany's Commission E recommends 6 g of the dried herb or its equivalent per day, usually divided into 3 doses.

Warning: Individuals with gallbladder disease should use artichoke only under medical supervision (see Safety Issues below).

SAFETY ISSUES

Artichoke leaf has not been associated with significant side effects in studies so far, but full safety testing has not been completed. For this reason, it should not be used by pregnant or nursing women. Safety in young children or in people with severe liver or kidney disease has also not been established.

In addition, because artichoke leaf is believed to stimulate gallbladder contraction, individuals with gallstones or other forms of gallbladder disease could be put at risk by using this herb. Such individuals should use artichoke leaf only under the supervision of a physician. It is possible that increased gallbladder contraction could lead to obstruction of ducts or even rupture of the gallbladder.

Individuals with known allergies to artichokes or related plants in the Asteraceae family, such as arnica or chrysanthemums, should avoid using artichoke or cynarin preparations.

ASHWAGANDHA *(Withania somniferum)*

Principal Proposed Uses   Adaptogen (Improve Ability to Withstand Stress)

Other Proposed Uses   Improve Exercise Ability, Immunity, Sexual Capacity, and Fertility; Reduce Cholesterol, Prevent Colds and Flus, Treat Insomnia and Anxiety

Ashwagandha is sometimes called "Indian ginseng," not because it's related botanically (it's closer to potatoes and tomatoes) but because its uses are similar. Like ginseng, ashwagandha is a "tonic herb" traditionally believed capable of generally strengthening the body. However, it is believed to be milder and less stimulating than ginseng.

WHAT IS ASHWAGANDHA USED FOR TODAY?

Modern herbalists classify ashwagandha as an adaptogen, a substance that increases the body's ability to withstand **stress** (see page 167) of all types. (See the chapter on **ginseng** for more information on adaptogens.)

Like other adaptogens, ashwagandha is said to improve physical energy, exercise capacity, and overall health; strengthen immunity against **colds** (see page 47), **flus** (see page 47), and other infections); increase sexual capacity and improve fertility; and normalize cholesterol. As its name "somniferum" suggests, it is also sometimes said to produce mild sedation (an effect potentially useful for those troubled by insomnia or anxiety). However, as yet the evidence for these and other potential benefits is limited to highly preliminary studies at best. [1–8]

DOSAGE

A typical dosage of ashwagandha is 1 teaspoon of powder twice a day, boiled in milk or water. Herbalists often recommend that those who are young or especially weak should take a lower dosage.

SAFETY ISSUES

Although formal scientific safety studies have not been completed, ashwagandha appears to be safe when taken in normal doses. However, because some of the constituents of ashwagandha can make you drowsy, it should not be combined with sedative drugs. The herb may also have some steroid-like activity at high dosages. Safety in young children, pregnant or nursing women, or those with severe liver or kidney disease has not been established.

⚠ INTERACTIONS YOU SHOULD KNOW ABOUT

If you are taking **sedative drugs,** you should not take ashwagandha at the same time.

ASTRAGALUS *(Astragalus membranaceus)*

Alternate or Related Names   Beg Kei, Bei Qi, Hwanggi, Membranous Milk Vetch, Astragali, Others

Principal Proposed Uses   Strengthen Immunity (Against Colds, Flus, and Other Illnesses)

Other Proposed Uses   Atherosclerosis, Hyperthyroidism, Hypertension (High Blood Pressure), Insomnia, Diabetes, Chronic Active Hepatitis, Genital Herpes, AIDS, Chemotherapy Side Effects

Dried and sliced thin, the root of the astragalus plant is a common component of traditional Chinese herbal formulas. According to Chinese medical theory, astragalus "strengthens the spleen, blood and Qi, raises the yang Qi of the spleen and stomach, and stabilizes the exterior."[1] Don't worry if you didn't understand what you just read, because without many months of training in the unique Chinese approach to illness, there's no way you could have. Suffice it to say that the traditional un-

derstanding of the way astragalus works is different from the way it tends to be presented today.

WHAT IS ASTRAGALUS USED FOR TODAY?

In the United States, astragalus has been presented as an immune stimulant useful for treating **colds and flus** (see page 47). Many people have come to believe that

Ashwagandha

they should take astragalus, like **echinacea** (see page 273), at the first sign of a cold.

The belief that astragalus can strengthen immunity has its basis in Chinese tradition. The expression "stabilize the exterior" means helping to create a "defensive shield" against infection.

However, according to Chinese healing tradition, astragalus formulas should not be taken during the early stage of infections. To do so is said to resemble "locking the chicken-coop with the fox inside," causing the infection to be "driven deeper."

Rather, astragalus is supposedly only appropriate for use while you're healthy, for the purpose of preventing future illnesses. Since it was the Chinese who first developed astragalus, perhaps these traditions should be taken seriously.

WHAT IS THE SCIENTIFIC EVIDENCE FOR ASTRAGALUS?

Although tradition suggests that astragalus should always be used in combination with other herbs, modern Chinese investigators have found various intriguing effects when astragalus is taken by itself. Extracts of astragalus have been shown to stimulate parts of the immune system in mice and humans, and to increase the survival time of mice infected with various diseases.[2,3] Preliminary research also suggests that astragalus might be useful in treating **atherosclerosis** (see page 16), hyperthyroidism, **hypertension** (see page 98), **insomnia** (see page 103), **diabetes** (see page 65), chronic active **hepatitis** (see page 189), genital **herpes** (see page 86), AIDS, and the side effects of cancer chemotherapy.[4–9]

However, none of these suggestions can be regarded as proven.

DOSAGE

A typical daily dosage of astragalus involves boiling 9 to 30 g of dried root to make tea. Newer products use an alcohol-and-water extraction method to produce an extract standardized to astragaloside content, although there is no consensus on the proper percentage.

SAFETY ISSUES

Astragalus appears to be relatively nontoxic. High one-time doses, as well as long-term administration, have not caused significant harmful effects.[10] Side effects are rare and generally limited to the usual mild gastrointestinal distress or allergic reactions. However, some Chinese herb manuals suggest that astragalus at 15 g or lower per day can raise blood pressure, while doses above 30 g may lower blood pressure.

As mentioned above, traditional Chinese medicine warns against using astragalus in cases of acute infections. Other traditional contraindications include "deficient yin patterns with heat signs" and "exterior excess heat patterns." Because understanding what these mean would require an extensive education in Chinese medicine, we recommend using astragalus only under the supervision of a qualified Chinese herbalist.

Safety in young children, pregnant or nursing women, or those with severe liver or kidney disease has not been established.

BCAAs

Supplement Forms/Alternate Names   Branched-Chain Amino Acids (Combined) or Leucine, Isoleucine, or Valine Separately

Principal Proposed Uses   Loss of Appetite (in Cancer Patients), Amyotrophic Lateral Sclerosis (ALS, Lou Gehrig's Disease)

Other Proposed Uses   Recovery from Surgery, Performance Enhancement, Muscular Dystrophy, Tardive Dyskinesia, Hepatic Encephalopathy

Branched-chain amino acids (BCAAs) are naturally occurring molecules (leucine, isoleucine, and valine) that the body uses to build proteins. The term "branched chain" refers to the molecular structure of these particular amino acids. Muscles have a particularly high content of BCAAs.

For reasons that are not entirely clear, BCAA supplements may improve appetite in cancer patients and slow the progression of amyotrophic lateral sclerosis (ALS, or Lou Gehrig's disease, a terrible condition that leads to degeneration of nerves, atrophy of the muscles, and eventual death).

BCAAs have also been proposed as a supplement to boost athletic performance.

BCAAs

Visit Us at TNP.com

BCAAs

REQUIREMENTS/SOURCES

Dietary protein usually provides all the BCAAs you need. However, physical stress and injury can increase your need for BCAAs to repair damage, so supplementation may be helpful.

BCAAs are present in all protein-containing foods, but the best sources are red meat and dairy products. Chicken, fish, and eggs are excellent sources as well. Whey protein and egg protein supplements are another way to ensure you're getting enough BCAAs. Supplements may contain all three BCAAs together or simply individual BCAAs.

THERAPEUTIC DOSAGES

The typical dosage of BCAAs is 1 to 5 g daily.

THERAPEUTIC USES

Preliminary evidence suggests that BCAAs may improve appetite in cancer patients.[1] There is also some evidence that BCAA supplements may reduce symptoms of **amyotrophic lateral sclerosis** (ALS, or Lou Gehrig's disease; see page 9); however, not all studies have had positive results.[2–5] Reports, but little real evidence, suggest that BCAAs may reduce muscle loss during recovery from **surgery** (see page 173).

Preliminary evidence suggests that BCAAs might decrease symptoms of **tardive dyskinesia** (see page 176), a movement disorder caused by long-term usage of antipsychotic drugs.[6]

Based on how they are metabolized in the body, there is some reason to believe that BCAAs might be helpful for individuals with **hepatic encephalopathy** (see page 112), a condition associated with severe liver disease.[7] However, the evidence that BCAAs actually help is not yet conclusive.

BCAAs have also been tried by athletes to build muscle; however, evidence suggests that they do not improve performance or enhance the muscle/fat ratio in the body (see the chapter on **sports performance** for more information).[8–15] BCAAs also do not appear to be helpful for muscular dystrophy.[16]

WHAT IS THE SCIENTIFIC EVIDENCE FOR BCAAs?

Appetite in Cancer Patients

A double-blind study tested BCAAs on 28 people with cancer who had lost their appetites due to either the dis-

ease itself or its treatment.[17] Appetite improved in 55% of those taking BCAAs (4.8 g daily) compared to only 16% of those who took placebo.

Amyotrophic Lateral Sclerosis (Lou Gehrig's Disease)

A small double-blind study suggested that BCAAs might help protect muscle strength in people with Lou Gehrig's disease.[18] Eighteen individuals were given either BCAAs (taken 4 times daily between meals) or placebo, and followed for 1 year. The results showed that people taking BCAAs declined much more slowly than those receiving placebo. In the placebo group, five of nine participants lost their ability to walk, two died, and another required a respirator. Only one of nine of those receiving BCAAs became unable to walk during the study period. This study is too small to give conclusive evidence, but it does suggest that BCAAs might be helpful for this disease.

However, other studies found no effect,[19,20] and one actually found a slight increase in deaths during the study period among those treated with BCAAs compared to placebo.[21]

Muscular Dystrophy

One double-blind placebo-controlled study found leucine ineffective at the dose of 0.2 g per kilogram body weight (15 g daily for a 75-kilogram woman) in 96 individuals with muscular dystrophy.[22] Over the course of 1 year, no differences were seen between the effects of leucine and placebo.

SAFETY ISSUES

BCAAs are believed to be safe; when taken in excess, they are simply converted into other amino acids. However, like other amino acids, BCAAs may interfere with medications for **Parkinson's disease** (see page 140).[23]

⚠ INTERACTIONS YOU SHOULD KNOW ABOUT

If you are taking **medication for Parkinson's disease** (such as **levodopa),** BCAAs may reduce its effectiveness.

Visit Us at TNP.com

BEE POLLEN

Principal Proposed Uses   There are no well-documented uses for bee pollen.

Other Proposed Uses   Allergies, Blood Purification, Respiratory Tract Infections, Endocrine Diseases, Colitis

Bee pollen is the pollen collected by bees as they gather nectar from flowers for making honey. Like honey, bee pollen is used as a food by the hive. The pollen granules are stored in pollen sacs on the bees' hind legs. Beekeepers who wish to collect bee pollen place a screen over the hive with openings just large enough for the bees to pass through. As the bees enter the hive, the screen compresses their pollen sacs, squeezing the pollen from them. The beekeepers can then collect the pollen from the screen.

Bee pollen is very high in protein and carbohydrates, and contains trace amounts of minerals and vitamins.[1] It is used in a number of Chinese herbal medicines and is sold as a nutritional supplement in the United States and other countries. Although it has been recommended for a variety of uses, particularly for improving sports performance and relieving allergies, little to no scientific evidence backs up any of the claims about the therapeutic value of bee pollen.

REQUIREMENTS/SOURCES

Bee pollen is not the sort of thing you will find in your everyday diet, unless you regularly eat the snack bars that include it. Tablets and some snack products containing bee pollen are available in pharmacies and health food stores.

THERAPEUTIC DOSAGES

Athletes using bee pollen report consuming 5 to 10 tablets per day. Tablets can contain variable amounts of bee pollen, usually between 200 to 500 mg. The manufacturer's recommendations may provide more guidance.

THERAPEUTIC USES

Bee pollen has been touted as an energy enhancer, and is sometimes used by athletes in the belief that it will improve their performance during competitions. However, like a number of the purported "sports supplements," there is no real evidence that bee pollen is effective and some evidence that it is not.[2]

Bee pollen is also commonly taken to try to prevent hay fever on the theory that eating pollens will help you build up resistance to them. When used for this purpose, locally grown bee pollen is usually recommended; however, be aware that it is possible to have a severe allergic reaction to the bee pollen itself. Other proposed uses of bee pollen include combating age-related memory loss[3] and other effects of aging, and treating diseases such as respiratory infections, endocrine disorders, colitis, and allergies. No scientific evidence supports any of these uses (see Safety Issues).

WHAT IS THE SCIENTIFIC EVIDENCE FOR BEE POLLEN?

A few clinical trials have tested bee pollen's ability to increase energy or improve memory.

Sports Performance

According to a 1977 article in the *New York Times*, two studies on the use of bee pollen to improve sports performance found it to be of no significant benefit.[4] Unfortunately, it has not been possible to obtain copies of the actual studies on which this article was based.

Both trials were said to be double-blind and placebo-controlled. The first, performed in 1975, involved 30 members of a university swim team. Participants were divided into 3 groups and given a daily dose of either 10 tablets of bee pollen, 10 placebo tablets, or 5 bee pollen and 5 placebo tablets. In 1976, the same experimental protocol was used, but this time with 60 participants: 30 swimmers and 30 long-distance runners. Bee pollen did not significantly improve performance in either trial. A third study on bee pollen's effects on sports performance, also difficult to obtain, reportedly found that breathing, heart rate, and perspiration returned to normal levels more quickly in track team members taking pollen than in those taking a placebo.[5] However, reviewers criticized the methods used in this study. The runners may have known who was taking placebo and who was taking pollen, and this could have influenced the results.

Memory

The effects of pure bee pollen on memory have not been investigated, but clinical trials of a Chinese herbal medicine containing bee pollen have been conducted in China and Denmark. The improvements in memory seen in the Chinese study were not significant, and in the more recent double-blind placebo-controlled crossover study in Denmark, no improvements were found at all.[6] The formula tested was only 14% bee pollen, so the results may not tell us very much about bee pollen's effectiveness.

Bee Pollen

Visit Us at TNP.com

SAFETY ISSUES

Several cases of serious allergic reactions to bee pollen have been reported in the medical literature, including anaphylaxis,[7,8] an acute allergic response which can be life threatening. The anaphylactic reactions occurred within 20 to 30 minutes of ingesting fairly small amounts of bee pollen—in one case less than a teaspoon.

The majority of these case reports involved people with known allergies to pollen.

BEE PROPOLIS

Supplement Forms/Alternate Names   Bee Glue, Bee Putty, Propolis

Principal Proposed Uses   There are no well-documented uses for bee propolis.

Other Proposed Uses
   Topical Uses: Genital Herpes, Skin Wounds, Oral Surgery, Tooth Decay Preventive, Eye Infections, Vaginal Infections
   Oral Uses: Treatment of Giardia, Cancer Prevention

Although honey is perhaps the most famous bee product of interest to human beings, bees also make propolis, another substance that humans have used for ages. Bees coat the hive with propolis in much the same way we use paint and caulking on our homes. People began using propolis more than 2,300 years ago for many purposes, the foremost of which was applying it to wounds to fight infection. It is a resinous compound made primarily from tree sap, and contains biologically active compounds called flavonoids, which come from its plant source. Propolis does indeed have antibiotic properties; the flavonoids in propolis may be responsible for its antimicrobial effects as well as other alleged health benefits.

REQUIREMENTS/SOURCES

Propolis is available in a wide assortment of products found in pharmacies and health food stores, including tablets, capsules, powders, extracts, ointments, creams, lotions, and other cosmetics.

THERAPEUTIC DOSAGES

Topical propolis ointments, creams, lotions, balms, and extracts are usually applied directly to the area being treated. However, we do not recommend applying bee propolis directly to the eyes (see Safety Issues).

Propolis intended for oral use comes in a wide variety of forms, including tablets, capsules, and extracts. Products vary so much that your best bet is to follow the directions on the label.

THERAPEUTIC USES

Test tube studies have found propolis to be active against a variety of microorganisms, including bacteria, viruses, and protozoans.[1–10] These findings have been the basis for most propolis research in humans and animals.

The results of a small controlled study suggests that propolis cream might cause attacks of **genital herpes** (see page 86) to heal faster.[11]

A preliminary controlled study found that propolis mouthwash following oral **surgery** (see page 173) significantly speeded healing time as compared to placebo.[12]

Animal studies also suggest that topical propolis may be of benefit in healing **wounds** (see page 123).[13,14]

One group of researchers compared a propolis extract against the standard antiprotozoal drug tinidazole in 138 people infected with the parasite giardia.[15] The extract appeared to work about as well as the drug therapy.

A number of clinical trials have tested the use of propolis for eye infections[16] and **vaginal infections** (see page 182).[17] However, these were poorly designed; better trials are necessary before we can say for sure that propolis is an effective treatment for any of these conditions.

In one interesting study, rats given propolis in their drinking water got fewer cavities than rats given regular water.[18] However, no human studies have been performed to see if we would also benefit.

Finally, test tube studies suggest that propolis has antioxidant, anti-inflammatory, and anticancer properties.[19–25] Again, without actual human studies, these results suggest the need for future research but do not prove propolis effective for any particular condition.

SAFETY ISSUES

Propolis is an ingredient commonly consumed in small quantities in honey. Safety studies have found it to be essentially nontoxic when taken orally; propolis also appears to be nonirritating when applied to the skin.[26]

However, allergic reactions to topical propolis occur relatively frequently, sometimes involving painful redness, swelling, and oozing sores.[27–38]

Propolis is also a known "sensitizing agent," meaning it can cause people to develop allergies to the propolis itself when it is used regularly.[39–42]

BETA-CAROTENE

Principal Proposed Uses   Heart Disease Prevention, Cataract Prevention, Macular Degeneration Prevention

Other Proposed Uses   Osteoarthritis, HIV Support, Sunburn Prevention, Photosensitivity, Alcoholism, Asthma, Depression, Epilepsy, Infertility, Headaches, Heartburn, Parkinson's Disease, Psoriasis, Rheumatoid Arthritis, Schizophrenia, Hypertension (High Blood Pressure)

Probably Ineffective Uses   Cancer Prevention, Nutritional Support for Smokers

Note: All the significant positive evidence for beta-carotene applies to food sources, not supplements.
Note: Beta-carotene and vitamin A are sometimes described as if they were the same thing. This is because the body converts beta-carotene into vitamin A. However, there are important differences between the two.

Beta-carotene belongs to a family of natural chemicals known as carotenes or carotenoids. Scientists have identified nearly 600 different carotenes (for information about other carotenes, see the chapters on **lycopene** and **lutein**). Widely found in plants, carotenes (along with another group of chemicals, the bioflavonoids) give color to fruits, vegetables, and other plants.

Beta-carotene is a particularly important carotene from a nutritional standpoint, because the body easily transforms it to **vitamin A** (see page 432). While vitamin A supplements themselves can be toxic when taken to excess, if you take beta-carotene, your body will make only as much vitamin A as you need. This built-in safety feature makes beta-carotene the best way to get your vitamin A.

Beta-carotene is also often recommended for another reason: it is an antioxidant, like **vitamin E** (see page 451) and **vitamin C** (see page 444). However, although there is a great deal of evidence that the carotenes found in food can provide a variety of health benefits (from reducing the risk of cancer to preventing heart disease), there is little to no evidence that high doses of purified beta-carotene supplements are good for you.

REQUIREMENTS/SOURCES

Although beta-carotene is not an essential nutrient, vitamin A is. Three mg (5,000 IU) of beta-carotene supplies about 5,000 IU of vitamin A. (See the chapter on **vitamin A** for requirements based on age and sex.)

Dark green and orange-yellow vegetables are good sources of beta-carotene. These include carrots, sweet potatoes, squash, spinach, romaine lettuce, broccoli, apricots, and green peppers.

THERAPEUTIC DOSAGES

We are not sure at the present time whether it is advisable to take dosages of beta-carotene much higher than the recommended allowance for nutritional purposes. It is probably much better to increase your intake of fresh fruits and vegetables.

THERAPEUTIC USES

It is difficult to recommend beta-carotene supplements for any use other than to supply nutritional levels of vitamin A.

Evidence suggests that mixed carotenes found in food can protect against **cancer** (see page 32) and **heart disease** (see page 16).[1–7] However, supplements that contain only purified beta-carotene may actually be harmful for these conditions.[8–12]

Similarly, although mixed carotenes found in food seem to slow the progression of **cataracts** (see page 42) and help prevent **macular degeneration** (see page 115), beta-carotene alone does not seem to work.[13–17] Dietary beta-carotene may also slow down the progression of **osteoarthritis** (see page 132), but we don't know whether beta-carotene supplements work for this purpose.[18]

Vitamin A deficiency may be linked to lower immune cell counts as well as higher death rates among people infected with **HIV** (see page 94).[19] A few preliminary studies have raised hopes that beta-carotene supplements might increase or preserve immune function or decrease symptoms among people with HIV.[20–23] However, not all studies have had positive results.[24,25]

Beta-carotene supplements may be helpful for protecting the skin from **sunburn** (see page 171), particularly in people with extreme **sensitivity to the sun**

Beta-Carotene

Visit Us at TNP.com

Beta-Carotene

Visit Us at TNP.com

(see page 144), but the evidence is somewhat contradictory.[26–36] Finally, beta-carotene has been proposed as a treatment for AIDS, alcoholism, **asthma** (see page 14), **depression** (see page 59), epilepsy, headaches, heartburn, **male** (see page 116) and **female infertility** (see page 79), **Parkinson's disease** (see page 140), **psoriasis** (see page 148), **rheumatoid arthritis** (see page 151), and schizophrenia, but there is little to no evidence that it works. Beta-carotene has sometimes been suggested as a treatment for **hypertension** (see page 98), but there is some evidence that it does not work.[37]

According to a double-blind placebo-controlled study of 141 women with **cervical dysplasia** (early cervical cancer; see page 43), beta-carotene, taken at a dosage of 30 mg daily, does *not* help to reverse the dysplasia.[38]

A double-blind placebo-controlled trial of 1,484 individuals with **intermittent claudication** (see page 106) found no benefit from beta-carotene (20 mg daily), vitamin E (50 mg daily), or a combination of the two.[39]

WHAT IS THE SCIENTIFIC EVIDENCE FOR BETA-CAROTENE?

Cancer Prevention

The story of beta-carotene and cancer is full of contradictions. It starts in the early 1980s, when the cumulative results of many studies suggested that people who eat a lot of fruits and vegetables are significantly less likely to get cancer.[40,41] A close look at the data pointed to carotenes as the active ingredients in fruits and vegetables. It appeared that a high intake of dietary carotene could dramatically reduce the risk of lung cancer,[42] bladder cancer,[43] breast cancer,[44] esophageal cancer,[45] and stomach cancer.[46]

The next step was to give carotenes to people and see if it made a difference. Researchers used purified beta-carotene instead of mixed carotenes, because it is much more readily available. They studied people in high-risk groups, such as smokers, because it is easier to see results when you look at people who are more likely to develop cancer to begin with. However, the results were surprisingly unfavorable.

The anticancer bubble burst for beta-carotene in 1994 when the results of the Alpha-Tocopherol, Beta-Carotene (ATBC) study came in.[47] These results showed that beta-carotene supplements did not prevent lung cancer, but actually increased the risk of getting it by 18%. This trial had followed 29,133 male smokers in Finland who took supplements of about 50 IU of vitamin E (alpha-tocopherol), 20 mg of beta-carotene, both, or placebo daily for 5 to 8 years. (In contrast, vitamin E was found to reduce the risk of cancer, especially prostate cancer. For more information, see the chapter on **vitamin E**.)

In January 1996, researchers monitoring the Beta-Carotene and Retinol Efficacy Trial (CARET) confirmed the prior bad news with more of their own: The beta-carotene group had 46% more cases of lung cancer deaths.[48] This study involved smokers, former smokers, and workers exposed to asbestos. Alarmed, the National Cancer Institute ended the $42 million CARET trial 21 months before it was planned to end.

At about the same time, the 12-year Physicians' Health Study of 22,000 male physicians was finding that 50 mg of beta-carotene taken every other day had no effect—good or bad—on the risk of cancer or heart disease. In this study, 11% of the participants were smokers and 39% were ex-smokers.[49,50]

Similarly, another study of beta-carotene supplements failed to find any effect on the risk of cancer or heart disease in women.[51]

Interestingly, some studies suggest that higher levels of carotene intake from diet *were* associated with lower levels of cancer.[52,53] What is the explanation for this apparent discrepancy? It could be that beta-carotene alone is not effective. The other carotenes found in fruits and vegetables may be more important for preventing cancer than beta-carotene. One researcher has suggested that taking beta-carotene supplements actually depletes the body of other beneficial carotenes.[54]

Heart Disease Prevention

The situation with beta-carotene and heart disease is rather similar to that of beta-carotene and cancer. Numerous studies suggest that carotenes as a whole can reduce the risk of heart disease.[55] However, isolated beta-carotene may not help prevent heart disease and could actually increase your risk.

The same double-blind intervention trial involving 29,133 Finnish male smokers (mentioned under the discussion of cancer and beta-carotene) found 11% *more* deaths from heart disease and 15 to 20% *more* strokes in those participants taking beta-carotene supplements.[56]

Similar poor results with beta-carotene were seen in another large double-blind study of smokers.[57] Beta-carotene supplementation was also found to increase the incidence of angina in smokers.[58]

The bottom line: as with cancer, the mixed carotenoids found in foods seem to be helpful for heart disease, but beta-carotene supplements do not.

Osteoarthritis

A high dietary intake of beta-carotene appears to slow the progression of osteoarthritis by as much as 70%, according to a study in which researchers followed 640 individuals over a period of 8 to 10 years.[59] However, again, we don't know if purified beta-carotene supplements work the same way as beta-carotene from food sources.[60]

HIV Support

One small double-blind study suggested that taking beta-carotene might raise white blood cell count in people with **HIV** (see page 94).[61] However, two subsequent larger controlled trials found no significant differences between those taking beta-carotene or placebo in white blood cell count, CD4+ count, or other measures of immune function.[62,63]

Two observational studies lasting 6 to 8 years suggest that higher intakes of vitamin A or beta-carotene may be helpful, but they also found that caution is in order with regard to dosage.[64,65] This group of researchers generally linked higher intake of vitamin A or beta-carotene to lower risk of AIDS and lower death rates, with an important exception: people with the highest intake of either nutrient (more than 11,179 IU per day of beta-carotene or more than 20,268 IU per day of vitamin A) did worse than those who took somewhat less.

SAFETY ISSUES

At recommended dosages, beta-carotene is very safe. The only side effects reported from beta-carotene overdose are diarrhea and a yellowish tinge to the hands and feet. These symptoms disappear once you stop taking beta-carotene or move to lower doses.

However, high-dose beta-carotene may slightly increase the risk of heart disease and cancer, especially in those who consume too much alcohol or **smoke cigarettes** (see page 131).[66–71] The solution: eat plenty of fresh fruits and vegetables, and get your beta-carotene that way.

BETAINE HYDROCHLORIDE

Principal Proposed Use   There are no well-documented uses for betaine hydrochloride.

Other Proposed Uses   Digestive Aid, Anemia, Asthma, Atherosclerosis, Diarrhea, Excess Candida (Yeast), Food Allergies, Gallstones, Hay Fever, Inner Ear Infections, Rheumatoid Arthritis, Thyroid Conditions, Ulcers, Heartburn

Betaine hydrochloride is a source of hydrochloric acid, a naturally occurring chemical in the stomach that helps us digest food by breaking up fats and proteins. Stomach acid also aids in the absorption of nutrients through the walls of the intestines into the blood and protects the gastrointestinal tract from harmful bacteria.

A major branch of alternative medicine known as *naturopathy* has long held that low stomach acid is a widespread problem that interferes with digestion and the absorption of nutrients. Betaine hydrochloride is one of the most common recommendations for this condition (along with the more folksy apple cider vinegar).

Betaine is also sold by itself, without the hydrochloride molecule attached. In this form, it is called trimethylglycine (TMG). TMG is not acidic, but recent evidence suggests that it may provide certain health benefits of its own (for more information, see **TMG**).

SOURCES

Betaine hydrochloride is not an essential nutrient, and no food sources exist.

THERAPEUTIC DOSAGES

Betaine hydrochloride is typically taken in pill form at dosages ranging from 325 to 650 mg with each meal.

THERAPEUTIC USES

Based on theories about the importance of stomach acid, betaine has been recommended for a wide variety of problems, including anemia, **asthma** (see page 14), **atherosclerosis** (see page 16), diarrhea, excess **candida** (see page 38) yeast, food allergies, **gallstones** (see page 83), hay fever and **allergies** (see page 2), inner ear infections, **rheumatoid arthritis** (see page 151), and thyroid conditions. When one sees such broadly encompassing uses, it is not surprising to find that there is as yet no real scientific research on its effectiveness for any of these conditions.

Many naturopathic physicians also believe that betaine hydrochloride can heal conditions such as **ulcers** (see page 180) and esophageal reflux (heartburn). This sounds paradoxical, since conventional treatment for those conditions involves reducing stomach acid, while betaine hydrochloride increases it. However, according to one theory, lack of stomach acid leads to incomplete digestion of proteins, and these proteins cause allergic reactions and other responses that lead to an increase in ulcer pain. Again, scientific evidence is lacking.

SAFETY ISSUES

Betaine hydrochloride should not be used by those with ulcers or esophageal reflux (heartburn) except on the advice of a physician. This supplement seldom causes any obvious side effects, but it has not been put through rigorous safety studies. In particular, safety for young children, pregnant or nursing women, or those with severe liver or kidney disease has not been established.

BILBERRY *(Vaccinium myrtillus)*

Alternate or Related Names   Whortleberry, Blueberry, Burren Myrtle, Dyeberry, Huckleberry, Others

Principal Proposed Uses
Eye Problems: Poor Night Vision, Diabetic Retinopathy, Prevention of Cataracts, Prevention and Treatment of Macular Degeneration
Strengthen Blood Vessels: Varicose Veins, Easy Bruising, Prevention of Post-Surgical Bleeding

Other Proposed Uses   Atherosclerosis, Diabetes (Leaf Rather Than Fruit)

Often called European blueberry, bilberry is closely related to American blueberry, cranberry, and huckleberry. Its meat is creamy white instead of purple, but it is traditionally used, like blueberries, in the preparation of jams, pies, cobblers, and cakes.

Bilberry fruit also has a long medicinal history. In the twelfth century, Abbess Hildegard of Bingen wrote of bilberry's usefulness for inducing menstruation. Over subsequent centuries, the list of uses for bilberry grew to include a bewildering variety of possibilities, from bladder stones to typhoid fever.

WHAT IS BILBERRY USED FOR TODAY?

The modern use of bilberry dates back to World War II, when British Royal Air Force pilots reported that a good dose of bilberry jam just prior to a mission improved their **night vision** (see page 128), often dramatically. After the war, medical researchers investigated the constituents of bilberry and subsequently recommended it for a variety of eye disorders.

Bilberry is used throughout Europe today for the treatment of poor night vision and day blindness, for which it is believed to be significantly helpful. However, the scientific evidence that it works is weak and contradictory.

Regular use of bilberry is also sometimes used in hopes that it can prevent or treat other eye diseases such as **macular degeneration** (see page 115), diabetic retinopathy, and **cataracts** (see page 42). However, there is no solid evidence that it works for any of these conditions.

Scientific research also found that bilberry contains biologically powerful substances known as anthocyanosides. Evidence suggests that anthocyanosides strengthen the walls of blood vessels, reduce inflammation, and generally stabilize all tissues containing collagen (such as tendons, ligaments, and cartilage).[1-5] Grape seed contains related substances with similar properties. However, bilberry's anthocyanosides appear to have numerous important effects on the eye.[6,7]

There is also some evidence that bilberry can be useful for **varicose veins** (see page 184). On the basis of this research, bilberry has often been recommended as a treatment for hemorrhoids, which are actually a type of varicose vein. European physicians additionally believe that bilberry's blood vessel–stabilizing properties also make it useful as a treatment before surgery to reduce bleeding complications, as well as for other blood-vessel problems such as **easy bruising** (see page 74), but the evidence as yet is only suggestive.

Animal studies also suggest that bilberry leaves (rather than the fruit) may be helpful for improving blood sugar control in **diabetes** (see page 65), and also in lowering blood **triglycerides** (see page 88).[8]

WHAT IS THE SCIENTIFIC EVIDENCE FOR BILBERRY?

Although bilberry is widely used by physicians in Europe based on research performed in the 1960s and earlier, all together the research into bilberry is not yet up to modern standards. However, this is an active area of research, and you can expect new information to be available soon.

Night Vision

A double-blind crossover trial of 15 individuals found no short- or long-term improvements in night vision attributable to bilberry.[9] Similarly negative results were seen in a double-blind placebo-controlled crossover trial of 18 subjects.[10]

In contrast, two much earlier controlled, but not double-blind, studies of bilberry found that the herb temporarily improved night vision.[11,12] However, the effect was not found to persist with continued use. A later double-blind placebo-controlled study on 40 healthy subjects found that a single dose of bilberry extract improved visual response for 2 hours.[13]

Visual benefits have also been reported in other small trials, but these studies did not use a placebo control group and are therefore not valid as evidence.[14,15,16]

Diabetic Retinopathy

A double-blind placebo-controlled trial of bilberry extract in 14 people with damage to the retina caused by diabetes and/or hypertension found significant improvements observable by ophthalmoscopic examination (looking in the eye with a machine) and angiography (examining the blood vessels).[17] However, this was a very preliminary study.

Other studies have found similar results, but they were not double-blind.[18,19]

Cataracts

Although antioxidants in general are believed to help prevent cataracts, direct research into bilberry's effects appears to be limited to one double-blind trial that combined the herb with vitamin E.[20] The combination slowed cataract growth, but whether it was the herb or the vitamin that helped most remains unclear.

Varicose Veins

In a placebo-controlled study that followed 60 people with varicose veins (technically, venous insufficiency) for 30 days, bilberry extract resulted in a significant decrease in pain and swelling.[21] Similar results were seen in a 30-day double-blind trial involving 47 individuals.[22] Numerous other studies have yielded similarly positive results, although they did not use a placebo group.[23,24] However, there is better evidence for **horse chestnut** (see page 325), **OPCs** (see page 373), and **gotu kola** (see page 315).

DOSAGE

The standard dosage of bilberry is 120 to 240 mg twice daily of an extract standardized to contain 25% anthocyanosides.

SAFETY ISSUES

Bilberry fruit is a food and as such is quite safe. Enormous quantities have been administered to rats without toxic effects.[25,26] One study of 2,295 people given bilberry extract found a 4% incidence of side effects such as mild digestive distress, skin rashes, and drowsiness.[27] Although safety in pregnancy has not been proven, clinical trials have enrolled pregnant women.[28] Safety in young children, nursing women, or those with severe liver or kidney disease is not known. There are no known drug interactions. Bilberry does not appear to interfere with blood clotting.[29]

Little is known about the safety of bilberry leaf. Based on animal evidence that it can reduce blood sugar levels in people with diabetes, it is possible that use of bilberry leaf by diabetics could require a reduction in drug dosage.[30]

BIOTIN

Supplement Forms/Alternate Names   Biocytin (Brewer's Yeast–Biotin Complex)

Principal Proposed Uses   There are no well-documented uses for biotin.

Other Proposed Uses   Diabetes, Brittle Nails, "Cradle Cap" in Children, Support for Individuals on Anticonvulsants

Biotin is a water-soluble B vitamin that plays an important role in metabolizing the energy we get from food. Biotin assists four essential enzymes that break down fats, carbohydrates, and proteins.

Very preliminary evidence suggests that biotin supplements may be helpful for people with diabetes.

REQUIREMENTS/SOURCES

Although biotin is a necessary nutrient, we usually get enough from bacteria living in the digestive tract. Actual biotin deficiency is uncommon, unless you frequently eat large quantities of raw egg white. (Raw egg white contains a protein that blocks the absorption of biotin. Fortunately, cooked egg white does not present this problem.)

The official U.S. and Canadian recommendations for daily intake of biotin are as follows:

- Infants 0–5 months, 5 mcg
     6–11 months, 6 mcg
- Children 1–3 years, 8 mcg
     4–8 years, 12 mcg
     9–13 years, 20 mcg
- Males and females 14–18 years, 25 mcg
     19 years and older, 30 mcg
- Pregnant women, 30 mcg
- Nursing women, 35 mcg

Good dietary sources of biotin include brewer's yeast, nutritional (torula) yeast, whole grains, nuts, egg yolks, sardines, legumes, liver, cauliflower, bananas, and mushrooms.

THERAPEUTIC DOSAGES

For people with diabetes, the usual recommended dosage of biotin is 7,000 to 15,000 mcg daily.

For treating "cradle cap" (a scaly head rash often found in infants), the usual dosage of biotin is 6,000 mcg daily, *given to the nursing mother* (not the child). A lower dosage of 3,000 mcg daily is used to treat brittle fingernails and toenails.

THERAPEUTIC USES

There is little hard evidence for any of the proposed uses of biotin. Highly preliminary evidence suggests that supplemental biotin can help reduce blood sugar levels in people with either type 1 (childhood onset) or type 2 (adult onset) **diabetes** (see page 65).[1,2] Biotin may also reduce the symptoms of diabetic neuropathy.[3] However, other supplements often recommended for diabetes have much better evidence behind them, such as **chromium** (see page 251), **lipoic acid** (see page 347), and **GLA** (see page 304) from evening primrose oil.

Even weaker evidence suggests that biotin supplements can promote healthy **nails**[4,5,6] (see page 31) and eliminate cradle cap.

Individuals taking antiseizure medications might benefit from biotin supplementation at nutritional doses.[7,8] However, it should be taken at least 2 hours before or after the medication dose. Note that excessive biotin supplementation should be avoided because it is possible that it might interfere with seizure control.

SAFETY ISSUES

Biotin appears to be quite safe. However, maximum safe dosages for young children, pregnant or nursing women, or those with severe liver or kidney disease have not been established.

⚠ INTERACTIONS YOU SHOULD KNOW ABOUT

If you are taking

- **Antiseizure medications:** You may need extra biotin, but take only a nutritional dose, and take it 2 to 3 hours apart from your antiseizure medication.
- **Alcohol:** You may need extra biotin.

BITTER MELON (*Momordica charantia*)

Principal Proposed Uses   Diabetes

Widely sold in Asian groceries as food, bitter melon is also a folk remedy for diabetes, cancer, and various infections.

WHAT IS BITTER MELON USED FOR TODAY?

Preliminary studies appear to confirm the first of these folk uses, suggesting that bitter melon may improve blood sugar control in people with adult-onset (type 2) **diabetes** (see page 65).[1–4] It appears to work by stimulating insulin release from the pancreas. If you have type 2 diabetes, you might consider adding bitter melon to your diet, but only under a doctor's supervision (see Safety Issues).

Bitter melon has also been suggested as a treatment for AIDS, but the evidence thus far is too weak to even mention. There is absolutely no evidence that it can treat cancer.

DOSAGE

The proper dosage is one small, unripe, raw melon or about 50 to 100 ml of fresh juice, divided into 2 or 3 doses over the course of the day. The only problem is that bitter melon tastes *extremely* bitter. Noted natur-

Bitter Melon

opath Michael Murray suggests that you should "simply plug your nose and take a 2-ounce shot."[5]

Tinctures of bitter melon have begun to arrive on the market, which may make the herb a bit easier to swallow. Follow the directions on the label for correct dosage.

SAFETY ISSUES

As a widely eaten food in Asia, bitter melon is generally regarded as safe. It can cause diarrhea and stomach pain if taken in excessive amounts, but the main risk of bitter melon comes from the fact that it may work! Combining it with standard drugs may reduce blood sugar too well, possibly leading to dangerously low levels.[6,7] For this reason, if you already take drugs for diabetes, you should add bitter melon to your diet only with a physician's supervision. And definitely don't stop your medication and substitute bitter melon instead. It is not as powerful as insulin or other conventional treatments.

Safety in young children, pregnant or nursing women, or those with severe liver or kidney disease has not been established.

⚠ INTERACTIONS YOU SHOULD KNOW ABOUT

If you are taking **medications to reduce blood sugar,** bitter melon might amplify the effect, and you may need to reduce your dose of medication.

BLACK COHOSH (*Cimicifuga racemosa*)

Alternate or Related Names   Black Snake Root, Rattleroot, Rattleweed, Squaw Root, Bugbane, Others

Principal Proposed Uses   Menopausal Symptoms

Other Proposed Uses   PMS, Dysmenorrhea (Painful Menstruation)

Black cohosh is a tall perennial herb originally found in the northeastern United States. Native Americans used it primarily for women's health problems, but also as a treatment for arthritis, fatigue, and snakebite. European colonists rapidly adopted the herb for similar uses, and in the late nineteenth century, black cohosh was the principal ingredient in the wildly popular Lydia E. Pinkham's Vegetable Compound for menstrual cramps. Migrating across the Atlantic, black cohosh became a popular European treatment for women's problems, arthritis, and high blood pressure.

WHAT IS BLACK COHOSH USED FOR TODAY?

Black cohosh has been approved by Germany's Commission E for use in treating **menopause** (see page 117), **dysmenorrhea** (see page 70), and **PMS** (see page 145). According to the results of a few studies, menopausal women report distinct improvements in hot flashes, sweating, headache, **vertigo** (see page 188), heart palpitations, **tinnitus** (see page 178), nervousness, irritability, sleep disturbance, anxiety, vaginal dryness, and depression. Black cohosh takes 4 to 6 weeks to produce its full benefits.

However, contrary to many reports, black cohosh does not work like estrogen. There is no evidence that it can prevent **osteoporosis** (see page 136) or **heart disease** (see page 16), two of estrogen's most famous benefits.

Black cohosh appears to be only mildly effective (if at all) for treating PMS and dysmenorrhea.

Some herbalists believe that black cohosh can prevent or treat mild **cervical dysplasia** (see page 43), but there is no evidence whatsoever that it really works.

WHAT IS THE SCIENTIFIC EVIDENCE FOR BLACK COHOSH?

The best evidence for black cohosh as a treatment for menopause comes from a double-blind study that followed 80 women for 12 weeks, comparing the benefits of black cohosh, conjugated estrogens (0.625 mg), and placebo.[1] According to the reported results, black cohosh was actually more effective than estrogen, both in relieving symptoms and in normalizing the appearance of vaginal cells under microscopic evaluation. Similar results were seen in open studies.[2,3]

Based on these and other results, black cohosh came to be described as a phytoestrogen—a plant that produces effects similar to estrogen. However, a recent, double-blind study that evaluated two different dosages of black cohosh did not find any change in vaginal-cell appearance or indeed any other objective measurements that would indicate an estrogen-like effect.[4] An animal study has also found no evidence that black cohosh works like estrogen.[5]

If it doesn't act like estrogen, how does black cohosh work? The answer is that we really don't know.

DOSAGE

The standard dosage of black cohosh is 1 or 2 tablets twice a day of a standardized extract, manufactured to contain 1 mg of 27-deoxyacteine per tablet.

Make sure not to confuse black cohosh with **blue cohosh** (*Caulophyllum thalictroides;* see page 225). Blue cohosh is potentially more dangerous since it contains chemicals that are toxic to the heart; one published case report documents profound heart failure in a child born to a mother who used blue cohosh to induce labor.[6]

SAFETY ISSUES

Black cohosh seldom produces any side effects other than occasional mild gastrointestinal distress. Studies in rats have found no significant toxicity when black cohosh was given at 90 times the therapeutic dosage for a period of 6 months.[7] Since 6 months in a rat corresponds to decades in a human, this study appears to make a strong statement about the long-term safety of black cohosh.

Unlike estrogen, black cohosh does not stimulate breast-cancer cells growing in a test tube.[8,9] However, black cohosh has not yet been subjected to large-scale studies similar to those conducted for estrogen. For this reason, safety for those with previous breast cancer is not known. Also, because of potential hormonal activity, black cohosh is not recommended for adolescents or pregnant or nursing women.

Black cohosh has been found to slightly lower blood pressure and blood sugar in certain animals.[10,11] For this reason, it's possible that the herb could interact with drugs for high blood pressure or diabetes, but there are no reports of any such problems.

Safety in young children or those with severe liver or kidney disease is not known.

COMBINING BLACK COHOSH WITH ERT

Some women on estrogen-replacement therapy (ERT) choose to take extremely low doses of estrogen (in the 0.312 mg range), hoping to somewhat alleviate the risk of osteoporosis without increasing the potential for breast cancer. Although there are no studies to tell us whether this will work, it is certainly a logical idea, and some gynecologists endorse it.

However, such a low dose of estrogen may not completely stop symptoms such as hot flashes. Black cohosh has been suggested as an addition to improve symptom control. While this technique has not been studied, it is again a logical idea that is probably safe (but don't ask us to guarantee it!).

TRANSITIONING FROM ERT TO BLACK COHOSH

Each woman is unique, but in general, many women successfully switch over from 0.625 mg of daily estrogen to the standard dosage of black cohosh without developing symptoms. However, transitioning from higher dosages of estrogen will frequently result in breakthrough hot flashes and other symptoms. Again, remember that black cohosh is not known to offer protection against cardiovascular disease and osteoporosis.

BLOODROOT (*Sanguinaria canadensis*)

Alternate or Related Names   Indian Paint, Tetterwort, Red Root, Paucon, Coon Root, Others

Principal Proposed Uses
   Oral Uses: Periodontal Disease Prevention (Used As a Toothpaste or Mouthwash)
   Topical Uses: Warts
   Internal Uses: Respiratory Illnesses

Bloodroot is a perennial flowering herb that was widely used by Native Americans both as a reddish-orange dye and as a medicine. Some tribes drank bloodroot tea as a treatment for sore throats, fevers, and joint pain, while others applied the somewhat caustic sap to skin cancers. European herbalists used bloodroot to treat respiratory infections, asthma, joint pain, warts, ringworm, and nasal polyps.

In the mid 1800s, a Dr. Fells of Middlesex Hospital in London developed a cancer treatment consisting of a paste of bloodroot, flour, water, and zinc chloride applied directly to breast tumors and other cancers. Similar formulations were used in various locales up through the turn of the century. Bloodroot was a common constituent of "drawing salves" believed capable of "pulling" tumors out of the body.

WHAT IS BLOODROOT USED FOR TODAY?

Herbalists frequently recommend bloodroot pastes and salves for the treatment of warts. Bloodroot is an *escharotic,* that is to say a scab-producing substance, and it functions much like commercial wart plasters containing salicylic acid. Although there has not been any real scientific study of the use of bloodroot for warts, based on its immediate effects it is likely to help at least somewhat.

One constituent of bloodroot, sanguinarine, appears to possess topical antibiotic properties.[1] On this basis, the FDA has approved the use of bloodroot in commercially available toothpastes and oral rinses to inhibit the development of dental plaque and **periodontal disease** (gingivitis; see page 142).

Bloodroot is also often combined with other herbs in cough syrups. Some herbalists recommend drinking bloodroot tea for respiratory ailments, but others consider the herb to be too unpredictable in its side effects.

DOSAGE

For the treatment of warts, bloodroot can be made into a paste and applied directly to the involved area. However,

start slowly to see how sensitive you are. Excessive application can lead to severe burns. Once you've discovered your tolerance, apply the herb for a day or so, then remove it and wait for the scab to develop and then drop off. This process can be repeated until the wart is gone.

Bloodroot tea for treating respiratory illnesses may be made by boiling 1 teaspoon of powdered root in a cup of water and taken 2 or 3 times daily.

SAFETY ISSUES

Oral bloodroot appears to be relatively safe and nontoxic.[2,3,4] However, in large doses, it causes nausea and vomiting, and even at lower dosages it has been known to cause peculiar side effects in some people, such as tunnel vision and pain in the feet. For this reason, many herbalists recommend that it be used only under the supervision of a qualified practitioner.

Topical applications of bloodroot can cause severe burns if used too vigorously and for too long a time. Despite some reassuring evidence from animal studies,[5] there are still theoretical concerns that bloodroot could be harmful during pregnancy.[6] Safety in young children, nursing women, or those with severe liver or kidney disease has also not been established.

BLUE COHOSH *(Caulophyllum thalictroides)*

Alternate or Related Names   Papoose Root, Squawroot, Blueberry Root, Beechdrops, Blue Ginseng, Others

Principal Proposed Uses   Regulating Menstrual Cycle, Inducing Labor

Warning: Blue cohosh is a toxic herb, and THE NATURAL PHARMACIST strongly recommends against using it.

Blue cohosh is a flowering herb native to North America, growing in forested areas from the southeastern United States to Canada. Sometimes known as squaw root or papoose root, the herb may have been used medicinally by native Americans, although this is controversial. Other common names for the herb include yellow ginseng and blue ginseng. Blue cohosh should not be confused with the similarly named (but unrelated and much safer) **black cohosh** (see page 223). Blue cohosh was used in the 1800s by European settlers and African Americans, primarily for gynecologic conditions.[1] Blue cohosh also has a reputation as an herb that can induce abortions, although concerns regarding its efficacy and safety make this use extremely ill-advised.[2] In addition, it has been used for the treatment of arthritis, cramps, epilepsy, inflammation of the uterus, hiccups, colic, and sore throat.

WHAT IS BLUE COHOSH USED FOR TODAY?

Blue cohosh is widely prescribed by herbalists and midwives today. A recent survey published in the *Journal of Nurse-Midwifery* found that 64% of certified nurse-midwives who prescribe herbal medicines use blue cohosh to induce labor.[3] It has also been used for a wide variety of menstrual problems, including several that it would not be logical to believe the same treatment could cure. For instance, blue cohosh has been used to start menstrual periods that were late in coming and to stop excessive or ongoing menstrual flow. However, there is little to no credible evidence that blue cohosh is effective for any of the conditions for which it has been used. Furthermore, several published reports cite cases of serious side effects to infants apparently caused by blue cohosh (see Safety Issues).

DOSAGE

Blue cohosh is usually used as a tincture. Dosages range from 5 to 10 drops taken every 2 to 4 hours.

SAFETY ISSUES

There are many serious safety concerns with blue cohosh.

Some of the compounds found in blue cohosh, such as caulophyllosaponin and caulosaponin, appear to constrict coronary vessels, limiting blood flow to the heart and re-ducing its ability to pump.[4] One published case report documents profound heart failure in a child born to a mother who used blue cohosh to induce labor.[5] Severe medical consequences were seen in another child as well.[6]

Blue cohosh also contains methylcytisine, a substance similar to nicotine, which can also cause constriction of coronary vessels. Another substance in blue cohosh, anagyrine, may cause birth defects.[7]

Given these reports, the availability of safe alterna-tives for stimulating labor, and the lack of studies to doc-ument the herb's efficacy and safety, use of blue cohosh is not recommended.

BLUE FLAG (*Iris versicolor,* or *Iris caroliniana Watson*)

Alternate or Related Names   Sweet Flag, Orris, Iris, Florentine Orris, White Flag Root, Others

Principal Proposed Uses   There are no well-documented uses for blue flag.

Other Proposed Uses   Constipation, Dermatitis, Menstrual Regulation

Grown throughout North America, the underground stem, or rhizome, of the eye-catching blue flag plant in the iris family was traditionally thought to have medicinal properties.

Historically, the plant has been used to treat constipa-tion, dermatitis, and skin disease. Late nineteenth-cen-tury medical literature also referenced the plant as an emmenagogue, a type of herb believed helpful for in-ducing labor, increasing menstrual flow or regulating the menstrual cycle.

Blue flag contains furfural, a known mucous membrane irritant.[1] It also contains isophthalic acid, iridin, beta-sitosterol, irigenin, irilone-4'-glucoside, and irisolone-4'-bioside.[2,3,4] Iridin reportedly can be poiso-nous to humans and animals; however, there is some uncertainty as to whether the chemical of that name cited as toxic is identical to the substance found in blue flag.[5]

WHAT IS BLUE FLAG USED FOR TODAY?

Blue flag has no established medical uses, and is not widely used today. However, some herbalists recom-mend it for skin diseases.

DOSAGE

Typical doses of blue flag are 0.6 to 2 g of the dried rhi-zome, or 1 to 2 ml of the liquid extract, 3 times daily.[6]

SAFETY ISSUES

Safety studies of blue flag have not been performed, and related species have been found toxic.[7] It is also said to cause nausea and vomiting when taken at higher doses.[8] For all these reasons, we recommend avoiding blue flag.

BOLDO (*Peumus boldus*)

Alternate or Related Names   Boldu, Boldus

Principal Proposed Uses   There are no well-documented uses for boldo.

Other Proposed Uses   Dyspepsia, Liver Protection, Anti-Inflammatory, Laxative

Boldo (*Peumus boldus*) is an evergreen shrub native to South America. It grows about 6 to 20 feet high and has thick waxy leaves. Although boldo has a long history of use as a culinary spice and medicinal herb, and is still one of the most common medicinal plants used in Chile, it has only recently become the subject of scientific research.

The leaves of the boldo plant have traditionally been used as a treatment for liver and bladder disorders as well as rheumatism. They have also been used for a wide variety of other ailments, including headache, earache, congestion, menstrual pain, and syphilis. Recent research suggests boldo may protect the liver from toxins, stimulate the gall bladder, and reduce inflammation.[1–4]

WHAT IS BOLDO USED FOR TODAY?

Germany's Commission E has approved boldo for "spastic gastrointestinal complaints and dyspepsia."[5] **Dyspepsia** (see page 71) is a rather vague term that corresponds to the common word "indigestion," indicating a wide variety of digestive problems including stomach discomfort, lack of appetite, and nausea.

In Europe, dyspepsia is commonly attributed to inadequate flow of bile from the gallbladder. Although this connection has not been proven, boldo has been used as a treatment for dyspepsia based on how it affects the gallbladder. Boldo does not seem to increase bile production, but it does cause gallbladder contraction.[6,7,8]

Boldo taken alone has not been well evaluated as a treatment for dyspepsia; however, a combination herbal treatment containing boldo (along with other herbs thought to stimulate the gallbladder) has been studied. In a double-blind trial, 60 individuals given either an artichoke leaf/boldo/celandine combination or placebo found improvements in symptoms of indigestion after 14 days of treatment.[9] How this combination might be effective for treating dyspepsia is unclear.

Note: Celandine can be liver toxic.[10,11,12]

Studies on animals have found that boldo may protect the liver from toxins,[13,14,15] perhaps due to the antioxidant effects of a boldo constituent called boldine.[16,17,18] Boldo also has anti-inflammatory properties,[19,20,21] and, in addition, may act as a laxative.[22] The essential oils found in boldo have antimicrobial properties.[23]

DOSAGE

Germany's Commission E recommends 3 g of the dried leaf or its equivalent per day for digestive complaints.

SAFETY ISSUES

Although comprehensive safety studies have not been completed, boldo appears to be safe at normal doses. No side effects were reported in any of the animal studies. However, the plant's essential oils are very toxic and can cause kidney damage if taken alone or if large amounts of the leaf are ingested. The safety of long-term use is also questionable.

Individuals with gallstones should only take boldo under a physician's supervision due to the risk of gallstones being expelled and becoming lodged in a bile duct or the intestines. Those with obstruction of the bile ducts should not use boldo at all, due to the risk of rupture.

Because of the potential toxicity of some of the constituents of boldo, pregnant women should not use it.[24] Safety in nursing women, young children, or individuals with severe liver or kidney disease has also not been established.

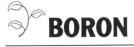

BORON

Supplement Forms/Alternate Names   Boron Chelate, Sodium Borate

Principal Proposed Uses   Osteoarthritis

Other Proposed Uses   Osteoporosis, Rheumatoid Arthritis

Plants need boron for proper health, but it's not known whether humans do. However, boron does seem to assist in the proper absorption of **calcium** (see page 234), **magnesium** (see page 351), and phosphorus from foods, and slows the loss of these minerals through urination. Very preliminary evidence suggests that boron may be helpful for arthritis and osteoporosis.

SOURCES

No dietary or nutritional requirement for boron has been established, and boron deficiency is not known to cause any disease. Good sources include leafy vegetables, raisins, prunes, nuts, non-citrus fruits, and grains. A typical American daily diet provides 1.5 to 3 mg of boron.

Boron

Visit Us at TNP.com

THERAPEUTIC DOSAGES

When used as a treatment for arthritis or osteoporosis, boron is often recommended at a dosage of 3 mg per day, an amount similar to the average daily intake from food. However, food sources may be safer (see Safety Issues).

THERAPEUTIC USES

Although boron is often added to supplements intended for the treatment of **osteoarthritis** (see page 132), the evidence that it helps is very weak.[1,2,3] Three other supplements—**glucosamine** (see page 308), **chondroitin** (see page 250), and **SAMe** (see page 403)—are much better researched treatments for osteoarthritis.

Boron has also been suggested as a treatment for **osteoporosis** (see page 136).[4] See the chapters on **isoflavones, calcium,** and **vitamin D** for more information on how to prevent or even reverse osteoporosis.

Finally, boron is sometimes recommended as a treatment for **rheumatoid arthritis** (see page 151), but there is no real evidence that it works.

WHAT IS THE SCIENTIFIC EVIDENCE FOR BORON?

Osteoarthritis

In areas of the world where people eat relatively high amounts of boron—between 3 and 10 mg per day—the incidence of osteoarthritis is below 10%. However, in regions where there is less boron in the diet—1 mg or less per day—the incidence of arthritis is higher.[5] This observation has given rise to the theory that boron supplements might be helpful for people who already have arthritis symptoms.

However, the only direct evidence that it works comes from one highly preliminary study.[6,7]

Osteoporosis

In one small study, 13 postmenopausal women were first fed a diet that provided 0.25 mg of boron for 119 days; then they were fed the same diet with a boron supplement of 3 mg daily for 48 days.[8] The results revealed that boron supplementation reduced the amount of calcium lost in the urine. This suggests (but certainly doesn't prove) that boron can help prevent osteoporosis. A more recent study failed to support this finding.[9]

SAFETY ISSUES

Since the therapeutic dosage of boron is about the same as the amount you can get from food, it is probably fairly safe. Unpleasant side effects, including nausea and vomiting, are only reported at about 50 times the highest recommended dose.

One potential concern with boron regards its effect on hormones. In at least two small studies, boron was found to increase the body's own estrogen levels, especially in women on estrogen-replacement therapy.[10,11] Because elevated estrogen increases the risk of breast and uterine cancer in women past menopause, this may be a matter of concern for those who wish to take supplemental boron. Further research is necessary to discover whether boron's apparent effects on estrogen is a real problem or not. At the present time, we would recommend getting your boron from fruits and vegetables: we know that they do not increase cancer risk (they reduce it).

⚠ INTERACTIONS YOU SHOULD KNOW ABOUT

If you are receiving **hormone-replacement therapy,** use of boron may not be advisable due to the risk of elevating estrogen levels excessively.

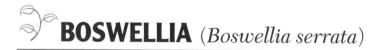

BOSWELLIA *(Boswellia serrata)*

Alternate or Related Names   Frankincense, Olibanum

Principal Proposed Uses   Rheumatoid Arthritis

Other Proposed Uses   Asthma, Osteoarthritis, Tendinitis, Bursitis, Ulcerative Colitis

The gummy resin of the boswellia tree has a long history of use in Indian herbal medicine as a treatment for arthritis, bursitis, respiratory diseases, and diarrhea.

WHAT IS BOSWELLIA USED FOR TODAY?

Boswellia is often recommended as a treatment for bursitis, **osteoarthritis** (see page 132), **rheumatoid arth-**

ritis (see page 151), and tendinitis, based on the recent work of Indian scientists. Of these possible uses, only rheumatoid arthritis has any scientific evidence behind it, and it is contradictory.

One small double-blind study suggests that boswellia might be helpful for **asthma** (see page 14).

In addition, a highly preliminary study suggests that boswellia may also be helpful for **ulcerative colitis** (see page 179).[1]

WHAT IS THE SCIENTIFIC EVIDENCE FOR BOSWELLIA?

Rheumatoid Arthritis

Investigations of boswellia have found that its constituents, including substances known as boswellic acids, possess anti-inflammatory properties.[2–5] Other preliminary research suggests that boswellia may protect cartilage from damage.[6] These properties could make boswellia useful in rheumatoid arthritis.

According to a recent review of unpublished studies, preliminary double-blind trials have found boswellia effective in relieving the symptoms of rheumatoid arthritis.[7] Two placebo-controlled studies, involving a total of 81 individuals with rheumatoid arthritis, found significant reductions in swelling and pain over the course of 3 months. Also, a comparative study of 60 people over 6 months found that boswellia extract produced symptomatic benefits comparable to oral gold therapy. However, this review was rather sketchy on details. It did not state whether or not boswellia could induce remission like gold shots, and not enough information was given to evaluate the quality of the research.

However, a recent double-blind placebo-controlled study that enrolled 78 patients found no benefit.[8] About half of the patients dropped out, which diminishes the significance of the results.

Asthma

A 6-week double-blind placebo-controlled study of 80 individuals with relatively mild asthma found that treatment with boswellia at a dose of 300 mg 3 times daily reduced the frequency of asthma attacks and improved objective measurements of breathing capacity.[9]

DOSAGE

A typical dose of boswellia is 400 mg 3 times a day of an extract standardized to contain 37.5% boswellic acids. The full effect may take 4 to 8 weeks to develop.

SAFETY ISSUES

Although comprehensive safety testing has not been completed, boswellia appears to be reasonably safe when used as directed. Reported side effects are rare and consist primarily of occasional allergic reactions or mild gastrointestinal distress. Safety in young children, pregnant or nursing women, or people with severe liver or kidney disease has not been established.

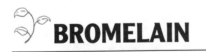

BROMELAIN

Principal Proposed Uses   Surgery, Athletic Injuries, Phlebitis, Sinusitis, Digestive Problems

Other Proposed Uses   Chronic Venous Insufficiency, Hemorrhoids, Easy Bruising, Gout, Arthritis, Ulcerative Colitis, Menstrual Pain

Bromelain is not actually a single substance, but rather a collection of protein-digesting enzymes found in pineapple juice and in the stem of pineapple plants. It is primarily produced in Japan, Hawaii, and Taiwan, and much of the original research was performed in the first two of those locations. Subsequently, European researchers developed an interest, and by 1995 bromelain had become the thirteenth most common individual herbal product sold in Germany.

WHAT IS BROMELAIN USED FOR TODAY?

In 1993, Germany's Commission E approved bromelain for "reducing swelling in the nose and sinuses caused by injuries and operations." However, bromelain is actually thought to be useful for other conditions as well, based on its apparent ability to reduce swelling and inflammation. In Europe, bromelain is used to aid in recovery from **surgery** (see page 173) and **athletic injuries** (see page 101), as well as to treat sinusitis and **phlebitis** (see page 143).

Bromelain

Visit Us at TNP.com

Other proposed uses of bromelain include chronic venous insufficiency (closely related to **varicose veins;** see page 184), **hemorrhoids** (see page 85), other diseases of the veins, **bruising** (see page 74), **osteoarthritis** (see page 132), **rheumatoid arthritis** (see page 151), **gout** (see page 84), **ulcerative colitis** (see page 179),[1] and **dysmenorrhea** (menstrual pain; see page 70). However, there is little real evidence that bromelain is effective for these conditions.

Bromelain is definitely useful as a digestive enzyme. Unlike most digestive enzymes, bromelain is active both in the acid environment of the stomach and the alkaline environment of the small intestine.[2,3] This may make it particularly effective as an oral digestive aid for those who do not digest food properly.[4,5,6]

Bromelain may also increase the absorption of various drugs, particularly antibiotics such as amoxicillin and tetracycline. This could offer both risks and benefits.[7–10]

WHAT IS THE SCIENTIFIC EVIDENCE FOR BROMELAIN?

While most large enzymes are broken down in the digestive tract, those found in bromelain appear to be absorbed whole to a certain extent.[11,12,13] This finding makes it reasonable to suppose that bromelain can actually produce systemic (whole body) effects. Once in the blood, bromelain appears to produce anti-inflammatory and "blood-thinning" effects.[14–30] These influences may be responsible for some of bromelain's therapeutic effects.

Injury and Surgery

In 1993, Germany's Commission E reviewed the evidence for bromelain's effectiveness in reducing the swelling caused by injury or surgery. They found five passable double-blind studies, of which three showed good results and two showed no benefit.[31] In their opinion, the best evidence was for surgery of the nose and sinuses. However, benefits have been seen for other forms of surgery as well.

A double-blind placebo-controlled study evaluated 160 women who received episiotomies (surgical cuts in the perineum) during childbirth.[32] Participants given 40 mg of bromelain 4 times daily for 3 days, beginning 4 hours after delivery, showed a statistically significant decrease in edema, inflammation, and pain. Ninety percent of patients taking bromelain demonstrated excellent or good responses compared to 44% in the placebo group. However, another double-blind study of 158 women who received episiotomies failed to find significant benefit.[33]

In a double-blind controlled trial, 95 patients undergoing treatment for cataracts were given 40 mg of bromelain or placebo (along with other treatments) 4 times daily for 2 days prior to surgery and 5 days post-operatively.[34] Overall, less inflammation was noted in the bromelain-treated group compared to the placebo group.

Benefits were also seen in a small double-blind placebo-controlled crossover study of people undergoing dental surgery.[35]

However, no significant benefits were seen in a double-blind placebo-controlled trial of 154 individuals undergoing plastic surgery of the face.[36]

A somewhat informal controlled study of 146 boxers suggested that bromelain helps bruises to heal more quickly.[37] Another study—this one without any type of control group—found that bromelain reduced swelling, pain at rest, and tenderness among 59 patients with blunt trauma injuries, including bruising.[38]

Sinusitis

Bromelain may be helpful for sinusitis.

In a double-blind trial, 48 patients with moderately severe to severe sinusitis received bromelain or placebo for 6 days.[39] All patients were placed on standard therapy for sinusitis, which included antihistamines, analgesics, and antibiotics. Upon completion of the study, inflammation was reduced in 83% of those taking bromelain compared to 52% of the placebo group. Breathing difficulty was relieved in 78% of the bromelain group and 68% of the placebo group. Overall, good to excellent results were observed in 87% of patients treated with bromelain compared to 68% on placebo.

Benefits were also seen in two other studies enrolling a total of more than 100 individuals with sinusitis.[40,41]

Phlebitis

Another double-blind study followed 73 people being treated for phlebitis, or inflammation of the veins of the leg.[42] Those who received bromelain in addition to standard treatments showed improved results.

Warning: Do not attempt to self-treat phlebitis.

DOSAGE

Recommended dosages of bromelain vary with the form used. Due to the wide variation, we suggest following label instructions.

SAFETY ISSUES

Bromelain appears to be essentially nontoxic, and it seldom causes side effects other than occasional mild gastrointestinal distress or allergic reactions.[43]

However, because bromelain "thins the blood" to some extent, it shouldn't be combined with drugs such as Coumadin (warfarin) without a doctor's supervision.

According to one small animal study, bromelain might interact with sedative medications, increasing their effect.[44] As noted above, it might also increase blood levels of various antibiotics, which could present risks in some cases. Safety in young children, pregnant or nursing women, or those with liver or kidney disease has not been established.

⚠ INTERACTIONS YOU SHOULD KNOW ABOUT

If you are taking medications that thin the blood such as **Coumadin (warfarin)** or **heparin,** sedative drugs such as **benzodiazepines,** or **antibiotics,** bromelain might amplify their effect.

BUGLEWEED (*Lycopus virginicus*)

Alternate or Related Names   Sweet Bugle, Water Bugle, Virginia Water Horehound, Gypsywort

Principal Proposed Uses   There are no well-documented uses for bugleweed.

Other Proposed Uses   Hyperthyroidism, Cyclic Mastalgia (Cyclic breast pain)

Bugleweed (*Lycopus virginicus*), from the mint family, is a native of North America. It is closely related to the European herb called gypsywort or gypsyweed (*L. europaeus*). For medicinal purposes, these two plants are often used interchangeably. The leaves of bugleweed are long and thin and grow in pairs from the stem. Small whitish flowers grow around the stem at the base of each pair of leaves.

The juice of bugleweed can be used as a fabric dye, and it was reportedly used by gypsies to darken their skin, which may be the origin of the common names applied to the European species of *Lycopus*.

Bugleweed also has a long-standing reputation as a medicinal plant. Herbalists have traditionally used bugleweed as a sedative, to treat mild heart conditions, and to reduce fever and mucus production in **flus and colds** (see page 47). More recently, bugleweed has been suggested as a treatment for hyperthyroidism and **mastodynia** (breast pain; see page 58).

WHAT IS BUGLEWEED USED FOR TODAY?

Several very preliminary studies suggest that bugleweed may be helpful for treating mild hyperthyroidism.

Hyperthyroidism is a condition in which the thyroid gland releases excessive amounts of thyroid hormone. Symptoms include weight loss, weakness, heart palpitations, and anxiety. Test tube and animal studies suggest that bugleweed may reduce thyroid hormone by decreasing levels of TSH (a hormone that stimulates the thyroid gland) and by impairing thyroid hormone synthesis.[1–5] In addition, bugleweed may block the action of thyroid-stimulating antibodies found in Grave's disease.[6]

Note: Self-treatment of hyperthyroidism can be dangerous. Physician supervision is necessary to determine why the thyroid is overactive to design a specific treatment plan.

Bugleweed may also reduce levels of the hormone prolactin, which is primarily responsible for the production of breast milk.[7] Elevated levels of prolactin may also cause breast pain in women; based on this finding, bugleweed has been recommended as a treatment for **cyclic mastalgia** (breast tenderness that comes and goes with the menstrual cycle; see page 58). However, due to its effects on thyroid hormone, we do not recommend that it be used for this purpose. The herb **chasteberry** (see page 245) also suppresses prolactin and is probably a safer option.

DOSAGE

The dosage of bugleweed must be adjusted by measuring thyroid hormone levels.

SAFETY ISSUES

The safety of bugleweed has not been established. Long-term or high-dose use of the herb may cause an enlarged thyroid. Bugleweed should not be used by individuals with hypothyroidism (low thyroid hormone) or an enlarged thyroid gland. Pregnant or nursing women should also avoid bugleweed because of potential effects on their children as well as on breast milk production.

Bugleweed should not be combined with thyroid medications. It may also interfere with diagnostic procedures that rely on radioactive isotopes to evaluate the thyroid.

⚠ INTERACTIONS YOU SHOULD KNOW ABOUT

If you are taking thyroid medications, do not use bugleweed.

If you are undergoing tests of your thyroid function, do not use bugleweed except on physician advice.

BURDOCK (*Arctium lappa*)

Alternate or Related Names   Bardana, Beggar's Buttons, Burr Seed, Clotbur, Cockle Buttons, Others

Principal Proposed Uses   Eczema, Psoriasis, Acne

Other Proposed Uses   Cancer?, Rheumatoid Arthritis

The common burdock, that well-known source of annoying burrs matted in dogs' fur, is also a medicinal herb of considerable reputation. Called *gobo* in Japan, burdock root is said to be a food that provides deep strengthening to the immune system. In ancient China and India, herbalists used it in the treatment of respiratory infections, abscesses, and joint pain. European physicians of the Middle Ages and later used it to treat cancerous tumors, skin conditions, venereal disease, and bladder and kidney problems.

Burdock was a primary ingredient in the famous (or infamous) Hoxsey cancer treatment. Harry Hoxsey was a former coal miner who parlayed a traditional family remedy for cancer into the largest privately owned cancer treatment center in the world, with branches in 17 states. (It was shut down in the 1950s by the FDA. Harry Hoxsey himself subsequently died of cancer.) Other herbs in his formula included **red clover** (see page 397), poke, prickly ash, **bloodroot** (see page 224), and barberry. Burdock is also found in the famous herbal cancer remedy Essiac.

Despite this historical enthusiasm, there is no significant evidence that burdock is an effective treatment for cancer or any other illness.

WHAT IS BURDOCK USED FOR TODAY?

Burdock is widely recommended for the relief of dry, scaly skin conditions such as **eczema** (see page 78) and **psoriasis** (see page 148). It is also used for treating **acne**

(see page 2). It can be taken internally as well as applied directly to the skin. Burdock is sometimes recommended for **rheumatoid arthritis** (see page 151). Unfortunately, there is as yet no real scientific evidence for any of these uses.

DOSAGE

A typical dosage of burdock is 1 to 2 g of powdered dry root 3 times per day.

SAFETY ISSUES

As a food commonly eaten in Japan (it is often found in sukiyaki), burdock root is believed to be safe. However, in 1978, the *Journal of the American Medical Association* caused a brief scare by publishing a report of burdock poisoning. Subsequent investigation showed that the herbal product involved was actually contaminated with the poisonous chemical atropine from an unknown source.[1] Safety in young children, pregnant or nursing women, or those with severe liver or kidney disease is not established.

⚠ INTERACTIONS YOU SHOULD KNOW ABOUT

If you are taking **insulin** or **oral medications to reduce blood sugar,** it is possible that burdock will increase its effect.[2,3]

BUTCHER'S BROOM (*Ruscus aculeatus*)

Alternate or Related Names   Kneeholm, Pettigree, Sweet Broom, Knee Holly, Jew's Myrtle

Principal Proposed Uses   Hemorrhoids, Varicose Veins

So named because its branches were a traditional source of broom straw used by butchers, this Mediterranean evergreen bush has a long history of traditional use in the treatment of urinary conditions.

WHAT IS BUTCHER'S BROOM USED FOR TODAY?

Butcher's broom has been approved by Germany's Commission E as supportive therapy for **hemorrhoids** (see page 85) and venous insufficiency, a condition closely related to **varicose veins** (see page 184).

Preliminary evidence from animal studies suggests that butcher's broom possesses anti-inflammatory properties and also constricts small veins.[1,2] One small, double-blind study in humans found improvements in vein function.[3]

DOSAGE

Butcher's broom is standardized to its ruscogenin content. A typical oral dose should supply 50 to 100 mg of ruscogenins daily.

For hemorrhoids, butcher's broom can also be applied as an ointment or in the form of a suppository.

SAFETY ISSUES

Butcher's broom is believed to be safe when used as directed, although detailed studies have not been performed. Noticeable side effects appear to be rare. Safety in young children, pregnant or nursing women, or those with liver or kidney disease has not been established.

BUTTERBUR *(Petasites hybridus)*

Alternate or Related Names   Bog Rhubarb, Petasites, Blatterdock, Bogshorns, Butter-Dock, Others

Principal Proposed Uses   Migraine Headaches (Prevention)

Other Proposed Uses   Pain, Asthma, Ulcer Protection

Butterbur can be found growing along rivers, ditches, and marshy areas in northern Asia, Europe, and parts of North America. It sends up stalks of reddish flowers very early in spring, before producing very large heart-shaped leaves with a furry gray underside. Once the leaves appear, butterbur somewhat resembles rhubarb—one of its common names is bog rhubarb. It is also sometimes referred to as "umbrella leaves" due to the size of its foliage. Other more or less descriptive common names abound, including blatterdock, bogshorns, butter-dock, butterly dock, capdockin, flapperdock, and langwort.

Butterbur is often described as possessing an unpleasant smell, but being malodorous hasn't protected it from harvesting by humans. The plant has a long medicinal history, including use for stomach cramps, whooping cough, and asthma.

Externally, butterbur has been applied as a poultice over wounds or skin ulcerations.

WHAT IS BUTTERBUR USED FOR TODAY?

Based on one double-blind trial, butterbur is becoming increasingly popular for preventing **migraine headaches** (see page 120).[1] For this purpose, it is taken in a special extract form (see Dosage below).

Migraine headaches are usually felt in the forehead or temples, often on one side only and typically accompanied by nausea and a preference for a darkened room. Headache attacks can last from several hours up to a day

or more. They are usually separated by completely pain-free intervals.

Individuals with frequent migraine attacks may wish to use medication on a daily basis to prevent them. The herb **feverfew** (see page 280) has become famous as a natural treatment for this purpose, and butterbur may be helpful as well. However, further study is needed to confirm this potential benefit.

Note: Serious diseases may occasionally first present themselves as migraine-type headaches. For this reason, proper medical diagnosis is essential if you suddenly start having migraines without a previous history, or if the pattern of your migraines changes significantly.

There is some evidence that butterbur has anti-inflammatory and anti-spasmodic effects.[2,3] This may make it useful for a variety of other painful conditions, including abdominal pain, tension headaches, back pain, bladder spasms, and gall bladder pain.[4,5,6]

Butterbur has also been investigated for asthma treatment.[7,8] However, the evidence that butterbur actually offers benefits for these conditions is weak to nonexistent.

Very weak evidence also suggests that butterbur might help protect the stomach lining from ulcers.[9,10]

WHAT IS THE SCIENTIFIC EVIDENCE FOR BUTTERBUR?

Migraines

Butterbur was tested as a migraine preventive in a double-blind placebo-controlled study involving 60 men and women who experienced at least 3 migraines per month.[11] After 4 weeks without any conventional medications, participants were randomly assigned to take either 50 mg of butterbur extract or placebo twice daily for 3 months.

The results were positive: both the number of migraine attacks and the total number of days of migraine pain were significantly reduced in the treatment group as compared to the placebo group. Three out of four individuals taking butterbur reported improvement, as compared to only one out of four in the placebo group. No significant side effects were noted.

However, these results need to be confirmed by an independent laboratory with another properly designed study before butterbur can be considered a proven treatment for migraine prevention.

DOSAGE

The usual dosage of butterbur as a migraine preventive is 50 mg twice daily of an extract that has been processed to remove potentially dangerous chemicals called pyrrolizidine alkaloids (see Safety Issues below).

Warning: Use of any butterbur product that still contains these alkaloids is definitely not recommended.

SAFETY ISSUES

No side effects from the use of butterbur have been reported. However, as mentioned above, butterbur contains liver-toxic and possibly carcinogenic components called pyrrolizidine alkaloids.[12] Fortunately, it is possible to remove these compounds from butterbur products.[13]

Safety in young children, pregnant or nursing women, or people with severe kidney or liver disease has not been established.

CALCIUM

Supplement Forms/Alternate Names   Calcium Carbonate, Dolomite, Oyster Shell Calcium, Calcium Citrate, Calcium Citrate Malate, Tricalcium Phosphate, Calcium Lactate, Calcium Gluconate, Calcium Aspartate, Calcium Orotate, Calcium Chelate, Bonemeal

Principal Proposed Uses   Osteoporosis, PMS (Premenstrual Syndrome)

Other Proposed Uses   Colon Polyps and Cancer Prevention, Hypertension (High Blood Pressure), High Cholesterol, Polycystic Ovary Syndrome, Preeclampsia, Attention Deficit Disorder, Migraine Headaches, Periodontal Disease

Calcium is the most abundant mineral in the body, making up nearly 2% of total body weight. More than 99% of the calcium in your body is found in your bones, but the other 1% is perhaps just as important for good health. Many enzymes depend on calcium in order to work properly, as do your nerves, heart, and blood-clotting mechanisms.

To build bone, you need to have enough calcium in your diet. But in spite of calcium-fortified orange juice and the best efforts of the dairy industry, most Americans are calcium deficient.[1] Calcium supplements are a simple way to make sure you're getting enough of this important mineral.

One of the most important uses of calcium is to prevent and treat osteoporosis, the progressive loss of bone mass to which postmenopausal women are especially vulnerable. Calcium works best when combined with vitamin D.

Recent evidence suggests that calcium may have another important use: dramatically reducing PMS symptoms.

REQUIREMENTS/SOURCES

Although there are some variations between recommendations issued by different groups, the official U.S. and Canadian recommendations for daily intake of calcium are as follows:

- Infants 0–6 months, 210 mg
    7–12 months, 270 mg
- Children 1–3 years, 500 mg
    4–8 years, 800 mg
- Males and females 9–18 years, 1,300 mg
    19–50 years, 1,000 mg
    51 years and older, 1,200 mg
- Pregnant women 1,000 mg (1,300 mg if under 19 years old)
- Nursing women 1,000 mg (1,300 mg if under 19 years old)

To absorb calcium, your body also needs an adequate level of vitamin D (for more information, see the chapter on **vitamin D**).

Milk, cheese, and other dairy products are excellent sources of calcium. Other good sources include orange juice or soy milk fortified with calcium, fish canned with its bones (e.g., sardines), dark green vegetables, nuts and seeds, and calcium-processed tofu.

If you wish to use calcium supplements, there are many forms available, each with its pros and cons. The most important ones include naturally derived forms of calcium, refined calcium carbonate, and chelated calcium.

Naturally Derived Forms of Calcium

These forms of calcium come from bone, shells, or the earth: bonemeal, oyster shell, and dolomite. Animals concentrate calcium in their shells, and calcium is found in minerals in the earth. These forms of calcium are economical, and you can get as much as 500 to 600 mg in one tablet. However, there are concerns that the natural forms of calcium supplements may contain significant amounts of lead.[2] Calcium supplements rarely list the lead content of their source, although they should. The lead concentration should always be less than 2 parts per million.

Refined Calcium Carbonate

This is the most common commercial calcium supplement, and it is also used as a common antacid. Calcium carbonate is one of the least expensive forms of calcium, but it can cause constipation and bloating, and it may not be well absorbed by people with reduced levels of stomach acid. Taking it with meals improves absorption, because stomach acid is released to digest the food.

Chelated Calcium

Chelated calcium is calcium bound to an organic acid (citrate, citrate malate, lactate, gluconate, aspartate, or orotate). The chelated forms of calcium offer some significant advantages and disadvantages compared with calcium carbonate.

On the plus side, certain forms of chelated calcium (calcium citrate and calcium citrate malate) appear to be better absorbed and more effective for osteoporosis treatment than calcium carbonate, although not all studies agree.[3–6] On the negative side, chelated calcium is much more expensive and bulkier than calcium carbonate. In other words, you have to take more and larger pills to get enough calcium. It is not at all uncommon to need to take five or six large capsules daily to supply the necessary amount, a quantity some people may find troublesome.

The form of calcium found in beverages is usually the chelated form, calcium citrate malate, or a slightly less well absorbed form, tricalcium phosphate.

THERAPEUTIC DOSAGES

Unlike some supplements, calcium is not taken at extra high doses for special therapeutic benefit. Rather, for all its uses it should be taken in the amounts listed under Requirements/Sources, along with the recommended level of vitamin D (see the chapter on **vitamin D** for proper dosage amounts).

Calcium absorption studies have found that your body can't absorb more than 500 mg of calcium at one time.[7] Therefore, it is most efficient to take your total daily calcium in two or more doses.

It isn't possible to put all the calcium you need in a single multivitamin/mineral tablet, so this is one supplement that should be taken on its own.

Furthermore, calcium may interfere with the absorption of **chromium** (see page 251) and **manganese** (see page 354).[8,9,10] Although the calcium present in some antacids or supplements may alter the absorption of **magnesium** (see page 351), this effect apparently has no significant influence on overall magnesium status.[11,12]

Also, if you take any of these supplements, it is best to do so at a different time from when you take calcium. This means that it is best to take your multivitamin and mineral pill at a separate time from your calcium supplement.

Calcium may also interfere with iron absorption.[13–18] However, you shouldn't take extra iron unless you know you are deficient. (For more information, see the chapter on **iron**.)

Some studies show that calcium may decrease **zinc** (see page 463) absorption when the two are taken together as supplements; however, studies have found that, in the presence of meals, zinc levels may be unaffected by increases of either dietary or supplemental calcium.[19–25]

Corticosteroids cause osteoporosis by decreasing intestinal absorption of calcium as well as through other mechanisms. Supplementation with calcium and vitamin D may help prevent the loss of bone density associated with long-term corticosteroid therapy.[26,27] Long-term or high-dose use of heparin might also cause osteoporosis, particularly in pregnant women. Again, supplemental calcium along with vitamin D maybe helpful.[28,29,30]

Another drug that may interfere with calcium absorption is isoniazid, mostly because of its interaction with vitamin D.[31,32,33]

Finally, carbamazepine and other anticonvulsant drugs may impair calcium[34,35] and vitamin D[36–40] absorption and thereby interfere with bone formation and maintenance. Calcium and vitamin D supplementation may be helpful in avoiding these side effects. However, since calcium carbonate might interfere with the effects of anticonvulsant drugs, if you use that form of calcium, you should take it at least 2 hours apart from your anticonvulsant drug.[41,42]

Calcium

Visit Us at TNP.com

THERAPEUTIC USES

There is little doubt that calcium supplementation is useful in helping prevent and slow down **osteoporosis** (see page 136).[43-48]

If you are a woman past menopause, this is true whether or not you are taking estrogen. Calcium supplements work best when combined with vitamin D.

A new and rather surprising use of calcium came to light recently when a large, well-designed study found that calcium is an effective treatment for **PMS** (premenstrual syndrome; see page 145).[49] Calcium supplementation reduced all major symptoms, including headache, food cravings, moodiness, and fluid retention. The benefits were so impressive that calcium should probably be considered the foremost treatment for PMS.

There may actually be a connection between these two uses of calcium: PMS may be an early sign of future osteoporosis.[50,51]

Recent evidence suggests that getting enough calcium may reduce the risk of developing colon **cancer** (see page 32) and colon polyps, a precancerous condition.[52]

Calcium deficiency may play a role in the development of **hypertension** (see page 98).[53,54] However, taking extra calcium does not appear to reduce blood pressure significantly.[55]

Calcium supplements might slightly improve **cholesterol** (see page 88) levels.[56,57]

One preliminary study suggests that supplementation with calcium and vitamin D may be helpful for women with polycystic ovary syndrome.[58]

Calcium supplementation has also been tried as a treatment to prevent preeclampsia in pregnant women. While the evidence from studies is conflicting,[59,60,61] calcium supplementation might be effective in women with low calcium levels to begin with.

Finally, calcium is also sometimes recommended for **attention deficit disorder** (see page 22), **migraine headaches** (see page 120), and **periodontal disease** (see page 142), but there is as yet little to no evidence that it is effective.

WHAT IS THE SCIENTIFIC EVIDENCE FOR CALCIUM?

Osteoporosis

Numerous studies indicate that calcium supplements are useful in preventing and slowing osteoporosis, the progressive loss of bone mass as we age. Calcium supplementation at the recommended dosages appears to reduce bone loss in postmenopausal women in every part of the body except the spine.[62,63] When vitamin D is taken along with calcium, it may be possible not only to slow down but actually reverse osteoporosis, in the spine as well as in other bones.[64]

If you are taking estrogen to keep your bones strong, additional calcium may provide even more benefit.[65] Calcium supplementation is also useful for adolescent girls as a way to "put calcium in the bank"—building up a supply for the future.[66] However, exercise may be even more important.[67]

One study found that in calcium-deficient pregnant women, calcium supplements can improve the bones of their unborn children.[68]

There is some good evidence that the use of calcium combined with vitamin D can help protect against the bone loss caused by corticosteroid drugs such as prednisone. In a 2-year double-blind placebo-controlled study of 130 individuals, daily supplementation with 1,000 mg of calcium and 500 IU of vitamin D actually reversed steroid-induced bone loss, causing a net bone gain.[69]

Premenstrual Syndrome (PMS)

According to a large and well-designed study published in a 1998 issue of *American Journal of Obstetrics and Gynecology,* calcium supplements are a simple and effective treatment for a wide variety of PMS symptoms.[70] In a double-blind placebo-controlled study of 497 women, 1,200 mg daily of calcium as calcium carbonate reduced PMS symptoms by half over a period of three menstrual cycles. These symptoms included mood swings, headaches, food cravings, and bloating. These results corroborate earlier, smaller studies.[71,72]

Colon Cancer

Recent evidence suggests that the use of calcium carbonate can inhibit the development of precancerous polyps in the colon and rectum. A double-blind placebo-controlled study followed 832 individuals with a history of polyps for 4 years.[73] Participants received either 3 g daily of calcium carbonate or placebo. The calcium group experienced 24% fewer polyps overall than the placebo group.

There is also evidence from observational studies that a high calcium intake is associated with a reduced incidence of colon cancer,[74] but not all studies have found this association.[75]

SAFETY ISSUES

In general, it's safe to take up to 2,000 mg of calcium daily, although this is more than you need.[76] Greatly excessive intake of calcium can cause numerous side effects, including dangerous or painful deposits of calcium within the body.

If you have cancer, hyperparathyroidism, or sarcoidosis, you should take calcium only under a physician's supervision.

People with kidney stones or a history of kidney stones are also often warned not to take supplemental calcium. The reason for this caution is that kidney stones are commonly made of calcium oxalate crystals. However, studies have found that increased intake of calcium from food actually reduces the risk of kidney stones.[77,78] Calcium supplements, on the other hand, might increase kidney stone risk, especially if they are not taken with meals.[79] The bottom line: Restriction of calcium—whether supplemental or dietary—may still be appropriate for certain people.[80] Ask your physician for advice specific to you.

Large observational studies have found that higher intakes of calcium are associated with a greatly increased risk of prostate cancer.[81,82,83] This seems to be the case whether the calcium comes from milk or from calcium supplements. However, without further research it is difficult to tell whether this is a cause-and-effect relationship or simply an accidental correlation.

Calcium supplements combined with high doses of vitamin D might interfere with some of the effects of calcium channel–blockers.[84] It is very important that you consult your physician before trying this combination.

Concerns have been raised that the aluminum in some antacids may not be good for you.[85] Since there is some evidence that calcium citrate supplements might increase the absorption of aluminum,[86–90] it might not be a good idea to take calcium citrate at the same time of day as aluminum-containing antacids. Another option is to use other forms of calcium, or to avoid antacids containing aluminum.

When taken over the long term, thiazide diuretics tend to increase levels of calcium in the body, by decreasing the amount excreted by the body.[91–94] It's not likely that this will cause a problem. However, since greatly increased calcium levels in the body can cause side effects such as calcium deposits, if you are using thiazide diuretics, you should consult with your physician on the proper doses of calcium and vitamin D for you.

Finally, calcium may interfere with the absorption of antibiotics in the tetracycline and fluoroquinolone families as well as thyroid hormone. If you are taking any of these drugs you should take your calcium supplements at least 2 hours before or after your medication dose.[95–100]

⚠ INTERACTIONS YOU SHOULD KNOW ABOUT

If you are taking

- **Corticosteroids, heparin,** or **isoniazid:** You may need more calcium.
- **Aluminum hydroxide:** You should take calcium citrate at least 2 hours apart to avoid increasing aluminum absorption.
- The anticonvulsants **phenytoin (Dilantin), carbamazepine, phenobarbital,** or **primidone:** You may need more calcium; however, it may be advisable to take your dose of anticonvulsant and your calcium supplement at least 2 hours apart because each interferes with the other's absorption.
- Antibiotics in the **tetracycline** or **fluoroquinolone (Cipro, Floxin, Noroxin)** families or **thyroid hormone:** You should take your calcium supplement at least 2 hours before or after your dose of medication, because calcium interferes with the absorption of these medications (and vice versa).
- **Thiazide diuretics:** Do not take extra calcium except on the advice of a physician.
- **Calcium channel–blockers:** Do not take calcium together with high-dose vitamin D except on the advice of a physician.
- **Calcium:** You may need extra **iron, manganese, zinc,** and **chromium.** Ideally, you should take calcium at a different time of day from these other minerals, because it may interfere with their absorption.
- **Soy:** A constituent of soy called phytic acid can interfere with the absorption of calcium, so it may be advisable to wait 2 hours after taking calcium supplements to eat soy (or vice versa).

CALENDULA

Alternate or Related Names   Marigold, Holligold, Goldbloom, Golds, Mary Bud, Others

Principal Proposed Uses
   Topical Uses: Skin Injuries (Cuts, Scrapes, Burns, Nonhealing Wounds, Etc.), Skin Inflammation (Eczema, Etc.), Hemorrhoids, Varicose Veins
   Oral Uses: Mouth Sores

Calendula, well known as one of the ornamental marigolds, blooms month after month from early spring to first frost. Because "calend" means month in Latin, the plant's lengthy flowering season is believed to have given calendula its name. The herb has been used to heal wounds and treat inflamed skin since ancient times.

An active ingredient that might be responsible for calendula's traditional medicinal properties has not been discovered. One theory suggests that volatile oils in the plant act synergistically with other constituents called *xanthophylls*.[1]

WHAT IS CALENDULA USED FOR TODAY?

Experiments on rats and other animals suggest that calendula cream exerts a **wound-healing** (see page 123) and anti-inflammatory effect,[2,3,4] but double-blind studies have not yet been reported.

Creams made with calendula flower are a nearly ubiquitous item in the German medicine chest, used for everything from children's scrapes to **eczema** (see page 78), **burns** (see page 123), and poorly healing wounds. These same German products are widely available in the United States as well.

Calendula cream is also used to soothe **hemorrhoids** (see page 85) and **varicose veins** (see page 184), and the tea reportedly reduces the discomfort of mouth sores. However, as yet there is no scientific evidence for these uses.

DOSAGE

Calendula cream should be applied 2 or 3 times daily to the affected area. For oral use as a mouthwash, pour boiling water over 1 to 2 teaspoons of calendula flowers and allow to steep for 10 to 15 minutes. Rinse your mouth with this liquid several times a day.

SAFETY ISSUES

Calendula is generally regarded as safe. Neither calendula cream nor calendula taken internally has been associated with any adverse effects other than occasional allergic reactions, and animal studies have found no significant toxic effects.[5] However, the same studies found that in high doses, calendula acts like a sedative and also reduces blood pressure. For this reason, it might not be safe to combine calendula with sedative or blood pressure medications.

⚠ INTERACTIONS YOU SHOULD KNOW ABOUT

If you are taking

- **Sleeping pills** or **antianxiety drugs:** Oral calendula might increase the sedative effect.
- **Medications to reduce blood pressure:** Oral calendula might amplify its effects.

CARNITINE

Supplement Forms/Alternate Names   L-Carnitine, L-Acetyl-Carnitine (LAC), L-Propionyl-Carnitine, Acetyl-L-Carnitine (ALC)

Principal Proposed Uses   Angina and Other Heart Conditions, Intermittent Claudication, Chronic Obstructive Pulmonary Disease, Alzheimer's Disease, Depression in the Elderly

Other Proposed Uses   High Cholesterol, Hyperactivity in Fragile X Syndrome, Chronic Fatigue Syndrome, Diabetic Cardiac Autonomic Neuropathy, Performance Enhancement, Irregular Heartbeat, Down's Syndrome, Muscular Dystrophy, Impaired Sperm Motility, Alcoholic Fatty Liver Disease, Toxicity Due to AZT (a Drug Used to Treat AIDS), Diabetes

---

Carnitine is an amino acid the body uses to turn fat into energy. It is not normally considered an essential nutrient, because the body can manufacture all it needs. However, supplemental carnitine may improve the ability of certain tissues to produce energy. This effect has led to the use of carnitine in various muscle diseases as well as heart conditions.

SOURCES

There is no dietary requirement for carnitine. However, a few individuals have a genetic defect that hinders the body's ability to make carnitine. In addition, diseases of the liver, kidneys, or brain may inhibit carnitine production. Certain medications, especially the antiseizure drugs Depakene (valproic acid) and Dilantin (phenytoin), may reduce carnitine levels; however, whether taking extra carnitine would be helpful has not been determined.[1–11] Heart muscle tissue, because of its high energy requirements, is particularly vulnerable to carnitine deficiency.

The principal dietary sources of carnitine are meat and dairy products, but to obtain therapeutic dosages a supplement is necessary.

THERAPEUTIC DOSAGES

Typical dosages for the diseases described here range from 500 to 1,000 mg 3 times daily. Carnitine is taken in three forms: L-carnitine (for heart and other conditions), L-propionyl-carnitine (for heart conditions), and acetyl-L-carnitine (for Alzheimer's disease). The dosage is the same for all three forms.

THERAPEUTIC USES

Carnitine is primarily used for heart-related conditions. Fairly good evidence suggests that it can be used along with conventional treatment for **angina** (see page 10), or chest pain, to improve symptoms and reduce medication needs.[12–17] When combined with conventional therapy, it may also reduce mortality rates after a heart attack.[18,19]

Lesser evidence suggests that it may be helpful for a condition called **intermittent claudication** (pain in the legs after walking due to narrowing of the arteries; see page 106),[20–28] as well as **congestive heart failure** (see page 54).[29–32] Also a few studies suggest that carnitine may be useful for **cardiomyopathy** (see page 40).[33,34]

Carnitine may also be helpful for improving exercise tolerance in people with **chronic pulmonary obstruction disease** (COPD; see page 45), more commonly known as emphysema.[35,36,37]

Warning: You should not attempt to self-treat any of these serious medical conditions, nor should you use carnitine as a substitute for standard drugs.

Evidence also suggests that one particular form of carnitine, acetyl-L-carnitine, may be helpful in **Alzheimer's disease** (see page 5),[38–44] although a recent large study found no benefit.[45] This form of carnitine may also be helpful for **depression** (see page 59) in the elderly.[46,47]

A genetic condition called fragile X syndrome can cause behavioral disturbances such as hyperactivity, along with mental retardation, autism, and alterations in appearance. A preliminary study of 17 boys found that acetyl-L-carnitine might help to reduce hyperactive behavior associated with this condition.[48]

Additionally, a preliminary study suggests that carnitine may be useful for improving blood sugar control in individuals with type 2 (adult onset) diabetes.[49] It also might help prevent diabetic cardiac autonomic neuropathy (injury to the nerves of the heart caused by diabetes).[50] Weak evidence suggests that carnitine may be able to improve **cholesterol** (see page 88) and triglyceride levels,[51] and also help individuals with degeneration of the cerebellum (the structure of the brain responsible for voluntary muscular movement).[52] One very small study suggests carnitine may be helpful for reducing symptoms of **chronic fatigue syndrome** (see page 44).[53]

Carnitine is widely touted as a physical **performance enhancer** (see page 158), but there is no real evidence that it is effective and some research indicates that it does not work.[54] Little to no evidence supports other claimed benefits such as treating irregular heartbeat, Down's syndrome, muscular dystrophy, impaired sperm motility, alcoholic fatty liver disease, and the toxicity of AZT (a drug used to treat AIDS).[55,56]

WHAT IS THE SCIENTIFIC EVIDENCE FOR CARNITINE?

Angina (Chest Pain)

Carnitine might be a good addition to standard therapy for angina. In one controlled study, 200 individuals with angina (the exercise-induced variety) took either 2 g daily of L-carnitine or were left untreated. All the study participants continued to take their usual medication for angina. Those taking carnitine showed improvement in several measures of heart function, including a significantly greater ability to exercise without chest pain.[57] They were also able to reduce the dosage of some of their heart medications (under medical supervision) as their symptoms decreased. Similarly positive results were seen in a double-blind trial.[58]

Other studies using L-propionyl-carnitine have also found benefits.[59–62]

Intermittent Claudication

People with advanced hardening of the arteries, or atherosclerosis, often have difficulty walking due to lack of blood flow to the legs. Pain may develop after walking less than half a block. Although carnitine does not increase blood flow, it appears to improve the muscle's ability to function under difficult circumstances.[63] In a double-blind study of 245 individuals with intermittent claudication, those treated with 2 g daily of L-propionyl-carnitine showed a 73% improvement in walking distance.[64] This result is not quite as good as it sounds, because there was a 46% improvement with placebo (the power of suggestion is always amazing!), but it was nonetheless significant.

Similar results have been seen in most but not all other studies.[65–72] Interestingly, nearly all the studies on carnitine for this condition have been performed by one investigator. L-propionyl-carnitine seems to be more effective for intermittent claudication than plain carnitine.

For another approach, see the discussion of inositol hexaniacinate in the chapter on **vitamin B₃** (page 437) and the chapter on **ginkgo** (page 298).

Congestive Heart Failure

Several small studies have found that carnitine, often in the form of L-propionyl-carnitine, can improve symptoms of congestive heart failure.[73–76] In one trial, benefits were maintained for 60 days after treatment with carnitine was stopped.[77]

After a Heart Attack

Carnitine may help reduce death rate after a heart attack. In a 12-month placebo-controlled study, 160 individuals who had experienced a heart attack received 4 g of L-carnitine daily or placebo, in addition to other conventional medication. The mortality rate in the treated group was significantly lower than in the placebo group, 1.2% versus 12.5%, respectively. There were also improvements in heart rate, blood pressure, angina (chest pain), and blood lipids.[78] A larger double-blind study of 472 people found that carnitine may improve the chances of survival if given within 24 hours after a heart attack.[79]

Note: Carnitine is used along with conventional treatment, not as a substitute for it.

Chronic Obstructive Pulmonary Disease (COPD)

Evidence from three double-blind placebo-controlled studies enrolling a total of 49 individuals suggests that L-carnitine can improve exercise tolerance in COPD, presumably by improving muscular efficiency in the lungs and other muscles.[80,81,82]

Alzheimer's Disease

Numerous double-blind or single-blind clinical studies involving a total of more than 1,400 people have evaluated the potential benefits of acetyl-L-carnitine in the treatment of Alzheimer's disease and other forms of dementia.[83–93] Most have found at least mildly positive results. However, the benefits are slight at most, and one of the best-designed studies found no benefit.

For example, one double-blind trial followed 130 individuals with mild to moderate Alzheimer's disease for 1 full year.[94] All participants worsened over that time, but according to 14 different measurements of mental function and behavior, the treated group deteriorated more slowly. However, the difference was not very large, and it was only statistically significant for a few of the rating scales used.

Some studies, however, have not found any benefit. In particular, a recent double-blind placebo-controlled trial that enrolled 431 participants for 1 year found no significant improvement at all in the group treated with acetyl-L-carnitine.[95]

The most likely explanation for the negative outcome in this well-designed study is that acetyl-L-carnitine produces only a small benefit at most.

Mild Depression

A double-blind study of 60 seniors with mild depression found that treatment with 3 g of carnitine daily over a 2-month period significantly improved symptoms as compared to placebo.[96] Positive results were seen in another study as well.[97]

Performance Enhancement

A 1996 review of clinical studies concluded that no scientific basis exists for the belief that carnitine supplements enhance athletic performance.[98] A few studies have found some benefit, but most have not.

SAFETY ISSUES

L-carnitine in its three forms appears to be safe, even when taken with medications. Individuals should take care, however, not to use forms of the supplement known as "D-carnitine" or "DL-carnitine," as these can cause angina, muscle pain, and loss of muscle function (probably by interfering with L-carnitine).

The maximum safe dosages for young children, pregnant or nursing women, or those with severe liver or kidney disease have not been established.

⚠ INTERACTIONS YOU SHOULD KNOW ABOUT

If you are taking antiseizure medications, particularly **valproic acid (Depakote, Depakene)** but also **phenytoin (Dilantin),** you may need extra carnitine.

CARTILAGE

Supplement Forms/Alternate Names   Shark Cartilage, Bovine Cartilage

Principal Proposed Uses   There are no well-documented uses for cartilage.

Other Proposed Uses   Cancer Treatment, Osteoarthritis, Minor Wounds, Psoriasis

Cartilage is a tough connective tissue found in many parts of the body. Your ears and nose are made from cartilage, and so is the gliding surface in your joints.

One constituent of cartilage, chondroitin, is widely used in Europe to treat arthritis (for more information, see the chapter on **chondroitin**). Cartilage itself has also been proposed as a treatment for arthritis.

The most commonly used forms of cartilage come from cows (bovine cartilage) and sharks. Provocative evidence suggests that shark cartilage might have some value in the treatment of cancer. However, properly designed studies have not yet been completed to tell us whether it really works.

SOURCES

Unless your uncle works at a slaughterhouse or you're brave enough to prepare your own cartilage from whole sharks, the preferred source of cartilage is your health food store or pharmacy, where you can purchase this supplement in pill or powdered form.

THERAPEUTIC DOSAGES

Various doses of cartilage have been used in different studies, ranging from 2.5 mg to 60 g daily.

THERAPEUTIC USES

Based on the belief that sharks don't get cancer, shark cartilage has been heavily marketed as a cure for cancer. While this is a myth (sharks do get cancer), shark cartilage has, in fact, shown some promise. Shark cartilage tends to inhibit the growth of new blood vessels (angiogenesis). Since cancers must build new blood vessels to feed themselves, this effect might be beneficial. Double-blind studies on shark cartilage for cancer are now under way.

Shark cartilage also inhibits substances called matrix metalloproteases (MMPs).[1] These little-understood enzymes affect the "extracellular matrix," the framework of substances that lie between cells in the body. MMPs are thought to play a role in diseases of the cornea, gums, skin, blood vessels, and joints, as well as cancer and illnesses that involve excessive fibrous tissue.

Weak evidence suggests that shark cartilage might be helpful for **psoriasis** (see page 148).[2]

Cartilage in general has been proposed as a treatment for the common "wear and tear" type of arthritis known as **osteoarthritis** (see page 132). The idea behind this is straightforward: Because osteoarthritis is a disease of the joints, and because cartilage is one of the elements that make up your joints, adding cartilage to the diet might help. This idea sounds a bit too simplistic to be real, but it is the same principle behind the use of **glucosamine** (see page 308) and **chondroitin** (see page 250) (specific substances found in the joints) for osteoarthritis. Since double-blind studies have found those treatments effective, perhaps cartilage itself will ultimately be proven to work. However, studies of cartilage have not yet been performed.

Highly preliminary studies suggest cartilage may help heal **minor wounds** (see page 123).[3]

WHAT IS THE SCIENTIFIC EVIDENCE FOR CARTILAGE?

A number of test tube experiments have found that shark cartilage extracts prevent new blood vessels from forming in chick embryos and other test systems.[4–9] As mentioned above, this effect could conceivably mean that shark cartilage might fight cancer. These findings have led to other test tube experiments, animal studies, and preliminary human trials to investigate the possible anticancer effects of shark cartilage. The results suggest that a particular liquid shark cartilage extract might be useful in the treatment of various cancers, including lung, prostate and breast cancer.[10–15] However, not all studies have been positive.[16,17]

Double-blind trials are needed to provide conclusive data. These are now under way in the United States and Canada.

SAFETY ISSUES

Because cartilage is just common, ordinary gristle, it is presumably safe to consume. However, for reasons that are not at all clear at this time, there is a report of an individual who developed liver inflammation after taking shark cartilage supplements.[18] He recovered fully when the supplements were discontinued.

Cartilage

Visit Us at TNP.com

CATNIP (*Nepeta cataria*)

Alternate or Related Names   Catnep, Catrup, Catmint, Catswort, Field Balm

Principal Proposed Uses   There are no well-documented uses for catnip.

Other Proposed Uses   Insomnia, Nervous Stomach, Indigestion, Irregular Menstruation, Colds

Although catnip has a stimulating effect on virtually all felines, in humans it is traditionally used as a sleep aid. It has also been used for digestive and menstrual problems, as a uterine stimulant in childbirth, and as a symptomatic treatment for colds. Publications from the late 1960s suggested that the plant, when smoked, produced a psychedelic high not unlike marijuana, but it was later discovered that the researchers had, in fact, mistaken the plant for cannabis.[1,2]

WHAT IS CATNIP USED FOR TODAY?

One ingredient of catnip, trans-cis-nepetalactone, is the active ingredient as far as cats are concerned. Most (but not all) cats respond to this substance with a complex reaction called the "catnip response" that can go on for about an hour.

Nepetalactone is similar to a class of substances called valepotriates, found in the sedative herb **valerian** (see page 428).[3] This has attracted some attention, as valerian also is used for insomnia and stomach discomfort (especially when caused by **stress;** see page 167). However, as valepotriates are no longer considered to be the active

ingredients in valerian, it is not clear that this relationship has any significance.

As yet, there is no real evidence that catnip produces any effect at all in humans. Tests conducted on chicks and rats have produced conflicting results, although high doses of catnip oil have increased sleeping times in the latter.[4,5]

DOSAGE

Catnip tea is most commonly made by mixing 1 to 2 teaspoons (1 to 2 g) of the dried herb, or half that amount of the liquid extract, per cup of water (240 ml),[6] and can be consumed up to 3 times a day.

SAFETY ISSUES

Although comprehensive safety studies have not been performed, catnip tea is generally regarded as safe. However, due to its traditional use as a uterine stimulant, pregnant women should not consume catnip except on the advice of a physician. Safety for young children or individuals with severe liver or kidney disease has not been established.

CAT'S CLAW (*Uncaria tomentosa*)

Alternate or Related Names   Una de Gato, Paraguaya, Garbato, Tambor hausca, Toron

Principal Proposed Uses
   Various Viral Diseases: Genital and Oral Herpes, Shingles (Herpes Zoster), AIDS, Feline Leukemia Virus
   Allergies, Arthritis, Ulcers

Cat's claw is a popular herb among the indigenous people of Peru, where it is used to treat cancer, diabetes, ulcers, arthritis, and infections, as well as assist in recovery from childbirth. It is also used as a contraceptive.

Scientific studies of cat's claw conducted in Peru, Italy, Austria, and Germany have yielded numerous intriguing findings but as yet no conclusive proof of any healing benefit. Nonetheless, with increasing international popularity, cultivation of cat's claw has become a major revenue source for the Ashaninka Indian tribe of Peru.

WHAT IS CAT'S CLAW USED FOR TODAY?

In Europe and Peru, cat's claw is considered a promising treatment for viral diseases such as **herpes** (see page 86), **shingles** (see page 156), AIDS, and feline leukemia virus. Its possible use for treating **allergies** (see page 2), stomach **ulcers** (see page 180), **rheumatoid arthritis** (see page 151), and **osteoarthritis** (see page 132) is also being studied.[1] However, the best description of the present state of affairs is that we don't yet know whether

Catnip

cat's claw really works. It certainly is not a proven treatment for cancer.

DOSAGE

The optimum dosage of cat's claw is not clear. Because of the wide variation in the forms and preparations sold, we recommend following the directions on the product's label.

SAFETY ISSUES

There have not been any reports of serious adverse effects from taking cat's claw. However, full safety studies have not been completed. Safety in young children, pregnant or nursing women, or those with severe liver or kidney disease has not been established.

CAYENNE (Capsicum frutescens, Capsicum annuum)

Alternate or Related Names   Capsicum, Grains of Paradise, African Pepper, Bird Pepper, Chili Pepper, Others

Principal Proposed Uses
Topical Uses: Post-Herpetic Neuralgia, Arthritis, Fibromyalgia, Other Forms of Pain
Oral Uses: Heart Disease, Protecting the Stomach from Irritation Due to Anti-Inflammatory Drugs, Dyspepsia

The capsicum family includes red peppers, bell peppers, pimento, and paprika, but the most famous medicinal member of this family is the common cayenne pepper. The substance capsaicin is the common "hot" ingredient in all hot peppers.

Cayenne and related peppers have a long history of use as digestive aids in many parts of the world, but the herb's recent popularity has, surprisingly, come through conventional medicine.

WHAT IS CAYENNE USED FOR TODAY?

Under the brand name Zostrix, a cream containing concentrated capsaicin has been approved by the FDA for the treatment of the pain that often lingers after an attack of **shingles** (technically, post-herpetic neuralgia; see page 156). There is also some evidence that capsaicin creams may be helpful for relieving various types of arthritis[1,2] as well as other forms of pain, such as **fibromyalgia** (see page 80).[3]

Cayenne pepper taken internally has recently been widely touted as a treatment for heart disease by those who have found it useful for themselves or others, but there is no scientific evidence that it is effective.

Some evidence suggests that oral use of cayenne can protect your stomach against damage caused by anti-inflammatory drugs.[4,5,6]

However, contrary to some reports, cayenne does not appear to be able to kill *Helicobacter pylori*, the stomach bacteria implicated as a major cause of ordinary **ulcers** (see page 180).[7]

Capsaicin, is sometimes recommended for indigestion; however, results from a small crossover placebo-controlled study of 11 individuals suggest that 5 mg capsaicin taken before a high-fat meal did not affect gastric function or **dyspepsia** (see page 71) symptoms.[8]

DOSAGE

Capsaicin creams are approved over-the-counter drugs and should be used as directed.

For internal use, cayenne may be taken at a dosage of 1 to 2 standard 00 gelatin capsules 1 to 3 times daily.

SAFETY ISSUES

As a commonly used food, cayenne is generally recognized as safe. Contrary to some reports, cayenne does not appear to aggravate stomach ulcers.[9]

⚠ INTERACTIONS YOU SHOULD KNOW ABOUT

If you are taking
- The asthma drug **theophylline:** Cayenne might increase the amount you absorb, possibly leading to toxic levels.[10]
- **Nonsteroidal anti-inflammatory drugs:** Cayenne might protect your stomach from damage.

CHAMOMILE German *(Matricaria recutita)*;
Roman *(Chamaemelum nobile)*

Alternate or Related Names
German: Pin Heads, Chamomilla, Chamomile, Single Chamomile, Hungarian Chamomile
Roman: Ground Apple, Whig Plant, English Chamomile

Principal Proposed Uses
Topical Uses: Skin Inflammation (Dermatitis, Eczema, Etc.), Wound Healing, Inflammation of the Mouth
Oral Uses: Gastrointestinal Discomfort, Tension and Stress

Probably Ineffective Uses   Mouth Sores Due to the Chemotherapy Drug 5-FU, Postradiation Skin Inflammation

Two distinct plants are known as chamomile and are used interchangeably: German and Roman chamomile. Although botanically far apart, they both look like miniature daisies and are traditionally thought to possess similar medicinal benefits.

Over a million cups of chamomile tea are drunk daily, testifying to its good taste at least. Chamomile was used by early Egyptian physicians for fevers, and by ancient Greeks, Romans, and Indians for headaches and disorders of the kidneys, liver, and bladder.

WHAT IS CHAMOMILE USED FOR TODAY?

The modern use of chamomile dates back to 1921, when a German firm introduced a topical form of chamomile named Kamillosan. This cream became a popular treatment for a wide variety of skin disorders, including eczema, bedsores, postradiation therapy skin inflammation, and contact dermatitis (e.g., poison ivy). Today, Germany's Commission E authorizes the use of various topical chamomile preparations for a variety of diseases of the skin and mouth.

The Commission E has also authorized oral chamomile as a treatment for pain and inflammation in the stomach and intestines, and inhaled chamomile vapor for **asthma** (see page 14) and other lung problems.

Chamomile tea remains popular for mild tension and **stress** (see page 167). It also might possibly help protect the stomach against irritation caused by alcohol or anti-inflammatory drugs, but this has not been proven.[1]

Concentrated alcohol extracts of chamomile are sometimes used to treat the pain caused by various types of arthritis. It has been suggested that chamomile's reported benefits are due to the constituents of its bright blue oil, including chamazulene, alpha-bisabolol, and bisaboloxides. However, the water-soluble part of chamomile may possess some relaxant properties.[2]

WHAT IS THE SCIENTIFIC EVIDENCE FOR CHAMOMILE?

Animal research suggests that chamomile extracts taken orally can relax the intestines and reduce inflammation.[3] Nonetheless, properly performed double-blind studies are largely lacking.

Numerous case reports and poorly designed or reported studies claim benefits of chamomile cream in inflammatory skin diseases and **wound healing** (see page 123).[4] For example, one double-blind study of 161 individuals found chamomile cream equally effective as 0.25% hydrocortisone cream for the treatment of eczema.[5] However, the report didn't state whether doctors or patients were blinded as to which treatment was which, so it isn't clear how reliable the results may be.

Another double-blind placebo-controlled trial by the same authors, involving 72 individuals with eczema, found somewhat odd results: In this trial, chamomile was not significantly more effective than placebo, but both were better than 0.5% hydrocortisone cream.[6] It is difficult to interpret what these results actually mean, but they certainly cannot be taken as proof that chamomile cream is effective.

A recent double-blind placebo-controlled trial of 164 individuals found that chamomile mouthwash was not effective for treating the mouth sores caused by chemotherapy with the drug 5-FU.[7] Negative results were also seen in a physician-blind trial of chamomile cream to reduce skin inflammation caused by radiation therapy.[8] Fifty women receiving radiation therapy for breast cancer were treated with either chamomile or placebo. No differences in radiation-induced skin damage between the two groups were seen.

DOSAGE

Chamomile cream is applied to the affected area 1 to 4 times daily.

Chamomile tea can be made by pouring boiling water over 2 to 3 heaping teaspoons of flowers and steeping for 10 minutes.

Chamomile tinctures and pills should be taken according to the directions on the label. Alcoholic tincture may be the most potent form for internal use.

SAFETY ISSUES

Chamomile is listed on the FDA's GRAS (generally recognized as safe) list.

Reports that chamomile can cause severe reactions in people allergic to ragweed have received significant media attention. However, when all the evidence is examined, it does not appear that chamomile is actually more allergenic than any other plant.[9] The cause of these reports may be products contaminated with "dog chamomile," a highly allergenic and bad-tasting plant of similar appearance.

Chamomile also contains naturally occurring coumarin compounds that can act as "blood thinners." Excessive use of chamomile is therefore not recommended when taking prescription anticoagulants.

Safety in young children, pregnant or nursing women, or those with liver or kidney disease has not been established, although there have not been any credible reports of toxicity caused by this common beverage tea.

⚠ INTERACTIONS YOU SHOULD KNOW ABOUT

If you are taking blood-thinning medications such as **Coumadin (warfarin), heparin,** or **Trental (pentoxifylline),** you should avoid using chamomile as it might increase their effect. This could potentially cause problems.

CHASTEBERRY (*Vitex agnus-castus*)

Principal Proposed Uses Cyclic Breast Discomfort (Often Associated with PMS), Other PMS Symptoms, Menstrual Irregularities, Female Infertility

Other Proposed Uses Menopausal Symptoms

Chasteberry is frequently called by its Latin names: *vitex* or, alternatively, *agnus-castus*. A shrub in the verbena family, chasteberry is commonly found on riverbanks and nearby foothills in central Asia and around the Mediterranean Sea. After its violet flowers have bloomed, a dark brown, peppercorn-size fruit with a pleasant odor reminiscent of peppermint develops. This fruit is used medicinally.

As the name implies, for centuries chasteberry was thought to counter sexual desire. A drink prepared from the plant's seeds was used by the Romans to diminish libido, and in ancient Greece, young women celebrating the festival of Demeter wore chasteberry blossoms to show that they were remaining chaste in honor of the goddess. Monks in the Middle Ages used the fruit for similar purposes, yielding the common name "monk's pepper."

WHAT IS CHASTEBERRY USED FOR TODAY?

The modern use of chasteberry dates back to the 1950s, when the German pharmaceutical firm Madaus Company first produced a standardized extract. This herb has become a standard European treatment for the cyclical breast tenderness that is often associated with PMS, which is sometimes called cyclic mastitis, **cyclic mastalgia** (see page 58), mastodynia, or fibrocystic breast disease. Chasteberry is also used for general **PMS** (see page 145) symptoms, as well as menstrual irregularities.

Research has shown that, unlike other herbs used for women's health problems, chasteberry does not contain any plant equivalent of estrogen or progesterone. Rather, it acts on the pituitary gland to suppress the release of prolactin.[1–4] Prolactin is a hormone that naturally rises during pregnancy to stimulate milk production. Inappropriately increased production of prolactin may be a factor in cyclic breast tenderness, as well as other symptoms of PMS. Elevated prolactin levels can also cause a woman's period to become irregular and even stop. For this reason, chasteberry is often tried for irregular or absent menstrual flow. However, we recommend that you do not attempt to self-treat significant menstrual irregularities without a full medical evaluation. There could be a serious medical condition causing the problem that you wouldn't want to miss.

High prolactin levels can also cause **infertility** (see page 79). For this reason, chasteberry is sometimes tried as a fertility drug;[5] however, the one double-blind study performed to evaluate this possible use was too small to return conclusive results.[6]

Finally, chasteberry is sometimes used for **menopausal symptoms** (see page 117), but there is no evidence that it is effective.

Chasteberry

Visit Us at TNP.com

Chasteberry

WHAT IS THE SCIENTIFIC EVIDENCE FOR CHASTEBERRY?

Despite its widespread use in Germany, the scientific record for chasteberry is not as strong as it should be.

Premenstrual Syndrome (PMS)

German gynecologists clearly believe that chasteberry is effective for PMS. In two rather informal studies enrolling about 3,000 women with PMS, doctors rated chasteberry as effective about 90% of the time.[7,8] Women reported significant or complete improvement in such symptoms as breast pain, fluid retention, headache, and fatigue.

However, this study did not involve a placebo group, and all the patients knew they were being treated. It is impossible to tell from the results what fraction of the benefit was due to the power of suggestion alone. It is a known fact that placebo treatment is highly effective for PMS, often reducing symptoms by as much as 70%.[9] Thus, the results of this study are more a survey of physicians' experiences with chasteberry than actual scientific evidence.

The opinion of experienced physicians is meaningful, but it's definitely not proof. Decades of experience have shown us how easy it is for even seasoned professionals to over- or underestimate the effectiveness of a treatment based on their preconceptions and the power of suggestion. When it comes to medical treatments, well-designed scientific studies are required to produce dependable evidence.

However, a search of medical literature failed to find any double-blind placebo-controlled studies that directly evaluated the benefits of chasteberry for PMS symptoms. One double-blind study has been performed, but unfortunately it compared chasteberry to **vitamin B$_6$** (pyridoxine; see page 439) instead of a placebo.[10]

Published in 1997, this study followed 175 women who were given either a standardized chasteberry extract or 200 mg of vitamin B$_6$ daily. Chasteberry proved to be at least as effective as vitamin B$_6$. Both treatments produced significant improvements in all major symptoms of PMS, including breast tenderness, edema, tension, headache, and depression.

Although this study has been widely described as evidence that chasteberry is effective for PMS, it doesn't ac-

tually prove anything at all. Vitamin B$_6$ itself has not been proven effective for PMS.[11] Therefore, the fact that chasteberry works just as well as vitamin B$_6$ establishes little! It is quite possible that much of the improvement seen in both groups was due to the placebo effect. We really need a good, large-scale, double-blind placebo-controlled study to discover just how effective chasteberry is, beyond the inevitable effects of suggestion.

Irregular Menstruation

One double-blind trial followed 52 women with a form of irregular menstruation known as *luteal phase defect*.[12] This condition is believed to be related to excessive prolactin release. After 3 months, the women who took chasteberry showed significant improvements.

DOSAGE

The typical dose of dry chasteberry extract is 20 to 40 mg given once a day. Chasteberry is sold often as a liquid extract to be taken at a dosage of 40 drops each morning. However, extracts that require higher or lower dosing are also available. We recommend following the label instructions.

SAFETY ISSUES

There haven't been any detailed studies of the safety of chasteberry. However, its widespread use in Germany has not led to any reports of significant adverse effects,[13] other than a single case of excessive ovarian stimulation possibly caused by chasteberry.[14]

Because it lowers prolactin levels, chasteberry is not an appropriate treatment for pregnant or nursing women. Safety in young children or those with severe liver or kidney disease has not been established.

There are no known drug interactions associated with chasteberry. However, it is quite conceivable that the herb could interfere with other hormonal medications.

⚠ INTERACTIONS YOU SHOULD KNOW ABOUT

If you are taking **hormones** or **drugs that affect the pituitary,** such as **bromocriptine,** it is possible that chasteberry might interfere with their action.

CHITOSAN

Supplement Forms/Alternate Names   Chitin (Chitosan is the deacetylated form)

Principal Proposed Uses   High Cholesterol

Other Proposed Uses   Kidney Failure, Salt-Induced Hypertension (when combined with Alginic Acid)
   Topical Uses: Wound Healing, Antimicrobial

Chitosan, a form of chitin chemically processed from crustacean shells, appears to reduce blood cholesterol levels. Like other forms of fiber such as oat bran, chitosan is not well digested by the human body. As it passes through the digestive tract, it seems to have an ability to bond with ingested fat and carry it out in the stool. This suggests a promising use for the supplement. Just imagine: if it worked, you could eat as much fatty, high cholesterol food as you wanted without the undesirable rise in cholesterol! An exaggeration, no doubt, but chitosan may prove to be useful in lowering cholesterol.

Chitosan has also been tried as an aid in kidney failure and wound healing.

Note: We do not recommend the use of chitosan in children or pregnant women due to concerns about possible growth retardation (see Safety Issues).

REQUIREMENTS/SOURCES

Chitosan can be extracted from the shells of shrimp, crab, or lobster. It is also found in yeast and some fungi. Another inexpensive source of chitin is "squid pens," a by-product of squid processing; these are small, plastic-like, inedible pieces of squid that are removed prior to eating.

THERAPEUTIC DOSAGES

The standard dosage of chitosan is 3 to 6 g per day, to be taken with food.

Chitosan can deplete the body of certain minerals (see Safety Issues). For this reason, when using chitosan, it may be helpful to take supplemental calcium, vitamin D, selenium, magnesium, and other minerals.

Also, according to a preliminary study in rats, taking **vitamin C** (see page 444) along with chitosan might provide additional benefit in lowering cholesterol.[1]

THERAPEUTIC USES

Evidence from animal studies and preliminary trials in humans suggests that chitosan can lower **cholesterol** (see page 88) levels.[2–5] In addition, it may raise levels of high-density lipoprotein, or HDL ("good") cholesterol.

Chitosan is thought to work against cholesterol by making it harder for the body to absorb fat.[6,7]

Chitosan may also be helpful in kidney failure.[8] In this case, it is thought to work by binding with toxins in the digestive tract and causing them to be excreted.

Studies in dogs have found that topically applied chitosan can help heal **wounds** (see page 123).[9] This effect might be due to stimulation of new tissue growth; in addition, topical chitosan appears to kill bacteria such as *Streptococcus* and yeast such as *Candida albicans,* which may also contribute to wound healing.[10]

Highly preliminary evidence suggests that oral chitosan may inhibit the expected rise in blood pressure after a high salt meal.[11] It has also been suggested that chitosan can stimulate the immune system and help fight tumors,[12] but there is no real evidence as yet that it works in these ways. Animal studies suggest that some forms of chitosan may help to prevent bone loss;[13] however, because chitosan also interferes with mineral absorption, the net effect in humans might actually be to increase bone loss (see Safety Issues below).

WHAT IS THE SCIENTIFIC EVIDENCE FOR CHITOSAN?

High Cholesterol

In one preliminary placebo-controlled crossover study (apparently blinded, but this was not stated), researchers gave chitosan in biscuits to 8 healthy adult men. The chitosan dose was 3 to 6 g daily during 2 ingestion periods equaling 14 days total over a 4-week time span.[14] Results showed a statistically significant reduction in total cholesterol and an increase in HDL ("good") cholesterol as compared to placebo. Cholesterol reduction was also seen in a controlled but unblinded study of 80 individuals with kidney failure.[15]

This research in humans supports evidence previously found in several animal studies.[16–21]

Kidney Failure

Individuals with kidney failure experience numerous health problems, including anemia, fatigue, and loss of appetite. In one unblinded study, researchers tested chitosan supplements in 80 people with kidney failure receiving ongoing hemodialysis treatment. Half the participants were given 45 mg tablets for a total of about 1,500 mg of chitosan daily for 12 weeks; the other half were not given a supplement.[22] Those in the treatment group showed a significant decrease in urea and creatinine levels. Further, they had a rise in hemoglobin levels and reported improved overall strength, appetite, and sleep as well. (Cholesterol levels were also reduced, as described above.)

SAFETY ISSUES

There is significant evidence that long-term, high-dose chitosan supplementation can result in malabsorption of some crucial vitamins and minerals including **calcium** (see page 234), **magnesium** (see page 351), **selenium** (see page 407) and **vitamins A** (see page 432), **D** (see page 449), **E** (see page 451), and **K** (see page 456).[23,24] In turn, this appears to lead to a risk of osteoporosis in adults and growth retardation in children. For this reason, adults taking chitosan should also take supplemental vitamins and minerals, making especially sure to get enough vitamin D, calcium, and magnesium.

Another possible risk of long-term ingestion of high doses of chitosan is that it could change the intestinal flora and allow the growth of unhealthful bacteria.[25]

Pregnant or nursing women and young children should probably avoid chitosan altogether.

CHOLINE

Principal Proposed Uses   There are no well-documented uses for choline.

Other Proposed Uses   Alzheimer's Disease, Other Neurological Conditions, High Cholesterol, HIV Support, Liver Disease, Cancer Prevention

Choline has only recently been recognized as an essential nutrient. Choline is part of the neurotransmitter acetylcholine, which plays a major role in the brain; for this reason, many studies have been designed to look at choline's role in brain function.

Choline functions as a part of a major biochemical process in the body called "methylation"; choline acts as a "methyl donor." Until recently, it was thought that the body could use other substances to substitute for choline, such as **folate** (see page 288), vitamins B_6 (see page 439) and B_{12} (see page 442), and the amino acid **methionine** (see page 360). But recent evidence has finally shown that, for many people, adequate choline supplies cannot be maintained by other nutrients, and must be obtained independently through diet or supplements.[1,2,3]

REQUIREMENTS/SOURCES

Choline is widespread in the foods we eat. The average diet provides about 500 to 1,000 mg of choline per day.[4,5] Lecithin, a fatty constituent in foods, is a major source of choline; it is comprised mostly of a type of choline called phosphatidylcholine (PC). (Lecithin and PC have been studied separately as treatments for a variety of illnesses; for more information on these supplements, see the full chapter on **lecithin**.)

According to U.S. and Canadian guidelines, the recommended daily intake of choline is as follows:

- Infants 0–5 months, 125 mg
    6–11 months, 150 mg
- Children 1–3 years, 200 mg
    4–8 years, 250 mg
    9–13 years, 375 mg
- Males 14 years and older, 550 mg
- Females 14–18 years, 400 mg
    19 years and older, 425 mg
- Pregnant women, 450 mg
- Nursing women, 550 mg
- Tolerable upper intake level (UL) for adults, 3.5 g°

°The "tolerable upper intake level" can be thought of as the highest daily intake over a prolonged time known to pose no risks to most members of a healthy population.

THERAPEUTIC DOSAGES

Most studies of choline as a treatment for diseases have used between 1 and 30 g of choline or choline-containing supplements per day. This wide range is due to the existence of several different types of choline supplements, all with varying amounts of the active ingredient.

THERAPEUTIC USES

Choline, as well as phosphatidylcholine and lecithin, has been studied quite extensively in people with **Alzheimer's disease** (see page 5) and other conditions

Choline

Visit Us at TNP.com

involving the brain. As noted above, this research is based on the fact that an important neurotransmitter, acetylcholine, is made from choline. We know that eating a lot of choline raises blood levels of choline, but we don't know the degree to which this enhances acetylcholine levels and, ultimately, brain function.[6–14]

Indeed, choline alone does not appear to diminish Alzheimer's symptoms in studies of people diagnosed with the disease,[15–19] nor does it appear to improve normal memory and cognition, or symptoms of **bipolar disorder** (see page 27), mania, or **tardive dyskinesia** (see page 176).[20–26]

Choline's reputation as a cholesterol-lowering agent has been extensively studied in trials involving lecithin. Studies showing a positive effect from choline were poorly controlled and lacked a placebo group;[27,28] well-designed studies do not support the claim that choline can reduce cholesterol levels.[29,30] However, preliminary evidence suggests choline—in concert with other methyl donors like folate, methionine, and vitamins B_{12} and B_6—may help to lower homocysteine levels, which could in turn help prevent **heart disease** (see page 16).[31,32]

Evidence suggests that individuals with HIV who are low in choline may experience more rapid disease progression.[33]

Numerous studies have found that diets very low in choline lead to impaired liver function.[34–39] But these diets are contrived: one would have to work very hard to get so little choline in the diet! To what degree additional choline may benefit people with pre-existing liver damage is an area of ongoing research. In one study, liver function improved in people with hepatitis who were given choline supplements,[40] but in another study, the same supplement failed to show improvements in individuals with hepatitis.[41] A study of malnourished hospitalized people with cirrhosis showed an improvement in several important measurements of liver function when choline supplements were given.[42]

Finally, there are theoretical reasons to believe that choline might have cancer-preventive properties. The notion stems from its function as a methyl donor. Methyl units are essential for RNA and DNA replication—a process ongoing in every cell of the body. The theory goes like this: diets lacking sufficient methyl donors (such as choline) may cause an error in RNA or DNA synthesis, leading to a mutated gene and, hypothetically, to cancer initiation.[43,44] Indeed, in rats fed diets very low in choline and other methyl donors, cancer rates increased.[45,46] However, as noted above in the discussion of liver disease, it is a long step from the effects of an artificially low-choline diet to taking choline supplements.

WHAT IS THE SCIENTIFIC EVIDENCE FOR CHOLINE?

Note: Many of the studies below used PC or lecithin instead of choline. However, because these substances break down to form choline, they are discussed here as well.

Several studies in the early 1980s examined supplemental lecithin in people diagnosed with Alzheimer's disease.[47,48,49] Although the groups studied were small (from 11 to 37 people), these were all double-blind placebo-controlled trials. After 3 to 6 months, no differences in cognitive function could be detected in those getting choline compared to placebo. More promising may be choline in combination with other drugs, or pharmaceutical derivatives of choline. A 1989 Canadian study combined lecithin with tetrahydroaminoacridine (THA), a drug that effectively improves symptoms associated with Alzheimer's disease but is toxic to the liver at high doses.[50] By combining THA with lecithin (3.4 g per day), researchers were able to use lower doses of the drug and achieve comparable improvements in symptoms of Alzheimer's.

Citicholine, a chemical related to choline, has also been studied for treating Alzheimer's disease, with some success.

In other areas of brain function, two studies showed some benefit from lecithin or pure choline in people with mania or bipolar disorder respectively, but these studies were small and poorly controlled.[51,52] Two other small double-blind placebo-controlled studies examined the effects of lecithin in people with tardive dyskinesia but found no substantial improvement in symptoms.[53,54]

Finally, studies in rats and mice found enhanced brain function in animals fed supplemental choline.[55,56] But in studies of healthy adults given lecithin as well as in observational trials evaluating dietary choline intake, little to no benefit was seen.[57,58]

SAFETY ISSUES

When taken at nutritional doses as recommended above (see Requirements/Sources), choline supplementation is safe. In higher dosages, minor but annoying side effects may occur, such as abdominal discomfort, diarrhea, and nausea. Maximum safe dosages for young children, pregnant or nursing women, or those with severe liver or kidney disease have not been determined.

Choline

Visit Us at TNP.com

CHONDROITIN

Supplement Forms/Alternate Names   Chondroitin Sulfate

Principal Proposed Uses   Osteoarthritis

Other Proposed Uses   Atherosclerosis, High Cholesterol

Chondroitin sulfate is a naturally occurring substance in the body. It is a major constituent of cartilage—the tough, elastic connective tissue found in the joints.

Based on the evidence of preliminary double-blind studies, chondroitin is widely used in Europe as a treatment for osteoarthritis, the "wear and tear" arthritis that many people suffer as they get older.

Furthermore, chondroitin may go beyond treating symptoms and actually protect joints from damage. Current medical treatments for osteoarthritis, such as NSAIDs (nonsteroidal anti-inflammatory drugs), treat the symptoms but don't actually slow the disease's progression, and they may actually make it get worse faster.[1–5] Chondroitin (along with glucosamine and SAMe) may take the treatment of osteoarthritis to a new level. However, more research needs to be performed to prove definitively that this exciting possibility is real.

SOURCES

Chondroitin is not an essential nutrient. Animal cartilage is the only dietary source of chondroitin. (When it's on your plate, animal cartilage is called gristle.) Unless you enjoy chewing gristle, you'd do best to obtain chondroitin in pill form from a health food store or pharmacy.

THERAPEUTIC DOSAGES

The usual dosage of chondroitin is 400 mg taken 3 times daily. Be patient! The results take weeks to develop. In commercial products it is often combined with **glucosamine** (see page 308). Preliminary information from one animal study suggests that this combination may be superior to either treatment alone.[6]

There are large differences between chondroitin products based on their chemical structure. This can be expected to lead to significant differences in absorption and hence effectiveness.[7] It may be advisable to use the exact products that were tested in double-blind trials.

THERAPEUTIC USES

Initially, chondroitin was primarily used in an injectable form. But in recent years, double-blind studies using the oral form of chondroitin for **osteoarthritis** (see page 132) have been reported.[8,9,10] The best evidence is for a pain-relieving effect, but some studies have found that it can also slow the progression of the disease.[11–14]

Chondroitin has also been proposed as a treatment for other conditions such as **atherosclerosis** (see page 16) and high **cholesterol** (see page 88), but as yet the evidence that it might help is quite preliminary.[15,16]

WHAT IS THE SCIENTIFIC EVIDENCE FOR CHONDROITIN?

For years, experts stated that oral chondroitin couldn't possibly work, because its molecules are so big that it seemed doubtful that they could be absorbed through the digestive tract. However, in 1995 researchers laid this objection to rest when they found evidence that up to 15% of chondroitin is absorbed intact.[17]

Reducing Symptoms of Osteoarthritis

Three recently published double-blind placebo-controlled studies involving a total of about 250 participants suggest that chondroitin can relieve symptoms of osteoarthritis. One enrolled 85 people with osteoarthritis of the knee and followed them for 6 months.[18] Participants received either 400 mg of chondroitin sulfate twice daily or placebo. At the end of the trial, doctors rated the improvement as good or very good in 69% of those taking chondroitin sulfate but in only 32% of those taking placebo.

Another way of comparing the results is to look at maximum walking speed among participants. Whereas individuals in the chondroitin group were able to improve their walking speed gradually over the course of the trial, walking speed did not improve at all in the placebo group. Additionally, there were improvements in other measures of osteoarthritis, such as pain level, with benefits seen as early as 1 month. This suggests that chondroitin was able to stop the arthritis from gradually getting worse (see also Slowing the Progression of Osteoarthritis).

Similar results were found in another study that was shorter (3 months) but followed more individuals (127 people).[19]

A third double-blind study involved only 42 participants; however, it followed them for a full year.[20] Chondroitin took months to reach its full effect but eventually relieved symptoms considerably better than placebo.

Chondroitin

Visit Us at TNP.com

Positive results were also seen in earlier studies, including one that found chondroitin about as effective as the anti-inflammatory drug dicoflenac.[21–24]

Slowing the Progression of Osteoarthritis

An interesting feature of the full-year study mentioned previously was that, whereas the placebo group showed progressive joint damage over the year, no worsening of the joints was seen in the group taking chondroitin. In other words, chondroitin seemed to protect the joints from damage, thus slowing or perhaps even halting the progression of the disease. Osteoarthritis tends to get worse with time.

As mentioned earlier, no conventional treatment for osteoarthritis protects joints from progressive damage, and some may actually accelerate the process. If further studies confirm that chondroitin prevents progressive damage to the joints, it would make chondroitin distinctly better than any conventional option. Unfortunately, this study was too small to prove anything on its own.

Another, larger study examined the progression of osteoarthritis in 119 people for 3 full years.[25] In this double-blind placebo-controlled trial, those who took 1,200 mg of chondroitin daily showed lower rates of severe joint damage. Only 8.8% of the chondroitin group developed severely damaged joints during the 3 years of the study, compared with almost 30% of the placebo group. This suggests that chondroitin was slowing the progression of osteoarthritis. Unfortunately, the researchers did not report whether this difference was statistically significant.

Additional evidence comes from animal studies. The effect of both oral and injected chondroitin was assessed in rabbits with damaged cartilage in the knee.[26] After 84 days of treatment, the rabbits that were given chondroitin had significantly more healthy cartilage remaining in the damaged knee than the untreated animals. Receiving chondroitin by mouth was as effective as taking it through an injection.

Putting all this information together, it appears quite likely that chondroitin can slow the progression of osteoarthritis. However, more studies are needed to confirm this very exciting possibility. It would also be wonderful if chondroitin could repair damaged cartilage and thus reverse arthritis, but none of the research so far shows such an effect. Chondroitin may simply stop further destruction from occurring.

How Does Chondroitin Work for Osteoarthritis?

Scientists are unsure how chondroitin sulfate works, but one of several theories (or all of them) might explain its mode of action.

At its most basic level, chondroitin may help cartilage by providing it with the building blocks it needs to repair itself. It is also believed to block enzymes that break down cartilage in the joints.[27,28] Another theory holds that chondroitin increases the amount of hyaluronic acid in the joints.[29] Hyaluronic acid is a protective fluid that keeps the joints lubricated. Finally, chondroitin may have a mild anti-inflammatory effect.[30]

SAFETY ISSUES

Chondroitin sulfate has not been associated with any serious side effects, which is not surprising when you consider that taking it by mouth is essentially the same as eating gristle. Subjects in clinical trials have found mild digestive distress to be the only real complaint.

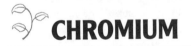

CHROMIUM

Supplement Forms/Alternate Names   Chromium Picolinate, Chromium Polynicotinate, Chromium Chloride, High-Chromium Brewer's Yeast

Principal Proposed Uses   Diabetes, Weight Loss

Other Proposed Uses   Performance Enhancement, High Cholesterol and Triglycerides, Syndrome X, Functional Hypoglycemia, Acne, Migraine Headaches, Psoriasis

Chromium is a mineral the body needs in very small amounts, but it plays an important role in human nutrition. Most of us are more familiar with chromium's industrial uses—for example, to make chrome-plated steel. Chromium's role in maintaining good health was discovered in 1957, when scientists extracted a substance known as *glucose tolerance factor* (GTF) from pork kid-

ney. GTF, which helps the body maintain normal blood sugar levels, contains chromium.

Chromium's most important function is to help regulate the amount of glucose (sugar) in the blood. Insulin plays a starring role in this fundamental biological process, by regulating the movement of glucose out of the blood and into cells. Scientists believe that insulin uses chromium as an assistant (technically, a *cofactor*) to "unlock the door" to the cell membrane, thus allowing glucose to enter the cell.

Based on chromium's close relationship with insulin, this trace mineral has been studied as a treatment for diabetes. The results have been positive: chromium supplements appear to improve blood sugar control in people with diabetes.

Recent evidence also suggests that chromium supplements might help dieters lose fat.

REQUIREMENTS/SOURCES

No official recommendation for daily intake has been established for chromium, but the Estimated Safe and Adequate Daily Dietary Intake is as follows:

- Infants 0–6 months, 10–40 mcg
  7–12 months, 20–60 mcg
- Children 1–3 years, 20–80 mcg
  4–6 years, 30–120 mcg
- Adults (and children 7 years and older), 50–200 mcg

Many Americans may be chromium-deficient.[1] Preliminary research done by the U.S. Department of Agriculture (USDA) in 1985 found low chromium intakes in a small group of people studied. Although large-scale studies are needed to show whether Americans as a whole are chromium deficient, we do know that many traditional sources of chromium, such as wheat, are depleted of this important mineral during processing.

Some researchers believe that inadequate intake of chromium may be one of the causes of the rising rates of adult-onset diabetes. However, the matter is greatly complicated by the fact that we lack a good test to determine chromium deficiency.[2]

Severe chromium deficiency has only been seen in hospitalized individuals receiving nutrition intravenously. Symptoms include problems with blood sugar control that cannot be corrected by insulin alone.

Another cause of chromium deficiency may be corticosteroid treatment. A very preliminary study found treatment with corticosteroids caused increased loss of chromium in the urine.[3] Perhaps this chromium loss is related to steroid-induced diabetes.

Chromium is found in drinking water, especially hard water, but concentrations vary so widely throughout the world that drinking water is not a reliable source. The most concentrated sources of chromium are brewer's yeast (not nutritional or torula yeast) and calf liver. Two ounces of brewer's yeast or 4 ounces of calf liver supply between 50 and 60 mcg of chromium. Other good sources of chromium are whole-wheat bread, wheat bran, and rye bread. Potatoes, wheat germ, green pep-

per, and apples offer modest amounts of chromium.

Calcium (see page 234) carbonate interferes with the absorption of chromium.[4]

THERAPEUTIC DOSAGES

The dosage of chromium used in studies ranges from 200 to 1,000 mcg daily. However, there may be potential risks in the higher dosages of chromium (see Safety Issues).

THERAPEUTIC USES

Chromium has principally been studied for its possible benefits in improving blood sugar control in people with **diabetes** (see page 65). Reasonably good evidence suggests that people with adult-onset (type 2) diabetes may show some improvement when given appropriate dosages of chromium.[5] One study suggests that chromium may be useful for diabetes that occurs during pregnancy.[6] Chromium also appears to help treat subtle problems with blood sugar control that are too mild to deserve the name "diabetes" but may cause an increased risk of heart disease.[7,8]

Chromium has been sold as a "fat burner" and is also said to help build muscle tissue. While studies evaluating its effects on weight loss are mostly negative, the largest study did find some benefit.[9–17] However, studies evaluating its benefits as a **performance enhancer** (see page 158) or aid to bodybuilding have yielded almost entirely negative results.[18–25]

Weak and contradictory evidence suggests that chromium may lower **cholesterol** (see page 88) and triglyceride levels.[26,27] In individuals taking beta-blockers, chromium may raise levels of HDL ("good") cholesterol.[28]

According to some authorities, impaired blood sugar control, high cholesterol, weight gain, and high blood pressure are all part of a bigger picture, given the mysterious-sounding name Syndrome X. Since chromium may be helpful for the first three of these conditions, chromium deficiency has been proposed as the cause of Syndrome X. However, the entire concept of Syndrome X is controversial, and many experts don't believe that it even exists.

Chromium is often suggested as a treatment for the opposite of diabetes, hypoglycemia (low blood sugar). In reality, this condition may not involve lower-than-normal levels of blood sugar at all but rather an abnormal response to normal changes in blood sugar levels. Possible symptoms include anxiety, sweating, and shakiness, which may develop between meals and are relieved by eating. However, there is no direct evidence that chromium is effective for this condition.

Chromium has also been proposed as a treatment for **acne** (see page 2), **migraine headaches** (see page 120), and **psoriasis** (see page 148), but there is as yet no real evidence that it works.

WHAT IS THE SCIENTIFIC EVIDENCE FOR CHROMIUM?

Diabetes

Moderately strong evidence supports the use of chromium for diabetes. In a recent double-blind placebo-controlled study, 180 people with type 2 diabetes were given placebo, 200 mcg of chromium picolinate daily, or a higher dosage of chromium picolinate—1,000 mcg daily. Individuals taking 1,000 mcg showed marked improvements in blood sugar levels. Lesser but still significant benefits were also seen in the 200-mcg group but not in the placebo group.[29]

Similarly positive results were seen in other small studies.[30,31] However, there have also been negative results.[32,33]

One placebo-controlled study of 30 women with pregnancy-related diabetes found that supplementation with chromium (at a dosage of 4 or 8 mcg chromium picolinate for each kilogram of body weight) significantly improved blood sugar control.[34]

Chromium might also be helpful for treating diabetes caused by corticosteroid treatment.[35,36]

Improved Blood Sugar Control in People Without Diabetes

Small double-blind trials have found that chromium supplementation can improve mild abnormalities in blood sugar control,[37,38,39] although one study found no benefit.[40] Another small double-blind trial found that chromium improved the body's response to insulin among overweight people at risk of developing diabetes.[41] There is growing evidence that mildly impaired blood sugar control increases the risk of heart disease.[42] Chromium supplementation may be appropriate.

Weight Loss

The evidence is mixed on whether chromium is an effective aid in weight loss. While the best-designed and largest study did find benefit, other studies did not.

A 3-month double-blind study of 122 moderately overweight individuals attempting to lose weight found that 400 mcg of chromium daily resulted in an average loss of 6.2 pounds of body fat, as opposed to 3.4 pounds in the placebo group. There was no loss of lean body mass.[43] These results suggest that chromium can help you lose body fat without losing muscle. It may work by helping the body process its insulin more effectively.

However, in one small double-blind placebo-controlled study, chromium picolinate at a dose of 400 mcg actually led to weight *gain* in young obese women.[44] When combined with exercise training, chromium picolinate produced no net effect. Interestingly, 400 mcg of chromium nicotinate combined with exercise did induce weight loss.

A 16-week double-blind placebo-controlled study of 95 Navy personnel found no weight loss or change in lean body mass with 400 mcg of chromium daily.[45]

Negative results were seen in other small double-blind trials as well.[46–49]

SAFETY ISSUES

Chromium appears to be safe when taken at a dosage of 50 to 200 mcg daily.[50] Side effects appear to be rare.

However, chromium is a heavy metal and might conceivably build up and cause problems if taken to excess. There is one report of kidney damage in a person who took 1,200 to 2,400 mcg of chromium for several months; in another report, as little as 600 mcg for 6 weeks was enough to cause damage.[51,52] While these may be relatively rare reactions, physician supervision is recommended when using more than the recommended nutritional intake.

For this reason, the dosage found most effective for individuals with type 2 diabetes—1,000 mcg daily—might present some health risks. It would be advisable to seek medical supervision if you want to take more than 200 mcg daily.

Also, keep in mind that if you have diabetes and chromium is effective, you may need to cut down your dosage of any medication you take for diabetes.[53] Medical supervision is advised.

There has been one report of a severe skin reaction caused by chromium picolinate.[54]

Concerns have also been raised over the use of the picolinate form of chromium in individuals suffering from affective or psychotic disorders, because picolinic acids can change the levels of neurotransmitters.[55] There are also concerns, still fairly theoretical, that chromium picolinate could cause adverse effects on DNA.[56]

The maximum safe dosages of chromium for young children, women who are pregnant or nursing, or those with severe liver or kidney disease have not been established.

⚠ INTERACTIONS YOU SHOULD KNOW ABOUT

If you are taking

- **Calcium carbonate supplements** or **antacids:** You may need extra chromium. You should also separate your chromium supplement and your doses of these substances by at least 2 hours, because they may interfere with chromium's absorption.
- **Corticosteroids:** You may need extra chromium.
- **Oral diabetes medications** or **insulin:** Seek medical supervision before taking chromium because you may need to reduce your dose of these medications.
- **Beta-blockers:** Chromium supplementation may improve levels of HDL ("good") cholesterol.

CINNAMON (*Cinnamomum zeylanicum*)

Alternate or Related Names   Ceylon Cinnamon

Principal Proposed Uses   Appetite Loss, Indigestion

Other Proposed Uses   Antimicrobial

Most Americans consider cinnamon a simple flavoring, but in traditional Chinese medicine, it's one of the oldest remedies, prescribed for everything from diarrhea and chills to influenza and parasitic worms. Cinnamon comes from the bark of a small Southeast Asian evergreen tree and is available as an oil, extract, or dried powder. It's closely related to cassia (*C. cassia*) and contains many of the same components, but the bark and oils from *C. zeyleanicum* have a better flavor.

WHAT IS CINNAMON USED FOR TODAY?

Germany's Commission E approves cinnamon for appetite loss and indigestion; however, these uses are backed by very little scientific evidence.[1]

Two animal studies suggest that an extract of cinnamon bark taken orally may help prevent stomach ulcers.[2,3]

Preliminary results from test tube and animal studies suggest that cinnamon oil and cinnamon extract have antifungal, antibacterial, and antiparasitic properties.[4–10] For example, cinnamon has been found to be active against *Candida albicans*, the fungus responsible for vaginal **yeast infections** (see page 38) and thrush (oral yeast infection), *Helicobacter pylori*, the bacteria that causes **stomach ulcers** (see page 180), and even head lice. However, it's a long way from studies of this type to actual proof of effectiveness. Until cinnamon is tested in double-blind human trials, we can't conclude that it can successfully treat these or any other infections.

Highly preliminary evidence also suggests that cinnamon might have antiallergic and antidiabetic properties.[11,12,13]

DOSAGE

Typical recommended dosages of cinnamon are 2 to 4 g daily of cinnamon bark or 0.05 to 0.2 g daily of essential oil.[14]

SAFETY ISSUES

As a widely used food, cinnamon is believed to be safe. However, cinnamon's essential oil is much more concentrated than the powdered bark commonly used for baking. There is some evidence that high doses of cinnamon oil might depress the central nervous system.[15] Germany's Commission E recommends that pregnant women should avoid taking cinnamon oil or high doses of the bark.[16] Maximum safe doses in young children, nursing women, or individuals with severe liver or kidney disease have not been determined.

When used topically, cinnamon bark oil may cause flushing and a burning sensation.[17] Some people have reported strong burning sensations or mouth ulcers after chewing cinnamon-flavored gum or candy.[18,19] However, these reactions disappeared within days of discontinuing the gum.

CITRUS BIOFLAVONOIDS

Supplement Forms/Alternate Names   Daflon, Diosmetin, Diosmin, Hesperidin, Naringin, Narirutin, Neohesperidin, Nobiletin, Rutin, Tangeretin

Principal Proposed Uses   Hemorrhoids

Other Proposed Uses   Chronic Venous Insufficiency, Easy Bruising, Nosebleeds, Lymphedema Following Breast Cancer Surgery

Cinnamon

Visit Us at TNP.com

Citrus fruits are well known for providing ample amounts of **vitamin C** (see page 444). But they also supply bioflavonoids, substances that are not required for life but that may improve health. The major bioflavonoids found in citrus fruits are diosmin, hesperidin, rutin, naringin, tangeretin, diosmetin, narirutin, neohesperidin, nobiletin, and quercetin.

This chapter addresses the first five bioflavonoids listed above. Please see the chapter on **quercetin** (page 396) for information on this supplement. A modified form of rutin, **oxerutin,** is also discussed in its own chapter.

Citrus bioflavonoids and related substances are widely used in Europe to treat diseases of the blood vessels and lymph system, including **hemorrhoids** (see page 85), **chronic venous insufficiency** (see page 184), **easy bruising** (see page 74), **nosebleeds** (see page 129), and lymphedema following breast cancer **surgery** (see page 173). These compounds are thought to work by strengthening the walls of blood vessels.

REQUIREMENTS/SOURCES

Citrus fruits contain citrus bioflavonoids in varying proportions. Even different brands of citrus juice may vary widely in their bioflavonoid concentrations and composition.[1] For use as a supplement, bioflavonoids are extracted either from citrus fruits or other plant sources, such as buckwheat.

THERAPEUTIC DOSAGES

A typical dosage of citrus bioflavonoids is 500 mg twice daily. The most studied citrus bioflavonoid treatment is a special combination of diosmin (90%) and hesperidin (10%).

THERAPEUTIC USES

Double-blind trials suggest that a micronized combination preparation of diosmin and hesperidin may be helpful for hemorrhoids.[2–6]

Diosmin and hesperidin, as well as the bioflavonoid rutin, may also be helpful for chronic venous insufficiency, a condition in which the veins in the legs begin to weaken.[7–10] The best evidence is for treatment of leg ulcers associated with this condition.[11,12]

At least one good double-blind trial found diosmin and hesperidin also to be helpful for individuals who develop bruises or nosebleeds easily.[13]

Citrus bioflavonoids have also been tried, with some success, for treating lymphedema (arm swelling) following breast cancer surgery.[14]

Note: Do not use bioflavonoid combinations containing tangeretin if you are taking tamoxifen for breast cancer.

In addition, highly preliminary evidence suggests that citrus bioflavonoids may help reduce **cholesterol** (see page 88) levels,[15,16] control inflammation,[17] benefit individuals with **diabetes** (see page 65),[18] reduce **allergic reactions** (see page 2),[19] and **prevent cancer** (see page 32).[20]

WHAT IS THE SCIENTIFIC EVIDENCE FOR CITRUS BIOFLAVONOIDS?

Hemorrhoids

A 2-month double-blind placebo-controlled trial of 120 individuals with recurrent hemorrhoid flare-ups found that treatment with combined diosmin and hesperidin significantly reduced the frequency and severity of hemorrhoid attacks.[21] Another double-blind placebo-controlled trial of 100 individuals had positive results with the same bioflavonoids in relieving symptoms once a flare-up of hemorrhoid pain had begun.[22] A 90-day double-blind trial of 100 individuals with bleeding hemorrhoids also found significant benefits for both treatment of acute attacks and prevention of new ones.[23] Finally, this bioflavonoid combination was found to compare favorably with surgical treatment of hemorrhoids.[24] However, less impressive results were seen in a double-blind placebo-controlled study in which all participants were given a fiber laxative with either combined diosmin and hesperidin or placebo.[25]

Chronic Venous Insufficiency

Unfortunately, most of the studies evaluating a combination of the bioflavonoids diosmin (90%) and hesperidin (10%) as a treatment for chronic venous insufficiency have not been placebo controlled. The best evidence that these bioflavonoids are effective in this condition comes from a 2-month double-blind placebo-controlled trial involving 107 individuals with nonhealing leg ulcers (sores) caused by poor circulation, which found that treatment with diosmin plus hesperidin significantly improved rate of healing.[26]

Also, a 3-month double-blind placebo-controlled trial of 67 individuals evaluated buckwheat tea (a good source of rutin) for chronic venous insufficiency.[27] The results showed less leg swelling in the treated group.

Easy Bruising

Some individuals bruise particularly easily due to fragile capillaries. A 6-week double-blind placebo-controlled study of 96 people with this condition found that combined diosmin and hesperidin decreased symptoms of capillary fragility, such as bruising and nosebleeds.[28]

Two rather poorly designed studies from the 1960s found benefits with a combination of vitamin C and citrus bioflavonoids for decreasing bruising in collegiate athletes.[29]

Coenzyme Q10

SAFETY ISSUES

Extensive investigations of diosmin and hesperidin have found them to be essentially nontoxic and free of drug interactions.[30] The combination has been given to 50 pregnant women in a research study, without apparent harm to mothers or babies.[31]

However, the citrus bioflavonoid tangeretin appears to interfere with the action of tamoxifen, a drug used to treat breast cancer.[32]

One highly preliminary study suggests that citrus bioflavonoids in the diet of pregnant women might increase the risk of infant leukemia; however, hesperidin did not produce this effect, and diosmin was not tested.[33]

⚠ INTERACTIONS YOU SHOULD KNOW ABOUT

If you are taking **tamoxifen** for breast cancer, you should avoid citrus fruits and juices and the citrus bioflavonoid tangeretin.

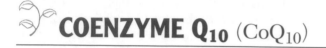

COENZYME Q_{10} (CoQ_{10})

Supplement Forms/Alternate Names   Ubiquinone

Principal Proposed Uses   Congestive Heart Failure, Cardiomyopathy, Other Forms of Heart Disease, Hypertension, Nutrient Depletion/Interference Caused by Various Medications

Other Proposed Uses   Periodontal Disease, Amyotrophic Lateral Sclerosis (Lou Gehrig's Disease), AIDS, Cancer, Diabetes, Male Infertility, Muscular Dystrophy, Obesity, Parkinson's Disease, Performance Enhancement

Coenzyme Q_{10} (CoQ_{10}), also known as ubiquinone, is a powerful antioxidant discovered by researchers at the University of Wisconsin in 1957. The name of this supplement comes from the word *ubiquitous*, which means "found everywhere." Indeed, CoQ_{10} is found in every cell in the body. It plays a fundamental role in the mitochondria, the parts of the cell that produce energy from food.

Japanese scientists first discovered the therapeutic properties of CoQ_{10} in the 1960s. Today, it is widely prescribed for heart conditions in Europe and Israel, as well as in Japan. CoQ_{10} appears to assist the heart during times of stress on the heart muscle, perhaps by helping it use energy more efficiently. While CoQ_{10}'s best-established use is for congestive heart failure, ongoing research suggests that it may also be useful for other types of heart problems and for a wide variety of additional illnesses.

CoQ_{10} supplementation might also be of value while using certain prescription medications.

SOURCES

Every cell in your body needs CoQ_{10}, but no U.S. Dietary Reference Intake (formerly known as the Recommended Dietary Allowance) has been established for this important substance because the body can manufacture CoQ_{10} from scratch.

Because CoQ_{10} is found in all animal and plant cells, we obtain small amounts of this nutrient from our diet. However, it would be hard to get a therapeutic dosage from food.

THERAPEUTIC DOSAGES

The typical recommended dosage of CoQ_{10} is 30 to 300 mg daily, often divided into 2 or 3 doses. CoQ_{10} is fat soluble and is better absorbed when taken in an oil-based soft gel form rather than in a dry form such as tablets and capsules.[1]

THERAPEUTIC USES

The best-documented use of CoQ_{10} is for treating **congestive heart failure** (see page 54).[2,3,4] Keep in mind that it is taken along with conventional medications, not instead of them.

Weaker evidence suggests that it may be useful for **cardiomyopathy** (see page 40) and other forms of **heart disease** (see page 16).[5,6,7] CoQ_{10} has been suggested as a treatment for **hypertension**[8–11] (see page 98) and to prevent the heart damage caused by certain types of cancer chemotherapy. Keep in mind that CoQ_{10} might conceivably interfere with the action of other chemotherapy drugs (although there is no good evidence that it does so). Therefore, if you are a cancer patient, check with your oncologist before using CoQ_{10}.

CoQ_{10} is sometimes claimed to be an effective treatment for **periodontal disease** (see page 142). However, the studies on which this idea is based are too flawed to be taken as meaningful.[12]

Highly preliminary studies suggest CoQ_{10} might be helpful for treating **amyotrophic lateral sclerosis** (see page 9).[13,14]

CoQ_{10} has additionally been proposed as a treatment for a wide variety of other conditions, including AIDS, **angina** (see page 10), cancer, **diabetes** (see page 65), **male infertility** (see page 116), muscular dystrophy, obesity, and **Parkinson's disease** (see page 140), but there is no solid evidence as yet that it is effective. It has also been used as a performance enhancer for athletes (see chapter on **sports performance** for more information). Although one double-blind study of 25 highly trained cross-country skiers found some benefit,[15] most studies evaluating this use have been negative rather than positive.[16–21]

Various medications either interfere with the body's production of CoQ_{10} or interfere with its action. It has been suggested (but not proven) that these effects on CoQ_{10} may play a role in the known side effects of these treatments, and that taking CoQ_{10} supplements might help. The best evidence is for the cholesterol-lowering drugs in the statin family, such as lovastatin (Mevacor), simvastatin (Zocor), and pravastatin (Pravachol).[22–25]

For several other categories of drugs, the evidence that they interfere with CoQ_{10} is provocative but less than solid. These include oral diabetes drugs (especially glyburide, phenformin, and tolazamide), beta-blockers (specifically propranolol, metoprolol, and alprenolol), antipsychotic drugs in the phenothiazine family, tricyclic antidepressants, methyldopa, hydrochlorothiazide, clonidine, and hydralazine.[26–31]

WHAT IS THE SCIENTIFIC EVIDENCE FOR COENZYME Q$_{10}$ (CoQ$_{10}$)?

Congestive Heart Failure

Very good evidence tells us that CoQ_{10} can be helpful for people with congestive heart failure (CHF). In this serious condition, the heart muscles become weakened, resulting in poor circulation and shortness of breath.

People with CHF have significantly lower levels of CoQ_{10} in heart muscle cells than healthy people.[32] This fact alone does not prove that CoQ_{10} supplements will help CHF; however, it prompted medical researchers to try using CoQ_{10} as a treatment for heart failure.

The results have been positive. Several double-blind studies have found that CoQ_{10} supplements can markedly improve symptoms and objective measurements of heart function when they are taken along with conventional medication.

In the largest of these studies, 641 individuals with moderate to severe congestive heart failure were monitored for 1 year.[33] Half were given 2 mg per kilogram body weight of CoQ_{10} daily; the rest were given placebo. Standard therapy was continued in both groups. The participants treated with CoQ_{10} experienced a significant reduction in the severity of their symptoms. No such improvement was seen in the placebo group. The people

who took CoQ_{10} also had significantly fewer hospitalizations for heart failure.

Similarly positive results were also seen in smaller studies involving a total of over 250 participants.[34,35]

However, one 6-month double-blind study of 45 individuals with congestive heart failure found no benefit.[36]

Cardiomyopathy

Cardiomyopathy is the general name given to conditions in which the heart muscle gradually becomes diseased. Several small studies suggest that CoQ_{10} supplements are helpful for some forms of cardiomyopathy.[37,38,39]

Hypertension

An 8-week double-blind placebo-controlled study of 59 men already taking medications for high blood pressure found that 120 mg daily of CoQ_{10} could reduce blood pressure by about 9% as compared to placebo.[40]

Similar results were seen in other trials, most of which were not double-blind.[41,42,43]

SAFETY ISSUES

CoQ_{10} appears to be extremely safe. No significant side effects have been found, even in studies that lasted a year.[44] However, individuals with severe heart disease should not take CoQ_{10} (or any other supplement) except under a doctor's supervision.

One study suggests that CoQ_{10} might reduce blood sugar levels in people with diabetes.[45] While this could potentially be helpful for treatment of diabetes, it might present a risk as well: Diabetics using CoQ_{10} might inadvertently push their blood sugar levels dangerously low. However, another trial in people with diabetes found no effect on blood sugar control.[46] The bottom line: If you have diabetes, make sure to track your blood sugar closely if you start taking CoQ_{10} (or, indeed, any herb or supplement).

Finally, CoQ_{10} might interfere with the anticoagulant effects of Coumadin (warfarin).[47] If you are taking Coumadin, you should not take CoQ_{10} unless under a doctor's supervision.

The maximum safe dosages of CoQ_{10} for young children, pregnant or nursing women, or those with severe liver or kidney disease have not been determined.

⚠ INTERACTIONS YOU SHOULD KNOW ABOUT

If you are taking

- **Cholesterol-lowering drugs** in the statin family, **red yeast rice** (which contains natural statin drugs), **beta-blockers** (specifically **propranolol, metoprolol,** and **alprenolol**), **antipsychotic** drugs in the **phenothiazine family, tricyclic antidepressants, methyldopa, hydrochlorothiazide, clonidine,** or **hydralazine:** You may need more coenzyme Q_{10}.

- **Coumadin (warfarin):** You should not take CoQ_{10} except on a physician's advice.

COLA NUT *(Cola acuminata and Cola nitida)*

Alternate or Related Names   Kola Tree, Guru Nut, Cola, Cola Seeds, Bissy Nut

Principal Proposed Uses   Stimulant

Indigenous to Western Africa, the cola tree is cultivated today in many tropical climates, including Central and South America, the West Indies, Sri Lanka, and Malaysia. Cola nuts are actually seeds removed from their seed coats. Traditionally, they are chewed raw or taken in pulverized or liquid extract form. Of the various species of cola nuts, the two most commonly edible kinds are *Cola acuminata* and *Cola nitida*.

Cola contains caffeine and related chemicals, and for this reason is a stimulant. For thousands of years, people in Africa have chewed the seeds to enhance mental alertness and fight fatigue. Centuries ago, Arabs traded gold dust for cola nuts before starting out on long treks across the Sahara.

Cola nut has been used in folk medicine as an aphrodisiac and an appetite suppressant, and to treat morning sickness, migraine headache, and indigestion. It has also been applied directly to the skin to treat **wounds** (see page 123) and inflammation. The tree's bitter twig has been used as well, to clean the teeth and gums.

WHAT IS COLA NUT USED FOR TODAY?

Based on the cola nut's caffeine content, Germany's Commission E has approved its use for the treatment of fatigue.[1]

Cola is ingested daily by millions as one of the main ingredients in cola soft drinks. It is also used in diet and "high-energy" products such as food bars and as a flavoring in alcoholic beverages, frozen dairy desserts, candy, baked goods, gelatins, and puddings.[2,3] However, the caffeine-containing cola nut, used in original recipes for Coca-Cola should not be confused with **gotu kola** (see full chapter for details).

Because of its caffeine content, cola nut would be expected to increase urination, stimulate the heart and lungs, and help analgesics such as aspirin to function more effectively.

DOSAGE

Germany's Commission E recommends the following daily dosage of cola: 2 to 6 g of cola nut, 0.25 to 0.75 g of cola extract, 2.5 to 7.5 g of cola liquid extract, 10 to 30 g of cola tincture, or 60 to 180 g of cola wine.[4]

SAFETY ISSUES

Although comprehensive safety studies have not been performed, moderate amounts of cola nut are generally regarded as safe. The Council of Europe and the U.S. Food and Drug Administration have approved it as a food additive. The typical side effects associated with cola nut are those of caffeine, including nervousness, heart irregularities, headaches, and sleeplessness.

Cola is not advised for individuals with stomach **ulcers** (see page 180) due both to its caffeine and its tannin content.[5,6] Tannins, found in many plants, are substances that can irritate the stomach.

Cola Nut

Visit Us at TNP.com

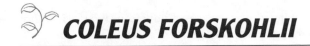

COLEUS FORSKOHLII

Principal Proposed Uses
Allergic Conditions: Asthma, Eczema, Allergies
Muscle Contraction: Asthma, Menstrual Cramps, Irritable Bowel Syndrome (Spastic Colon), Bladder Pain, Hypertension, Glaucoma

Other Proposed Uses   Psoriasis

A member of the mint family, *Coleus forskohlii* grows wild on the mountain slopes of Nepal, India, and Thailand. In traditional Asian systems of medicine, it was used for a variety of purposes, including treating skin rashes, asthma, bronchitis, insomnia, epilepsy, and angina. But modern interest is based almost entirely on the work of a drug company, Hoechst Pharmaceuticals.

Like other drug manufacturers, Hoechst regularly screens medicinal plants in hopes of discovering new medications. In 1974, work performed in collaboration with the Indian Central Drug Research Institute found that the rootstock of *Coleus forskohlii* could lower blood pressure and decrease muscle spasms. Intensive study identified a substance named forskolin that appeared to be responsible for much of this effect.

Like certain drugs used for asthma, forskolin increases the levels of a fundamental natural compound known as cyclic AMP.[1,2] Cyclic AMP plays a major role in many cellular functions, and some drugs that affect it relax the muscles around the bronchial tubes.

WHAT IS *COLEUS FORSKOHLII* USED FOR TODAY?

Herb manufacturers have begun to offer extracts of *Coleus forskohlii* that have been specially manufactured to contain high levels of forskolin.

Forskolin has been found to stabilize the cells that release histamine and other inflammatory compounds.[3] This suggests that *Coleus forskohlii* may be a useful treatment for **asthma** (see page 14), **eczema** (see page 78), and other allergic conditions.

Studies have also found that forskolin relaxes smooth muscle tissue.[4,5] For this reason, *Coleus forskohlii* has been suggested as a treatment for asthma, menstrual cramps or **dysmenorrhea** (see page 70), **angina** (see page 10), **irritable bowel syndrome** (spastic colon; see page 108), crampy bladder pain (as in **bladder infections;** see page 28), and **hypertension** (high blood pressure; see page 98).

Coleus forskohlii has also been proposed as a treatment for **psoriasis** (see page 148), because that disease appears to be at least partly related to low levels of cyclic AMP in skin cells.

WHAT IS THE SCIENTIFIC EVIDENCE FOR *COLEUS FORSKOHLII*?

The scientific evidence for the herb *Coleus forskohlii* as a treatment for any disease is weak. What is known relates to the substance forskolin rather than the whole herb.

Animal studies and open studies in humans suggest that forskolin can reduce blood pressure and dilate bronchial tubes.[6-9] A tiny double-blind study indicates that forskolin taken by inhalation may be as effective as standard asthma inhalers,[10] and forskolin eyedrops appear to improve glaucoma.[11]

DOSAGE

A common dosage recommendation is 50 mg 2 or 3 times a day of an extract standardized to contain 18% forskolin.

However, because such an extract provides significant levels of forskolin, a drug with wide-ranging properties, we recommend that *Coleus forskohlii* extracts be taken only with a doctor's supervision.

SAFETY ISSUES

The safety of *Coleus forskohlii* and forskolin has not been fully evaluated, although few significant risks have been noted in studies performed thus far. Caution should be exercised when combining this herb with blood-pressure medications and "blood thinners." Safety in young children, pregnant or nursing women, or those with severe liver or kidney disease has not been established.

Colostrum

Visit Us at TNP.com

⚠ INTERACTIONS YOU SHOULD KNOW ABOUT

If you are taking blood pressure medications such as **beta-blockers, clonidine,** or **hydralazine,** or blood-thinning drugs such as **Coumadin (warfarin), heparin,** or **Trental (pentoxifylline),** *Coleus forskohlii* should only be used under the supervision of a physician.

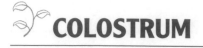

COLOSTRUM

Principal Proposed Uses   Prevention and Treatment of Infectious Diarrhea

Other Proposed Uses   Ulcer Prevention

Colostrum is the fluid that new mothers' breasts produce during the first day or two after birth. It gives newborn infants a rich mixture of antibodies and growth factors that help them get a good start.

Although colostrum has been available since the first mammals walked the earth, it is relatively new as a nutritional supplement. The resurgence of breast-feeding in the 1970s sparked a revival of interest in colostrum for both infants and adults. However, most commercial colostrum preparations come from cows, not humans. Although cows are quite different from humans, bovine colostrum contains a number of substances that can affect the human digestive tract, and can be prepared to contain antibodies against human diseases.

REQUIREMENTS/SOURCES

Breast-feeding is the healthiest way to nourish a newborn, and a mother's colostrum is undoubtedly good for a baby. But don't believe claims (by at least one manufacturer) that most babies would die without colostrum. Colostrum is good for health, but it's not essential for life.

Colostrum has just become available in capsules that contain its immune proteins in dry form.

THERAPEUTIC DOSAGES

The usual recommended dosage of colostrum is 10 g daily.

Note: Most of the studies of colostrum for infectious conditions used colostrum prepared by immunizing cows against specific diseases (hyperimmune colostrum). This form is not generally available as a dietary supplement.

THERAPEUTIC USES

Many, but not all, studies have found that hyperimmune or ordinary colostrum might be able to help prevent or treat various forms of infectious diarrhea.[1–10]

For years, people with **ulcers** (see page 180) were advised to eat a bland diet and drink lots of milk. Although this treatment was eventually found to be ineffective, it does seem that colostrum (although not milk) might help protect the stomach from damage caused by anti-inflammatory drugs, at least according to one study in rats and a small human trial.[11,12] Presumably, the growth factors found in colostrum help stimulate the stomach to regenerate.

Colostrum might also be helpful for short bowel syndrome (a condition following digestive tract surgery), chemotherapy-induced mouth ulcers, and inflammatory bowel disease (**Crohn's disease;** see page 57, and **ulcerative colitis;** see page 179), but as yet there is no real evidence that it is effective.[13]

WHAT IS THE SCIENTIFIC EVIDENCE FOR COLOSTRUM?

Infectious Diarrhea

Preliminary evidence suggests that colostrum might help prevent or possibly treat infectious diarrhea. Most of these studies used colostrum from cows exposed to organisms that cause disease in humans (hyperimmune colostrum).

In a controlled, but not blinded, trial, cows were immunized with rotavirus, a virus that causes diarrhea in children.[14] Colostrum from these cows was then given to 10 infants, while 10 others were not treated. The results indicated that colostrum prepared in this way could help prevent diarrhea. However, once diarrhea started, treatment with colostrum was not helpful.

In contrast, a double-blind placebo-controlled trial of 80 children with rotavirus diarrhea did find that similarly prepared colostrum could reduce symptoms and shorten recovery time.[15] Colostrum prepared by immunizing cows with a monkey form of rotavirus was found ineffective for treating rotavirus in a double-blind trial of 135 children.[16] The difference between these results may lie in the level and type of antibodies found in the colostrum.

Both hyperimmune and normal colostrum have been tried for prevention or treatment of Cryptosporidium infection in people with AIDS, but the evidence that it works is weak at best.[17,18,19]

Other studies suggest that hyperimmune colostrum might help prevent infections with the Shigella parasite,[20] as well as *E. coli* (a common cause of traveler's diarrhea).[21] However, a study looking at Bangladeshi children infected with *Helicobacter pylori* (the organism that causes digestive ulcers) found no benefits with hyperimmune colstrum.[22]

SAFETY ISSUES

Colostrum does not seem to cause any significant side effects. However, comprehensive safety studies have not been performed. Safety in young children or women who are pregnant or nursing has not been established.

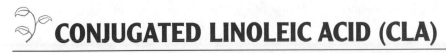

CONJUGATED LINOLEIC ACID (CLA)

Principal Proposed Uses   There are no well-documented uses for conjugated linoleic acid.

Other Proposed Uses   Reducing Body Fat, Diabetes, Cancer Prevention

Conjugated linoleic acid (CLA) is a mixture of different isomers, or chemical forms, of linoleic acid. This is an essential fatty acid—a type of fat that your body needs as much as it needs vitamins. Although it has become popular as a "fat-burning" supplement, we don't really know how or even whether CLA really works.

REQUIREMENTS/SOURCES

Although linoleic acid itself is an important nutritional source of essential fatty acids, there is no evidence that you need to get *conjugated* linoleic acid in your diet. CLA does occur in food, but it would be very difficult to get the recommended dose that way. Supplements are the only practical source.

THERAPEUTIC DOSAGES

The typical dosage of CLA ranges from 3 to 5 g daily. As with all supplements taken at this high a dosage, it is important to purchase a reputable brand, as even very small amounts of a toxic contaminant could quickly mount up.

THERAPEUTIC USES

The evidence that CLA can help you lose fat while retaining muscle is highly preliminary at best.[1–4]

During the course of investigations into its effect on fat, CLA was found to act somewhat similarly to a drug used for **diabetes** (see page 65), thiazolidinedione. This led to research into the possible usefulness of CLA as a treatment for diabetes. In one study, CLA reduced blood sugar levels in diabetic rats as effectively as standard diabetes medications.[5] The same researchers also performed a small double-blind placebo-controlled trial in humans. The results showed that CLA improved insulin responsiveness in people with type 2 (adult onset) diabetes. Although this study is far too preliminary to prove that CLA is effective, it does point to a direction for future research.

Numerous animal and test tube studies suggest that CLA might help prevent cancer.[6]

SAFETY ISSUES

CLA appears to be a safe nutritional substance. However, maximum safe dosages for young children, pregnant or nursing women, or those with severe liver or kidney disease have not been determined.

Conjugated Linoleic Acid (CLA)

Visit Us at TNP.com

COPPER

Supplement Forms/Alternate Names   Copper Sulfate, Copper Picolinate, Copper Gluconate, Copper Complexes of Various Amino Acids

Principal Proposed Uses   There are no well-documented uses for copper.

Other Proposed Uses   Osteoporosis, High Cholesterol, Heart Disease, Osteoarthritis, Rheumatoid Arthritis

The human body contains only 70 to 80 mg of copper, but it's an essential part of many important enzymes. Copper's possible role in treating disease is based on the fact that these enzymes can't do their jobs without it. However, there is little direct evidence that taking extra copper can treat any disease.

REQUIREMENTS/SOURCES

Although a precise dietary requirement for copper has not been determined, the Estimated Safe and Adequate Daily Dietary Intake is as follows:

- Infants 0–6 months, 0.4–0.6 mg
    7–12 months, 0.6–0.7 mg
- Children 1–3 years, 0.7–1.0 mg
    4–6 years, 1.0–1.5 mg
    7–10 years, 1.0–2.0 mg
    11–18 years, 1.5–2.5 mg
- Adults 19 years and older, 1.5–3.0 mg

Excessive **zinc** (see page 463) intake reduces copper stores in the body.[1,2] In addition, if you are taking **iron** (see page 333) or large doses of **vitamin C** (see page 444), you may need extra copper.[3–7] Ideally, you should take copper at least 2 hours apart from these two nutrients, so that they don't interfere with each other's absorption.

Oysters, nuts, legumes, whole grains, sweet potatoes, and dark greens are good sources of copper. Drinking water that passes through copper plumbing is a good source of this mineral, and sometimes it may even provide too much.

THERAPEUTIC DOSAGES

The typical adult supplemental dosage of copper is 1 to 3 mg daily.

THERAPEUTIC USES

Copper has been proposed as a treatment for **osteoporosis** (see page 136), based primarily on studies that found benefit using mixtures of various trace minerals.[8,9]

One researcher, L. M. Klevay, has claimed in more than a dozen papers that copper deficiencies increase the risk of high **cholesterol** (see page 88) and **heart disease** (see page 16), but he has failed to supply any real evidence that this idea is true. A double-blind clinical trial of copper supplements for reducing heart disease risk found no benefit.[10]

Similarly, copper has long been mentioned as a possible treatment for **osteoarthritis** (see page 132) and **rheumatoid arthritis** (see page 151), but there is as yet no real evidence that it works.

SAFETY ISSUES

Copper is safe when taken at nutritional dosages, but these should not be exceeded. As little as 10 mg of copper daily produces nausea, and 60 mg may cause vomiting.

Oral contraceptives might increase levels of copper in the body. Women taking oral contraceptives should consult a physician before taking copper supplements.[11,12,13]

Maximum safe dosages of copper for young children, pregnant or nursing women, or those with severe liver or kidney disease have not been determined.

⚠ INTERACTIONS YOU SHOULD KNOW ABOUT

If you are taking

- **Zinc:** You need to make sure to get enough copper.
- **Iron** supplements, **manganese,** or high doses of **vitamin C:** You may need extra copper. If you do take a copper supplement, it might be ideal to take it either 2 hours before or after these other substances.
- **Oral contraceptives:** It might not be advisable to take extra copper.

CRANBERRY *(Vaccinium macrocarpon)*

Principal Proposed Uses   Bladder Infections (Prevention and Possible Treatment)

Other Proposed Uses   Periodontal Disease

The cranberry plant is a close relative of the common blueberry. Native Americans used it both as food and for the treatment of bladder and kidney diseases. The Pilgrims learned about cranberry from local tribes and quickly adopted it for their own use. Subsequent physicians used it for bladder infections, for "bladder gravel" (small bladder stones), and to remove "blood toxins."

In the 1920s, researchers observed that drinking cranberry juice makes the urine more acidic. Because common urinary tract–infection bacteria such as *E. coli* dislike acidic surroundings, physicians concluded that they had discovered a scientific explanation for the traditional uses of cranberry. This discovery led to widespread medical use of cranberry juice for treating bladder infections. Cranberry fell out of favor with physicians after World War II, but it became popular again during the 1960s—as a self-treatment.

WHAT IS CRANBERRY USED FOR TODAY?

Cranberry is widely used today to prevent **bladder infections** (see page 28). Contrary to the research from the 1920s, it now appears that acidification of the urine is not so important as cranberry's ability to block bacteria from adhering to the bladder wall.[1,2,3] If the bacteria can't hold on they will be washed out with the stream of urine.

Cranberry juice is believed to be most effective as a form of prevention. When taken regularly, it appears to reduce the frequency of recurrent bladder infections in women prone to develop them. Cranberry may also be helpful during a bladder infection but not as reliably.

Cranberry juice may also be useful for treating or preventing **gum disease** (see page 142).[4]

WHAT IS THE SCIENTIFIC EVIDENCE FOR CRANBERRY?

Bladder Infection

One double-blind study followed 153 women with an average age of 78.5 years for a period of 6 months.[5] Half were given a standard commercial cranberry cocktail drink, the other a placebo drink prepared to look and taste the same. Both treatments contained the same amount of vitamin C to eliminate the possible antibacterial influence of that supplement.

Despite the weak preparation of cranberry used, the results showed a 58% decrease in the incidence of bacteria and white blood cells in the urine.

Interestingly, studies have found that in women who frequently develop bladder infections, bacteria seem to have a particularly easy time holding on to the bladder wall.[6] This suggests that cranberry juice can actually get to the root of their problem, but more research is needed.

Another double-blind placebo-controlled study evaluated the effectiveness of cranberry extract in children with bladder paralysis (neurogenic bladder) who needed to use a catheter.[7] The results showed no benefit.

Gum Disease

Preliminary evidence suggests that cranberry juice might be useful for treating or preventing gum disease.[8] However, there is one kink to work out before cranberry could be practical for this purpose: the sweeteners added to cranberry juice aren't good for your teeth, but without them cranberry juice is very bitter.

DOSAGE

The proper dosage of dry cranberry juice extract is 300 to 400 mg twice daily. For people who prefer juice, 8 to 16 ounces daily should suffice. Pure cranberry juice, not sugary cranberry juice cocktail with its low percentage of cranberry, should be used for best effect.

SAFETY ISSUES

There are no known risks of this food for adults, children, or pregnant or nursing women. However, cranberry juice may allow the kidneys to excrete certain drugs more rapidly, thereby reducing their effectiveness. All weakly alkaline drugs may be affected, including many antidepressants and prescription painkillers.

⚠ INTERACTIONS YOU SHOULD KNOW ABOUT

If you are taking **weakly alkaline drugs,** which include many **antidepressants** and **prescription painkillers,** cranberry might decrease their effectiveness.

CREATINE

Supplement Forms/Alternate Names   Creatine Monohydrate

Principal Proposed Uses   Performance Enhancement

Other Proposed Uses   Weight Loss, Improved Ratio of Body Fat to Muscle, High Triglycerides, Congestive Heart Failure, Amyotrophic Lateral Sclerosis (ALS, Lou Gehrig's Disease), Huntington's Disease, Mitochondrial Illnesses

Creatine is a naturally occurring substance that plays an important role in the production of energy in the body. The body converts it to phosphocreatine, a form of stored energy used by muscles.

In recent years, many athletes have tried supplemental creatine as a performance enhancer. If you're a U.S. baseball fan, you probably know that Mark McGwire, the all-time single-season home run champ, takes creatine (along with many other supplements).

Although the evidence for creatine is not definitive, of all sports supplements, it has the most evidence behind it. Numerous small double-blind studies suggest that it can increase athletic performance in sports that involve intense but short bursts of activity.

The theory behind its use is that supplemental creatine can build up a reserve of phosphocreatine in the muscles, to help them perform on demand. Supplemental creatine may also help the body make new phosphocreatine faster when it has been used up by intense activity.

SOURCES

Although some creatine exists in the daily diet, it is not an essential nutrient because your body can make it from the amino acids **L-arginine** (see page 208), glycine, and **L-methionine** (see page 360). Provided you eat enough protein (the source of these amino acids), your body will make all the creatine you need for good health.

Meat (including chicken and fish) is the most important dietary source of creatine and its amino acid building blocks. For this reason, vegetarian athletes may potentially benefit most from creatine supplementation.

THERAPEUTIC DOSAGES

For bodybuilding and exercise enhancement, a typical dosage schedule starts with a "loading dose" of 15 to 30 g daily (divided into 2 or 3 separate doses) for 3 to 4 days, followed by 2 to 5 g daily. Some authorities recommend skipping the loading dose. (By comparison, we typically get only about 1 g of creatine in the daily diet.)

Creatine's ability to enter muscle cells can be increased by combining it with glucose, fructose, or other simple carbohydrates. Caffeine appears to block the effects of creatine.[1]

THERAPEUTIC USES

Creatine is one of the bestselling and best-documented supplements for enhancing athletic performance, but the scientific evidence that it works is far from complete (see chapter on **sports performance** for more information). The best evidence we have points to benefits in forms of exercise that require repeated short-term bursts of high-intensity exercise, such as soccer and basketball.[2–5]

Creatine has also been proposed as an aid to promote weight loss and to reduce the proportion of fat to muscle in the body, but there is little evidence that it is effective for this purpose.[6] Better evidence exists for **chromium** (see page 251) in this regard.

Preliminary evidence suggests that creatine supplements may be able to reduce levels of triglycerides in the blood.[7] (Triglycerides are fats related to cholesterol that also increase risk of heart disease when elevated in the body.)

Finally, preliminary studies, including small double-blind trials, suggest that creatine may be helpful for various muscle illnesses, including **amyotrophic lateral sclerosis** (Lou Gehrig's disease; see page 9), **congestive heart failure** (see page 54), Huntington's disease, mitochondrial illnesses, and muscular dystrophy.[8–17] Although the evidence is still not strong, creatine seems to be able to reduce fatigue and increase strength in these conditions.

WHAT IS THE SCIENTIFIC EVIDENCE FOR CREATINE?

Exercise Performance

Several small double-blind studies suggest that creatine can improve performance in exercises that involve repeated short bursts of high-intensity activity.[18]

For example, a double-blind study investigated creatine and swimming performance in 18 men and 14 women.[19] Men taking the supplement had significant increases in speed when doing 6 bouts of 50-meter swims started at 3-minute intervals, as compared with men taking placebo. However, their speed did not improve when swimming 10 sets of 25-yard lengths started at 1-minute intervals. It may be that the shorter rest time between laps was not enough for the swimmers' bodies to resynthesize phosphocreatine.

Interestingly, none of the women enrolled in the study showed any improvement with the creatine supplement. The authors of this study noted that women normally have more creatine in their muscle tissue than men do, so perhaps creatine supplementation (at least at this level) is not of benefit to women, as it appears to be for men. Further research is needed to fully understand this gender difference in response to creatine.

In another double-blind study, 16 physical education students exercised 10 times for 6 seconds on a stationary cycle, alternating with a 30-second rest period.[20] The results showed that individuals who took 20 g of creatine for 6 days were better able to maintain cycle speed. Similar results were seen in many other studies, although there have been negative results as well.[21–25]

Isometric exercise capacity (pushing against a fixed resistance) also seems to improve with creatine.[26] In addition, two double-blind placebo-controlled studies, each lasting 28 days, provide some evidence that creatine and creatine plus HMB can increase lean muscle and bone mass.[27] The first enrolled 52 college football players during off-season training, and the other followed 40 athletes engaged in weight training.

However, studies of endurance or nonrepeated exercise have *not* shown benefits.[28–31] Therefore, creatine probably won't help you for marathon running or single sprints.

High Triglycerides

A 56-day double-blind placebo-controlled study of 34 men and women found that creatine supplementation can reduce levels of triglycerides in the blood by about 25%.[32] Effects on other blood lipids such as total cholesterol were insignificant.

Congestive Heart Failure

Easy fatigability is one unpleasant symptom of congestive heart failure. Creatine supplementation has been tried as a treatment for this symptom, with some positive results.

A double-blind study examined 17 men with congestive heart failure who were given 20 g of creatine daily for 10 days.[33] Exercise capacity and muscle strength increased in the creatine-treated group. Similarly, muscle endurance improved in a double-blind placebo-controlled crossover study of 20 men with chronic heart failure.[34] Treatment with 20 g of creatine for 5 days increased the amount of exercise they could complete before they reached exhaustion.

These results are promising, but further study is needed.[35]

SAFETY ISSUES

Creatine appears to be safe, at least in healthy athletes. No significant side effects have been found with the regimen of several days of a high dosage (15 to 30 g daily) followed by 6 weeks of a lower dosage (2 to 3 g daily). A placebo-controlled study of 100 football players found no adverse consequences during 10 months to 5 years of creatine supplementation.[36]

However, there are some potential concerns with creatine. Because it is metabolized by the kidneys, fears have been expressed that creatine supplements could cause kidney injury, and there are two worrisome case reports.[37,38] However, evidence suggests that creatine is safe for people whose kidneys are healthy to begin with, and who don't take excessive doses.[39,40] Nonetheless, individuals with kidney disease, especially those on dialysis, should avoid creatine.

Another concern revolves around the fact that creatine is metabolized in the body to the toxic substance formaldehyde.[41] However, it is not clear whether the amount of formaldehyde produced in this way will cause any harm. Three deaths have been reported in individuals taking creatine, but other causes were most likely responsible.[42]

As with all supplements taken in very high doses, it is important to purchase a high-quality form of creatine, as contaminants present even in very low concentrations could conceivably build up and cause problems.

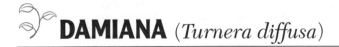

DAMIANA (*Turnera diffusa*)

Principal Proposed Uses   Male Sexual Capacity

Other Proposed Uses
Respiratory Diseases: Asthma
Depression, Digestive Problems, Impotence in Men, Difficulty Achieving Orgasm in Women, Menstrual Disorders

The herb damiana has been used in Mexico for some time as a male aphrodisiac.[1] Classic herbal literature of the nineteenth century describes it as a "tonic," or general body strengthener.

WHAT IS DAMIANA USED FOR TODAY?

Damiana continues to be a popular aphrodisiac for males. However, if it works at all, the effect appears to be rather mild. No scientific trials have been reported.

Damiana is also sometimes said to be helpful for treating **asthma** (see page 14) and other respiratory diseases, **depression** (see page 59), digestive problems, menstrual disorders, and various forms of **sexual dysfunction** (see page 155)— for example, **impotence** (see page 100) in men and inability to achieve orgasm in women.[2,3]

Like the herb **uva ursi** (see page 427), damiana contains arbutin, although at a concentration about 10 times lower. Arbutin is a urinary antiseptic, but the levels present in damiana are probably too small to make this herb a useful treatment for **bladder infections** (see page 28).

DOSAGE

The proper dosage of damiana is 2 to 4 g taken 2 to 3 times daily, or as directed on the label.

SAFETY ISSUES

Damiana appears to be safe at the recommended dosages. It appears on the FDA's GRAS (generally recognized as safe) list and is widely used as a food flavoring. However, because damiana contains low levels of cyanide-like compounds, excessive doses may be dangerous. Safety in young children, pregnant or nursing women, or those with severe liver or kidney disease is not established. The only common side effect of damiana is occasional mild gastrointestinal distress.

DANDELION (*Taraxacum officinale*)

Alternate or Related Names   Blowball, Cankerwort, Lion's Tooth, Priest's Crown, Swine Snout, Others

Principal Proposed Uses   Fluid Retention (Leaves), Nutritional Supplement (Leaves), Liver/Gallbladder Disease (Root), Various Forms of Arthritis (Root), Constipation (Root)

The common dandelion, enemy of suburban lawns, is an unusually nutritious food. Its leaves contain substantial levels of vitamins A, C, D, and B complex as well as iron, magnesium, zinc, potassium, manganese, copper, choline, calcium, boron, and silicon.

Worldwide, the root of the dandelion has been used for the treatment of a variety of liver and gallbladder problems. Other historical uses of the root and leaves include the treatment of breast diseases, water retention, digestive problems, joint pain, fever, and skin diseases.

The most active constituents in dandelion appear to be eudesmanolide and germacranolide, substances unique to this herb. Other ingredients include taraxol, taraxerol, and taraxasterol, along with stigmasterol, beta-sitosterol, caffeic acid, and p-hydroxyphenylacetic acid.[1]

WHAT IS DANDELION USED FOR TODAY?

Dandelion leaves are widely recommended as a food supplement for pregnant and also postmenopausal women because of the many nutrients they contain. They also appear to produce a mild diuretic effect, which may be appreciated by those who suffer from fluid retention.

In the folk medicine of many countries, dandelion root is regarded as a "liver tonic," a substance believed to benefit the liver in an unspecified way. This led to its use for many illnesses traditionally believed to be caused by a "sluggish" or "congested" liver, including constipation, headaches, eye problems, gout, skin problems, fatigue, and boils.

Building on this traditional thinking, some modern naturopathic physicians believe that dandelion can help "detoxify" or clean out the liver and gallbladder.[2] This concept has led to the suggestion that dandelion can reduce the side effects of medications processed by the liver, as well as relieve symptoms of diseases in which impaired liver function plays a role. However, there is as yet no real evidence for any of these uses.

Dandelion root is also used like other bitter herbs to improve appetite and treat minor digestive disorders. When dried and roasted, it is sometimes used as a coffee substitute. Finally, dandelion root has been used for the treatment of "rheumatism" (arthritis) and mild **constipation** (see page 56).

Dandelion

Visit Us at TNP.com

The scientific basis for the use of dandelion is scanty. Preliminary studies suggest that dandelion root stimulates the flow of bile.[3,4,5] Dandelion leaves have also been found to produce a mild diuretic effect.[6]

DOSAGE

A typical dosage of dandelion root is 2 to 8 g 3 times daily of dried root; 250 mg 3 to 4 times daily of a 5:1 extract; or 5 to 10 ml 3 times daily of a 1:5 tincture in 45% alcohol. The leaves may be eaten in salad or cooked.

SAFETY ISSUES

Dandelion root and leaves are believed to be quite safe, with no side effects or likely risks other than rare allergic reactions.[7–10] It is on the FDA's GRAS (generally recognized as safe) list and approved for use as a food flavoring by the Council of Europe.

However, based on dandelion root's effect on bile secretion, Germany's Commission E has recommended that it not be used at all by individuals with obstruction of the bile ducts or other serious diseases of the gallbladder, and only under physician supervision by those with gallstones.[11]

Some references state that dandelion root can cause hyperacidity and thereby increase ulcer pain, but this concern has been disputed.[12]

Because the leaves contain so much **potassium** (see page 390), they probably resupply any potassium lost due to dandelion's mild diuretic effect, although this has not been proven.

People with known allergies to related plants, such as **chamomile** (see page 244) and **yarrow** (see page 460), should use dandelion with caution.

There are no known drug interactions with dandelion. However, based on what we know about dandelion root's effects, there might be some risk when combining it with pharmaceutical diuretics or drugs that reduce blood sugar levels.

Safety in young children, pregnant or nursing women, or those with severe liver or kidney disease has not been established.

⚠ INTERACTIONS YOU SHOULD KNOW ABOUT

If you are taking **diuretic drugs** or **insulin** and **oral medications that reduce blood sugar levels,** use dandelion only under doctor's supervision.

DEVIL'S CLAW (*Harpagophytum procumbens*)

Alternate or Related Names   Grapple Plant, Wood Spider

Principal Proposed Uses
   Pain and Inflammation: Rheumatoid Arthritis, Osteoarthritis, Back Pain, Gout
   Digestive Problems: Loss of Appetite, Mild Stomach Upset

Devil's claw is a native of South Africa, so named because of its rather peculiar appearance. Its large tuberous roots are used medicinally, after being chopped up and dried in the sun for 3 days.

Native South Africans used the herb to reduce pain and fever and stimulate digestion. European colonists brought devil's claw back home, where it became a popular treatment for arthritis.

WHAT IS DEVIL'S CLAW USED FOR TODAY?

In modern Europe, devil's claw is used to treat all types of joint pain, including **osteoarthritis** (see page 132), **rheumatoid arthritis** (see page 151), and **gout** (see page 84). Devil's claw is also used for soft-tissue pain, such as back pain.

Like other bitter herbs (and this is one of the bitterest!), devil's claw is said to improve appetite and relieve mild stomach upset.

WHAT IS THE SCIENTIFIC EVIDENCE FOR DEVIL'S CLAW?

One double-blind study followed 89 individuals with rheumatoid arthritis for a 2-month period. The group given devil's claw showed a significant decrease in pain intensity and improved mobility.[1]

Another double-blind study of 50 people with various types of arthritis found that 10 days of treatment with devil's claw provided significant pain relief.[2]

A double-blind study of 197 individuals with chronic back pain found devil's claw only marginally effective at best.[3] Similarly unimpressive results were seen in a

Devil's Claw

Visit Us at TNP.com

previous double-blind study of 118 individuals with back pain.[4]

We don't know how devil's claw works. Some studies have found an anti-inflammatory effect but others have not.[5,6] Apparently, the herb doesn't produce the same changes in prostaglandins as standard anti-inflammatory drugs.[7]

DOSAGE

A typical dosage of devil's claw is 750 mg 3 times daily of a preparation standardized to contain 3% iridoid glycosides.

SAFETY ISSUES

Devil's claw appears to be quite safe, with no evidence of toxicity at doses many times higher than recommended.[8]

A 6-month open study of 630 people with arthritis showed no side effects other than occasional mild gastrointestinal distress. Devil's claw is not recommended for people with ulcers. According to one case report, the herb devil's claw might increase the potential for bleeding while taking Coumadin (warfarin).[9] Safety in young children, pregnant or nursing women, or those with severe liver or kidney disease has not been established.

⚠ INTERACTIONS YOU SHOULD KNOW ABOUT

If you are taking blood-thinning medications such as **Coumadin (warfarin)** or **heparin,** devil's claw might enhance their effect, possibly producing a risk of bleeding.

DHEA (Dehydroepiandrosterone)

Supplement Forms/Alternate Names   DHEA Sulfate

Principal Proposed Uses   Lupus, Osteoporosis, Adrenal Failure

Other Proposed Uses   Sexual Dysfunction in Women, Impotence, Depression, Chronic Fatigue Syndrome, HIV Support, Immune Support, Performance Enhancement, Fighting Aging, Preventing Heart Disease

Dehydroepiandrosterone (DHEA), a hormone produced by the adrenal glands, is the most abundant hormone in the *steroid* family found in the bloodstream. Your body uses DHEA as the starting material for making the sex hormones testosterone and estrogen.

Exciting evidence tells us that DHEA might be helpful for the autoimmune disease lupus, at least in women. DHEA might also help prevent osteoporosis (again, in women). Additionally, DHEA appears to be beneficial when taken along with standard treatment for women with adrenal failure.

Other uses with some evidence include improving sexual function in men and women and alleviating depression. However, keep in mind that DHEA is not a natural supplement. The DHEA you can buy at the store is made by a synthetic chemical process, and it is a hormone, not a nutrient. Although DHEA appears to be safe to use in the short term, its safety when taken for prolonged periods is unknown.

SOURCES

The body makes its own DHEA; we get very little in our diets. DHEA production peaks early in life and begins to decline as we reach adulthood. By age 60, our bodies produce just 5 to 15% as much as when we were 20. It's not clear whether this decline in DHEA is a bad thing, but some believe that it may contribute to the aging process.

For use as a dietary supplement, DHEA is manufactured synthetically from substances found in soybeans. Contrary to popular belief, there is no DHEA in **wild yam** (see page 459).

THERAPEUTIC DOSAGES

A typical therapeutic dosage of DHEA is 50 to 200 mg daily, although some studies used dosages above and below this range. A cream containing 10% DHEA may also be used; it is typically applied to the skin at a dosage of 3 to 5 g daily.

Physicians sometimes check DHEA levels and adjust the daily dose to achieve blood levels of 20 to 30 nmol/L.

THERAPEUTIC USES

Most of the evidence for DHEA involves benefits in women.

Exciting evidence suggests that DHEA might help reduce symptoms in women with lupus.[1,2,3]

Increasing evidence suggests that DHEA may also be helpful for preventing or treating **osteoporosis** (see page 136), especially in women over 70.[4,5,6] In addition, there are good theoretical reasons (but little direct evidence) to believe that individuals taking corticosteroids such as prednisone might be protected from osteoporosis and other drug side effects by taking DHEA at the same time.[7,8]

In some individuals, the adrenal glands fail to work, typically due to illness (or surgical removal of the adrenal glands). Traditionally, such people are given a variety of hormonal medications to make up for what their own adrenal glands are not producing. These hormones preserve the lives of individuals with adrenal failure, but they don't completely restore health. This may be due to the fact that the normal adrenal gland makes DHEA, a hormone not usually supplied in standard treatment. One double-blind study of women with adrenal failure found that adding DHEA supplements to the usual treatment improved feelings of well-being, sexual function, and even cholesterol levels.[9] Although this study was small, it was published in a major journal and will likely influence medical practice.

However, keep in mind that the vague concept of "adrenal weakness," widely discussed in natural medicine circles, is not the same as adrenal failure, and there is no reason to believe that DHEA would make a difference in those circumstances.

Evidence from a large double-blind trial suggests that DHEA might improve **libido in women** (see page 155) over 70.[10] However, not all studies have had positive results.[11,12]

A small double-blind study suggests that DHEA might be helpful for men who find it difficult to achieve an erection, when blood tests show they are low in this hormone.[13]

DHEA is also sometimes proposed for **depression** (see page 59), on the basis of one small double-blind study and one observational study.[14,15]

Highly preliminary evidence suggests that DHEA might be helpful for **chronic fatigue syndrome** (see page 44).[16]

According to very preliminary evidence, DHEA might help improve the immune response to vaccinations,[17,18] and strengthen immunity following **burns** (see page 123).[19,20]

DHEA seems to decrease in people with AIDS, possibly because of malnutrition[21] and/or stress.[22] However, a trial examining whether supplemental DHEA can improve mood and fatigue among people with **HIV** (see page 94) returned inconclusive results.[23]

Athletes have used DHEA on the belief that it might limit the body's response to cortisol and thereby cause an increase in muscle tissue growth. However, study results have been mixed, so it's uncertain whether DHEA really interferes with cortisol or not.[24,25] In any case, most (but not all), studies have found no performance benefits from taking DHEA.[26,27,28]

Primarily because DHEA naturally decreases with age, this hormone has been widely hyped as a kind of fountain of youth. However, there is no real evidence that taking DHEA will slow down any of the effects of aging. Two studies found that DHEA supplementation does not increase the general sense of well-being in older women;[29,30] another found no benefit in older men.[31] However, indirect evidence suggests that DHEA might help prevent heart disease.[32–37] In this case, it seems likely to be more beneficial for men than for women.

DHEA has also been proposed as a treatment for **Alzheimer's disease** (see page 5) and **weight loss** (see page 192), but the little evidence that is available appears more negative than positive.[38,39]

WHAT IS THE SCIENTIFIC EVIDENCE FOR DHEA (DEHYDROEPIANDROSTERONE)?

Lupus (Systemic Lupus Erythematosus, or SLE)

A 12-month double-blind placebo-controlled trial of 381 women with mild or moderate **lupus** (see page 114) evaluated the effects of DHEA at a dose of 200 mg daily.[40] While participants in both groups improved (the power of placebo is amazing!), DHEA was more effective, reducing many symptoms of the disease. However, DHEA was found to adversely affect cholesterol levels (specifically, the ratio of total cholesterol to HDL cholesterol) and raise levels of testosterone. For this reason, study authors recommend the monitoring of serum cholesterol and keeping watch for adverse effects caused by increased testosterone.

Similarly positive results were seen in earlier small studies.[41,42]

Even if DHEA is not strong enough to completely control symptoms of SLE on its own, it might allow a reduction in dosage of the more dangerous standard medications. In addition, it might directly help offset some of the side effects of corticosteroid treatment, such as accelerated osteoporosis.[43,44] (**Calcium**, **vitamin D**, and **ipriflavone** might also help prevent corticosteroid-induced osteoporosis. See these chapters for more information.)

Osteoporosis

DHEA appears to be helpful for osteoporosis in older women. A double-blind placebo-controlled trial of 280 men and women ranging in age from 60 to 79 years evaluated the effects of 50 mg of DHEA daily for 1 year.[45] The results suggest that DHEA can fight osteoporosis in women over 70. However, neither men nor younger women responded.

Additional evidence that DHEA might help osteoporosis comes from previous smaller clinical trials and observational studies.[46,47,48]

Adrenal Insufficiency

A study published in the *New England Journal of Medicine* supports adding DHEA to the usual hormone regimen for adrenal failure.[49] This double-blind placebo-controlled trial evaluated the effects of DHEA in 24 women with this condition. The results showed that DHEA improved sexual function, feelings of overall well-being, and cholesterol levels.

Improving Libido in Women

The double-blind placebo-controlled trial of 280 men and women described under Osteoporosis also looked for effects on sexual function.[50] The results indicate that for women over 70, DHEA might improve libido. Neither men nor younger women responded.

Impotence

A double-blind placebo-controlled study enrolled 40 men with difficulty achieving or maintaining an erection, who also had low measured levels of DHEA.[51] The results showed that DHEA at a dose of 50 mg daily significantly improved sexual performance.

Performance Enhancement

A small double-blind study found no benefit with DHEA at a dose of 150 mg per day for men undergoing weight training.[52] In addition, a 12-week double-blind study of 40 trained male athletes given either DHEA or androstenedione at 100 mg daily found no improvement in lean body mass or strength, or change in testosterone levels.[53]

A 12-month double-blind placebo-controlled crossover trial of 16 individuals aged 50 to 65 found some evidence of fat loss and strength improvement in the male participants during the period in which they received 100 mg of DHEA daily.[54] No improvement was seen in female participants.

SAFETY ISSUES

DHEA appears to be safe when taken in therapeutic doses, at least in the short term. One study found no significant side effects in 50 women who took up to 200 mg daily for up to 1 year.[55]

However, DHEA, even at the low dose of 25 mg per day, may decrease levels of HDL ("good") cholesterol.[56,57] In addition, DHEA may cause acne and male pattern hair growth.[58,59]

Concerns have been raised by one study in rats and another in trout that linked DHEA to liver cancer.[60,61] However, at least four other animal studies suggest that DHEA may have some anticancer effects.[62,63]

A 15-year human observational trial looking for a connection between naturally occurring DHEA levels and breast cancer found no relationship, either positive or negative.[64] However, another study found a relationship between higher levels of DHEA and ovarian cancer.[65] Overall, the long-term safety of DHEA supplements remains unknown. This is the case with many supplements, but because there are animal studies suggesting that DHEA might increase the risk of liver cancer, caution is warranted. Estrogen is one example of a hormone that increases the risk for certain forms of cancer, and it took years for researchers to discover that risk. Keep in mind also that the body converts DHEA into other hormones, including estrogen and testosterone. This could be dangerous for women with hormone-influenced diseases such as breast cancer.

The safety of DHEA in young children, pregnant or nursing women, and individuals with severe liver or kidney disease has not been established. We also don't know whether DHEA interacts with other hormone treatments, such as estrogen, although it certainly stands to reason that it might.

⚠ INTERACTIONS YOU SHOULD KNOW ABOUT

If you are taking **corticosteroids** (such as prednisone), you might be protected from some side effects by taking DHEA at the same time.

DMAE

Supplement Forms/Alternate Names   2-Dimethylaminoethanol, Deanol

Principal Proposed Uses   Attention Deficit Disorder

Other Proposed Uses   Alzheimer's Disease, Tardive Dyskinesia, Huntington's Chorea

DMAE (2-dimethylaminoethanol) is a chemical that has been used to treat a number of conditions affecting the brain and central nervous system. Like other such treatments, it is thought to work by increasing production of the neurotransmitter acetylcholine, although this has not been proven.

REQUIREMENTS/SOURCES

DMAE is sold in pharmacies and health food stores, as well as on the Internet, as a nutritional supplement.

THERAPEUTIC DOSAGES

Manufacturers' recommended dosages and those used in clinical studies vary between 400 and 1,800 mg daily.

THERAPEUTIC USES

Preliminary evidence suggests that DMAE may be helpful for attention deficit hyperactivity disorder (ADHD).[1,2]

More widely marketed today as a memory and mood enhancer, DMAE is said to improve intellectual functioning; however, there are no clinical studies that support its use for those purposes. The basis for such claims probably stems from its purported ability to increase levels of a neurotransmitter called acetylcholine. Drugs and supplements called "cholinergics" that increase acetylcholine have been used to treat Alzheimer's dementia, tardive dyskinesia, and Huntington's chorea. Because DMAE was believed to be a cholinergic, it has been tried for all of these disorders. However, well-designed placebo-controlled studies have yielded almost entirely negative results.[3–9] In addition, there is some controversy over whether DMAE really increases acetylcholine at all.[10]

WHAT IS THE SCIENTIFIC EVIDENCE FOR DMAE?

ADHD (Attention Deficit Hyperactivity Disorder)

There is some evidence that DMAE may be helpful for ADHD, according to studies performed in the 1970s. Two such studies were reported in a review article on DMAE.[11] Fifty children aged 6 to 12 years who had been diagnosed with hyperkinesia (their diagnosis today would likely be ADHD) participated in a double-blind study comparing DMAE to placebo. The dose was increased from 300 mg daily to 500 mg daily by the third week, and continued for 10 weeks. Evaluations revealed statistically significant test score improvements in the treatment group compared to the placebo group.

Another double-blind study compared DMAE with both methylphenidate (Ritalin) and placebo in 74 children described as having unspecified "learning disabilities" (also probably what we would call ADD today).[12] It found significant test score improvement for both treatment groups over a 10-week period. Positive results were also seen in a small open study.[13]

Alzheimer's Disease

Most people over the age of 40 experience some memory loss, but **Alzheimer's disease** (see page 5) is much more serious, leading to severe mental deterioration (dementia) in the elderly. Microscopic examination shows that in the areas of the brain involved in higher thought processes, nerve cells have died and disappeared, particularly cells that release the chemical acetylcholine. Drugs such as tacrine and danazol, and supplements such as huperzine A, are used for Alzheimer's based on their ability to increase acetylcholine levels. Because DMAE is also thought to increase acetylcholine, trials have been performed to test its effectiveness for the same purpose. However, there is no real evidence as yet that it works.

A double-blind placebo-controlled study involving 27 patients with Alzheimer's disease tested DMAE as a treatment.[14] Thirteen participants were placed in the group receiving DMAE; however, 6 of them had to drop out of the study because of side effects such as drowsiness, increased confusion, and elevated blood pressure. In those completing the trial, no differences were seen between the treatment group and those taking placebo.

An open trial enrolling 14 patients found no improvement in either memory or cognitive function. The researchers did note improvements in symptoms of depression, but in the absence of a placebo group this observation means little.[15]

Tardive Dyskinesia

Tardive dyskinesia (TD) (see page 176) is a potentially permanent side effect of drugs used to control schizophrenia. This late-developing (tardy, or tardive) complication consists of annoying, uncontrollable movements (dyskinesias), particularly in the face.

Based on its supposed cholinergic effect, DMAE has been proposed as a treatment for TD. Although some case reports and open studies seemed to suggest that DMAE might be useful for this purpose,[16,17] properly designed studies using double-blind methods and placebo control groups have not borne this out. Of 12 double-blind studies reviewed, only one found DMAE to be significantly effective when compared with placebo.[18] A meta-analysis of proposed treatments for TD found DMAE to be no more effective than placebo.[19] It seems likely, though not entirely certain, that the benefits seen in open studies and individual cases were the result of a placebo effect. However, it is also possible that some particular individuals respond well to DMAE, even if most don't.

Dong Quai

Visit Us at TNP.com

Huntington's Chorea

Huntington's chorea is a genetically inherited disease that results in personality changes and, somewhat similarly to TD, uncontrolled spastic movements. It doesn't usually become symptomatic until a person's age reaches the late thirties or older, although about 10% of people with Huntington's will begin to show signs of the disorder in childhood or adolescence.

DMAE was not found to be an effective treatment for Huntington's chorea in double-blind placebo-controlled trials, although mixed results have been obtained using DMAE in open trials.[20,21,22]

SAFETY ISSUES

Although most clinical investigations using DMAE report that the participants experienced no side effects, enough researchers have found adverse reactions to suggest that some caution is appropriate in using this supplement. One study, as noted above, reported increased confusion, drowsiness, and elevated blood pressure;[23] another reports headache and muscle tension as possible adverse effects;[24] and another paper suggests that weight loss and insomnia may accompany use of DMAE.[25] There is also one case report of a woman who developed severe TD after taking DMAE for 10 years for a hand tremor.[26] Besides this, a number of manufacturers warn against the use of DMAE by people with epilepsy or a history of convulsions.

Maximum safe dosages for young children, pregnant or nursing women, or people with severe liver or kidney disease have not been established.

DONG QUAI (Angelica sinensis)

Principal Proposed Uses
    Menstrual Disorders: Dysmenorrhea, PMS, Irregular Menstruation

Probably Ineffective Uses   Menopausal Symptoms (When Taken Alone)

One of the major herbs in the Chinese repertoire, *Angelica sinensis* is closely related to European *Angelica archangelica,* a common garden herb and the flavoring in Benedictine and Chartreuse liqueurs. The carrot-like roots of this fragrant plant are harvested in the fall after about 3 years of cultivation and stored in airtight containers prior to processing.

Traditionally, dong quai is said to be one of the most important herbs for strengthening the "xue." The Chinese term "xue" is often translated as "blood," but it actually refers to a complex concept of which the blood itself is only a part. In the late 1800s, an extract of dong quai known as *Eumenol* became popular in Europe as a "female tonic," and this is how most people still understand it in the West.

WHAT IS DONG QUAI USED FOR TODAY?

Dong quai is often recommended as a treatment for menstrual cramps or **dysmenorrhea** (see page 70) and **PMS** (see page 145), as well as hot flashes and other **menopausal symptoms** (see page 117). The scientific evidence regarding these uses is very weak, consisting primarily of test tube and animal studies, as well as a few uncontrolled studies of people.[1–5] Furthermore, a recent 24-week study compared the effects of dong quai against a placebo in 71 postmenopausal women.[6] According to the results, dong quai does not reduce menopausal symptoms at all.

Dong quai may be more effective when used in traditional herbal formulas. Two of the most common are Dong Quai and Paeonia, and Bupleurum and Dong Quai. These herbal combinations are frequently used for treating certain types of menopausal symptoms, as well as menstrual pain, fibrocystic breast disease, PMS, abnormal fetal movements, and pelvic inflammatory disease.[7,8,9] However, there is no scientific evidence that they are effective.

Another popular herbal formula is Dong Quai 4, so named because of the total number of herbs involved. This combination, with variations tailored to the individual, is traditionally used to treat certain forms of menstrual irregularity, menstrual pain, anemia, and **insomnia** (see page 103).[10,11] A competent Chinese herbalist can tell you which formula would be best for you (according to tradition), as well as adjust the constituents to exactly match your personal needs.

DOSAGE

We recommend using dong quai under the supervision of a qualified Chinese herbalist, not because the herb is dangerous, but because it is difficult to self-prescribe Chinese herbal formulas.

If you wish to self-treat with dong quai, a typical dosage is 10 to 40 drops of dong quai tincture 1 to 3 times daily, or 1 standard 00 gelatin capsule 3 times daily.

SAFETY ISSUES

Dong quai is believed to be generally nontoxic. Very large amounts have been given to rats without causing harm.[12] Side effects are rare and primarily consist of mild gastrointestinal distress and occasional allergic reactions (such as rash).

Certain constituents of dong quai can cause increased sensitivity to the sun, but this has not been observed to occur in people using the whole herb.

According to traditional beliefs, inappropriate long-term use of dong quai (such as taking it as a single herb rather than in a combination) can damage the digestive tract and cause other disturbances in overall health. Dong quai is also generally contraindicated during the first 3 months of pregnancy and during acute respiratory infections, and in women with excessively heavy menstruation. However, there is no scientific evidence for these concerns. Safety in young children, pregnant or nursing women, or those with severe liver or kidney disease has not been established. One case report suggests that dong quai usage by a nursing mother caused elevated blood pressure in both the mother and child.[13]

Dong quai may interact with the blood-thinning drug Coumadin (warfarin), increasing the risk of bleeding, according to one case report.[14] Dong quai might also conceivably interact with other blood-thinning drugs, such as heparin, aspirin, and Trental (pentoxifylline). Additionally, dong quai could conceivably interact with natural products with blood-thinning properties, such as **garlic** (see page 291), **ginkgo** (see page 298), or high-dose **vitamin E** (see page 451).

⚠ INTERACTIONS YOU SHOULD KNOW ABOUT

If you are taking blood-thinning drugs such as **Coumadin (warfarin), heparin, Trental (pentoxifylline),** or **aspirin,** dong quai might interact and increase the risk of bleeding.

ECHINACEA *(Echinacea purpurea, E. angustifolia, E. pallida)*

Alternate or Related Names   Black Sampson, Rudbeckia, Sampson Root, Purple Coneflower, Hedgehog, Others

Principal Proposed Uses   Colds and Flus (Shortening the Duration, Reducing Symptoms)

Other Proposed Uses
   Stimulating Immunity: "Aborting" a Cold That Has Just Started, Preventing Colds, Helping the Body Fight Off
   Other Infections
   Ear Infections

The decorative plant *Echinacea purpurea*, or purple coneflower, has been one of the most popular herbal medications in both the United States and Europe for over a century.

Native Americans used the related species *Echinacea angustifolia* for a wide variety of problems, including respiratory infections and snakebite. Herbal physicians among the European colonists quickly added the herb to their repertoire. Echinacea became tremendously popular toward the end of the nineteenth century, when a businessman named H. C. F. Meyer promoted an herbal concoction containing *E. angustifolia*. The garish, exaggerated, and poorly written nature of his labeling helped define the characteristics of a "snake oil" remedy.

However, serious manufacturers developed an interest in echinacea as well. By 1920, the respected Lloyd Brothers Pharmaceutical Company of Cincinnati, Ohio, counted echinacea as its largest selling product. In Europe, physicians took up the American interest in *E. angustifolia* with enthusiasm. Demand soon outstripped the supply coming from America, and, in an attempt to rapidly plant echinacea locally, the German firm Madeus and Company mistakenly purchased a quantity of *Echinacea purpurea* seeds. This historical accident is the reason why most echinacea today belongs to the *purpurea* species instead of *angustifolia*. Another family member, *Echinacea pallida,* is also used.

Echinacea was the number one cold and flu remedy in the United States until it was displaced by sulfa antibiotics. Ironically, antibiotics are not effective for colds, while echinacea appears to offer some real help. Echinacea remains the primary remedy for minor respiratory infections in Germany, where over 1.3 million prescriptions are issued each year.

Echinacea

WHAT IS ECHINACEA USED FOR TODAY?

Germany's Commission E authorizes the use of echinacea juice for "supportive treatment of recurrent infections of the upper respiratory tract and lower urinary tract" and echinacea root extracts for "supportive treatment of flu-like infections." Echinacea has become a popular treatment for **colds and flus** (see page 47) in the United States as well, nearing the top of the charts for several years running.

This herb is thought to be an immune stimulant, a type of treatment not found in conventional medicine. Drugs attack infections, but echinacea appears to activate the body's infection-fighting capacity. However, there is no evidence that echinacea strengthens or "nourishes" the immune system when taken over the long term. It probably just stimulates it into action in the short term. Long-term use of echinacea has not proved effective.

The best scientific evidence about echinacea concerns its ability to help you recover from colds and minor flus more quickly. The old saying goes that a "cold lasts seven days, but if you treat it, it will be over in a week." However, good evidence tells us that echinacea can actually help you get over colds much faster. It also appears to significantly reduce symptoms while you are sick.

Echinacea may also be able to "abort" a cold, if taken at the first sign of symptoms, but taking echinacea regularly throughout cold season is probably not a great idea. Evidence suggests that it does not work for this purpose, and might actually slightly impair your immunity.

Echinacea is also sometimes tried for other infectious illnesses, such as **ear infections** (see page 73) in children, but there is no direct evidence as yet that it works.

WHAT IS THE SCIENTIFIC EVIDENCE FOR ECHINACEA?

Reasonably large and well-designed double-blind placebo-controlled studies involving a total of about 650 individuals have found echinacea effective for reducing the symptoms and duration of colds. These studies have used all three species of the herb. We don't know which one is better, or whether they are all equivalent.

Reducing the Symptoms and Duration of Colds

Clinical studies with various species of echinacea have found benefits in lessening the symptoms and duration of colds. One double-blind study of 100 individuals with acute flu-like illnesses found that echinacea could significantly reduce cold symptoms.[1] Half of the group received a combination herb product containing *E. angustifolia*, the other half took placebo. The participants rated the severity of symptoms of headache, lethargy, cough, and limb pain. In the treated group, symptoms were significantly less severe.

Another double-blind study of echinacea's effect on flu-like illnesses followed 180 people who were given either 450 mg or 900 mg of *E. purpurea* daily or placebo.[2] By about the third day, those participants receiving the higher dose of echinacea (900 mg) were doing significantly better than those in the placebo or low-dose echinacea groups. Reduction of symptoms was also seen in another double-blind study of *E. purpurea* involving about 200 participants.[3]

Echinacea has also been found to reduce the time needed to get well. A double-blind placebo-controlled study using the *E. pallida* species followed 160 adults with recent onset of cold-like illnesses.[4] The results showed that treatment reduced the average period of illness from 13 days to about 9.5 days, compared to placebo. (These must have been bad colds to last so long!)

Evidence from a double-blind study involving 120 people tells us that *E. purpurea* can cut in half the time it takes for your cold to "turn the corner" and start to get better. This study is described in the next section, "Aborting" a Cold.

Finally, a double-blind study of 263 individuals with colds found that a special combination herbal treatment containing echinacea, wild indigo, and wormwood significantly relieved cold symptoms and reduced time to recovery.[5] **Note:** Do not attempt to mix these ingredients yourself. Wild indigo and wormwood can be dangerous if used improperly.

"Aborting" a Cold

A double-blind study suggests that echinacea can not only make colds shorter and less severe, it can sometimes stop a cold that is just starting.[6] In this study, 120 people were given *E. purpurea* or a placebo as soon as they started showing signs of getting a cold.

Participants took either echinacea or placebo at a dosage of 20 drops every 2 hours for 1 day, then 20 drops 3 times a day for 9 more days. The results over the 10-day study period were promising. Fewer people in the echinacea group felt that their initial symptoms actually developed into "real" colds (40% of those taking echinacea versus 60% taking the placebo actually became ill). Also, among those who did come down with "real" colds, improvement in the symptoms started sooner in the echinacea group (4 days instead of 8 days). Both of these results were statistically significant. However, echinacea's ability to shorten the duration of colds was more dramatic.

Preventing Colds

Several studies have attempted to discover whether the daily use of echinacea can prevent colds from even starting, but the results have not been promising.

Visit Us at TNP.com

In one double-blind placebo-controlled trial, 302 healthy volunteers were given an alcohol tincture containing either *E. purpurea* root, *E. angustifolia* root, or placebo for 12 weeks.[7] The results showed that *E. purpurea* was associated with perhaps a 20% decrease in the number of people who got sick, and *E. angustifolia* with a 10% decrease. However, the difference was not statistically significant. This means that the benefit, if any, was so small that it could have been due to chance alone.

Another double-blind placebo-controlled study enrolled 109 individuals with a history of four or more colds during the previous year, and gave them either *E. purpurea* juice or placebo for a period of 8 weeks.[8] No benefits were seen in the frequency, duration, or severity of colds. (Note: this paper is actually a more detailed look at a 1992 study widely misreported as providing evidence of benefit.)[9]

Another study, not yet published, found indications that regular use of echinacea might actually increase the risk of colds.[10] For a period of 6 months, 200 people were given either echinacea or placebo. Use of the herb was associated with a 20% higher incidence of sore throat, runny nose, and sinusitis. This suggests that long-term use of echinacea might actually slightly impair immune function.

Another double-blind placebo-controlled trial followed 117 individuals, each given echinacea for 14 days and then inoculated with a cold virus.[11] No difference in rate or severity of infection was seen.

One double-blind placebo-controlled study did find that long-term use of echinacea offered some help, but only for those especially prone to colds.[12] The study involved 609 students at the University of Cologne. Half of the participants were treated with a German product containing *E. angustifolia* for at least 8 weeks; the other half received placebo.

In the group as a whole, echinacea did not significantly decrease the number of colds. However, of the 609 participants, 363 students were rated as particularly prone to infection, based on the number of colds each had developed the winter before. This relatively high-risk group did show a reduction in the number of colds they caught, compared to the control group: the infection-prone students developed on average 20% fewer colds (a statistically significant, although small, improvement).

The bottom line: echinacea is probably not worth using as a long-term preventive treatment. It is better used directly at the onset of a cold to reduce its severity and duration.

Immune Stimulation

Both test-tube and animal studies have found that polysaccharides found in echinacea can increase antibody production, raise white blood cell counts, and stimulate the activity of key white blood cells.[13–18] However, it's not clear how meaningful these studies really are.

DOSAGE

Echinacea is usually taken at the first sign of a cold and continued for 7 to 14 days. The three species of echinacea are used interchangeably. The typical dosage of echinacea powdered extract is 300 mg 3 times a day. Alcohol tincture (1:5) is usually taken at a dosage of 3 to 4 ml 3 times daily, echinacea juice at a dosage of 2 to 3 ml 3 times daily, and whole dried root at 1 to 2 g 3 times daily. There is no broad agreement on what ingredients should be standardized in echinacea tinctures and solid extracts.

Many herbalists feel that liquid forms of echinacea are more effective than tablets or capsules, because they feel part of echinacea's benefit is due to activation of the tonsils through direct contact.[19]

Echinacea should only be used as a short term "boost" to your immunity. It does not appear to strengthen your immunity when taken for months. See the chapters on **ginseng** (see page 301) and **vitamin E** (see page 451) for treatments that might strengthen immunity.

Finally, **goldenseal** (see page 314) is frequently combined with echinacea in cold preparations. However, there is not a shred of evidence that oral goldenseal stimulates immunity, nor did traditional herbalists use it for this purpose.[20]

SAFETY ISSUES

Echinacea appears to be safe. Even when taken in very high doses, it has not been found to cause any toxic effects.[21,22] Reported side effects are also uncommon and usually limited to minor gastrointestinal symptoms, increased urination, and mild allergic reactions.[23] However, severe allergic reactions have occurred occasionally, some of them life threatening.[24] Studies dating back to the 1950s suggest that echinacea is safe in children.[25]

Germany's Commission E warns against using echinacea in cases of autoimmune disorders such as multiple sclerosis, lupus, and rheumatoid arthritis, as well as tuberculosis or leukocytosis. There are also rumors that echinacea should not be used by people with AIDS. These warnings are theoretical, based on fears that echinacea might actually activate immunity in the wrong way. But there is no evidence that echinacea use has actually harmed anyone with these diseases.

The Commission E monograph also recommends against using echinacea for more than 8 weeks.

One study raised questions about possible antifertility effects of echinacea. When high concentrations of echinacea were placed in a test tube with hamster sperm and

Elderberry

ova, the sperm were less able to penetrate the ova.[26] However, since we have no idea whether this much echinacea can actually come in contact with sperm and ova when they are in the body rather than a test tube, these results may not be meaningful in real life.

The safety of echinacea in young children, pregnant or nursing women, or those with severe liver or kidney disease has not been established. There are no known drug interactions.

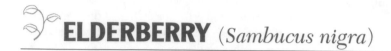

ELDERBERRY (*Sambucus nigra*)

Alternate or Related Names   Black Elder, Black-Berried Alder, Boor Tree, Elder, Bountry, Others

Principal Proposed Uses   Colds and Flus

Other Proposed Uses   HIV Support, Herpes

Native Americans used tea made from elderberry flowers to treat respiratory infections. They also used the leaves and flowers in poultices applied to wounds, and the bark, suitably aged, as a laxative. The berries are frequently made into beverages, pies, and preserves, but they have also been used to treat arthritis.

WHAT IS ELDERBERRY USED FOR TODAY?

Elderberry flowers are a potential rival for echinacea. Many clinicians feel that elderberry is actually more effective at shortening **colds and flus** (see page 47) than the latter, far more famous (and better-studied) herb. According to a preliminary double-blind study performed in Israel, a standardized elderberry extract reduced almost by half the recovery time from a particular strain of epidemic influenza.[1] Elderberry is being studied for potential activity against other viral illnesses as well, including **HIV**[2] (see page 94) and **herpes** (see

page 86).[3] Standardized elderberry extracts are seeing increasing use throughout Europe.

DOSAGE

Elderberry-flower tea is made by steeping 3 to 5 g of dried flowers in 1 cup of boiling water for 10 to 15 minutes. A typical dosage is 1 cup 3 times daily. Standardized extracts should be taken according to the directions on the product's label.

SAFETY ISSUES

Elderberry flowers are generally regarded as safe. Side effects are rare and consist primarily of occasional mild gastrointestinal distress or allergic reactions. Nonetheless, safety in young children, pregnant or nursing women, or those with severe liver or kidney disease has not been established.

ELECAMPANE (*Inula helenium*)

Alternate or Related Names   Alant, Elfdock, Elfwort, Horse-Elder, Horseheal, Others

Principal Proposed Uses
Chronic Respiratory Diseases: Asthma
Poor Digestion

The Latin name of elecampane comes from Helen of Troy, who was supposed to have carried elecampane with her while being abducted from Sparta. Revered by the ancient Greeks and Romans, this herb was recommended for treating such diverse problems as indigestion, melancholy, sciatica, bronchitis, and asthma.

WHAT IS ELECAMPANE USED FOR TODAY?

Modern herbalists primarily regard elecampane as a long-term treatment for respiratory diseases such as

Visit Us at TNP.com

asthma (see page 14) and bronchitis, especially when excessive mucus is a notable feature. Animal studies suggest that the oil of elecampane may help suppress coughs.[1] Unfortunately, no human trials of elecampane have been reported.

Elecampane is also sometimes recommended as a daily supplement to improve general digestion.

One of elecampane's constituents, alantolactone, has been used in concentrated form as a treatment for intestinal parasites,[2] but it isn't clear whether the whole herb is particularly effective for this purpose.

DOSAGE

A typical dosage of elecampane root is 1.5 to 4 g 3 times daily, either in capsule form or boiled in water as tea.

SAFETY ISSUES

The only reported adverse effects of elecampane are occasional allergic reactions. However, safety in young children, pregnant or nursing women, or those with severe liver or kidney disease has not been established.

EPHEDRA (Ephedra sinica)

Alternate or Related Names   Ma Huang, Desert Herb, Ephedrine

Principal Proposed Uses   Asthma*, Sinus Congestion*

Questionable Uses   Stimulant, Weight-Loss Aid

*Ephedra is effective for these conditions but not recommended due to safety concerns.

The Chinese herb ma huang is a member of a primitive family of plants that look like thin, branching, connected straws. A related species, *Ephedra nevadensis*, grows wild in the American Southwest and is widely called "Mormon tea." However, only the Asian species of ephedra contains the active compounds ephedrine and pseudoephedrine.

Ma huang was traditionally used by Chinese herbalists during the early stages of respiratory infections and also for the short-term treatment of certain kinds of asthma, eczema, hay fever, narcolepsy, and edema. However, ma huang was not supposed to be taken for an extended period of time, and people with less than robust constitutions were warned to use only low doses or avoid ma huang altogether. If these warnings had been heeded, perhaps some of the current problems with ephedra could have been avoided (see the discussion under What Is Ephedra Used for Today?).

Japanese chemists isolated ephedrine from ma huang at the turn of the century, and it soon became a primary treatment for asthma in the United States and abroad. Ephedra's other major ingredient, pseudoephedrine, became the decongestant Sudafed.

WHAT IS EPHEDRA USED FOR TODAY?

Although it can still be found in a few over-the-counter drugs for **asthma** (see page 14), physicians seldom prescribe ephedrine anymore. The problem is that ephedrine mimics the effects of adrenaline and causes symptoms such as rapid heartbeat, high blood pressure, agitation, insomnia, nausea, and loss of appetite. The newer asthma drugs are much safer and easier to tolerate.

Recently, pills containing ephedrine have been sold as **weight-loss** (see page 192) aids and "natural" stimulants. Unfortunately, these products have been overused and combined with other stimulants, such as caffeine, resulting in severe overstimulation and even death in some people.[1] In 1997, the FDA proposed stiff limits on dietary supplements containing ephedrine, but they are presently under appeal by manufacturers who say they go too far. The FDA's intervention stemmed from unscrupulous manufacturers, who (mostly via the Internet) promoted ma huang as a natural hallucinogen ("herbal ecstasy") and not as a bronchial decongestant. Dosages of ephedrine required to produce psychoactive effects are exceedingly toxic to the heart; the FDA has documented 38 deaths of otherwise healthy young people who reportedly used ephedrine for psychedelic purposes.

When used properly, ephedra may still be useful as a short-term treatment for sinus congestion and mild asthma, but we would not recommend it as conventional treatments are safer and cause fewer side effects.

DOSAGE

The dosage of ephedra should be adjusted according to the amount of the ephedrine it provides. For adults, no more than 25 mg should be taken at one time, and a total daily intake of 100 mg should not be exceeded.[2] However, because there is no way to know whether the labeling of ephedra sold as a dietary supplement is correct, we do not recommend using ephedra at all.

SAFETY ISSUES

According to a 7-member expert panel convened to review the safety of ephedra, when taken in appropriate doses and by healthy individuals, ephedra is probably safe.[3] However, as mentioned above, there is no ready way to be sure of the dose you are getting, leading to potential risk of overdosage.

In addition, ephedra should not be taken by those with enlargement of the prostate, high blood pressure, heart disease, diabetes, hardening of the arteries, glau-

coma, or hyperthyroidism.[4] Furthermore, never combine ephedra with monoamine-oxidase inhibitors (MAO inhibitors) such as Nardil (phenelzine), or fatal reactions may develop. If symptoms such as a rapid heart rate or a marked increase in blood pressure develop, reduce the dosage or simply stop taking it altogether.

Ephedra is not recommended for young children, pregnant or nursing women, or those with severe liver, heart, or kidney disease.

⚠ INTERACTIONS YOU SHOULD KNOW ABOUT

If you are taking **MAO inhibitors,** do not take ephedra.

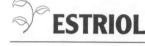

ESTRIOL

Supplement Forms/Alternate Names   Oestriol, Tri-Estrogen

Principal Proposed Uses   Menopausal Symptoms

There are many forms of estrogen in the body. The ovary produces a form named estradiol, which is converted into another important estrogen called estrone. Estriol is yet another form of estrogen metabolized from estradiol, weaker than the other two, but still active.

The estrogen tablets prescribed for menopausal symptoms usually contain estradiol, estrone, or a combination of the two. Some alternative medicine physicians have popularized the use of estriol as an alternative, and there is no doubt that estriol is also effective for symptoms of menopause. However, despite claims that it is safer than other forms of estrogen, the balance of evidence suggests that, in fact, estriol presents precisely the same risks (see Safety Issues below).

REQUIREMENTS/SOURCES

Estriol is manufactured in the body from estrone, estradiol, and **androstenedione** (see page 206). When taken as a drug, it is manufactured synthetically, or extracted from animal products.

THERAPEUTIC DOSAGES

The usual dose of estriol is 2 to 8 mg taken once daily. Estriol is also commonly sold in combination with other forms of estrogen.

THERAPEUTIC USES

Like more common forms of estrogen, estriol is used for the treatment of **menopausal symptoms** (see page 117). Double-blind and other controlled trials have found oral or vaginal estriol effective for reducing hot flashes, night sweats, insomnia, **osteoporosis** (see page 136), vaginal dryness, and recurrent **urinary tract infections** (see page 28).[1–9]

Estriol may cause less vaginal bleeding as a side effect than other forms of estrogen, although this has not been proven.[10,11]

Claims that estriol has an anticancer effect are based on exaggerated interpretations of very weak studies.[12,13,14] It is more likely that estriol increases cancer risk, just like other forms of estrogen (see Safety Issues, below).

SAFETY ISSUES

Like other forms of estrogen, oral estriol stimulates the growth of uterine tissue. This leads to risk of uterine cancer. In a placebo-controlled study of 1,110 women, uterine tissue stimulation was seen among women given estriol orally (1–2 mg daily) as compared to those given placebo.[15] Another large study found that oral estriol increased the risk of uterine cancer.[16] In another study of 48 women given estriol (1 mg twice daily), uterine tissue stimulation was seen in the majority of cases.[17] In contrast, a 12-month double-blind trial of oral estriol (2 mg daily) in 68 Japanese women found no effect on the

Estriol

uterus.[18] It may be that the high levels of soy in the Japanese diet altered the results.

For this reason, to protect the uterus estriol, like other forms of estrogen, needs to be balanced with progesterone. Additionally, one study suggests that estriol is less likely to affect the uterus when taken in a once-daily dose rather than in multiple daily doses.[19]

However, the uterus isn't the only organ at risk of cancer. Test tube studies suggest that estriol is just as likely to cause breast cancer as any other form of estrogen.[20] While this doesn't constitute proof, it does raise an alarm. Until proven otherwise, estriol must be regarded as increasing breast cancer risk.

As with other forms of estrogen, vaginal estriol preparations are safer than oral preparations.[21,22]

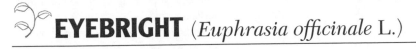

EYEBRIGHT (*Euphrasia officinale* L.)

Alternate or Related Names Euphrasia

Principal Proposed Uses Eye Infections

The herb eyebright has been used since the Middle Ages as an eyewash for infections and irritations. However, as much as one would like to believe that all traditions are wise, eyebright appears to have been selected for treating eye diseases not because it works particularly well, but because its petals look bloodshot.[1] This follows from the classic medieval philosophic attitude known as the *Doctrine of Signatures,* which states that herbs show their proper use by their appearance.

WHAT IS EYEBRIGHT USED FOR TODAY?

Like many herbs, eyebright contains astringent substances and volatile oils that are probably at least slightly antibacterial. But there's no evidence that eyebright is particularly effective for treating eye diseases; Germany's Commission E recommends against using it. Warm compresses consisting of nothing but water (or ordinary black tea) are probably equally effective under the same conditions.

Eyebright tea is also sometimes taken internally to treat jaundice, respiratory infections, and memory loss. However, there is no evidence that it is effective for these conditions.

DOSAGE

Traditionally, eyebright tea is made by boiling 1 tablespoon of the herb in a cup of water. This is then used as an eyewash or taken internally up to 3 times daily.

SAFETY ISSUES

Eyebright can cause tearing of the eyes, itching, redness, and many other symptoms, probably due to direct irritation.[2] It appears to be safe when taken internally, but not many studies have been performed. Safety in young children, pregnant or nursing women, or those with severe liver or kidney disease has not been established.

FENUGREEK (*Trigonella foenumgraecum*)

Alternate or Related Names Greek Hay Seed, Bird's Foot

Principal Proposed Uses
Diabetes: Blood Sugar Control, Cholesterol Levels
Constipation

For millennia, fenugreek has been used both as a medicine and as a food spice in Egypt, India, and the Middle East. It was traditionally recommended for the treatment of wounds, bronchitis, digestive problems, arthritis, kidney problems, and male reproductive conditions.

WHAT IS FENUGREEK USED FOR TODAY?

Present interest in fenugreek focuses on its benefits for people with **diabetes** (see page 65) or high **cholesterol** (see page 88). Numerous animal studies and preliminary

Fenugreek

Visit Us at TNP.com

trials in humans have found that fenugreek can reduce blood sugar and serum cholesterol levels in people with diabetes. Like other high-fiber foods, it may also be helpful for **constipation** (see page 56).

WHAT IS THE SCIENTIFIC EVIDENCE FOR FENUGREEK?

Small studies, none of which were double-blind, suggest that fenugreek can be helpful both for type 1 (childhood onset) and type 2 (adult onset) diabetes.

In one open study of 60 people with type 2 diabetes, 25 g per day of fenugreek led to significant improvements in overall blood sugar control, blood sugar elevations in response to a meal, and cholesterol levels.[1] Another open study found benefits with only 15 g of fenugreek daily.[2]

Finally, in a small single-blind controlled study, people with type 1 diabetes were randomly prescribed either fenugreek at a dose of 50 g twice daily as part of their lunch and dinner, or the same meals without the powder, each for 10 days. Those on the fenugreek diet had significant decreases in their fasting blood sugar.[3]

DOSAGE

Because the seeds of fenugreek are somewhat bitter, they are best taken in capsule form. The typical dosage is 5 to 30 g of defatted fenugreek taken 3 times a day with meals.

SAFETY ISSUES

As a commonly eaten food, fenugreek is generally regarded as safe. The only common side effect is mild gastrointestinal distress when it is taken in high doses.

Because fenugreek can lower blood sugar levels, it is advisable to seek medical supervision before combining it with diabetes medications.

Extracts made from fenugreek have been shown to stimulate uterine contractions in guinea pigs.[4] For this reason, pregnant women should not take fenugreek in dosages higher than is commonly used as a spice, perhaps 5 g daily. Besides concerns over pregnant women, safety in young children, nursing women, or those with severe liver or kidney disease has also not been established.

⚠ INTERACTIONS YOU SHOULD KNOW ABOUT

If you are taking **diabetes medications** such as **insulin** or **oral hypoglycemics,** fenugreek may enhance their effect. This may cause excessively low blood sugar, and you may need to reduce your dose of medication.

FEVERFEW (*Tanacetum parthenium*)

Alternate or Related Names   Featherfew, Featherfoil, Midsummer Daisy

Principal Proposed Uses   Migraine Headaches (Prevention and Treatment)

Other Proposed Uses   Arthritis

Originally native to the Balkans, this relative of the common daisy was spread by deliberate planting throughout Europe and the Americas. Feverfew's feathery and aromatic leaves have long been used medicinally to improve childbirth, promote menstruation, induce abortions, relieve rheumatic pain, and treat severe headaches.

Contrary to popular belief, feverfew is not used for lowering fevers. Actually, "feverfew" is a corruption of the name "featherfoil."[1] Featherfoil became featherfew and ultimately feverfew. In a weird historical reversal, this name then led to a widespread belief among herbalists that feverfew could lower fevers. After a while they noticed that it didn't work, and then angrily rejected feverfew as a useless herb! Feverfew remained

out of fashion until a serendipitous event occurred in the late 1970s.

At that time, the wife of the chief medical officer of the National Coal Board in England suffered from serious migraine headaches. When workers in the industry learned of this fact, a sympathetic miner suggested she try a folk treatment he had used. She followed his advice and chewed feverfew leaves. The results were dramatic: her migraines disappeared almost completely.

Her husband was impressed, too. He used his high office to gain the ear of a physician who specialized in migraine headaches, Dr. E. Stewart Johnson of the London Migraine Clinic. Johnson subsequently tried feverfew on 10 of his patients. The results were so good that he subsequently gave the herb to 270 of his patients. A whopping 70% reported considerable relief.

Thoroughly excited now, Dr. Johnson enrolled 17 feverfew-using patients in an interesting type of double-blind study: Half continued to use feverfew, and the other half were transferred, without their knowledge, to a placebo.[2] Over a period of 6 months, the patients withdrawn from feverfew demonstrated a dramatic increase in headaches, nausea, and vomiting.

Unfortunately, this study didn't prove much. It was too small, and because the patients were already feverfew users, it didn't say anything about the effectiveness of feverfew in the population at large. (Presumably, the participants used feverfew because they already knew that the herb worked for them.) Nonetheless, the study brought a flood of response from the public, and ultimately led to the properly performed double-blind experiments described below.

For many years, it was assumed that the active ingredient in feverfew was a substance named parthenolide. Numerous articles were published explaining exactly how parthenolide prevented migraines, stating that it caused platelets to release serotonin and reduce the synthesis of prostaglandins, leukotrienes, and thromboxanes.[3–6] Based on this premature explanation, indignant authors complained that samples of feverfew on the market varied as much as 10 to 1 in their parthenolide content. No less an authority than herbal expert Varro Tyler said, "Standardization of the herbal material on the basis of its parthenolide content is urgently required if this potentially valuable herb is to be used effectively." [7]

However, everyone was jumping the gun. A recent study found that an extract of feverfew standardized to a high-parthenolide content is entirely ineffective.[8] Apparently, this high-parthenolide extract lacked some essential substance or group of substances present in the whole leaf. What those substances may be, however, remains mysterious.

WHAT IS FEVERFEW USED FOR TODAY?

Feverfew is primarily used for prevention of chronic, recurrent **migraine headaches** (see page 120). It must be taken religiously every day for best results.

Feverfew is also sometimes used at the onset of a migraine attack. It is not believed to be effective for cluster or tension headaches.

It is important to remember that serious diseases may occasionally first present themselves as migraine-type headaches. For this reason, proper medical diagnosis is essential if you suddenly start having migraines without a previous history, or if the pattern of your migraines changes significantly.

Feverfew is sometimes recommended for various forms of arthritis, but there is no evidence that it works.

WHAT IS THE SCIENTIFIC EVIDENCE FOR FEVERFEW?

Three double-blind studies have been performed to evaluate feverfew's effectiveness as a preventive treatment for migraines. Two returned positive results, the other negative.

The Nottingham trial followed 59 individuals for 8 months.[9] For 4 months, half received a daily capsule of powdered feverfew leaf; the other half took placebo. The groups were then switched and followed for an additional 4 months. Treatment with feverfew produced a 24% reduction in the number of migraines and a significant decrease in nausea and vomiting during the headaches.

A recent Israeli study of 57 people with migraines found a significant decrease in severity of migraine headaches.[10] Unfortunately, it did not report whether there was any change in the frequency of migraines. This study also used powdered feverfew leaf.

However, a Dutch study involving 50 people showed no difference whatsoever between placebo and a special feverfew extract standardized to parthenolide content.[11] As mentioned above, the explanation appears to be that parthenolide is not the active ingredient in feverfew.

DOSAGE

Given the recent confusion surrounding parthenolide, previous dosage recommendations for feverfew based on parthenolide content have been cast in doubt. At the present time, the best recommendation is probably to take 80 to 100 mg of powdered whole feverfew leaf daily.

When taken at the onset of a migraine headache, higher amounts of feverfew are often used. However, the optimum dosage has not been determined.

SAFETY ISSUES

Among the many thousands of people who use feverfew as a folk medicine in England, there have been no reports of serious toxicity. Animal studies suggest that feverfew is essentially nontoxic.[12]

In the 8-month Nottingham trial, there were no significant differences in side effects between the treated and control groups.[13] There were also no changes in measurements on blood tests and urinalysis.

In a survey involving 300 people, 11.3% reported mouth sores from chewing feverfew leaf, occasionally accompanied by general inflammation of tissues in the mouth.[14] A smaller percentage reported mild gastrointestinal distress.[15] However, mouth sores do not seem to occur in people who use encapsulated feverfew leaf powder, the usual form.

In view of its use as a folk remedy to promote abortions, feverfew should probably not be taken during pregnancy.

Because feverfew might slightly inhibit the activity of blood-clotting cells known as platelets,[16] it should not be combined with strong anticoagulants, such as Coumadin (warfarin) or heparin, except on medical advice. Feverfew might also increase the risk of stomach problems if combined with anti-inflammatory drugs such as aspirin.[17,18,19]

Safety in young children, pregnant or nursing women, or those with severe kidney or liver disease has not been established.

⚠ INTERACTIONS YOU SHOULD KNOW ABOUT

If you are taking **Coumadin (warfarin), heparin, aspirin** or other **nonsteroidal anti-inflammatory drugs:** Do not use feverfew except on medical advice.

🌱 FISH OIL

Supplement Forms/Alternate Names   Eicosapentaenoic Acid (EPA), Omega-3 Oil(s), Docosahexaenoic Acid (DHA), Omega-3 Fatty Acids

Principal Proposed Uses   Heart Disease Prevention, Rheumatoid Arthritis

Other Proposed Uses   Dysmenorrhea (Menstrual Pain), Bipolar Disorder (Manic-Depressive Illness), Raynaud's Phenomenon, Psoriasis, Osteoporosis, Lupus, Crohn's Disease, Depression, Prevention of Premature Birth, Vision Improvement in Premature Babies, Kidney Stones, Chronic Fatigue Syndrome, Diabetic Neuropathy, Allergies, Gout, Hypertension, Migraine Headaches, Ulcerative Colitis, Asthma, HIV Support, Prostate Cancer Prevention, IgA Nephropathy, Male Infertility, Multiple Sclerosis

If you're old enough, you may remember your mother giving you cod liver oil. This practice actually began when the smoke-filled skies of nineteenth-century England deprived youngsters of exposure to the sun. Without sun, their bodies couldn't make vitamin D, and they developed rickets. Because cod liver oil contains large amounts of vitamin D, it cured rickets and made a great contribution to public health. Today, however, other constituents of cod liver and other fish oils have become of interest: the omega-3 fatty acids.

Omega-3 fatty acids are one type of *essential fatty acids,* special fats that the body needs as much as it needs vitamins. (The other type is the omega-6 fatty acids. For more information, see the chapter on **GLA**.) Much of the research into the potential therapeutic benefits of omega-3 fatty acids began when studies of the Inuit (Eskimo) people found that although their diets contain an enormous amount of fat from fish, seals, and whales, they seldom suffer heart attacks or develop rheumatoid arthritis. This is presumably because those sources of fat are very high in omega-3 fatty acids.

Subsequent investigation found that the omega-3 fatty acids found in fish oil can lower blood triglyceride levels, "thin" the blood, and also decrease inflammation in various parts of the body. These effects, as well as others, may explain many of fish oil's apparent benefits.

REQUIREMENTS/SOURCES

There is no daily requirement for fish oil. However, a healthy diet should provide at least 5 g of essential fatty acids daily.

Many grains, fruits, vegetables, and vegetable oils contain significant amounts of essential omega-6 and/or omega-3 fatty acids. Some authorities believe that it is important to consume several times more omega-3 fatty acids than omega-6 fatty acids. If this theory is true, taking fish oil supplements might help ensure the proper balance.

Cod liver oil is the most common form of fish oil, but it may not be the best for reasons of safety (see Safety Issues). Salmon oil, mackerel oil, halibut oil, and the oils from other coldwater fish might be better choices.

THERAPEUTIC DOSAGES

Typical dosages of fish oil are 3 to 9 g daily, but this is not the upper limit. In one study, participants ingested 60 g daily.

The most important omega-3 fatty acids found in fish oil are called EPA (eicosapentaenoic acid) and DHA (docosahexaenoic acid). In order to match the dosage used in several major studies, you should probably take enough fish oil to supply about 1.8 g of EPA (1,800 mg) and 0.9 g of DHA daily (900 mg).

Some manufacturers add vitamin E to fish oil capsules to keep the oil from becoming rancid. Another method is to remove all the oxygen from the capsule.

Flaxseed oil also contains omega-3 fatty acids, although of a different kind. It has been suggested as a less smelly substitute for fish oil. However, there is no evidence that it is effective when used for the same therapeutic purposes as fish oil.[1]

THERAPEUTIC USES

There has been a great deal of excitement about the possibility of using fish oil to help prevent **heart disease** (see page 16). Fish or fish oil appears to lower triglyceride levels, raise HDL ("good") cholesterol, "thin" the blood, reduce levels of homocysteine, slow down atherosclerosis, and perhaps also treat **hypertension** (see page 98).[2–13]

Fish oil has also become recognized as an effective treatment for early stages of **rheumatoid arthritis** (see page 151). It appears to significantly reduce symptoms without side effects and may magnify the benefits of standard arthritis drugs.[14] However, we have no evidence that fish oil slows the progress of the disease. Consult your rheumatologist to determine what treatment is best for you.

Various essential fatty acids, including fish oil, **flaxseed oil** (see page 285), and **GLA (gamma-linolenic acid)** (see page 304), are widely recommended for **dysmenorrhea** (menstrual pain; see page 70), and two studies suggest that fish oil may indeed be effective.[15,16]

A study suggests that fish oil can be very helpful for **bipolar disorder** (see page 27), more commonly known as manic-depressive illness.[17] More research is needed, but this appears to be a potential breakthrough for this devastating condition, whose conventional treatment causes a great many side effects.

Small studies also suggest that fish oil may be helpful in **Raynaud's phenomenon** (a condition in which a person's hands and feet show abnormal sensitivity to cold temperatures) (see page 149),[18,19] **psoriasis** (see page 148),[20] **osteoporosis** (see page 136),[21,22] the autoimmune disease **lupus** (see page 114),[23] and a form of kidney disease called IgA nephropathy.[24]

Evidence is mixed on whether fish oil can help prevent flare-ups of **Crohn's disease** (see page 57), a condition in which parts of the digestive tract are highly inflamed. A 1-year double-blind trial involving 78 participants with Crohn's disease in remission who were at high risk for relapse found that fish oil supplements helped keep the disease from flaring up.[25] However, a double-blind placebo-controlled trial that followed 120 individuals for 1 year found that fish oil did not reduce the relapse rate as compared to placebo.[26] Negative results were also seen in a smaller double-blind trial.[27]

Interesting, but highly preliminary, evidence suggests that fish oil, or its constituents, might be helpful for treating **depression** (see page 59), preventing premature birth, improving vision in premature babies, treating **kidney stones** (see page 109), alleviating the symptoms of **chronic fatigue syndrome** (see page 45), and reducing the risk of prostate **cancer** (see page 32).[28–34] Fish oil has also been proposed as a treatment for many other conditions, including **diabetic neuropathy** (see page 65),[35] **allergies** (see page 2), **gout** (see page 84), and **migraine headaches** (see page 120), but there has been little real scientific investigation of these uses.

Small double-blind trials suggest that fish oil might be helpful for reducing symptoms of **ulcerative colitis** (see page 179).[36–40] However, another small double-blind placebo-controlled trial found no such benefit.[41] Larger studies will be necessary to discover for certain whether fish oil helps or not. Regular use of fish oil does not appear to help prevent disease flare-ups.[42,43]

Despite widely publicized claims that fish oil helps **asthma** (see page 14), preliminary studies have not found it effective, and one study found that fish oil can actually worsen aspirin-related asthma.[44,45,46]

Fish oil is also sometimes recommended for enhancing immunity in **HIV infection** (see page 94). However, one 6-month double-blind study found that a combination of the omega-3 fatty acids in fish oil plus the amino acid arginine was no more effective than placebo in improving immune function in people with HIV.[47] Fish oil, however, might help individuals with HIV gain weight.[48]

Finally, preliminary studies suggest fish oil may help symptoms of **multiple sclerosis** (see page 124); however, one double-blind study found no difference between people taking fish oil and those taking olive oil (used as a placebo).[49–53]

Docosahexaenoic acid (DHA), a component of fish oil, has been evaluated as a possible treatment for **male infertility** (see page 116), but a double-blind trial of 28 men with impaired sperm activity found no benefit.[54]

WHAT IS THE SCIENTIFIC EVIDENCE FOR FISH OIL?

Heart Disease Prevention

There is some evidence that fish oil can help prevent heart disease, but it is not definitive.

An open trial of 11,324 individuals followed for 3 to 5 years did find that fish oil could significantly reduce the risk of death from heart attack, and that it was more effective for this purpose than vitamin E.[55] However, because this was not a double-blind study, the results can't be taken as fully reliable.

We do know that fish oil can lower serum triglycerides.[56] Like cholesterol, triglycerides are a type of fat in the blood that tends to damage the arteries, leading to heart disease. Reducing triglyceride levels should help prevent heart disease to some extent.

Fish oil also appears to modestly raise the levels of HDL ("good") cholesterol.[57,58] Additionally, it may help the heart by "thinning" the blood and by reducing blood levels of homocysteine.[59] Blood clots play a major role in heart attacks, and homocysteine is an amino acid that appears to raise the risk of heart disease.

Studies contradict one another on whether fish oil can lower blood pressure.[60–65] A 6-week double-blind placebo-controlled study of 59 overweight men suggests that the DHA in fish oil, but not the EPA, can reduce blood pressure.[66]

Rheumatoid Arthritis

The omega-3 fatty acids in fish oil can help reduce the symptoms of rheumatoid arthritis, according to 12 double-blind placebo-controlled studies involving a total of over 500 people.[67] This evidence is so strong that it has impressed many conventional physicians. However, unlike some conventional treatments, fish oil probably does not slow the progression of rheumatoid arthritis.

Menstrual Pain

Regular use of fish oil may reduce the pain of menstrual cramps.

In a 4-month study of 42 young women aged 15 to 18, half the participants received a daily dose of 6 g of fish oil, providing 1,080 mg of EPA and 720 mg of DHA daily.[68] After 2 months, they were switched to placebo for another 2 months. The other group received the same treatments in reverse order. The results showed that these young women experienced significantly less menstrual pain while they were taking fish oil.

Another double-blind study followed 78 women, who received either fish oil, seal oil, fish oil with vitamin B_{12} (7.5 mcg daily), or placebo for three full menstrual periods.[69] Significant improvements were seen in all treatment groups, but the fish oil plus B_{12} proved most effective, and its benefits continued for the longest time after treatment was stopped (3 months). The researchers offered no explanation why B_{12} should be helpful.

Bipolar Disorder

A 4-month double-blind placebo-controlled study of 30 individuals suggests that fish oil can produce striking benefits in bipolar disorder, preventing relapse and improving emotional state.[70] Eleven of the 14 individuals who took fish oil improved or remained well during the course of the study, while only 6 out of the 16 given placebo responded similarly.

The study will now be repeated by Baylor University and Harvard Medical School/McLean Hospital, enrolling 120 people for a period of 3 years.

Raynaud's Phenomenon

In small double-blind studies, high dosages of fish oil have been found to reduce the severe finger and toe responses to cold temperatures that occur in Raynaud's phenomenon.[71,72] However, these studies suggest that a very high dosage must be used to get results, perhaps 12 g daily. Gamma-linolenic acid (GLA), an omega-6 fatty acid, may work as well.

Psoriasis

There is some evidence that eicosapentaenoic acid (EPA) from fish oil may be helpful in psoriasis. One double-blind study followed 28 people with chronic psoriasis for 8 weeks.[73] Half received 1.8 g of EPA daily (supplied by 10 capsules of fish oil), and the other half received placebo. By the end of the study, researchers saw significant improvement in itching, redness, and scaling, but not in the size of the psoriasis patches. However, another double-blind study followed 145 people with moderate to severe psoriasis for 4 months and found no benefit as compared to placebo.[74]

Osteoporosis

Essential fatty acids may also help prevent osteoporosis when taken along with calcium. In one study, 65 postmenopausal women were given calcium along with either placebo or a combination of omega-6 fatty acids (GLA) and omega-3 fatty acids (from fish oil) for a period of 18 months. At the end of the study, the treated groups had denser bones and fewer fractures than the placebo group.[75] Similar results were seen in another study of 40 women.[76]

Lupus

Lupus is a serious autoimmune disease that can cause numerous problems, including fatigue, joint pain, and kidney disease. One small 34-week double-blind placebo-controlled crossover study compared placebo against daily doses of EPA (20 g) from fish oil.[77] A total of 17 individuals completed the trial. Of these, 14 showed improvement when taking EPA, while only 4 did so when treated with placebo. However, evidence suggests that fish oil is specifically not effective for lupus nephritis (kidney damage caused by lupus).[78,79]

SAFETY ISSUES

Fish oil appears to be safe. The most common problem is fishy burps.

Because fish oil has a mild "blood-thinning" effect, it should not be combined with powerful blood-thinning medications, such as Coumadin (warfarin) or heparin, except on a physician's advice. However, contrary to some reports, fish oil does not seem to cause bleeding problems when it is taken by itself.[80]

Also, fish oil does not appear to raise blood sugar levels in people with diabetes.[81] Nonetheless, if you have diabetes, you should not take any supplement except on the advice of a physician.

Fish oil may temporarily raise the level of LDL ("bad") cholesterol, but this effect seems to be short-lived, and levels return to normal with continued use.[82,83]

If you decide to use cod liver oil as your fish oil supplement, make sure you do not exceed the safe maximum intake of **vitamin A** (see page 432) and **vitamin D** (see page 449). These vitamins are fat soluble, which means that excess amounts tend to build up in your body, possibly reaching toxic levels. Pregnant women should not take more than 2,667 IU of vitamin A daily because of the risk of birth defects; 5,000 IU per day is a reasonable upper limit for other individuals. Look at the bottle label to determine how much vitamin A you are receiving. (It is less likely that you will get enough vitamin D to produce toxic effects.)

⚠ INTERACTIONS YOU SHOULD KNOW ABOUT

If you are taking **Coumadin (warfarin)** or **heparin,** do not take fish oil except on the advice of a physician.

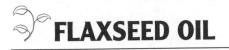

FLAXSEED OIL

Supplement Forms/Alternate Names   Linseed Oil

Principal Proposed Uses   There are no well-documented uses for flaxseed oil.

Other Proposed Uses   Heart Disease Prevention, Rheumatoid Arthritis, Bipolar Disorder, Cancer Prevention

Note: Flaxseed oil contains alpha-linolenic acid.

Flaxseed oil is derived from the hard, tiny seeds of the flax plant. It has been proposed as a less smelly alternative to fish oil. Like fish oil, flaxseed oil contains omega-3 fatty acids, a type of fat your body needs as much as it needs vitamins.

However, it's important to realize that the omega-3 fatty acids in flaxseed oil aren't identical to what you get from fish oil. Flaxseed oil contains alpha-linolenic acid (ALA), while fish oil contains eicosapentaenoic acid (EPA) and docosahexaenoic acid (DHA). The effects and potential benefits may not be the same.

Flaxseeds contain another important group of chemicals known as *lignans*. **Lignans** (see page 345) are being studied for use in preventing cancer. However, contrary to some reports, flaxseed *oil* has no lignans.[1]

REQUIREMENTS/SOURCES

Flaxseed oil contains both omega-3 and omega-6 fatty acids, which are essential to health. Although the exact daily requirement of these essential fatty acids is not known, deficiencies are believed to be fairly common.[2] Flaxseed oil may be an economical way to ensure that you get enough essential fatty acids in your diet.

The essential fatty acids in flax can be damaged by exposure to heat, light, and oxygen (essentially, they become rancid). For this reason, you shouldn't cook with flaxseed oil. A good product should be sold in an opaque container, and the manufacturing process should keep the temperature under 100 degrees Fahrenheit. Some manufacturers combine the product with vitamin E because it helps prevent rancidity.

THERAPEUTIC DOSAGES

A typical dosage is 1 to 2 tablespoons of flaxseed oil daily. It can be taken in capsule form or made into salad dressing. Some people find the taste pleasant, although others would politely disagree.

For whole flaxseed, a typical dose is 1 tablespoon of the seed (not ground) with plenty of liquid 2 to 3 times daily.

THERAPEUTIC USES

The best use of flaxseed oil is as a general nutritional supplement to provide essential fatty acids. There is little evidence that it is effective for any specific therapeutic purpose.

Flaxseed oil has been proposed as a less smelly alternative to fish oil for the prevention of **heart disease** (see page 16). Although fish oil is much better studied,

Flaxseed Oil

Visit Us at TNP.com

there is some evidence that flaxseed oil or whole **flaxseed** (see page 286) may reduce LDL ("bad") **cholesterol** (see page 88), perhaps slightly reduce **hypertension** (see page 98), and, overall, slow down **atherosclerosis** (see page 16).[3,4,5]

In addition, one study found that a diet high in ALA (from sources other than flaxseed oil) was associated with a reduced risk of heart disease.[6] However, there were so many other factors involved that it is hard to say what caused what.[7]

Although fish oil appears to be effective for reducing symptoms of **rheumatoid arthritis** (see page 151), flaxseed oil does not seem to work.[8]

One very preliminary study suggests that flaxseed oil may be helpful for controlling **bipolar disorder** (see page 27) when combined with conventional medications.[9]

Finally, although flaxseed or flaxseed oil are sometimes recommended as prevention or treatment for **cancer** (see page 32), the evidence is still extremely preliminary.[10–13]

SAFETY ISSUES

Flaxseed oil appears to be a safe nutritional supplement when used as recommended.

FLAXSEED

Alternate or Related Names   Linseed, Lint Bells, Flax, Winterlien

Principal Proposed Uses   Constipation, Irritable Bowel Syndrome

Other Proposed Uses   Diverticulitis, Atherosclerosis Prevention, Elevated Cholesterol, Cancer Prevention, Menopausal Symptoms, Kidney Disease, Gastritis, Gastroenteritis, Painful Skin Inflammation (topical)

Flaxseeds are the hard, tiny seeds of *Linum usitatissimum*, the flax plant that has been widely used for thousands of years as a source of food and clothing. So far, scientists have isolated at least three flaxseed components with potential health benefits. The first is fiber, valuable in treating **constipation** (see page 56). The benefits of the other two substances, alpha-linolenic acid (a type of **omega-3 fatty acid;** see page 285) and lignans, are not yet fully confirmed; still, preliminary research suggests that these components may be helpful in prevention of cancer and heart disease and perhaps in treatment of chronic kidney disease and menopausal symptoms.

The oil made from flaxseed has no appreciable amounts of lignans but it does contain alpha-linolenic acid. See **flaxseed oil** (page 285) and **lignans** (page 345) for more information on these substances.

WHAT IS FLAXSEED USED FOR TODAY?

Germany's Commission E authorizes the use of flaxseed for various digestive problems, such as chronic constipation, irritable bowel syndrome, diverticulitis, and general stomach discomfort.[1] The fiber in flaxseed binds with water, swelling to form a soothing gel which helps soften the stool and move it along in the intestines. The natural action of fiber-containing foods such as flaxseed can be particularly helpful when constipation is chronic. At least one study has found that flaxseed can help with chronic constipation in irritable bowel disease.[2]

Like other high-fiber foods, flaxseed may also be helpful in reducing cholesterol.[3,4,5] It's possible that besides the effects of its fiber, other components of flax, such as its lignans or oil, may help lower cholesterol and prevent atherosclerosis.[6–10]

Flaxseed, its lignans, and its oil are also being investigated for potential cancer prevention or even treatment.[11–18] In addition, very preliminary research indicates potential benefits in treating menopausal symptoms and certain kidney diseases.[19,20,21]

Warning: Do not use flaxseed to treat kidney disease or cancer without a doctor's supervision, because these conditions are potentially quite serious.

Because of its soothing nature, flaxseed is routinely used in Europe for symptomatic relief of short-term inflammation of the stomach and intestines (gastritis or gastroenteritis) as well as applied externally for painful skin inflammations.[22] However, research on these uses is fairly minimal.

WHAT IS THE SCIENTIFIC EVIDENCE FOR FLAXSEED?

Constipation

In a double-blind study, 55 people with chronic constipation caused by irritable bowel syndrome received either ground flaxseed or psyllium seed (a well-known treatment for constipation) daily for 3 months.[23] Those taking flaxseed had significantly fewer problems with constipation, abdominal pain, and bloating than those taking psyllium. The flaxseed group had even further improvements in constipation and bloating while continuing their treatment in the 3 months after the double-blind study ended. The researcher concluded that flaxseed relieved constipation more effectively than psyllium.

Cholesterol and Atherosclerosis

Several human studies have found that flaxseed lowers cholesterol.[24,25,26] In one double-blind study, 38 older women with high cholesterol ate bread or muffins containing either flaxseed or sunflower seed for 6 weeks, later switching to the opposing treatment for another 6 weeks.[27] Total cholesterol dropped with both regimens, but only those on the flaxseed regimen had significantly lower LDL, the "bad" cholesterol. In another investigation, 29 men and older women with high cholesterol ate muffins with either partially defatted flaxseed or a wheat bran placebo for 3 weeks each.[28] Those eating flaxseed showed significant decreases in both total and LDL cholesterol, compared to little change with placebo.

Finally, in the double-blind study on constipation mentioned earlier, both treatments—flaxseed and psyllium—led to a 10% reduction in total cholesterol and a 14% reduction in LDL cholesterol.[29] In none of these studies did flaxseed lower HDL ("good") cholesterol.

Flaxseed may also have a direct effect in preventing atherosclerosis, a condition in which arteries become lined with fatty deposits. Two rabbit studies found that both flaxseed and one of its lignans prevented atherosclerosis.[30,31] The lignan also lowered the rabbits' cholesterol, but flaxseed by itself did not.

The oil from flaxseeds has been suggested as an alternative to fish oil in prevention of heart disease. Fish oil, however, lowers blood triglyceride levels as its main effect, and flaxseed oil does not affect triglyceride levels.[32]

Cancer

Scientists are investigating whether flaxseed or its lignans can help prevent or treat cancer, particularly cancer of the breast and colon. Observational studies suggest that people who eat more lignan-containing foods have a lower incidence of breast and perhaps colon cancer.[33] However, other factors may have been responsible for these outcomes.

The lignans in flaxseed are phytoestrogens, plant chemicals mimicking the effects of estrogen in the body: phytoestrogens hook onto the same spots on cells where estrogen attaches. If there is little estrogen in the body, for example after menopause, lignans may act like weak estrogen. However, when natural estrogen is abundant, lignans may reduce the hormone's effects by displacing it from cells; displacing estrogen in this manner may help prevent those cancers that depend on estrogen, such as breast cancer, from starting and developing. This is also how **soy** (see page 411) is believed to work in breast cancer prevention, although the phytoestrogens in soy are **isoflavones** (see page 335).

Some preliminary research indicates that these lignans may also fight cancer in other ways, perhaps by acting as antioxidants.[34,35,36]

Animal investigations using flaxseed and its lignans offer supporting evidence for a potential cancer preventive or even cancer treatment effect; several found that one or the other inhibited breast and colon cancer in animals[37,38,39] and reduced metastases from melanoma (a type of skin cancer) in mice.[40] Test tube studies found that flaxseed or one of its lignans inhibited the growth of human breast cancer cells,[41] and that the lignans enterolactone and enterodiol inhibited the growth of human colon tumor cells.[42] This preliminary research is promising, but much more is needed before we can draw any conclusions.

Although much of this anticancer work has focused on the lignans in flaxseed, one study also found that flaxseed oil—which contains no appreciable amounts of lignans—slowed the growth of malignant breast tumors in rats.[43]

THERAPEUTIC DOSAGES

According to the European Scientific Cooperative on Phytotherapy, the usual dose of flaxseed for constipation is 5 g of whole, cracked, or freshly crushed seeds soaked in water and taken with a glassful of liquid 3 times a day.[44] Expect effects to begin 18 to 24 hours later. Because of this time delay, it's recommended to take flaxseed for a minimum of 2 to 3 days. Children aged 6 to 12 should be given half the adult dose, while children younger than 6 should be treated only under the guidance of a physician.[45]

In one study, people received 6 to 24 g per day of flaxseed for 6 months for constipation caused by irritable bowel syndrome.[46]

To soothe an upset stomach, soak 5 to 10 g of whole flaxseed in a half cup of water, strain after 20 to 30 minutes, then drink.[47] For painful skin inflammations, the recommended dose is 30 to 50 g of crushed or powdered seed applied externally as a warm poultice or compress.[48]

Like other sources of fiber, flaxseed should be taken with plenty of fluids, or it may actually worsen constipation. Also, it's best to start with smaller doses and then increase.

SAFETY ISSUES

Don't take flaxseed or other laxatives if you have significant abdominal pain. Talk with your doctor.

Flaxseed appears to be safe when used as directed. Because of its potential effects on estrogen, however, avoid taking large amounts of flaxseed if you are pregnant or breast-feeding. One study found that pregnant rats who ate large amounts of flaxseed (5% or 10% of their diet), or one of its lignans, gave birth to offspring with altered reproductive organs and functions[49]—in humans, eating 25 g of flaxseed per day amounts to about 5% of the diet.[50] Lignans were also found to be transferred to baby rats during nursing.[51]

There are no reports that lignans cause or worsen cancer when taken in usual amounts. However, a few sensitive test tube studies have found that cancer cells were stimulated by lignans such as those present in flaxseed[52]—in contrast to other studies in which lignans inhibited cancer cell growth.[53] Like estrogen, lignans' positive or negative effects on cancer cells may depend on dose, type of cancer cell, and levels of hormones in the body. If you have cancer, particularly breast cancer, talk with your doctor before consuming large amounts of flaxseeds.

As with many substances, there have been reports of life-threatening allergic reactions to flaxseed.

If you have diabetes, flaxseed (like other high-fiber foods) may delay glucose absorption,[54] potentially leading to better blood sugar control and changes in the need for hypoglycemic drugs. Talk with your doctor about appropriate use.

Finally, flaxseeds contain tiny amounts of cyanide-containing substances, which can be a problem among livestock eating large amounts of flax.[55] While normal cooking and baking of whole flaxseeds or flour eliminates any detectable amounts of cyanide,[56] it is at least theoretically possible that eating huge amounts of raw or unprocessed flaxseeds or flaxseed meal could pose a problem. However, most authorities are not concerned about this possibility.[57]

FOLATE

Supplement Forms/Alternate Names   Folic Acid, Folacin

Principal Proposed Uses   Prevention of Birth Defects of the Brain and Spinal Cord, Heart Disease Prevention, Cancer Prevention

Other Proposed Uses   Gout, Bipolar Disorder, Depression, Osteoarthritis, Osteoporosis, Restless Legs Syndrome, Rheumatoid Arthritis, Seborrheic Dermatitis, Vitiligo, Migraine Headaches, Periodontal Disease

Folate, a B vitamin, plays a critical role in many biological processes. It participates in the crucial biological process known as methylation, and plays an important role in cell division: without sufficient amounts of folate, cells cannot divide properly. Adequate folate intake can reduce the risk of heart disease and prevent serious birth defects, and it may lessen the risk of developing certain forms of cancer.

Because the chances are good that you don't get enough folate in your diet, this is one vitamin really worth paying attention to.

REQUIREMENTS/SOURCES

Folate requirements rise with age. The official U.S. and Canadian recommendations for daily intake are as follows:

- Infants 0–5 months, 65 mcg
    6–11 months, 80 mcg
- Children 1–3 years, 150 mcg
    4–8 years, 200 mcg

- Males 9–13 years, 300 mcg
    14 years and older, 400 mcg
- Females 9–13 years, 300 mcg
    14 years and older, 400 mcg
- Pregnant women, 600 mcg
- Nursing women, 500 mcg

Folate deficiency is very common, and authorities have suggested adding folate to common foods, such as bread, at higher dosages than what is presently required.[1,2,3]

Various drugs may impair your body's ability to absorb or utilize folate, including antacids, bile acid sequestrants (such as cholestyramine and colestipol), H_2 blockers, methotrexate, various antiseizure medications (carbamazepine, phenobarbital, phenytoin, primidone, or valproate), sulfasalazine and possibly other certain NSAID-type drugs, high-dose triamterene, nitrous oxide, and the antibiotic trimethoprim-sulfamethoxazole.[4–29] Oral contraceptives may also affect folate slightly, but there doesn't appear to be a need for supplementation.[30,31,32]

Good sources of folate include dark green leafy veg-etables, oranges, other fruits, rice, brewer's yeast, beef liver, beans, asparagus, **kelp** (see page 340), soybeans, and soy flour.

THERAPEUTIC DOSAGES

For most uses, folate should be taken at nutritional doses, about 400 mcg daily for adults. However, higher dosages—up to 10 mg daily—have been used to treat specific diseases. Before taking more than 400 mcg daily, it is important to make sure that you don't have a vitamin B_{12} deficiency (see Safety Issues).

A particular kind of digestive enzyme, pancreatin (see the chapter on **proteolytic enzymes**) may interfere with the absorption of folate.[33] You can get around this by taking the two supplements at different times of day.

THERAPEUTIC USES

The use of folate supplements by pregnant women dra-matically decreases the risk that their children will be born with a serious birth defect called neural tube de-fect.[34,35] This congenital problem consists of problems with the brain or spinal cord.

Folate also lowers blood levels of homocysteine, a suspected risk factor in **heart disease** (see page 16).[36–41] According to some experts, increased folate supplementation of foods could reduce heart disease deaths in the United States by as much as 50,000 people annually.[42]

Studies suggest that a deficiency in folate might pre-dispose people to develop **cancer** (see page 32) of the cervix,[43] colon,[44] lung,[45] breast,[46] and mouth.[47] Large observational studies suggest that folate supplements may help prevent colon cancer, especially when taken for many years.[48,49,50] This is yet another reason to make sure you get enough folate daily. High-dose folate (10 mg daily) might be helpful for normalizing abnormalities in the appearance of the cervix (as seen under a micro-scope) in women taking oral contraceptives, but it does not appear to reverse actual cervical dysplasia.[51,52]

Folate deficiency may also increase the risk of Alzheimer's disease, although this has not yet been proven.[53]

Very high dosages of folate may be helpful for **gout** (see page 84),[54] although some authorities suggest that it was actually a contaminant of folate that caused the ben-efit seen in some studies.[55] Furthermore, other studies have found no benefit at all.[56,57]

Based on intriguing but not yet definitive evidence, folate in various dosages has been suggested as a treat-ment for **bipolar disorder** (see page 27), **depression** (see page 59), **osteoarthritis** (in combination with vita-min B_{12}; see page 132), **osteoporosis** (see page 136), **restless legs syndrome** (see page 150), **rheumatoid arthritis** (see page 151), **seborrheic dermatitis** (see page 154), and **vitiligo** (splotchy loss of skin pigmenta-tion; see page 191).[58–74] Other conditions for which it has been suggested include **migraine headaches** (see page 120) and **periodontal disease** (see page 142).

WHAT IS THE SCIENTIFIC EVIDENCE FOR FOLATE?

Neural Tube Defect

Very strong evidence tells us that regular use of folate by pregnant women can reduce the risk of neural tube de-fect by 50 to 80%.[75,76]

Heart Disease Prevention

According to a recent study that examined data on 80,000 women, a high intake of folate may cut the risk of heart disease in half.[77]

Folate is thought to work by reducing blood levels of a substance called homocysteine. Individuals with high homocysteine levels appear to have more than twice the risk of developing heart disease than those with low ho-mocysteine levels,[78] and folate supplements, alone or in combination with **vitamin B_6** (see page 439) and **vita-min B_{12}** (see page 442), effectively reduce the level of homocysteine in the blood.[79–82]

SAFETY ISSUES

Folate at nutritional doses is extremely safe. The only se-rious potential problem is that folate supplementation can mask the early symptoms of vitamin B_{12} deficiency (a special type of anemia), potentially allowing more ir-reversible symptoms of nerve damage to develop. For this reason, when taking more than 400 mcg daily, it is important to get your B_{12} level checked. See the chapter on vitamin B_{12} for more information.

Very high dosages of folate, greater than 5 mg (5,000 mcg) daily, can cause digestive upset. Maximum safe dosages have not been established for young children or pregnant or nursing women.

As mentioned previously, the antiseizure drug pheny-toin may interfere with folate absorption. Conversely, fo-late may reduce the effectiveness of phenytoin.[83–88] If you are taking phenytoin, you should consult with a physician about the proper dosage of folate for you.

Contrary to some reports, individuals who are taking the drug methotrexate for rheumatoid arthritis, juvenile rheumatoid arthritis, or psoriasis can safely take folate supplements at the same time.[89,90,91] In fact, supple-mental folate may actually be helpful under these condi-tions.[92,93] However, if you are taking methotrexate for any other purpose, do not take folate except on the ad-vice of a physician.

⚠ INTERACTIONS YOU SHOULD KNOW ABOUT

If you are taking

- **Aspirin**, other **anti-inflammatory medications, drugs that reduce stomach acid** (such as **antacids**, and **H₂ blockers**), **sulfa antibiotics, oral contraceptives, estrogen-replacement therapy, valproic acid, carbamazepine, phenobarbital, primidone, triamterene, nitrous oxide**, or **bile acid sequestrants** (such as **cholestyramine and colestipol**): You may need to take extra folate.

- **Phenytoin:** You may need more folate. However, too much folate can interfere with this medication and cause seizures! Physician supervision is essential.
- **Pancreatin** (a proteolytic enzyme): It may be advisable to separate your dose of pancreatin from your dose of folate by at least 2 hours in order to avoid absorption problems.
- **Methotrexate** for rheumatoid arthritis, juvenile rheumatoid arthritis, or psoriasis: You may do well to take a folate supplement. You can use folate without fear of decreasing the medication's effects. However, if you are taking methotrexate for other purposes, do not take folate except on the advice of a physician.

GAMMA ORYZANOL

Principal Proposed Uses   Menopausal Symptoms ("Hot Flashes"), High Cholesterol

Other Proposed Uses   Anxiety, Stomach Distress, Bodybuilding

Gamma oryzanol is a mixture of substances derived from rice bran oil, including sterols and ferulic acid. It has been approved in Japan for several conditions, including menopausal symptoms, mild anxiety, stomach upset, and high cholesterol. Each year Japan manufactures 7,500 tons of gamma oryzanol from 150,000 tons of rice bran. Not surprisingly, most of the research on oryzanol has been performed in Japan and few studies have been translated into English.

Scientists are not certain how gamma oryzanol works. For menopause, it may affect a key hormone, luteinizing hormone (LH). Gamma oryzanol may also interfere with the absorption of cholesterol into the body from food, thus reducing cholesterol levels in the blood.

SOURCES

There is no daily requirement for gamma oryzanol.

Rice bran oil is the principal source of gamma oryzanol, but it is also found in the bran of wheat and other grains, as well as various fruits, vegetables, and herbs. However, to get enough gamma oryzanol to reach recommended therapeutic dosages, you will need to take supplements.

THERAPEUTIC DOSAGES

The typical dosage of gamma oryzanol is 300 mg daily.

THERAPEUTIC USES

Despite the widespread use of gamma oryzanol for **menopausal symptoms** (see page 117), the studies available provide little evidence that it is effective. The most commonly cited Japanese study was very small and did not have a control group.[1]

Gamma oryzanol may be useful for elevated **cholesterol** (see page 88), although the principal evidence appears to be limited to a few animal studies.[2,3] No serious evidence has been presented in English for using gamma oryzanol as a treatment for **anxiety** (see page 11) or stomach distress.

Very preliminary evidence suggests that gamma oryzanol may increase endorphin release and aid muscle development.[4,5] These findings have created an interest in using gamma oryzanol as a **sports supplement** (see page 158). However, one double-blind study found it not effective.[6]

WHAT IS THE SCIENTIFIC EVIDENCE FOR GAMMA ORYZANOL?

Menopausal Symptoms

Gamma oryzanol may be effective in treating hot flashes associated with menopause. An early study examined 21 women, 8 who were experiencing menopause and 13 who had had their ovaries surgically removed. Each woman was given 300 mg daily of gamma oryzanol.[7] After 38 days, more than 67% of the women improved significantly. However, because this study had no control group, there's no way to know whether the benefit was caused by gamma oryzanol or merely the power of suggestion. Keep in mind that at least 50% of menopausal women given placebo experience significant relief from symptoms.[8]

High Cholesterol

The best evidence that gamma oryzanol can lower cholesterol levels comes from animal studies. In one such study, 32 hamsters with experimentally induced high cholesterol were given a high-saturated-fat diet containing 5% coconut oil and 0.1% cholesterol, with or without 1% oryzanol, for 7 weeks.[9] Despite the unhealthy diet, the hamsters that were given oryzanol absorbed 25% less cholesterol from their food than the control group, and experienced a significant (28%) drop in total cholesterol

in the blood. A small, uncontrolled study in people found similar reductions in cholesterol.[10]

Bodybuilding

A 9-week, double-blind placebo-controlled trial of 22 weight-trained males found no difference between placebo or 500 mg daily of gamma oryzanol in terms of performance, body composition, or hormone levels.[11]

SAFETY ISSUES

No significant side effects have been reported with gamma oryzanol. However, the maximum safe dosages for young children, pregnant or nursing women, or those with severe liver or kidney disease have not been established.

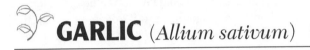

GARLIC (*Allium sativum*)

Alternate or Related Names   Poor Man's Treacle, Clove Garlic, Common Garlic, Allium, Stinking Rose

Principal Proposed Uses   Atherosclerosis, (Lowering Cholesterol, Reducing Blood Pressure, "Thinning the Blood"), Heart Attack Prevention

Other Proposed Uses   Cancer Prevention, Topical Antibiotic and Antifungal, Athlete's Foot, Immune Stimulant, Asthma, Candida, Colds, Diabetes, Vaginal Infections

Probably Ineffective Uses   Oral Antibiotic, Ear Infections

The story of garlic's role in human history could fill a book, as indeed it has, many times. Its species name, *sativum*, means cultivated, indicating that garlic does not grow in the wild. So fond have humans been of this herb that garlic can be found almost everywhere in the world, from Polynesia to Siberia. Interestingly, as far back as the first century A.D., Dioscorides wrote of garlic's ability to "clear the arteries."

From Roman antiquity through World War I, garlic poultices were used to prevent wound infections. The famous microbiologist, Louis Pasteur, performed some of the original work showing that garlic could kill bacteria. In 1916, the British government issued a general plea for the public to supply it with garlic in order to meet wartime needs. Garlic was called "Russian penicillin" during World War II because, after running out of antibiotics, the Russian government turned to this ancient treatment for its soldiers.

Conventional doctors in the United States continued to use garlic even when they had abandoned nearly all other herbs. After World War II, Sandoz Pharmaceuticals manufactured a garlic compound for intestinal spasms, and the Van Patten Company produced another for lowering blood pressure.

In the 1950s, garlic finally fell completely out of favor with American physicians. European physicians continued to investigate garlic.

WHAT IS GARLIC USED FOR TODAY?

In Europe, garlic has come to be seen as an all-around treatment for preventing **atherosclerosis** (see page 16), the cause of heart disease and strokes. As we'll see in the following discussion, many (but not all) studies have found that certain forms of garlic can lower total **cholesterol** (see page 88) levels by about 9 to 12%, as well as possibly improve the ratio of good and bad cholesterol. Garlic also appears to slightly improve **hypertension** (see page 98), protect against free radicals, and slow blood coagulation. Putting all these benefits together, garlic may be a broad-spectrum treatment for arterial disease. Indeed, a double-blind placebo-controlled study that followed 152 individuals for 4 years found that garlic significantly reduced the development of atherosclerosis.[1]

Preliminary evidence suggests that regular use of garlic may help prevent **cancer** (see page 32). While eating garlic is commonly stated to raise immunity, there is no real evidence that this is the case.

Garlic is an effective antibiotic when it contacts the tissue directly, but there is no evidence that it will work in this way if you take it by mouth.

Garlic has known antifungal properties,[2-5] and there is highly preliminary evidence suggesting that ajoene, a compound derived from garlic, might help treat **athlete's foot** (see page 21).[6]

Garlic has also been proposed as a treatment for **asthma** (see page 14), **candida** (see page 38), **colds** (see page 47), **diabetes** (see page 65), and **vaginal infections** (see page 182).[7,8]

Garlic oil products are often recommended for children's ear infections. While these products may reduce pain, it is very unlikely that they have any actual effect on the infection because the eardrum is in the way.

Contrary to some reports, garlic does not appear to be able to kill *Helicobacter pylori*, the stomach bacteria implicated as a major cause of **ulcers** (see page 180).[9,10]

WHAT IS THE SCIENTIFIC EVIDENCE FOR GARLIC?

The science behind using garlic to prevent atherosclerosis is moderately strong, although there are some contradictions in the research record.

Garlic preparations have been found to slow hardening of the arteries in animals, reducing the size of plaque deposits by nearly 50%.[11,12] Garlic appears to function somewhat like prescription drugs by interfering with the manufacture of cholesterol.[13,14,15]

Garlic extracts have been found to reduce blood pressure in dogs and rats.[16] Numerous test tube, animal, and human studies suggest that various forms of garlic can reduce blood clotting and neutralize free radicals.[17-23]

High Cholesterol

At least 28 controlled clinical studies of using garlic to treat elevated cholesterol were published between 1985 and 1995. Together, they suggest that garlic can lower cholesterol by about 9 to 12%.[24,25] Virtually all of these studies used garlic standardized to alliin content (see the discussion under Dosage). Garlic oil does not seem to be effective.

One of the best of these studies was conducted in Germany and published in 1990.[26] A total of 261 patients at 30 medical centers were given either 800 mg of standardized garlic daily or placebo. Over the course of 16 weeks, patients in the treated group experienced a 12% drop in total cholesterol and a 17% decrease in triglyceride levels. The greatest benefits occurred in patients with initial cholesterol levels of 250 to 300 mg/dL.

Another double-blind study, reported in 1996, followed 41 men with cholesterol readings of 220 to 290 mg/dL.[27] The men received either placebo or 7.2 g of aged garlic extract daily for 6 months; then their treatments were switched for 4 months. The results showed a 7% decrease in total serum cholesterol and a 4% decrease in LDL ("bad") cholesterol in the garlic-treated group. There was also a 5.5% decrease in blood pressure.

One widely quoted study compared garlic to the standard cholesterol-lowering drug bezafibrate.[28] Although the results showed them to be equally effective, the study was not designed properly, so the results mean little. Both groups in the study were asked to improve their diets. The effects of the dietary change could have easily overshadowed real differences between the treatments.

In contrast to these positive results, a couple of other studies have shown no benefit with garlic powder. One study, published in 1996, followed 115 individuals with total cholesterol concentrations of 231 to 328 mg/dL, half of whom received 900 mg daily of a standard garlic extract standardized to contain 1.3% allicin.[29] The results showed no significant difference between the treated and placebo groups. Other studies have also found no benefit.[30,31,32]

However, just as in the bezafibrate study, all participants in these two studies were asked to make dietary changes, which may have overwhelmed garlic's antihypercholesterolemic effects.

It can be said with some certainty that garlic oil is not effective for lowering cholesterol.[33]

Hypertension (High Blood Pressure)

Numerous studies have found that garlic lowers blood pressure slightly, usually in the neighborhood of 5 to 10% more than placebo.[34,35] However, all of these studies suffered from significant flaws, and most were performed on people without high blood pressure.

One of the best studies followed 47 subjects with an average starting blood pressure of 171/101.[36] Over a period of 12 weeks, half were treated with 600 mg of garlic powder daily standardized to 1.3% alliin, the other half were given placebo. The results showed a statistically significant drop of 11% in the systolic blood pressure and 13% in the diastolic pressure. (Blood pressure also fell in the placebo group, by 5% and 4%, respectively, so the actual improvement due to garlic is somewhat less than it first appears.) Some garlic studies have been criticized on the basis of the participants being able to tell whether they were being given real garlic or placebo by detecting the garlic odor, but the study authors state that regular questioning of the participants revealed that they could not tell which group they were in.

Another study suggests that garlic's effects increase if it is given a longer time to act. In a 16-week open trial, about 40 subjects with mild hypertension were given 600 mg 3 times daily of a garlic preparation standardized to 1.3% alliin (an unusually high dose).[37] The participants started with an average blood pressure of 151/96. At 4 weeks, there was a 10% drop in systolic blood pressure, and at 16 weeks the improvement reached 19%. Similar progressive changes occurred in the diastolic blood pressure.

Overall Effects on Hardening of the Arteries

In a double-blind placebo-controlled study that followed 152 individuals for 4 years, standardized garlic powder at a dosage of 900 mg daily significantly slowed the development of atherosclerosis as measured by ultrasound.[38] Although this study suffered from some statistical flaws, it nonetheless provides direct evidence that all of garlic's effects combine to protect against hardening of the arteries.

A recent observational study of 200 individuals suggests that garlic affects hardening of the arteries not only by lowering cholesterol or blood pressure, but also through other effects.[39] The study measured the flexibility of the aorta, the main artery exiting the heart. Even in individuals with the same blood pressure and cholesterol levels, those who took garlic showed less evidence of damage to their arteries.

Heart Attack Prevention

In one study, 432 individuals who had suffered a heart attack were given either garlic oil or no treatment at all over a period of 3 years.[40] The results showed a significant reduction of second heart attacks and about a 50% reduction in death rate among those taking garlic.

Cancer Prevention

Several large studies strongly suggest that a diet high in garlic can prevent cancer. In one of the best, the Iowa Women's Study, a group of 41,837 women were questioned as to their lifestyle habits in 1986, and then followed continuously in subsequent years. At the 4-year follow-up, questionnaires showed that women whose diets included significant quantities of garlic were approximately 30% less likely to develop colon cancer.[41]

The interpretations of studies like this one are always a bit controversial. For example, it's possible that the women who ate a lot of garlic also made other healthy lifestyle choices. While researchers looked at this possibility very carefully and concluded that garlic was a common factor, it is not clear that they are right. What is really needed to settle the question is an intervention trial, where some people are given garlic and others are given a placebo. However, none has yet been performed.[42]

Antimicrobial

There is no question that raw garlic can kill a wide variety of microorganisms by direct contact, including fungi, bacteria, viruses, and protozoa.[43,44] A double-blind study reported in 1999 found that a cream made from the garlic constituent ajoene was just as effective for fungal skin infections as the standard drug terbinafine.[45] These findings may explain why garlic was traditionally applied directly to **wounds** (see page 123) in order to prevent infection (but keep in mind that it can burn the skin). But there is no real evidence that taking garlic orally can kill organisms throughout the body. Thus, it's not an antibiotic in the usual sense. It's more like Bacitracin ointment.

DOSAGE

A typical dosage of garlic is 900 mg daily of a garlic powder extract standardized to contain 1.3% alliin, providing about 12,000 mcg of alliin daily. However, a great deal of controversy exists over the proper dosage and form of garlic. Most everyone agrees that one or two raw garlic cloves per day are adequate for most purposes, but virtual trade wars have taken place over the potency and effectiveness of various dried, aged, or deodorized garlic preparations. The problem has to do with the way garlic is naturally constructed.

A relatively odorless substance, alliin, is one of the most important compounds in garlic. When garlic is crushed or cut, an enzyme called allinase is brought in contact with alliin, turning it into allicin. The allicin itself then rapidly breaks down into entirely different compounds. Allicin is most responsible for garlic's strong odor. It can also blister the skin and kill bacteria, viruses, and fungi. Presumably the garlic plant uses allicin as a form of protection from pests and parasites. It also may provide much of the medicinal benefits of garlic.

When you powder garlic to put it in a capsule, it acts like cutting the bulb. The chain reaction starts: Alliin contacts allinase, yielding allicin, which then breaks down. Unless something is done to prevent this process, garlic powder won't have any alliin or allicin left by the time you buy it.

Some garlic producers declare that alliin and allicin have nothing to do with garlic's effectiveness and simply sell products without it. This is particularly true of aged powdered garlic and garlic oil. But others feel certain that allicin is absolutely essential. However, in order to make garlic relatively odorless, they must prevent the alliin from turning into allicin until the product is consumed. To accomplish this feat, they engage in marvelously complex manufacturing processes, each unique and proprietary. How well each of these methods work is a matter of finger-pointing controversy.

The best that can be said at this point is that in most of the studies that found cholesterol-lowering powers in garlic, the daily dosage supplied at least 10 mg of alliin. This is sometimes stated in terms of how much allicin will be created from that alliin. The number you should look for is 4 to 5 mg of "allicin potential."

Garlic

Visit Us at TNP.com

Genistein

Alliin-free aged garlic also appears to be effective when taken at a dose of 1 to 7.2 g daily.

SAFETY ISSUES

As a commonly used food, garlic is on the FDA's GRAS (generally recognized as safe) list. Rats have been fed gigantic doses of aged garlic (2,000 mg per kilogram body weight) for 6 months without any signs of negative effects.[46] Unfortunately, there do not appear to be any animal toxicity studies on the most commonly used form of garlic—powdered garlic standardized to alliin content.

The only common side effect of garlic is unpleasant breath odor. Even "odorless garlic" produces an offensive smell in up to 50% of those who use it.[47]

Other side effects occur only rarely. For example, a study that followed 1,997 people who were given a normal dose of deodorized garlic daily over a 16-week period showed a 6% incidence of nausea, a 1.3% incidence of dizziness on standing (perhaps a sign of low blood pressure), and a 1.1% incidence of allergic reactions.[48] These are very low percentages in comparison to those usually reported in drug studies. There were also a few reports of bloating, headaches, sweating, and dizziness.

When raw garlic is taken in excessive doses, it can cause numerous symptoms, such as stomach upset, heartburn, nausea, vomiting, diarrhea, flatulence, facial flushing, rapid pulse, and insomnia.

Topical garlic can cause skin irritation, blistering, and even third-degree burns, so be very careful about applying garlic directly to the skin.[49]

Since garlic "thins" the blood, it is not a good idea to take high-potency garlic pills immediately prior to or after surgery or labor and delivery, due to the risk of excessive bleeding.[50] Similarly, garlic should not be combined with blood-thinning drugs, such as Coumadin (warfarin), heparin, aspirin, or Trental (pentoxifylline). In addition, garlic could conceivably interact with natural products with blood-thinning properties, such as **ginkgo** (see page 298) or high-dose **vitamin E** (see page 457).

Garlic may also combine poorly with certain HIV medications. Two people with **HIV** (see page 94) experienced severe gastrointestinal toxicity from the HIV drug ritonavir after taking garlic supplements.[51]

Garlic is presumed to be safe for pregnant women (except just before and immediately after delivery) and nursing mothers, although this has not been proven.

⚠ INTERACTIONS YOU SHOULD KNOW ABOUT

If you are taking

- Blood-thinning drugs such as **Coumadin (warfarin), heparin, aspirin,** or **Trental (pentoxifylline):** Do not use garlic except on medical advice.
- **Ginkgo** or high-dose **vitamin E:** Taking garlic at the same time might conceivably cause a risk of bleeding problems.

GENISTEIN

Principal Proposed Uses   Osteoporosis Prevention, Cancer Prevention

Other Proposed Uses   Cholesterol Reduction, Improving Menopausal Symptoms, Amyotrophic Lateral Sclerosis (Lou Gehrig's Disease)

Genistein, a naturally occurring chemical present in soy, has attracted scientific interest for its possible benefits in cancer and heart disease prevention. Genistein is a type of chemical called a phytoestrogen—an estrogen-like substance present in some plants. There are two main types of phytoestrogens: **isoflavones** (see page 335) and **lignans** (see page 345). **Soy** (see page 411) is the most abundant source of isoflavones, with genistein the most abundant isoflavone in soy.

Like other phytoestrogens, genistein can work in two ways: either by increasing or decreasing the effects of estrogen. This happens because genistein binds to special sites on cells called estrogen receptors. Genistein stimu-

lates these receptors, but not as strongly as real estrogen; at the same time, it blocks estrogen itself from attaching. The net result is that when there is a lot of estrogen in the body, such as before menopause, genistein may partly block its effects. Since estrogen appears to increase the risk of various forms of cancer, regular use of genistein by pre-menopausal women might help reduce this risk. On the other hand, if there is little human estrogen present, such as after menopause, genistein can partly make up for it. This is one rationale for using genistein to prevent osteoporosis.

Genistein may have many other beneficial effects as well. In test tube studies, genistein has been found to in-

Visit Us at TNP.com

hibit the growth of cancers—not only those that feed on estrogen (such as some types of breast cancer) but also those that do not.[1,2] In addition, it is a potent antioxidant. Along with other soy isoflavones, it appears to lower cholesterol and may help prevent the development of atherosclerosis.

There is a possibility that genistein may also reduce symptoms of menopause, although most of the evidence we have for this effect involves mixed isoflavones from soy.

REQUIREMENTS/SOURCES

Genistein is found in high quantities in soy and in negligible quantities in a few other foods. Most soy foods contain about 1 to 2 mg of genistein per gram of protein.[3]

THERAPEUTIC DOSAGES

The optimum dosage of genistein is unknown. In Asia, population groups who eat soy foods daily containing 20 to 80 mg of genistein have lower rates of breast and prostate cancer than do groups in the West with less genistein in their diets.[4] However, we don't know whether genistein alone is responsible for this lower rate of cancer. Other factors besides isoflavones may be involved.

THERAPEUTIC USES

Scientists are studying genistein as a possible treatment or preventive for **osteoporosis** (see page 136), **cancer** (see page 32), **heart disease** (see page 16), and **amyotrophic lateral sclerosis** (see page 9). Most of the evidence for genistein comes from test tube studies and animal studies, with the best evidence for benefit in osteoporosis. Human studies have tended to focus on soy foods and soy isoflavones in general, not specifically on genistein.

WHAT IS THE SCIENTIFIC EVIDENCE FOR GENISTEIN?

Osteoporosis

Estrogen has a powerfully protective effect on bone. In women, osteoporosis (bone loss) most often occurs after menopause when the ovaries stop putting out estrogen. Surgical removal of the ovaries (sometimes called surgical menopause) also causes osteoporosis.

In 1996, a study in rats found that eating soy decreased the bone loss resulting from ovary removal. Since then, three more rat studies have found that oral or injected genistein also significantly protected bone after the ovaries were removed.[5,6,7] The exact way in which genistein protects bone is not yet clear. Unlike estrogen, which helps prevent the destruction of bone

cells, two studies found that genistein seemed to assist in creating new bone cells.[8,9]

Interestingly, in one of the different rat studies, a small dose of genistein helped protect the rats' bones, while a larger dose of genistein seemed to have the opposite effect—causing increasing bone destruction.[10] Studies in humans are needed to determine whether genistein is truly effective, and to find the optimum dose.

Cancer

Scientists have found multiple mechanisms by which genistein may inhibit cancer. In the test tube, genistein has been found to suppress the growth of a wide range of cancer cells.[11,12] In other test tube studies, genistein seemed to enhance the effects of other chemotherapy drugs.[13]

In two animal studies, genistein inhibited skin cancer when applied to the skin of mice or fed to rats.[14,15] In another study, newborn female rats treated with genistein had less breast cancer later in life than those treated with placebo.[16]

Heart Disease

Soy protein has been found to lower cholesterol in numerous trials. In an animal study, for example, rats fed genistein had significantly decreased cholesterol compared to the control group.[17] A recent double-blind study of 156 people suggests that the isoflavones in soy, including genistein, may be responsible for much of this effect.[18] However, this conclusion isn't certain; another double-blind study found no change in cholesterol among 21 women given soy isoflavones isolated from soy protein.[19]

Genistein may have other means of preventing heart disease. Test tube studies suggest that genistein may help keep cholesterol in the blood from depositing on blood vessel walls, as occurs in atherosclerosis.[20] Finally, very early test tube research suggests genistein may also inhibit the formation of blood clots, which are a major cause of heart attacks.[21]

Other Conditions

Most of the studies on menopausal symptoms such as hot flashes have involved soy protein or a combination of soy isoflavones rather than pure genistein. (Refer to the chapter on **soy** for a discussion of studies on menopause.)

Preliminary animal studies suggest genistein may be helpful for treating amyotrophic lateral sclerosis.[22]

SAFETY ISSUES

Studies in animals have found soy isoflavones including genistein essentially nontoxic.[23]

Gentian

However, because of its effects on estrogen, there are at least theoretical concerns that genistein may not be safe for women who have already had breast cancer. While most test tube and animal studies have found that genistein inhibits cancer, evidence from one highly preliminary study in humans found changes suggestive of increased breast cancer risk after women took a commercial soy protein product.[24]

There are also concerns that use of soy products by pregnant women could exert a hormonal effect that impacts unborn fetuses.[25,26]

Finally, while fears have been expressed by some experts that soy isoflavones might interfere with the action of oral contraceptives, one study of 40 women suggests that such concerns are groundless.[27] Another trial found that soy does not interfere with the action of estrogen-replacement therapy in menopausal women.[28]

Talk with your doctor before taking genistein or huge amounts of soy while pregnant or nursing.

Soy products may impair thyroid function or reduce absorption of thyroid medication, at least in children.[29,30,31] For this reason, individuals with impaired thyroid function should use soy with caution.

GENTIAN (*Gentiana lutea*)

Alternate or Related Names   Bitter Root, Bitterwort, Gentian Root, Pale Gentian

Principal Proposed Uses   Poor Appetite, Poor Digestion

For reasons that aren't entirely clear, bitter plants have the capacity to stimulate appetite, and gentian ranks high on the scale of bitterness. Two of its constituents, gentiopicrin and amarogentin, taste bitter even when diluted by a factor of 50,000![1]

In traditional European herbology, gentian and other bitter herbs are believed to strengthen the digestive system when taken over a period of time. However, in Chinese medicine, gentian is regarded as a rather intense herb that should seldom be taken over the long term. We are not sure which view is right, although we tend to lean toward the Chinese viewpoint, and recommend gentian only for short-term use.

WHAT IS GENTIAN USED FOR TODAY?

Gentian extracts are widely sold in liquor stores under the name "bitters," for the purpose of increasing appetite. Tinctures are also sold medicinally for the same purpose.

DOSAGE

A typical dosage of gentian is 20 drops of tincture 15 minutes before meals. To make the intensely bitter taste more tolerable, you can mix the tincture in juice or water.

SAFETY ISSUES

Gentian is somewhat mutagenic, meaning that it can cause changes in the DNA of bacteria.[2] For this reason, gentian should not be taken during pregnancy. Safety in young children, nursing women, or those with severe liver or kidney disease is also not established.

In the short term, gentian rarely causes any side effects, except for occasional worsening of ulcer pain and heartburn. (For some people, it relieves stomach problems.)

GINGER (*Zingiber officinale*)

Principal Proposed Uses   Nausea (Motion Sickness, Morning Sickness in Pregnancy), Post-Surgical Nausea

Other Proposed Uses   Osteoarthritis, Atherosclerosis, Migraine Headaches, Rheumatoid Arthritis

Native to southern Asia, ginger is a 2- to 4-foot perennial that produces grass-like leaves up to a foot long and almost an inch wide. Ginger root, as it is called in the grocery store, actually consists of the under-

ground stem of the plant, with its bark-like outer covering scraped off.

Ginger has been used as food and medicine for millennia. Arabian traders carried ginger root from China and India to be used as a food spice in ancient Greece and Rome, and tax records from the second century A.D. show that ginger was a delightful source of revenue to the Roman treasury. Presently, the annual production of ginger exceeds 2 million pounds.

Chinese medical texts from the fourth century B.C. suggest that ginger is effective in treating nausea, diarrhea, stomachaches, cholera, toothaches, bleeding, and rheumatism. Ginger was later used by Chinese herbalists to treat a variety of respiratory conditions, including coughs and the early stages of colds.

Ginger's modern use dates back to the early 1980s, when a scientist named D. Mowrey noticed that ginger-filled capsules reduced his nausea during an episode of flu. Inspired by this, he performed the first double-blind study of ginger. Germany's Commission E subsequently approved ginger as a treatment for indigestion and motion sickness.

One of the most prevalent ingredients in fresh ginger is the pungent substance gingerol. However, when ginger is dried and stored, its gingerol rapidly converts to the substances shogaol and zingerone. Which, if any, of these substances is most important has not been determined.

WHAT IS GINGER USED FOR TODAY?

Ginger has become widely accepted as a treatment for **nausea** (see page 126). Even some conventional medical texts suggest ginger for the treatment of the nausea and vomiting of pregnancy, although others are more cautious.

Ginger is also used for motion sickness. Medications, such as meclizine, are usually more effective, but they can cause drowsiness. Some conventional physicians recommend ginger over other motion-sickness drugs for older people who are unusually sensitive to drowsiness or loss of balance.

European physicians sometimes give their patients ginger before and just after **surgery** (see page 173) to prevent the nausea that many people experience on awakening from anesthesia. However, this treatment should only be attempted with a doctor's approval.

Weak evidence suggests ginger might be helpful for **osteoarthritis** (see page 132).[1]

Ginger has been suggested as a treatment for numerous other conditions, including **atherosclerosis** (see page 16), **migraine headaches** (see page 120), **rheumatoid arthritis** (see page 151), **high cholesterol** (see page 88), **burns** (see page 123), **ulcers** (see page 180), **depression** (see page 59), **impotence** (see page 100), and liver toxicity. However, there is negligible evidence for these uses.

In traditional Chinese medicine, hot ginger tea taken at the first sign of a **cold** (see page 47) is believed to offer the possibility of averting the infection. However, once more there is no scientific evidence for this use.

WHAT IS THE SCIENTIFIC EVIDENCE FOR GINGER?

The evidence for ginger's effectiveness is mixed. It has been suggested that, in some negative studies, poor-quality ginger powder might have been used.[2] In general, while most antinausea drugs influence the brain and the inner ear, ginger appears to act only on the stomach.[3]

Motion Sickness

The first ginger study followed 36 college students with a known tendency toward motion sickness.[4] They were treated with either ginger or the standard nausea drug dimenhydrinate, and then placed in a rotating chair to see how much they could stand. Both treatments seemed about equally effective.

Another study also found equivalent benefit between ginger and dimenhydrinate in a group of 60 passengers on a cruise through rough seas.[5] A later study of 79 Swedish naval cadets found that ginger could decrease vomiting and cold sweating, but didn't significantly decrease nausea and **vertigo** (see page 188).[6]

However, a 1984 study funded by NASA found that ginger was not any more effective than placebo.[7] Two other small studies have also failed to find any benefit.[8,9] The reason for the discrepancy may lie in the type of ginger used, or the severity of the stimulant used to bring on motion sickness.

Nausea and Vomiting of Pregnancy

A preliminary double-blind study performed in Denmark concluded that ginger can significantly reduce the nausea and vomiting often associated with pregnancy. Effects became apparent in 19 of 27 women after 4 days of treatment, although the relief was far from total.[10]

Post-Surgical Nausea

A British double-blind study compared the effects of ginger, placebo, and metoclopramide in the treatment of nausea following gynecological **surgery** (see page 173).[11] The results in 60 women indicated that both treatments produced similar benefits as compared to placebo.

A similar British study followed 120 women receiving elective laparoscopic gynecological surgery.[12] Whereas nausea and vomiting developed in 41% of the participants given placebo, in the groups treated with ginger or metoclopramide (Reglan) these symptoms developed in only 21% and 27%, respectively.

However, a double-blind study of 108 people undergoing similar surgery found no benefit with ginger as

Ginger

Visit Us at TNP.com

compared to placebo.[13] Negative results were also seen in another recent study of 120 women.[14]

DOSAGE

For most purposes, the standard dosage of powdered ginger is 1 to 4 g daily taken in 2 to 4 divided doses.

To prevent motion sickness, it is probably best to begin treatment 1 or 2 days before the trip and continue it throughout the period of travel.

In the nausea and vomiting of pregnancy, the best form of ginger is probably freshly brewed tea, made from boiled ginger root and diluted to taste. If chilled, carbonated, and sweetened, this would become the original form of ginger ale, a famous antinausea beverage. Powdered ginger can be used as well.

SAFETY ISSUES

Ginger is on the FDA's GRAS (generally recognized as safe) list as a food, and the treatment dosages of ginger are comparable to dietary usages.

Like onions and **garlic** (see page 291), extracts of ginger inhibit blood coagulation in test-tube experiments.[15,16,17] This has led to a theoretical concern that ginger should not be combined with drugs such as Coumadin (warfarin), heparin, Trental (pentoxifylline), or even aspirin. European studies with actual oral ginger taken alone in normal quantities have not found any significant effect on blood coagulation,[18,19,20] but it is still possible that combination treatment could cause problems.

No side effects have been observed with ginger at recommended dosages.

⚠ INTERACTIONS YOU SHOULD KNOW ABOUT

If you are taking strong blood-thinning drugs such as **Coumadin (warfarin), heparin, Trental (pentoxifylline),** or even **aspirin,** ginger might possibly increase the risk of bleeding problems.

GINKGO (*Ginkgo biloba*)

Alternate or Related Names   Maidenhair-Tree

Principal Proposed Uses
   Memory and Mental Function: Alzheimer's Disease, Non-Alzheimer's Dementia, and Normal Age-Related Memory Loss

Other Proposed Uses   Impaired Circulation in the Legs (Intermittent Claudication), PMS Symptoms, Altitude Sickness, Vertigo, Tinnitus, Sexual Dysfunction in Women Due to Antidepressant Drugs, Macular Degeneration, Assisting Antipsychotic Medications, Depression, Complications of Diabetes, Raynaud's Phenomenon, Assisting Chemotherapy

Traceable back 300 million years, the ginkgo is the oldest surviving species of tree. Although it died out in Europe during the Ice Age, ginkgo survived in China, Japan, and other parts of East Asia. It has been cultivated extensively for both ceremonial and medical purposes, and some particularly revered trees have been lovingly tended for over 1,000 years.

In traditional Chinese herbology, tea made from ginkgo seeds has been used for numerous problems, most particularly asthma and other respiratory illnesses. The leaf was not used. But in the 1950s, German researchers started to investigate the medical possibilities of ginkgo leaf extracts rather than remedies using the seeds. Thus, modern ginkgo preparations are not the same as the traditional Chinese herb, and the comparisons often drawn are incorrect.

WHAT IS GINKGO USED FOR TODAY?

Presently, ginkgo is the most widely prescribed herb in Germany, reaching a total prescription count of over 6 million in 1995.[1] German physicians consider it to be as effective as any drug treatment for **Alzheimer's disease** (see page 5) and other severe forms of memory and mental function decline. A growing body of evidence also suggests that ginkgo is helpful for ordinary age-related memory loss.

Germany's Commission E also recommends ginkgo for the treatment of restricted circulation in the legs due to hardening of the arteries known as **intermittent claudication** (see page 106).

Recently, ginkgo has attracted interest for possibly reversing the **impotence** (see page 100) or **difficulty achieving orgasm** (see page 155) caused by certain antidepressant drugs.[2–5] Preliminary Chinese research suggests that ginkgo might be able to improve the effectiveness of medications used for schizophrenia and perhaps reduce their side effects as well.[6]

One study suggests that ginkgo may be helpful in relieving the bloating and fluid retention as well as the emotional disturbance of **PMS** (see page 145).[7]

An intriguing double-blind placebo-controlled study suggests that ginkgo extracts may be helpful for preventing **altitude sickness** (see page 4) and reducing symptoms of cold hands and feet.[8]

Ginkgo may also be effective for **vertigo**[9] (see page 188) as well as **tinnitus** (ringing in the ear; see page 178).[10]

Additionally, ginkgo is used to treat **macular degeneration** (see page 115), **depression** (see page 59), complications of **diabetes** (see page 65), and **Raynaud's phenomenon** (see page 149), although as yet there is little evidence that it is effective for these purposes.

One study evaluated combination therapy with ginkgo extract and the chemotherapy drug 5FU for the treatment of pancreatic cancer, on the theory that ginkgo might enhance blood flow to the tumor and thereby help 5FU penetrate better.[11] The results were promising.

WHAT IS THE SCIENTIFIC EVIDENCE FOR GINKGO?

The scientific record for ginkgo is extensive and impressive.

Numerous studies have found that ginkgo extracts can improve circulation.[12,13] We don't know exactly how ginkgo does this, but unknown constituents in the herb appear to make the blood more fluid, reduce the tendency toward blood clots, extend the life of a natural blood vessel–relaxing substance, and act as an antioxidant.[14,15] However, ginkgo's influence on mental function and other conditions may or may not have anything to do with its effects on circulation.

Impaired Mental Function in the Elderly

In the past, European physicians believed that the cause of mental deterioration with age (senile dementia) was reduced circulation in the brain due to atherosclerosis. Since ginkgo can improve circulation, they assumed that ginkgo was simply getting more blood to brain cells and thereby making them work better.

However, the contemporary understanding of age-related memory loss and mental impairment no longer considers chronically restricted circulation the primary issue. Ginkgo (and other drugs used for dementia) may instead function by directly stimulating nerve-cell activity and protecting nerve cells from further injury,[16] although improvement in circulatory capacity may also play a role.

According to a 1992 article published in *Lancet*, over 40 double-blind controlled trials have evaluated the benefits of ginkgo in treating age-related mental decline.[17] Of these, eight were rated of good quality, involving a total of about 1,000 people and producing positive results in all but one study. The authors of the *Lancet* article felt that the evidence was strong enough to conclude that ginkgo extract is an effective treatment for this condition.

Studies since 1992 have verified this conclusion, both in people with Alzheimer's disease and those without the disorder.[18,19] Interestingly, European physicians are so certain that ginkgo is effective that it's become hard for them to perform scientific studies of the herb. To them, it's unethical to give Alzheimer's patients a placebo when they could take ginkgo instead and have additional months of useful life.[20]

This objection does not apply in the United States, where ginkgo is not an approved treatment. A recent study published in the *Journal of the American Medical Association* reported on the results of a year-long double-blind trial of *Ginkgo biloba* in over 300 individuals with Alzheimer's disease or other forms of severe age-related mental decline.[21] Participants were given either 40 mg of the ginkgo extract or placebo 3 times daily. The results showed significant (but not miraculous) improvements in the treated group.

Ordinary Age-Related Memory Loss

The results of four double-blind studies suggest that ginkgo might be useful for ordinary age-related memory loss.

In a double-blind placebo-controlled trial, 241 seniors complaining of mildly impaired memory were given either placebo or low-dose or high-dose ginkgo for 24 weeks.[22] The results showed modest improvements in certain types of memory, especially in the low-dose ginkgo group.

A double-blind placebo-controlled trial examined the effects of ginkgo extract in 40 men and women (ages 55 to 86) who did not suffer from any mental impairment.[23] Over a 6-week period, the results showed improvements in measurements of mental function.

A third trial followed 60 individuals aged 61 to 88 years who suffered from mild to moderate mental impairment.[24] They were divided into three groups: placebo, 120 mg of ginkgo daily, or 240 mg of ginkgo daily. Over a period of 3 months, participants treated with the 120 mg of standardized ginkgo extract showed distinct and significant improvement in mental function as compared to placebo. Interestingly, the higher dose of ginkgo did not prove any better than the placebo.

Finally, a double-blind trial of 26 individuals found that a single dose of 120 mg of ginkgo extract improved short-term memory, especially in people over 50.[25]

Impaired Circulation in the Legs (Intermittent Claudication)

In intermittent claudication, impaired circulation can cause a severe, cramp-like pain in one's legs after walking only a short distance. According to Germany's Commission E, at least four reasonably good double-blind studies have found that ginkgo can increase pain-free walking distance by 75 to 500 feet.[26]

One double-blind study enrolled 111 people for 24 weeks.[27] Subjects were measured for pain-free walking distance by walking up a 12% slope on a treadmill at 3 kilometers per hour (about 2 miles per hour). At the beginning of treatment, both the placebo and ginkgo (120 mg daily) groups were able to walk about 350 feet without pain. By the end of the trial, both groups had improved (the power of placebo is amazing!), although the ginkgo group improved significantly more: Participants taking ginkgo showed about a 40% increase in pain-free walking distance as compared to only a 20% improvement in the placebo group.

Similar improvements were also seen in a double-blind placebo-controlled trial of 60 individuals who had achieved maximum benefit from physical therapy.[28]

A 24-week double-blind placebo-controlled study of 74 individuals with intermittent claudication found that ginkgo at a dose of 240 mg per day was more effective than 120 mg per day.[29]

PMS Symptoms

One double-blind placebo-controlled study evaluated the benefits of *Ginkgo biloba* extract for women with PMS symptoms.[30] This trial enrolled 143 women, 18 to 45 years of age, and followed them for two menstrual cycles. Each woman received either the ginkgo extract (80 mg twice daily) or placebo on day 16 of the first cycle. Treatment was continued until day 5 of the next cycle, and resumed again on day 16 of that cycle.

The results were impressive. As compared to placebo, ginkgo significantly relieved major symptoms of PMS, especially breast pain and emotional disturbance.

Macular Degeneration

One preliminary double-blind study suggests that ginkgo may improve macular degeneration.[31]

Sexual Dysfunction

Although there is no double-blind evidence at the time of this writing, case reports and open studies suggest that ginkgo can reverse the sexual dysfunction (impotence in men, inability to achieve orgasm in women) caused by drugs in the Prozac family as well as other types of antidepressant medications.[32-36]

Altitude Sickness

Exposure to high altitudes and cold conditions can cause headache, insomnia, vertigo, nausea, shortness of breath, as well as pain, numbness, and stiffness in the fingers and toes.

A double-blind placebo-controlled study of 44 mountaineers on a Himalayan expedition found that 160 mg daily of standardized ginkgo extract helped prevent many of these symptoms.[37]

Vertigo

A 3-month double-blind trial of 70 individuals with a variety of vertiginous syndromes found that ginkgo extract given at a dose of 160 mg twice daily produced results superior to placebo.[38] By the end of the trial, 47% of the individuals given ginkgo had significantly recovered versus only 18% in the placebo group.

Tinnitus

There is growing evidence that ginkgo may be helpful for tinnitus.

In a 12-week controlled, randomized, double-blind study of 99 people experiencing tinnitus (ringing in the ears), the participants receiving *Ginkgo biloba* extract experienced a significant reduction in loudness of tinnitus as compared to the placebo group.[39]

In another double-blind study, 103 individuals who had experienced tinnitus for less than 1 year were given *Ginkgo biloba* extract or placebo.[40] Individuals in the treated group showed a marked improvement in symptoms.

Altogether there have been five placebo-controlled trials of *Ginkgo biloba* extract for treating tinnitus, of which only one found ginkgo ineffective.[41-45] That trial was small and used an unusual form of ginkgo extract.[46]

DOSAGE

The standard dosage of ginkgo is 40 to 80 mg 3 times daily of a 50:1 extract standardized to contain 24% ginkgo-flavone glycosides.

SAFETY ISSUES

Ginkgo appears to be safe. Extremely high doses have been given to animals for long periods of time without serious consequences.[47] Safety in young children, pregnant or nursing women, or those with severe liver or kidney disease, however, has not been established.

In all the clinical trials of ginkgo up through 1991 combined, involving a total of almost 10,000 participants, the incidence of side effects produced by ginkgo extract was extremely small. There were 21 cases of gastrointestinal discomfort, and even fewer cases of headaches, dizziness, and allergic skin reactions.[48]

One study found that when high concentrations of ginkgo were placed in a test tube with hamster sperm and ova, the sperm were less able to penetrate the ova.[49] However, since we have no idea whether this much ginkgo can actually come into contact with sperm and ova when they are in the body rather than a test tube, these results may not be meaningful in real life.

Contact with live ginkgo plants can cause severe allergic reactions, and ingestion of ginkgo seeds can be dangerous.

German medical authorities do not believe that ginkgo possesses any serious drug interactions.[50] However, because of ginkgo's "blood-thinning" effects, some experts warn that it should not be combined with blood-thinning drugs such as Coumadin (warfarin), heparin, aspirin, and Trental (pentoxifylline), and use of such drugs was prohibited in most of the double-blind trials of ginkgo. It is also possible that ginkgo could cause bleeding problems if combined with natural blood thinners, such as **garlic** (see page 291) and high-dose **vitamin E** (see page 451). There have been two case reports in highly regarded journals of subdural hematoma (bleeding in the skull) and hyphema (spontaneous bleeding into the iris chamber) in association with ginkgo use.[51,52]

⚠ INTERACTIONS YOU SHOULD KNOW ABOUT

If you are taking

- Blood-thinning drugs such as **Coumadin (warfarin), heparin, aspirin,** or **Trental (pentoxifylline):** Simultaneous use of ginkgo might cause bleeding problems.
- Natural substances with blood-thinning properties, such as **garlic, phosphatidylserine,** or high-dose **vitamin E:** It is possible that, again, simultaneous use of ginkgo might cause bleeding problems.
- **Antidepressant drugs,** especially in the **SSRI** family: Ginkgo might remedy sexual side effects such as impotence or inability to achieve orgasm.
- **Antipsychotics:** Ginkgo might help them work better with fewer side effects.

GINSENG (*Panax ginseng, Panax quinquefolius, Eleutherococcus senticosus*)

Alternate or Related Names   Five-Fingers, Red Berry, American Ginseng, Chinese Ginseng, Korean Ginseng, Others

Principal Proposed Uses   Adaptogen (Improving Resistance to Stress), Strengthening Immunity Against Colds and Flus, Improving Blood Sugar Control in People with Diabetes, Enhancing Mental Function, Preventing Herpes Attacks, Improving General Well-Being

Other Proposed Uses   Performance Enhancement, Preventing Cancer, Reversing Impotence

Probably Ineffective Uses   Menopause

There are actually three different herbs commonly called ginseng: Asian or Korean ginseng (*Panax ginseng*), American ginseng (*Panax quinquefolius*), and Siberian "ginseng" (*Eleutherococcus senticosus*). The last herb is actually not ginseng at all, but the Russian scientists responsible for promoting it believe that it functions identically.

Asian ginseng is a perennial herb with a taproot resembling the human body. It grows in northern China, Korea, and Russia; its close relative, *Panax quinquefolius*, is cultivated in the United States. Because ginseng must be grown for 5 years before it is harvested, it commands a high price, with top-quality roots easily selling for more than $10,000. Dried, unprocessed ginseng root is called "white ginseng," and steamed, heat-dried root is "red ginseng." Chinese herbalists believe that each form has its own particular benefits.

Ginseng is widely regarded by the public as a stimulant, but according to everyone who uses it seriously that isn't the right description. In traditional Chinese herbology, *Panax ginseng* was used to strengthen the digestion and the lungs, calm the spirit, and increase overall energy. When the Russian scientist Israel I. Brekhman became interested in the herb prior to World War II, he came up with a new idea about ginseng: He decided that it was an adaptogen.

The term *adaptogen* refers to a hypothetical treatment described as follows: An adaptogen should help the body adapt to stresses of various kinds, whether heat, cold, exertion, trauma, sleep deprivation, toxic exposure, radiation, infection, or psychological stress. Furthermore, an adaptogen should cause no side effects, be effective in treating a wide variety of illnesses, and help return an organism toward balance no matter what may have gone wrong.

Ginseng

Visit Us at TNP.com

Perhaps the only indisputable example of an adaptogen is healthy lifestyle. By eating right, exercising regularly, and generally living a life of balance and moderation, you will increase your physical fitness and ability to resist illnesses of all types. Whether there are any substances that can do as much remains unclear. However, Brekhman felt certain that ginseng produced similarly universal benefits.

Interestingly, traditional Chinese medicine (where ginseng comes from) does not entirely agree. There is no one-size-fits-all in Chinese medical theory. Like any other herb, ginseng is said to be helpful for those people who need its particular effects, and neutral or harmful for others. But in Europe, Brekhman's concept has taken hold, and ginseng is widely believed to be a universal adaptogen.

In the 1940s, Brekhman decided that a much less expensive herb, *Eleutherococcus senticosus*, was just as good as ginseng. A thorny bush that grows much more rapidly than true ginseng, this later received the misleading name of "Siberian" or "Russian ginseng." Contrary to some reports, its chemical makeup is completely unrelated to that of *Panax ginseng*.

WHAT IS GINSENG USED FOR TODAY?

If Brekhman is right, ginseng (whether *Eleutherococcus* or *Panax*) should be the right treatment for most of us. Modern life is tremendously stressful, and if an herb could help us withstand it, it would be a terrifically useful herb indeed. Ginseng is widely used for this purpose in Russia and Eastern Europe. However, the scientific basis for this use is largely limited to animal studies.

There have been a few studies of ginseng for certain more specific purposes: strengthening immunity against **colds and flus** (see page 47) and other infections (including **herpes**; see page 86), helping to control **diabetes** (see page 65), stimulating the mind, increasing a general sense of well-being, and improving physical performance capacity (**sports performance**; see page 158), with some positive results.

Ginseng is also said to help prevent **cancer** (see page 32), fight chemical dependency, and improve sexual performance, but there is as yet little direct evidence that it really works.[1,2,3] Highly preliminary evidence suggests that American ginseng might help breast cancer chemotherapy drugs work better.[4]

However, *Panax ginseng* does not appear to be helpful for menopausal symptoms.[5]

WHAT IS THE SCIENTIFIC EVIDENCE FOR GINSENG?

Adaptogenic Effects

Numerous studies have evaluated the effects of oral ginseng on animals under conditions of extreme **stress** (see page 167). The results suggest that ginseng increases physical endurance and causes physiological changes that may help the body adapt to adverse conditions.[6–12] In addition, studies in mice found that consuming ginseng before exposure to a virus significantly increased the survival rate and the number of antibodies produced.[13,14]

Immune Stimulation

A double-blind placebo-controlled study suggests that *Panax ginseng* can improve immunity.[15] This trial enrolled 227 participants at three medical offices in Milan, Italy. Half were given ginseng at a dosage of 100 mg daily, the other half placebo. Four weeks into the study, all participants received influenza vaccine.

The results showed a significant decline in the frequency of colds and flus in the treated group compared to the placebo group (15 versus 42 cases). Also, antibody measurements in response to the vaccination rose higher in the treated group than in the placebo group.

Two other studies found evidence that ginseng increases the number of immune cells in the blood,[16,17] although a third did not.[18]

Diabetes

A double-blind study evaluated the effects of *Panax ginseng* (at dosages of 100 mg or 200 mg daily) on 36 people with adult-onset diabetes.[19] The results showed improvements in blood sugar control. The authors attributed this benefit to a spontaneously increased level of physical activity in the ginseng group.

Improved blood sugar control was also seen in two small double-blind placebo-controlled trials using American ginseng (*Panax quinquefolius*).[20,21]

Mental Function

A recent study found that *Panax ginseng* can improve some aspects of mental function.[22] Over a period of 2 months, 112 healthy, middle-aged adults were given either ginseng or placebo. The results showed that ginseng improved abstract thinking ability. However, there was no significant change in reaction time, memory, concentration, or overall subjective experience between the two groups. Another double-blind trial of 16 healthy males found favorable changes in ability to perform mental arithmetic in those given ginseng extract for 12 weeks.[23]

Herpes Infection

A 6-month double-blind trial of 93 men and women with recurrent herpes infections found that treatment with *Eleutherococcus* (2 g daily) reduced the frequency of infections by almost 50%.[24]

Sports Performance

The evidence for *Panax ginseng* as a sports supplement is mixed. An 8-week double-blind placebo-controlled trial evaluated the effects of *Panax ginseng* with and without exercise in 41 individuals.[25] The participants were given either ginseng or placebo, and then underwent exercise training or remained untrained throughout the study. The results showed that ginseng improved aerobic capacity in individuals who did not exercise, but offered no benefit in those who did exercise. In a 9-week double-blind placebo-controlled trial of 30 highly trained athletes, treatment with *Panax ginseng* or *Panax ginseng* plus vitamin E produced significant improvements in aerobic capacity.[26] Another double-blind placebo-controlled trial of 37 individuals also found some benefit.[27]

However, negative results were seen with *Panax ginseng* in an 8-week double-blind trial that followed 31 healthy men in their twenties.[28] Negative results have been seen in other small trials of *Panax ginseng* as well.[29–34]

A double-blind study of 20 athletes over an 8-week period found that a standard *Eleutherococcus* formulation produced no improvement in physical performance.[35]

General Well-Being

The results of a double-blind study of 625 individuals suggests that *Panax ginseng* improves general sense of well-being.[36]

Preventing Cancer

A recent observational study on ginseng and cancer prevention has been widely publicized, but a close look at the data arouses some suspicions. This study was performed in South Korea and followed a total of 4,587 men and women aged 39 years and older from 1987 to 1991.[37] People who regularly consumed *Panax ginseng* were compared with otherwise similar individuals (matched in sex, age, alcohol use, smoking, education, and economic status) who did not.

The reported results were impressive. Those who used ginseng showed a 60% decrease in risk of death from cancer. Lung cancer and gastric cancer were particularly reduced. The more ginseng consumed, the greater the effect.

However, there is something a bit fishy about this study. Use of ginseng less than three times per year caused a 54% reduction in risk. It seems difficult to believe that so occasional a use of ginseng could reduce cancer mortality by more than half!

Menopause

A double-blind placebo-controlled study of 384 postmenopausal women found no significant benefit, and no evidence of hormonal effects.[38]

DOSAGE

The typical recommended daily dosage of *Panax ginseng* is 1 to 2 g of raw herb, or 200 mg daily of an extract standardized to contain 4 to 7% ginsenosides. In one study of American ginseng *(Panax quinquefolius)* for diabetes, the dose used was 3 g.[39] *Eleutherococcus* is taken at a dosage of 2 to 3 g whole herb or 300 to 400 mg of extract daily.

Ordinarily, a 2- to 3-week period of using ginseng is recommended, followed by a 1- to 2-week "rest" period. Russian tradition suggests that ginseng should not be used by those under 40.

Finally, because *Panax ginseng* is so expensive, some products actually contain very little of it. Adulteration of ginseng supplements with other herbs and even caffeine is not unusual.[40,41]

SAFETY ISSUES

The various forms of ginseng appear to be nontoxic, both in the short and long term, according to the results of studies in mice, rats, chickens, and dwarf pigs.[42–45] Ginseng also does not seem to be carcinogenic.

Side effects are rare. Occasionally women report menstrual abnormalities and/or breast tenderness when they take ginseng. However, a large double-blind trial found no estrogen-like effects.[46]

Unconfirmed reports suggest that highly excessive doses of ginseng can cause insomnia, raise blood pressure, increase heart rate, and possibly cause other significant effects. Whether some of these cases were actually caused by caffeine mixed in with ginseng remains unclear. Ginseng allergy can also occur, as can allergy to any other substance.

In 1979, an article was published in the *Journal of the American Medical Association* claiming that people can become addicted to ginseng and develop blood pressure elevation, nervousness, sleeplessness, diarrhea, and hypersexuality.[47] This report has since been thoroughly discredited and should no longer be taken seriously.[48,49]

However, there is some evidence that ginseng can interfere with drug metabolism, specifically drugs processed by an enzyme called "CYP 3A4."[50] Ask your physician or pharmacist whether you are taking any medications of this type. There have also been specific reports of ginseng interacting with MAO inhibitor drugs[51] and also with a test for digitalis,[52] although again it is not clear whether it was the ginseng or a contaminant that caused the problem. There has also been one report of ginseng reducing the anticoagulant effects of Coumadin (warfarin).[53]

Safety in young children, pregnant or nursing women, or people with severe liver or kidney disease has not been established. Interestingly, Chinese tradition suggests that ginseng should not be used by pregnant or nursing mothers.

Ginseng

Visit Us at TNP.com

⚠ INTERACTIONS YOU SHOULD KNOW ABOUT

If you are taking

- **Drugs** processed by an enzyme called "CYP 3A4": Ginseng might interfere. Ask your physician or pharmacist whether you are taking any medications of this type.

- **MAO inhibitor drugs** or **digitalis:** It is possible that ginseng might cause problems.
- **Insulin** or **oral hypoglycemics:** Ginseng may reduce your dosage need.
- **Coumadin (warfarin):** Ginseng might decrease its effect.
- **Influenza vaccine:** Ginseng might help it work better.

GLA (Gamma-Linolenic Acid)

Supplement Forms/Alternate Names   Omega-6 Oil(s), Omega-6 Fatty Acids, Sources of GLA include Black Currant Seed Oil, Borage Oil, Evening Primrose Oil

Principal Proposed Uses   Cyclic Mastalgia (Cyclic Mastitis, Fibrocystic Breast Disease, Mastodynia), General PMS Symptoms, Diabetic Neuropathy, Eczema

Other Proposed Uses   Rheumatoid Arthritis, Raynaud's Phenomenon, Osteoporosis, Weight Loss, Ulcerative Colitis, Kidney Stones, Multiple Sclerosis, Chronic Fatigue Syndrome, Tardive Dyskinesia, Asthma, and Many Others

GLA (gamma-linolenic acid) is one of the two main types of *essential fatty acids.* These are "good" fats that are as necessary for your health as vitamins. Specifically, GLA is an omega-6 fatty acid. (For more information on the other major category of essential fatty acids, omega-3, see the chapter on **fish oil**.)

The body uses essential fatty acids to make various prostaglandins and leukotrienes. These substances influence inflammation and pain; some of them increase symptoms, while others decrease them. Taking GLA may swing the balance over to the more favorable prostaglandins and leukotrienes, making it helpful for diseases that involve inflammation.

GLA is widely used in Europe to treat diabetic neuropathy and eczema. Both European and U.S. physicians use GLA to treat cyclic mastalgia, a condition marked by breast pain associated with the menstrual cycle. It may also be useful for other PMS symptoms.

GLA has also been proposed as a treatment for many other conditions.

REQUIREMENTS/SOURCES

The body ordinarily makes all the GLA it needs from linoleic acid, an omega-6 essential fatty acid found in many foods. In certain circumstances, however, the body may not be able to convert linoleic acid to GLA efficiently. These include advanced age, diabetes, high alcohol intake, eczema, cyclic mastitis, viral infections, excessive saturated fat intake, elevated cholesterol levels,

and deficiencies of vitamin B_6, zinc, magnesium, biotin, or calcium.[1–5] In such cases, taking GLA supplements may make up for a genuine deficiency.

Very little GLA is found in the diet. Borage oil is the richest supplemental source (17 to 25% GLA), followed by black currant oil (15 to 20%) and evening primrose oil (7 to 10%). Borage and evening primrose are the most common sources.

THERAPEUTIC DOSAGES

The usual dosage of GLA used to treat cyclic mastalgia or eczema is about 200 to 400 mg daily (about 2 to 4 g of evening primrose oil or 1 to 2 g of borage oil). Diabetic neuropathy is typically treated with about 400 to 600 mg daily (about 4 to 6 g of evening primrose or 2 to 3 g of borage oil), and rheumatoid arthritis may require as much as 2,000 to 3,000 mg (best obtained from purified GLA).

GLA should be taken with food. Don't forget that full benefits may take over 6 months to develop, so be patient.

THERAPEUTIC USES

Most commonly in the form of evening primrose oil, GLA has become a standard treatment for **cyclic mastalgia** (see page 58), breast pain that cycles with the menstrual period.[6–9] It is widely used for this purpose by conventional physicians in both Europe and North America, and as a mark of its acceptance it is even mentioned in the AMA's official *Drug Evaluations* textbook.[10]

Evening primrose oil is also said to be useful for other **PMS** (see page 145) symptoms, although the evidence is not strong.[11]

Evening primrose oil also appears to be effective for diabetic neuropathy,[12,13] a complication of **diabetes** (see page 65). This condition, which develops in many people with diabetes, consists of pain and/or numbness due to progressive nerve damage.

Additionally, evening primrose oil is widely used in Europe as a treatment for **eczema** (see page 78). Unfortunately, the scientific evidence that it works is mixed at best, and the most recent studies have not found it to be effective.[14–18] GLA has also been suggested for the treatment of itching due to kidney dialysis.[19,20]

Very high doses of purified GLA may be of some benefit in treating **rheumatoid arthritis** (see page 151), especially when combined with conventional treatments.[21-24] GLA may also help in **Raynaud's phenomenon** (a condition in which the fingers and toes react to cold in an exaggerated way; see page 149),[25,26] and in **osteoporosis** (see page 136).[27,28]

GLA has also been tried as a treatment for **weight loss** (see page 192), with mixed results. One double-blind study of 74 women found that evening primrose oil failed to produce any weight loss as compared to placebo, however, another investigation that restricted treatment to 47 people with a family history of obesity found it produced a small but significant loss of weight.[29,30]

A preliminary study found high doses of GLA may increase the effectiveness of tamoxifen in the treatment of breast cancer.[31] **Note:** Individuals undergoing treatment for cancer should not take GLA (or any other supplement) except under physician supervision.

A small double-blind placebo-controlled trial found some benefit in **ulcerative colitis** (see page 179) with evening primrose oil.[32]

GLA is sometimes recommended for **kidney stones** (see page 109), however the evidence supporting this use is very preliminary.[33,34]

Some researchers have suggested that gamma-linolenic acid (GLA) might be beneficial in **multiple sclerosis** (see page 124).[35] So far, however, little evidence suggests that it helps, and one uncontrolled study found it ineffective.[36,37,38]

GLA combined with fish oil may be helpful for treating **chronic fatigue syndrome** (see page 44); however, the results of double-blind trials have been mixed.[39,40]

Although GLA is sometimes suggested as a treatment for **tardive dyskinesia** (see page 176), two double blind studies have found it ineffective for this disorder.[41]

Thus far, we've mentioned only a fraction of the conditions for which GLA has been proposed as a treatment. Others include asthma, allergies, bursitis, endometriosis, heart disease, irritable bowel syndrome, prostate cancer, prostate enlargement or benign prostatic hyperplasia (BPH), Sjögren's disease, and many more. However, none of these potential uses has as yet been scientifically evaluated to any significant extent.

WHAT IS THE SCIENTIFIC EVIDENCE FOR GLA (GAMMA-LINOLENIC ACID)?

Cyclic Mastalgia

Cyclic mastalgia, also known as fibrocystic breast disease, cyclic mastitis, and mastodynia, is a condition in which a woman's breasts become painful during the week or two before her menstrual period. The discomfort is accompanied by swelling, inflammation, and sometimes actual cysts that form in the breasts. It is often associated with other symptoms of premenstrual syndrome (PMS).

We do not know the cause of cyclic mastalgia, but researchers have found that it seems to be associated with an imbalance of fatty acids in the body.[42]

Evidence suggests that GLA relieves cyclic mastalgia, perhaps by restoring the balance of essential fatty acids.[43] One report published in 1985 compared the effectiveness of four different therapies in women with severe, painful mastalgia: GLA from evening primrose oil and the pharmaceuticals danazol, bromocriptine, and progestins (often, but not quite accurately, called progesterone).[44]

The results suggest that evening primrose oil was effective in just under 50% of participants. However, this was not actually a study in the usual sense; it was more a collation of records from the Cardiff Clinic, a medical center that specializes in the treatment of breast pain. Contrary to how this study is sometimes reported, it did not have a placebo group.

To really know whether a treatment is effective, you need double-blind placebo-controlled studies to eliminate the power of suggestion. One such study was reported in 1981. This trial followed 73 women suffering from cyclic mastalgia.[45] The results were consistent with the Cardiff Clinic's results, finding that evening primrose oil reduced pain in almost 50% of the women taking it, while only 19% of the women improved in the placebo group.

However, this study was reported only in a very brief form, and many details are missing. We really need better-designed and better-reported studies to know for sure how effective evening primrose oil really is for cyclic mastalgia.

If you have a severe form of cyclic mastalgia with actual breast cysts, there is some evidence that evening primrose oil will not be completely effective. In a double-blind study of 200 women treated for 1 year, evening primrose oil had no effect on recurrent breast cysts.[46,47] The conclusion appears to be that evening primrose oil relieves breast pain but cannot make breast cysts go away.

Other PMS Symptoms

Although several small studies suggest that GLA as evening primrose oil is helpful in reducing overall PMS symptoms, all of them suffer from serious flaws.[48]

Diabetic Neuropathy

Diabetic neuropathy is a gradual degeneration of nerves caused by diabetes. There is some evidence that GLA can be helpful, if you give it long enough to work. In one double-blind placebo-controlled study, 111 people with mild diabetic neuropathy received either 480 mg daily of GLA or placebo.[49] After 12 months, the group taking GLA was doing significantly better than the placebo group. Good results were seen in a smaller study as well.[50]

In addition, numerous studies in animals have found that evening primrose oil can protect nerves from diabetes-induced nerve injury.[51,52]

There is some preliminary evidence that GLA may be more effective for this condition when it is combined with **lipoic acid** (see page 347).[53,54]

Eczema

Despite the fact that GLA (evening primrose oil) is widely used in Europe to treat eczema, the evidence that it works is mixed at best.

A 1989 review of the literature found significant benefit in the nine double-blind controlled studies performed to that date.[55] Evening primrose oil seemed especially effective in relieving itching. However, this review has been sharply criticized for including poorly designed studies and possibly misinterpreting study results.[56]

Improvements in symptoms other than itching were seen in a double-blind study of 48 children with eczema.[57]

However, other research has failed to find any benefit. For example, a 16-week double-blind study involving 58 children with eczema found no difference between the effects of evening primrose oil and placebo.[58] A 24-week double-blind study of 160 adults with eczema, who were given either placebo or GLA from borage oil, also found no benefit.[59] In addition, negative results were seen in a 16-week double-blind placebo-controlled study of 102 individuals with eczema.[60] Another double-blind trial followed 39 people with hand dermatitis for 24 weeks. Evening primrose oil at a dosage of 6 g daily produced no significant improvement as compared to the placebo.[61]

Itching Due to Kidney Dialysis

GLA has been tried for improving itching in individuals undergoing kidney dialysis. However, one small double-blind placebo-controlled trial failed to find benefit.[62] Another trial compared GLA-rich evening primrose oil to linoleic acid and found itching relieved equally; but due to the lack of a placebo control, these results are difficult to interpret.[63]

Rheumatoid Arthritis

According to many studies, fish oil, a source of omega-3 essential fatty acids, definitely improves symptoms of rheumatoid arthritis. A few studies suggest that GLA may also work. One double-blind study followed 56 people with rheumatoid arthritis for 6 months.[64] Participants received either 2.8 g daily of GLA or placebo. The group taking GLA experienced significantly fewer symptoms than the placebo group, and the improvements grew over time.

Other small studies have found similar results.[65,66] The overall conclusion appears to be that purified GLA may offer some benefit for rheumatoid arthritis, especially when used along with standard treatment for rheumatoid arthritis.[67]

Raynaud's Phenomenon

High dosages of evening primrose oil may be useful for Raynaud's phenomenon, a condition in which a person's hands and feet show abnormal sensitivity to cold temperature. A small double-blind study found that GLA produced significantly better results than placebo.[68,69] Similar results have been obtained with the omega-3 fatty acids found in fish oil.

Osteoporosis

Essential fatty acids, when combined with calcium, may help prevent osteoporosis. In one study, 65 postmenopausal women were given calcium along with either placebo or a combination of omega-6 fatty acids (from evening primrose oil) and omega-3 fatty acids (from fish oil) for a period of 18 months. At the end of the study period, both treated groups had higher bone density and fewer fractures than the placebo group.[70] Similar results were seen in another study of 40 women.[71]

Weight Loss

In a 12-week double-blind study of 100 obese women, treatment with evening primrose oil failed to produce any weight loss as compared to placebo.[72]

SAFETY ISSUES

Most of the safety information we have regarding GLA comes from experience with evening primrose oil.

Animal studies suggest that evening primrose oil is completely nontoxic and noncarcinogenic.[73] Over 4,000 people have taken GLA or evening primrose oil in scientific studies, and no significant adverse effects have ever been noted.

Early reports suggested the possibility that GLA might worsen temporal lobe epilepsy, but there has been no later confirmation.[74]

The maximum safe dosage of GLA for young children, pregnant or nursing women, or those with severe liver or kidney disease has not been established.

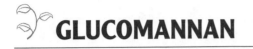

GLUCOMANNAN

Principal Proposed Uses   High Cholesterol

Other Proposed Uses   High Blood Pressure, Weight Loss, Diabetes, Constipation

Glucomannan is a dietary fiber derived from the tubers of *Amorphophallus konjac*. Konjac flour (made from these tubers) is used to make a jelly called konyaku, a common food product in Japan.

Fiber containing foods such as oats are known to help reduce cholesterol and improve constipation, and may also help regulate blood sugar and assist in weight reduction by creating a feeling of fullness. However, many people have a hard time consuming enough fiber from food, and turn to fiber supplements such as guar gum and pectin, to help fulfill their daily requirements. Glucomannan offers one advantage over these forms of fiber: much smaller doses are necessary. When glucomannan is placed in water, it can swell up to 17 times its original volume. These qualities make it potentially quite convenient as a fiber supplement.

SOURCES

Although glucomannan can be derived from other sources such as yeast, most studies have used glucomannan purified from the konjac root.

THERAPEUTIC DOSAGES

Most of the studies described here used 3 to 5 g per day in divided doses before meals. However, there are concerns regarding the form of glucomannan used (see Safety Issues below).

THERAPEUTIC USES

Several small controlled studies have found glucomannan to be effective for reducing total **cholesterol** (see page 88).[1–7] Glucomannan appears to reduce LDL ("bad") cholesterol and, according to some studies, increase HDL ("good") cholesterol. In addition, glucomannan may improve other risk factors for **heart disease** (see page 16), such as high triglyceride levels and **high blood pressure** (see page 98).

By expanding in the stomach, glucomannan might be useful for people trying to lose weight. Many people report a feeling of fullness after taking glucomannan and some studies found a significant **weight loss** (see page 192) among those taking glucomannan compared to those on placebo.[8–12] However, not all studies of glucomannan for weight loss have had positive results.[13,14]

Glucomannan may also help the body to regulate blood sugar levels, and therefore could be helpful in treating **diabetes** (see page 65).[15,16] Additionally, glucomannan might be helpful for individuals who experience episodes of low blood sugar.[17]

Like other dietary fibers, glucomannan may help to reduce **constipation** (see page 56).[18,19]

WHAT IS THE SCIENTIFIC EVIDENCE FOR GLUCOMANNAN?

High Cholesterol and High Blood Pressure

In a double-blind study, 63 people were given either 3.9 g per day of glucomannan or placebo for 4 weeks and then switched to the other treatment.[20] While taking glucomannan, participants showed significant reductions in total cholesterol, LDL cholesterol, and triglycerides, as compared to placebo. In addition, their systolic blood pressure (the upper number in the blood pressure reading) was also reduced. However, there was no significant increase in HDL cholesterol and no improvement in the ratio of LDL to HDL cholesterol.

Participants in another study were given either 3 g per day of glucomannan or placebo over an 8-week period.[21] The glucomannan group showed improvements in total and HDL cholesterol as well as a reduction in systolic blood pressure. Those taking glucomannan also lost weight, whereas the placebo group gained weight over the length of the trial.

Several other controlled studies have found similar results.[22–25]

Glucomannan

Visit Us at TNP.com

Weight Loss

A few small double-blind studies suggest that glucomannan may be helpful for people trying to lose weight; however, in other studies, no such benefit was seen.[26–29]

One double-blind placebo-controlled trial of 20 women who were more than 20% over their ideal weight found glucomannan to be more effective than placebo at promoting weight loss.[30] All participants were instructed not to change their eating or exercise habits while on the treatment. Those in the treatment group took 1 g of glucomannan 3 times a day for 8 weeks and lost an average of 5.5 pounds during that period; in comparison, those in the placebo group gained an average of 1.5 pounds, a significant difference. The glucomannan group also had a reduction of total and LDL cholesterol as well as triglyceride levels.

However, another double-blind trial of 60 obese children did not find a significant difference in weight loss between the glucomannan and the placebo groups.[31] In this study, the children received either 1 g of glucomannan or placebo twice a day for 8 weeks.

Diabetes

A study of individuals with diabetes tested the effectiveness of glucomannan fiber-enriched biscuits against wheat bran biscuits for blood sugar control.[32] While using the glucomannan biscuits, people had a significant improvement in glucose control as compared to the wheat bran biscuits.

Other studies have also found evidence that glucomannan can improve blood sugar control.[33]

However, while this evidence is promising, much larger studies need to be performed before glucomannan can be considered an effective treatment for diabetes.

SAFETY ISSUES

In Japan, food products containing glucomannan have a long history of use and are believed to be safe. However, there are some concerns about taking glucomannan as a supplement.

Some people taking glucomannan complain of excess gas, stomach distension, or mild diarrhea. These symptoms usually abate within a couple of days of treatment or with a reduction of the dosage.

In a few cases, glucomannan tablets have caused obstruction of the esophagus when they expanded before reaching the stomach.[34,35] In response to these reports, tablets of this type have been banned. Capsules, however, do not seem to pose the same risk because their casing prevents the glucomannan from contacting water until it reaches the stomach. The dramatic expansion of glucomannan has also raised some concerns that it could cause an obstruction in the intestines; nonetheless, as of yet, there have been no reports of this actually happening.

One option to offset all expansion risk is to mix glucomannan powder in water so that it expands before it is ingested; however, this strategy defeats the convenience of this form of fiber.

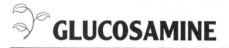

GLUCOSAMINE

Supplement Forms/Alternate Names   Glucosamine Sulfate, Glucosamine Hydrochloride, N-Acetyl Glucosamine

Principal Proposed Uses   Osteoarthritis (Relieving Symptoms and Slowing the Course of the Disease)

Other Proposed Uses   Tendinitis, Muscle Injury Prevention

Glucosamine, most commonly used in the form glucosamine sulfate, is a simple molecule derived from glucose, the principal sugar found in blood. In glucosamine, one oxygen atom in glucose is replaced by a nitrogen atom. The chemical term for this modified form of glucose is *amino sugar*.

Glucosamine is produced naturally in the body, where it is a key building block for making cartilage. In Europe, glucosamine is widely used to treat osteoarthritis. Studies show that glucosamine supplements relieve pain and other arthritis symptoms. Interestingly, these improvements seem to last for several weeks after glucosamine supplements are discontinued.

This observation has led to the exciting idea that glucosamine may actually make a deep change in osteoarthritis, rather than simply relieving symptoms. Conventional treatments for arthritis reduce the symptoms but don't slow the actual progress of the disease; in fact, nonsteroidal anti-inflammatory drugs, such as indomethacin, may actually speed the progression of osteoarthritis by interfering with cartilage repair and promoting cartilage destruction.[1–5]

In contrast, glucosamine appears to go beyond treating the symptoms to actually slowing the disease itself. (Chondroitin sulfate and SAMe may do the same.) If this is true, it would represent a revolutionary breakthrough in the treatment of arthritis.

Glucosamine

Visit Us at TNP.com

Some athletes use glucosamine, in the (unproved) belief that it can prevent muscle injuries, relieve tendinitis, and repair damaged cartilage.

REQUIREMENTS/SOURCES

There is no U.S. Dietary Reference Intake (formerly known as the Recommended Dietary Allowance) for glucosamine. Your body makes all the glucosamine it needs from building blocks found in foods.

Glucosamine is not usually obtained directly from food. Glucosamine supplements are derived from chitin, a substance found in the shells of shrimp, lobsters, and crabs.

THERAPEUTIC DOSAGES

For osteoarthritis, a typical dosage of glucosamine is 500 mg 3 times daily. A 1,500-mg dose taken once daily may also be effective.[6] Be patient: results take weeks to develop. Glucosamine is available in three forms: glucosamine sulfate, glucosamine hydrochloride, and N-acetyl glucosamine. All three forms are sold as tablets or capsules. There is some dispute over which form is best.

Glucosamine is often sold in combination with **chondroitin** (see page 250). Preliminary information from one animal study suggests that this mixture may be superior to either treatment alone.[7]

THERAPEUTIC USES

Glucosamine is used to treat **osteoarthritis** (see page 132). The research indicates that it is effective, and about equal in strength to low dosages of nonsteroidal anti-inflammatory drugs such as ibuprofen.[8–12] It reduces pain and swelling and improves mobility with results that continue for weeks after treatment stops. It also appears to help prevent progressive joint damage, thereby slowing the course of the disease.[13]

Glucosamine has also been proposed to treat tendinitis, to prevent muscle injuries, and to repair damaged cartilage, but there is as yet no evidence that it is effective.

WHAT IS THE SCIENTIFIC EVIDENCE FOR GLUCOSAMINE?

Osteoarthritis

Symptom Relief

Solid evidence indicates that glucosamine supplements effectively relieve pain and other symptoms of osteoarthritis. Two types of studies have been performed, those that compared glucosamine against placebo and those that compared it against standard medications.

A recent double-blind study compared glucosamine sulfate against placebo in 252 people with osteoarthritis of the knee.[14] After 4 weeks, the group that was given glucosamine experienced significantly reduced pain and improved movement, to a greater extent than the improvements seen in the placebo group.

Another double-blind study followed 329 people who were divided into four groups. One group was given the standard antiarthritis drug piroxicam (Feldene), a second was given glucosamine, a third received both treatments, and the fourth received placebo only.[15,16] Over 90 days, piroxicam and glucosamine proved equally effective at reducing symptoms. Interestingly, the combination treatment (piroxicam plus glucosamine) didn't produce significantly better results than either treatment taken alone.

After 90 days, treatment was stopped and the participants were followed for an additional 60 days. The benefits of piroxicam rapidly disappeared, but the benefits of glucosamine lasted for the full 60 days.

Similar results have been seen in other studies that compared glucosamine against ibuprofen.[17,18]

However, not every study has been positive. A recent 2-month double-blind placebo-controlled trial of 98 individuals with osteoarthritis of the knee found no benefit.[19] The authors suggest that the relatively advanced osteoarthritis found in these participants was responsible for the negative outcome. Negative results were also seen in a double-blind placebo-controlled trial of glucosamine chloride.[20]

Slowing the Course of the Disease

A 3-year double-blind placebo-controlled study of 212 individuals found that glucosamine can protect joints from further damage.[21] Over the course of the study, individuals given glucosamine showed some actual improvement in pain and mobility, while those given placebo worsened steadily. Even more importantly, x rays showed that glucosamine treatment prevented progressive damage to the knee joint.

We don't know exactly how glucosamine works. However, besides serving as a basic building block for cartilage, glucosamine appears to stimulate cartilage cells in your joints to make proteoglycans and collagen, two proteins essential for the proper function of joints.[22–26]

Glucosamine may also help prevent collagen from breaking down.[27]

SAFETY ISSUES

Glucosamine appears to be extremely safe for people of all ages. No significant side effects have been reported in any of the studies of glucosamine. However, recent case reports and animal studies have raised concerns that glucosamine might be harmful for individuals with diabetes. It may raise blood sugar levels[28–32] and also increase the risk of long-term diabetes side effects such as cataracts.[33]

Glucosamine

Visit Us at TNP.com

GLUTAMINE

Supplement Forms/Alternate Names   L-Glutamine

Principal Proposed Uses   There are no well-documented uses for glutamine.

Other Proposed Uses   Post-Exercise Colds, Recovery from Critical Illness, Food Allergies
   Digestive Disorders: Irritable Bowel Syndrome, Crohn's Disease, Ulcerative Colitis
HIV Support, Overtraining Syndrome, Attention Deficit Disorder, Ulcers, "Brain Booster"

Glutamine, or L-glutamine, is an amino acid derived from another amino acid, glutamic acid. Glutamine plays a role in the health of the immune system, digestive tract, and muscle cells, as well as other bodily functions. It appears to serve as a fuel for the cells that line the intestines. Heavy exercise, infection, surgery, and trauma can deplete the body's glutamine reserves, particularly in muscle cells.

The fact that glutamine does so many good things in the body has led people to try glutamine supplements as a treatment for various conditions, including preventing the infections that often follow endurance exercise, reducing symptoms of overtraining syndrome, improving nutrition in critical illness, alleviating allergies, and treating digestive problems.

SOURCES

There is no daily requirement for glutamine, because the body can make its own supply. As mentioned earlier, various severe stresses may result in a temporary glutamine deficiency.

High-protein foods such as meat, fish, beans, and dairy products are excellent sources of glutamine.

THERAPEUTIC DOSAGES

Therapeutic dosages of glutamine range from 1.5 to 6 g daily, divided into several separate doses.

THERAPEUTIC USES

Endurance athletes frequently catch an infectious illness after completing a marathon or similar forms of exercise. Preliminary evidence suggests that glutamine (like **vitamin C**; see page 444) might help prevent such infections (see the chapter on **sports performance** for more information).[1–4]

Glutamine (often combined with other nutrients) might be useful as a nutritional supplement for people undergoing recovery from critical illness.[5]

It has also been suggested as a treatment for **food allergies** (see page 82), based on a theory called "leaky gut syndrome." This theory holds that in some people whole proteins leak through the wall of the digestive tract and enter the blood, causing allergic reactions. Preliminary evidence suggests that glutamine supplements might reduce leakage through the intestinal walls.[6,7] On the same principle, glutamine supplements have been suggested for people with other digestive problems, such as **irritable bowel syndrome** (see page 108), **Crohn's disease** (see page 57), **ulcerative colitis** (see page 179), and the digestive distress caused by cancer chemotherapy.[8–14] However, there is no real evidence that it works for these conditions. Preliminary evidence suggests glutamine combined with antioxidants or other nutrients may help people with **HIV** (see page 94) to gain weight.

Based on glutamine's role in muscle, it has been suggested that glutamine might be useful for athletes experiencing overtraining syndrome. As the name suggests, this syndrome is the cumulative effect of a training regimen that allows too little rest and recovery between workouts. Symptoms include depression, fatigue, reduced performance, and physiological signs of stress. Glutamine supplements have additionally been proposed as treatment for **attention deficit disorder** (see page 22), **ulcers** (see page 180), and as a "brain booster." However, there is little to no scientific evidence for any of these uses.

WHAT IS THE SCIENTIFIC EVIDENCE FOR GLUTAMINE?

Infections in Athletes

A double-blind placebo-controlled study evaluated the benefits of supplemental glutamine (5 g) taken at the end of exercise in 151 endurance athletes.[15] The result showed a significant decrease in infections among treated athletes. Only 19% of the athletes taking glutamine got sick, as compared to 51% of those on placebo. Although we don't know how glutamine works to prevent these infections, there is some evidence that it may function by stimulating certain aspects of the immune system.[16]

Recovery from Critical Illness

One small double-blind study found that glutamine supplements might have significant nutritional benefits for

Glutamine

seriously ill people.[17] In this study, 84 critically ill hospital patients were divided into two groups. All the patients were being fed through a feeding tube. One group received a normal feeding-tube diet, whereas the other group received this diet plus supplemental glutamine. After 6 months, 14 of the 42 patients receiving glutamine had died, compared with 24 of the control group. The glutamine group also left both the intensive care ward and the hospital significantly sooner than the patients who did not receive glutamine.

HIV Related Weight Loss

Although research is still preliminary, one double-blind placebo-controlled study found that a combination of glutamine and antioxidants (vitamins C and E, beta-carotene, selenium, and N-acetyl cysteine) led to significant weight gain in people with HIV who had lost weight.[18] Another small double-blind trial found that combination treatment with glutamine, arginine and beta-hydroxy beta-methylbutyrate (HMB) could increase muscle mass and possibly improve immune status.[19]

Cancer Chemotherapy

A double-blind trial of 65 women undergoing chemo therapy for advanced breast cancer sought to discover whether glutamine at a dose of 30 g per day could reduce chemotherapy-induced diarrhea.[20] The results did not show any benefit from glutamine treatment.

Crohn's Disease

Because glutamine is the major fuel source for cells of the small intestine, glutamine has been proposed as a treatment for Crohn's disease, a disease of the small intestine.[21] However, two double-blind trials enrolling a total of 30 people found no benefit.[22,23]

SAFETY ISSUES

As a naturally occurring amino acid, glutamine is thought to be a safe supplement when taken at recommended dosages. However, those who are hypersensitive to monosodium glutamate (MSG) should use glutamine with caution, as the body metabolizes glutamine into glutamate. Also, because many anti-epilepsy drugs work by blocking glutamate stimulation in the brain, high dosages of glutamine may overwhelm these drugs and pose a risk to people with epilepsy.

Finally, in one case report high doses of the supplement L-glutamine (more than 2 g per day) may have triggered episodes of mania in two people not previously known to have **bipolar disorder** (see page 27).[24]

Maximum safe dosages for young children, pregnant or nursing women, or those with severe liver or kidney disease have not been determined.

⚠ INTERACTIONS YOU SHOULD KNOW ABOUT

If you are taking **antiseizure medications,** including **carbamazepine, phenobarbital, Dilantin (phenytoin), Mysoline (primidone),** and **valproic acid (Depakene),** use glutamine only under medical supervision.

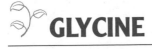

GLYCINE

Principal Proposed Uses   Schizophrenia

Other Proposed Uses   Stroke, Genetic Abnormalities, Prostate Enlargement (BPH), Wound Healing, Liver and Kidney Protection, Cancer Prevention

---

Glycine is the simplest of the 20 different amino acids used as building blocks to make proteins for your body. It is one of several amino acids known to act as neurotransmitters, helping to pass signals from one brain cell to another. For this reason, it is not entirely surprising that glycine supplements may affect brain chemistry. Glycine has shown considerable promise for the treatment of schizophrenia, and may have other uses as well.

REQUIREMENTS/SOURCES

Your body is able to make glycine using another amino acid, serine. Because you can manufacture glycine, you don't really have to consume any, so it's called a "nonessential amino acid." Most of us get about 2 g of glycine a day from the foods we regularly eat anyway. This dietary glycine comes mostly from high-protein foods like meat, fish, dairy products, and legumes. For treating certain disease conditions, however, much larger amounts than are normally consumed might be helpful; such high doses can only be obtained by taking supplements.

THERAPEUTIC DOSAGES

Dosages of oral glycine used in clinical trials for therapeutic purposes range from 2 g to 60 g daily.

THERAPEUTIC USES

Glycine has been tried as a supportive treatment for schizophrenia.[1-5] Preliminary evidence suggests that high doses of glycine (from 15 to 60 g daily) combined with standard therapy can help with some aspects of this disease.

Note: Although glycine appears to be helpful when combined with older drugs for schizophrenia, it might interfere with the action of newer antipsychotic medications.[6] (See Safety Issues.)

One large double-blind study suggests that low doses of glycine may be helpful for limiting the spreading brain damage that occurs during stroke.[7] However, there are also theoretical concerns that glycine could increase such damage, so you should not try this treatment except under physician supervision.

Very preliminary clinical studies have found that glycine may be useful for treatment of two relatively rare genetic abnormalities: 3-phosphoglycerate dehydrogenase deficiency and isovaleric acidemia.[8,9,10]

Studies performed in the 1950s and 1960s suggested that a combination of glycine, alanine, and glutamic acid may be helpful for prostate enlargement.[11,12] However, as this work does not meet modern research standards, the results can't be taken as reliable.

Glycine alone and in combination with other amino acids has been studied as a topical treatment for **wounds** (see page 123). A randomized, double-blind placebo-controlled study with 22 participants showed improvements in healing time and pain control.[13] However, larger studies are necessary to validate these preliminary findings.

Animal studies suggest that dietary glycine may protect against chemically-induced damage to the liver or kidneys, and possibly speed recovery from injury.[14,15,16]

Other studies in laboratory animals suggest that dietary glycine may prevent tumor formation and growth in the livers of mice and rats.[17,18] However, it is too early to say whether glycine will prevent cancer in humans.

Manufacturers advertising glycine supplements have made a number of additional claims for it, including prevention of epileptic seizures, reducing acid in the stomach, treating muscle spasticity (as in **multiple sclerosis**, MS; see page 124), boosting the immune system, and calming the mind. It is also proposed as a **sports supplement** (see page 158), said to work in this capacity by

increasing release of human growth hormone (HGH). As yet, there is no real scientific evidence that glycine works for any of these purposes.

Because it has a sweet taste, glycine has also been recommended as a sugar substitute both for people with diabetes and hypoglycemia. It is not known to have any sort of therapeutic effect for these conditions; the advantage lies only in that the person is not using sugar.

WHAT IS THE SCIENTIFIC EVIDENCE FOR GLYCINE?

Schizophrenia

Schizophrenia is not, as many people believe, a "multiple personality" disorder. Rather, it is a severe and probably genetic condition that causes such symptoms as hallucinations, delusions, thought disorders, social withdrawal, and blunted emotions.

Various medications are used for schizophrenia with reasonably good results. However, they tend to be most effective for the "positive" symptoms of schizophrenia, such as hallucinations and delusions—these symptoms are called "positive" because they are the presence of abnormal mental functions, rather than the absence of normal mental functions. Medications are less helpful for the "negative" symptoms of schizophrenia, such as apathy, depression, and social withdrawal: glycine may be of benefit here.

A clinical trial enrolled 22 participants with schizophrenic symptoms that were not well managed by medications alone.[19] In this placebo-controlled double-blind crossover study, volunteers were randomly assigned to receive either 0.8 g per kilogram of body weight (about 60 g per day) of glycine or placebo for 6 weeks, along with their regular medications. The groups were then switched after a 2-week "wash-out" period during which they all received placebo.

Significant improvements (about 30%) in symptoms such as depression and apathy were seen with glycine when compared to placebo. As a bonus, glycine also reduced some of the side effects caused by the prescription drugs. Furthermore, the benefits appeared to continue for another 8 weeks after the glycine was discontinued.

No changes were seen in positive symptoms (for instance, hallucinations), but we don't know if that is because these symptoms were already being controlled by prescription medications or if glycine simply has no effect on that aspect of schizophrenia.

Three earlier double-blind placebo-controlled clinical trials of glycine together with standard drugs for schizophrenia also found it to be helpful for negative symptoms.[20-23] All of these studies used very small groups (from 12 to 18 people), so much larger trials are still needed to verify glycine's effectiveness.

Glycine does not appear to be helpful for individuals using the newer antipsychotic drug clozapine, presumably because clozapine is very different from previous generation antipsychotics.[24]

Stroke

Glycine's usefulness for treating stroke victims was investigated in a double-blind placebo-controlled study with 200 participants.[25] The results suggest that glycine can protect against the spreading damage to the brain that usually follows a stroke. Stroke victims who were treated within 6 hours following the event were given either 1 to 2 g of glycine sublingually (dissolved under the tongue) or placebo treatment for a period of 5 days. Participants in the study who were given glycine suffered significantly less extensive neural damage than those receiving placebo. This appears to be an impressive result.

Although other researchers using glycine for brain disorders have reported that such small doses of glycine would not be sufficient to cross the blood-brain barrier,[26] measurements of amino acids in the cerebrospinal fluid during the above study suggest that it did enter the brain. There are potential concerns that high dose glycine could *increase* stroke damage (see Safety Issues below).

SAFETY ISSUES

No serious adverse effects from using glycine have been reported, even at doses as high as 60 g per day. One par-

ticipant in the 22-person trial described above developed stomach upset and vomiting, but it ceased when the glycine was discontinued.

Based on theoretical concerns, it is possible that glycine could actually increase brain damage in strokes by increasing levels of glutamate, a neurotransmitter thought to be responsible for some of the injury.[27] Although the clinical trial that tested glycine as a therapy for stroke victims found it to be protective rather than damaging, it is possible that higher doses could be harmful.[28]

While glycine seems to work well with standard antipsychotic drugs, a double-blind placebo-controlled trial suggests that it is not helpful and may even be harmful when combined with the newer medication clozapine.[29] In this study, glycine was found to reduce the benefits of clozapine without helping to relieve the participants' negative symptoms. Comparable problems might occur with medications similar to clozapine.

Maximum safe doses for young children, pregnant or nursing women, or people with liver or kidney disease are not known.

⚠ INTERACTIONS YOU SHOULD KNOW ABOUT

If you are taking **newer antipsychotic medications** such as **clozapine**, do not take glycine.

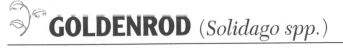

GOLDENROD (*Solidago spp.*)

Alternate or Related Names   Aaron's Rod, Woundwort

Principal Proposed Uses   Mild Bladder Infections, Bladder/Kidney Stones

---

Goldenrod is often falsely accused of being an intensely allergenic plant, because of its unfortunate tendency to bloom brightly at the same time and often in locations quite near to the truly allergenic ragweed. However, actual allergic reactions to this gorgeous plant are unusual.

There are numerous species of goldenrod (27 have been collected in Indiana alone) but all seem to possess similar medicinal properties, and various species are used interchangeably in Europe.[1]

WHAT IS GOLDENROD USED FOR TODAY?

In Europe, goldenrod is used as a supportive treatment for **bladder infections** (see page 28), irritation of the

urinary tract, and bladder/kidney stones. Goldenrod increases the flow of urine, helping to wash out bacteria and **kidney stones** (see page 109), and may also directly soothe inflamed tissues and calm muscle spasms in the urinary tract.[2] It isn't used as a cure in itself, but rather as a support to other, more definitive treatments such as antibiotics.

We don't really know how well the herb works. Several studies have found that goldenrod increases urine flow,[3] but there is no direct evidence that the herb is effective in resolving bladder infections or bladder/kidney stones. Its active ingredients are not known.

Warning: Since urinary conditions are potentially serious, seek a doctor's supervision.

Goldenseal

Visit Us at TNP.com

DOSAGE

A typical dosage is 3 to 4 g of dried herb 2 to 3 times daily. Make sure to drink plenty of water while taking goldenrod, to help it do its job.

SAFETY ISSUES

The safety of goldenrod hasn't been fully evaluated. However, no significant reactions or side effects have been reported.[4] Safety in young children, pregnant and nursing women, or those with severe liver or kidney disease has not been established.

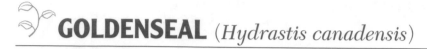

GOLDENSEAL (Hydrastis canadensis)

Alternate or Related Names   Orange Root, Yellow Root, Yellow Puccoon, Ground Raspberry, Wild Curcuma, Others

Principal Proposed Uses
   Topical Uses: Poorly Healing Sores, Fungal Infections, Inflamed Mucous Membranes
   Internal Uses: Minor Digestive Problems, Sore Throat

Other Proposed Uses
   Urinary Tract Infections

Incorrect Uses   "Immune Stimulant," "Antibiotic" for Common Cold, Masking Positive Findings on Drug Screens

Although goldenseal root is one of the most popular herbs sold today, it is taken almost entirely for the wrong reasons (see What Is Goldenseal Used for Today?). Originally, it was used by Native Americans both as a dye and as a treatment for skin disorders, digestive problems, liver disease, diarrhea, and eye irritations. European settlers learned of the herb from the Iroquois and other tribes and quickly adopted goldenseal as a part of early colonial medical care.

In the early 1800s, a flamboyant herbalist named Samuel Thompson created a wildly popular system of medicine (some would say personality cult) that swept the country. Thompson spoke of goldenseal in glowing terms, as a nearly magical cure for many conditions. His evangelism led to a dramatic upsurge in demand, followed by overcollection and decimation of the wild plant. Prices skyrocketed and then collapsed when Thompsonianism faded away.

Goldenseal has passed through several more booms and busts. Today, it is again in great demand, but now it is under intentional cultivation.

WHAT IS GOLDENSEAL USED FOR TODAY?

Contemporary herbalists use goldenseal primarily as a topical antibiotic for **wounds** (see page 123) that are not healing well. In practice, goldenseal salves, creams, ointments, and powders appear to speed wound healing.

Unfortunately, there are no reliable scientific studies to verify this strong clinical impression. What we do know is that one of goldenseal's constituents, berberine, possesses strong activity against a wide variety of bacteria and fungi.[1,2] Another factor may be that goldenseal seems to have a soothing effect on inflamed mucous membranes.

Goldenseal is most effective by direct contact. It does not seem to be an effective oral antibiotic, probably because the blood levels of berberine that can be achieved by taking goldenseal orally are far too low to matter.[3] However, goldenseal may also be beneficial in treating sore throats and diseases of the digestive tract because it can contact the affected area directly. Since berberine is concentrated in the bladder, goldenseal may be useful in resolving **bladder infections** (see page 28). It may be helpful for treating fungal infections of the skin as well.

Strangely, goldenseal is most commonly used inappropriately. Goldenseal is frequently combined with echinacea to be taken as an "immune booster" and "antibiotic" for the prevention and treatment of **colds** (see page 47). However, as the noted herbalist Paul Bergner has pointed out, there are three things wrong with this packaging: (1) there is no credible evidence that goldenseal increases immunity; (2) the herb was never used historically as an early treatment for colds; and (3) antibiotics aren't effective against colds anyway.[4] Nevertheless, the echinacea in these products may be helpful (see the chapter on **echinacea**).

Tradition suggests that goldenseal may help relieve the clogged sinuses and chest congestion that can linger after the acute phase of a cold, although there is no scientific evidence to turn to.

The other myth that has helped drive the sales of goldenseal is the widespread street belief that it can block a positive drug screen. The origin of this false idea dates back to a work of fiction published in 1900 by a pharmacist and author named John Uri Lloyd. In *Stringtown on the Pike,* Lloyd's most successful novel, a dead man is found to have traces of goldenseal in his stomach. In fact, he had taken goldenseal regularly (and correctly) as a digestive aid, but a toxicology expert mistakes the goldenseal for strychnine, and deduces intentional murder.

This work of fiction sufficed to create a folkloric connection between goldenseal and drug testing. Although the goldenseal in the story actually made a drug test come out falsely positive, this has been turned around to become a belief that goldenseal can make urine drug screens come out negative. A word to the wise: It doesn't work.

DOSAGE

When used as a topical for skin wounds, a sufficient quantity of goldenseal cream, ointment, or powder should be applied to cover the wound. Make sure to clean the wound at least once a day to prevent goldenseal particles from being trapped in the healing tissues.

For mouth sores and sore throats, goldenseal tincture may be swished or gargled. Goldenseal may also be used as strong tea for this purpose, made by boiling 0.5 to 1 g in a cup of water. Goldenseal tea can also be used as a douche for vaginal candidiasis.

For oral use, to aid the digestive tract or loosen clogged sinuses, a typical dosage of goldenseal is 250 to 500 mg 3 times daily. Goldenseal is generally only taken for a couple of weeks at most.

SAFETY ISSUES

Goldenseal appears to be safe when used as directed. One widespread rumor claims that goldenseal can disrupt the normal bacteria of the intestines. However, there is no scientific evidence that this occurs, and many herbalists believe that such concerns are unwarranted.[5] Another fallacy is that small overdoses of goldenseal are toxic, causing ulcerations of the stomach and other mucous membranes. This idea is based on a misunderstanding of old literature.[6]

However, because berberine has been reported to cause uterine contractions and to increase levels of bilirubin, goldenseal should not be used by pregnant women.[7,8] Safety in young children, nursing women, or those with severe liver or kidney disease is also not established.

Side effects of oral goldenseal are uncommon, although there have been reports of gastrointestinal distress and increased nervousness in people who take very high doses.

GOTU KOLA *(Centella asiatica)*

Alternate or Related Names   Indian Pennywort, Marsh Penny, Indian Hydrocotyle, White Rot, Thick-Leaved Pennywort, Others

Principal Proposed Uses   Varicose Veins

Other Proposed Uses   Hemorrhoids, Keloid Scars, Burn Healing, Wound Healing, Anal Fissures, Bladder Ulcers, Perineal Lesions, Liver Cirrhosis, Scleroderma, Improving Mental Performance

Gotu kola is a creeping plant native to subtropical and tropical climates. In India and Indonesia, gotu kola has a long history of use to promote wound healing and slow the progress of leprosy. It was also reputed to prolong life, increase energy, and enhance sexual potency.[1] Other uses of gotu kola included treating skin diseases, diarrhea, menstrual disorders, vaginal discharge, and venereal disease.

Based on these many traditional indications, gotu kola was accepted as a drug in France in the 1880s. British physicians in Africa used a special extract to treat leprosy.

WHAT IS GOTU KOLA USED FOR TODAY?

In the 1970s, Italian and other European researchers found evidence that gotu kola could significantly improve symptoms of **varicose veins** (see page 184), particularly overall discomfort, tiredness, and swelling. However, the herb is not believed to do much to reduce the unsightliness of veins that are already badly damaged. Some clinicians suggest that regular use of gotu kola can prevent the development of visible varicose veins, but this hasn't been proven. Gotu kola has also been suggested as a treatment for **hemorrhoids** (see page 85) because they are a type of varicose vein.

Like other herbs used for the treatment of varicose veins, gotu kola appears to have a generally beneficial effect on connective tissues. Along these lines, it has been used to prevent the development of keloid (bulging, enlarged) scars following **surgery** (see page 173), as well as to soften existing keloids. Gotu kola has also been tried as a treatment for improving **burn** (see page 123) and

Gotu Kola

Visit Us at TNP.com

wound (see page 123) healing and to alleviate the symptoms of the connective tissue disease scleroderma.

Gotu kola has a reputation for improving memory, and the positive results from a study of rats performed in 1992 produced a temporary rush of public interest.[2] However, the benefits in humans, if any, are far from impressive.

Gotu kola should not be confused with the caffeine-containing kola nut (see page 258), used in original recipes for Coca-Cola.

WHAT IS THE SCIENTIFIC EVIDENCE FOR GOTU KOLA?

There is significant scientific evidence for the effectiveness of gotu kola in varicose veins/venous insufficiency.

A vacuum suction chamber has been used in some gotu kola studies to evaluate the rate of fluid leakage in venous insufficiency. It produces swelling when applied to the skin of the ankle. When leg veins are leaking a lot of fluid, this swelling takes longer to disappear.

In one study of people with venous insufficiency, 2 weeks of treatment with gotu kola extracts was shown to reduce the time necessary for the swelling to disappear.[3]

A placebo-controlled study (whether it was double-blind was not stated) of 52 patients with venous insufficiency compared the effects of gotu kola extract at 180 mg daily and 90 mg daily against placebo.[4] After 4 weeks of treatment, researchers observed improvement in various measurements of vein function in all treated patients, but not in the placebo group. They also found that the higher dose was more effective than the lower dose. This kind of dose responsiveness is generally taken as good evidence that a treatment is actually effective.

Another study of double-blind design followed 87 people with varicose veins and compared the benefits of gotu kola at 60 mg and 30 mg daily against placebo.[5] Again, the results showed improvements in both treated groups, but greater improvement at the higher dose.

A double-blind study of 94 individuals with venous insufficiency of the lower limb compared the benefits of gotu kola extract at 120 mg daily and 60 mg daily against a placebo.[6] The results also showed a significant dose-related improvement in the treated groups in symptoms such as subjective heaviness, discomfort, and edema.

A 1992 review of all the gotu kola studies available concluded that gotu kola extract provides a dose-related improvement in venous insufficiency symptoms, reducing foot swelling, ankle edema, and fluid leakage from the veins.[7]

Although the subject is far from completely understood, it appears that gotu kola may improve the structure and function of the connective tissue in the body, keeping veins stronger and also possibly reducing the symptoms of other connective-tissue diseases. Along these lines, numerous clinical reports and preliminary studies suggest that gotu kola extracts may be useful in treating keloids, burns, wounds, anal fissures, bladder ulcers, dermatitis, hemorrhoids, perineal lesions, periodontal disease, cellulite, liver cirrhosis, and scleroderma.[8,9] Animal studies of purified asiaticoside, one of gotu kola's constituents, have also found a wound healing effect.[10] While some of these studies are intriguing and make a good case for further research, none can be regarded as definitive.

DOSAGE

The usual dosage of gotu kola is 20 to 60 mg 3 times daily of an extract standardized to contain 40% asiaticoside, 29 to 30% asiatic acid, 29 to 30% madecassic acid, and 1 to 2% madecassoside. Be patient, because gotu kola takes at least 4 weeks to work.

For the prevention of keloid scars, the herb is usually taken for 3 months prior to surgery, and for another 3 months afterwards.

SAFETY ISSUES

Orally, gotu kola appears to be nontoxic.[11] It seldom causes any side effects other than the occasional allergic skin rash. However, there are some concerns that gotu kola may be carcinogenic if applied topically to the skin.[12]

Although gotu kola has not been proven safe for pregnant or nursing women, studies in rabbits suggest that it does not harm fetal development,[13] and Italian physicians have given it to pregnant women.[14] Safety in young children and those with severe liver or kidney disease has not been established.

GRASS POLLEN EXTRACT

Alternate or Related Names   Rye Pollen Extract, Timothy Pollen Extract

Principal Proposed Uses   Prostate Enlargement (BPH)

Other Proposed Uses   Prostate Cancer, Prostatitis, Lowering Blood Lipids and Cholesterol

Like the more famous saw palmetto, grass pollen extract is used to treat prostate enlargement (BPH). The grasses used for this preparation are 92% rye, 5% timothy, and 3% corn.[1] Grass pollen has also been investigated for its potential to treat prostatitis and prostate cancer, and for reducing cholesterol.

Related grass pollen extracts are used for allergy shots. The grass pollen extracts described here have their allergenic component removed, and so can't possibly work to treat hay fever (see Safety Issues below). Grass pollen is also an entirely different product than **bee pollen** (see page 215).

SOURCES

Grass pollen extract tablets for prostate disease are available in pharmacies and health food stores or can be ordered from a number of sources on the Internet.

THERAPEUTIC DOSAGES

The recommended dosage for grass pollen extract tablets is between 80 and 120 mg per day.[2]

THERAPEUTIC USES

Two double-blind placebo-controlled studies tell us that grass pollen extract can help reduce symptoms of prostate enlargement (see What is the Scientific Evidence for Grass Pollen Extract).[3,4] Technically called benign prostatic hyperplasia (BPH), this common problem of middle-aged and older men can result in difficulties with urination, ranging in severity from inconvenient to life-threatening, in the absence of treatment.

Grass pollen has also been investigated for its usefulness in treating prostatitis (inflammation of the prostate) and prostatodynia (pain in the prostate with an unknown cause),[5,6,7] prostate cancer,[8,9,10] and **high cholesterol** (see page 88).[11] Animal studies also suggest that it may protect the liver from damage by some types of poisons.[12] However, the scientific evidence for all of these proposed uses is weak to nonexistent.

WHAT IS THE SCIENTIFIC EVIDENCE FOR GRASS POLLEN EXTRACT?

Two double-blind placebo-controlled studies found that grass pollen extract can improve symptoms of prostate enlargement. There have also been open studies that compared grass pollen to different treatments for BPH.

In the first double-blind placebo-controlled study, 103 BPH sufferers were assigned to take either placebo or 2 capsules of a standardized grass pollen extract 3 times daily for a period of 12 weeks.[13] At the end of the study, 69% of the participants who had been taking the grass pollen had reduced the number of trips they had to make to the bathroom at night. In the placebo group, only 37% reported improvement in this symptom. The amount of urine remaining in the bladder following urination was reduced in the treatment group by 24 ml and by 4 ml for the placebo group. Both of these were statistically significant improvements for those taking grass pollen.

The second double-blind placebo-controlled study lasted longer but enrolled fewer participants.[14] Fifty-seven men with prostate enlargement were enrolled in the study, with 31 taking 92 mg of the grass pollen extract daily for 6 months and the remaining 26 taking placebo. As with the previous study, statistically significant improvements in nighttime frequency of urination and emptying of the bladder were found with use of grass pollen extract. Additionally, 69% of the participants receiving treatment reported overall improvement, while only 29% of the group taking the placebo felt they had improved—another statistically significant difference.

An important finding in this study was that the prostates of the men taking grass pollen significantly decreased in size according to ultrasound measurements taken. Not all treatments for BPH can reduce prostate size. It may be that treatments, which shrink the prostate, can reduce the need for surgery—such is the case, at least, with the prescription drug finasteride. Whether grass pollen offers this same potential benefit is not yet known.

Two additional studies compared grass pollen to other alternative treatments for prostate enlargement, rather than to placebo.[15,16] An unblinded study pitted grass pollen against **pygeum** (see page 395).[17] Although pygeum is considered a more established treatment for prostate enlargement, grass pollen appeared to work better. The pollen extract was found to be significantly more effective in improving the flow of urine, emptying of the bladder, and the participants' perceptions of relief. Those in the grass pollen group also had a significant reduction in prostate size while there was no reduction of size in the pygeum group. It appears from this that grass pollen is a more effective treatment than pygeum, but since the study was not blinded, the results are somewhat questionable.

A double-blind comparison study pitted grass pollen against an amino acid preparation and found no significant difference between the two.[18] Unfortunately, since we don't know how well the amino acid medication works, the result has little meaning.

A number of animal and uncontrolled studies of grass pollen's effects on prostate enlargement and its symptoms also found it to be helpful, but such uncontrolled studies prove little.[19–27]

No one is certain how the grass pollen extract causes the beneficial results seen in the studies. One theory is that it inhibits the body's manufacturing of prostaglandins and leukotrienes, which might relieve congestion and act as an anti-inflammatory.[28] This, however, probably would not explain the reduction in prostate size, meaning that there may be more than one mechanism at work.

SAFETY ISSUES

No serious side effects have been reported with the use of grass pollen extract. No adverse reactions were observed in any of the clinical trials discussed above, although one review author mentioned rare reports of stomach upset and skin rash.[29]

Although many people are allergic to grass pollen, the grass pollen products discussed in this chapter are processed to remove allergenic proteins.[30] For this reason, it is unlikely that grass-allergic individuals will have an allergic reaction.

Maximum safe doses for young children, pregnant or nursing women, or those with liver or kidney disease are not known.

GREEN TEA (Camellia sinensis)

Alternate or Related Names   Black Tea, Chinese Tea

Principal Proposed Uses   Cancer Prevention

Other Proposed Uses   Heart Disease Prevention, Liver Disease Prevention, Sun Damage/Sunburn Prevention

People have been drinking tea for thousands of years, but only in the last couple of decades have we begun to document the potential health benefits of this ancient beverage. Both black and green tea are made from the same plant, but more of the original substances endure in the less-processed green form. Green tea contains high levels of substances called polyphenols, known to possess strong antioxidant, anticarcinogenic, antitumorigenic, and even antibiotic properties.[1,2]

A growing body of evidence in both human and animal studies suggests that regular consumption of green tea can reduce the incidence of a variety of cancers, including colon, pancreatic, and stomach cancers. Green tea might also help prevent heart disease and liver disease.

WHAT IS GREEN TEA USED FOR TODAY?

Based on the widely publicized results of observational studies, as well as basic research on its constituents, green tea has become popular as a daily drink for **cancer prevention** (see page 32).[3,4] There is some evidence that it may be helpful for preventing **heart disease** (see page 16) as well.[5–8] However, the observational studies used to draw these conclusions can be misleading, and not everyone who examines the data concludes that green tea has been proven effective.[9]

A lesser-known potential benefit of green tea is the possibility that it might prevent liver disease.[10] Researchers found that on average individuals with high intake of green tea had lower levels of "liver enzymes." Elevated liver enzymes occur with various liver diseases, so this data suggests that green tea might be preventing such problems as **hepatitis** (see page 189) and alcoholic liver disease.

Preliminary studies suggest that polyphenols from green tea might also help protect the skin from sun damage and **sunburn** (see page 171).[11,12]

Very preliminary evidence suggests that black tea, which is quite similar but not identical to green tea, may help protect against **osteoporosis**[13] (see page 136) and may help prevent **atherosclerosis** (see page 16).[14]

DOSAGE

Studies suggest that 3 cups of green tea daily provide protection against cancer. However, because not everyone wants to take the time to drink green tea, manufacturers have offered extracts that can be taken in pill form. A typical dosage is 100 to 150 mg 3 times daily of a green tea extract standardized to contain 80% total polyphenols and 50% epigallocatechin gallate. Whether these extracts work as well as the real thing remains unknown.

SAFETY ISSUES

As a widely consumed beverage, green tea is generally regarded as safe. It does contain caffeine, although at a lower level than black tea or coffee, and can therefore cause insomnia, nervousness, and the other well-known symptoms of excess caffeine intake. Green tea should not be given to infants and young children.

⚠ INTERACTIONS YOU SHOULD KNOW ABOUT

If you are taking

- **MAO inhibitors:** The caffeine in green tea could cause serious problems.
- **Coumadin (warfarin):** Large doses of green tea could interfere with its effectiveness, because green tea contains **vitamin K**, which directly counteracts Coumadin's blood-thinning action.[15]

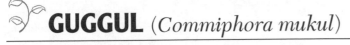

GUGGUL (*Commiphora mukul*)

Principal Proposed Uses　High Cholesterol

Guggul, the sticky gum resin from the mukul myrrh tree, plays a major role in the traditional herbal medicine of India. It was traditionally combined with other herbs for the treatment of arthritis, skin diseases, pains in the nervous system, obesity, digestive problems, infections in the mouth, and menstrual problems.

WHAT IS GUGGUL USED FOR TODAY?

In the early 1960s, Indian researchers discovered an ancient Sanskrit medical text that appears to clearly describe the symptoms and treatment of high cholesterol.[1] One of the main recommendations was guggul. Subsequent tests in animals found that guggul gum both lowered cholesterol levels and also separately protected against the development of hardening of the arteries.

Numerous research trials followed this discovery, culminating in preliminary studies examining guggul's effectiveness in humans.[2-5] The evidence was strong enough for the Indian government to approve guggul as a treatment for high cholesterol.

It appears that guggul can lower **cholesterol** (see page 88) by about 11 to 12% and triglycerides by 12.5 to 17%.[6,7,8] The full benefits may take several months to develop.

WHAT IS THE SCIENTIFIC EVIDENCE FOR GUGGUL?

A double-blind placebo-controlled study of guggul for reducing cholesterol enrolled 61 individuals and followed them for 24 weeks.[9] After 12 weeks of following a healthy diet, half the participants received placebo and the other half received guggul at a dose providing 100 mg of guggulsterones daily. The results after 24 weeks of treatment showed that the treated group experienced an 11.7% decrease in total cholesterol, along with a 12.7% decrease in LDL ("bad") cholesterol, a 12% decrease in triglycerides, and an 11.1% decrease in the total cholesterol/HDL ("good") cholesterol ratio. These improvements were significantly greater than what was seen in the placebo group.

Similar results were seen in a placebo-controlled trial of 40 individuals (the study report didn't state whether or not it was double-blind).[10]

Another double-blind study of 228 individuals given either guggul or the standard drug clofibrate found approximately equal efficacy between the two treatments.[11]

DOSAGE

Guggul is manufactured in a standardized form that provides a fixed amount of guggulsterones, the presumed active ingredients in guggul. The typical daily dose should provide 100 mg of guggulsterones.

Guggul

Visit Us at TNP.com

SAFETY ISSUES

In clinical trials of standardized guggul extract, no significant side effects other than occasional mild gastrointestinal distress have been seen.[12,13,14] Laboratory tests conducted in the course of these trials did not reveal any alterations in liver or kidney function, blood cell numbers and appearance, heart function, or blood chemistry.

However, safety in young children, pregnant or nursing women, or those with severe liver or kidney disease has not been established.

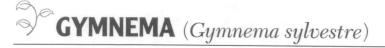

GYMNEMA (*Gymnema sylvestre*)

Principal Proposed Uses   Diabetes (Blood Sugar Control)

Native to the forests of India, *Gymnema sylvestre* has a coincidental double relationship to sugar: When placed on the tongue, it blocks the sensation of sweetness, and when taken internally, it appears to help control blood sugar levels in diabetes. There doesn't seem to be any connection between these two effects.

Indian physicians first used gymnema to treat diabetes almost 2,000 years ago. In the 1920s, preliminary scientific studies found that gymnema leaves do indeed reduce blood sugar levels,[1] but nothing much came of this discovery for decades.

WHAT IS GYMNEMA USED FOR TODAY?

With the recent revival of interest in herbs, gymnema has become increasingly popular in the United States as a supportive treatment for **diabetes** (see page 65). A few animal and preliminary human studies suggest that gymnema can increase insulin secretion and also enhance insulin's effectiveness.[2,3] Gymnema is most likely to be helpful in mild cases of adult-onset diabetes when insulin injections are not yet required. However, it is also used as a supportive treatment in more serious forms of the disease.

Warning: Diabetes is a dangerous illness, thus gymnema should only be used under medical supervision.

Under no circumstances should you try to replace insulin with gymnema alone.

DOSAGE

Gymnema is usually taken at a dosage of 400 to 600 mg daily of an extract standardized to contain 24% gymnemic acid.

SAFETY ISSUES

When used in appropriate dosages, gymnema appears to be fairly safe, although extensive studies have not been performed. One obvious risk is that if gymnema is successful, it may lower blood sugar levels too far, causing a dangerous hypoglycemic reaction. For this reason, medical supervision is essential.

Safety in young children, pregnant or nursing women, or those with severe kidney or liver disease has not been established.

⚠ INTERACTIONS YOU SHOULD KNOW ABOUT

If you are taking **insulin** or **oral medications** to reduce blood sugar levels, gymnema might cause them to work even better, potentially causing hypoglycemia. Therefore, you may need to reduce your dose of medication.

HAWTHORN (*Crataegus oxyacantha*)

Alternate or Related Names   Haw, May, Whitethorn

Principal Proposed Uses   Early Stages of Congestive Heart Failure, Benign Heart Palpitations, Hypertension
(High Blood Pressure)

Other Proposed Uses   Angina, Atherosclerosis

The name "hawthorn" is derived from "hedgethorn," reflecting this spiny tree's use as a living fence in much of Europe. Besides protecting estates from trespassers, hawthorn has also been used medicinally since ancient times. Roman physicians used hawthorn as a heart drug in the first century A.D., but most of the literature from that period focuses on its symbolic use for religious rites and political ceremonies.

During the Middle Ages, hawthorn was used for the treatment of dropsy, a condition we now call congestive heart failure. It was also used for treating other heart ailments as well as for sore throat.

WHAT IS HAWTHORN USED FOR TODAY?

Hawthorn is widely regarded in modern Europe as a safe and effective treatment for the early stages of **congestive heart failure** (CHF; see page 54). Although not as potent as that other famous heart herb of the Middle Ages, foxglove, hawthorn is much safer. The active ingredients in foxglove are the drugs digoxin and digitoxin. However, hawthorn does not appear to have any single active ingredient. This has prevented it from being turned into a drug.

Like foxglove and the drugs made from it, hawthorn appears to improve the heart's pumping ability. But it offers one very important advantage. Digitalis and some other medications that increase the power of the heart also make it more irritable and liable to dangerous irregularities of rhythm. In contrast, hawthorn has the unique property of both strengthening the heart and stabilizing it against arrhythmias by lengthening what is called the *refractory period.*[1,2,3] This term refers to the short period following a heartbeat during which the heart cannot beat again. Many irregularities of heart rhythm begin with an early beat. Digitalis shortens the refractory period, making such a premature beat more likely, while hawthorn protects against such potentially dangerous breaks in the heart's even rhythm. Also, with digitalis the difference between the proper dosage and the toxic dosage is very small. Hawthorn has an enormous range of safe dosing.[4]

Nevertheless, we don't recommend self-treating congestive heart failure! The disease is simply too dangerous. There are also medical treatments (such as ACE inhibitors) that have been proven to save lives in CHF, a benefit that hawthorn may not provide. You need a physician versed in both conventional and alternative medicine to guide you if you wish to use hawthorn for this condition.

There is one condition in which you may be able to safely use hawthorn as a self-treatment: annoying heart palpitations that have been thoroughly evaluated and found to be benign. Common symptoms include occasional thumping as well as episodes of racing heartbeat. These may occur without any identifiable medical cause and may not require any medical treatment, except for purposes of comfort. Although there is little scientific evidence to support it, many people use hawthorn for this condition.

However, because there are many dangerous kinds of heart palpitations, it is absolutely necessary to get a thorough checkup first. You should only self-treat with hawthorn after a doctor tells you that you have no medically significant heart problems. Full benefits may take a month or two to develop.

Finally, hawthorn sometimes lowers blood pressure a little, but seldom enough to make a significant difference.[5,6] It may be helpful for other heart-related conditions, such as **angina** (see page 10) and **atherosclerosis** (see page 16) in general, but there is as yet little direct evidence.

WHAT IS THE SCIENTIFIC EVIDENCE FOR HAWTHORN?

There has been a significant amount of solid research regarding the use of hawthorn as a treatment for congestive heart failure. Between 1981 and 1994, 14 controlled clinical studies of hawthorn were performed, most of them double-blind.[7,8] In all, 741 people participated in these trials. The cumulative results strongly suggest that hawthorn is an effective treatment for congestive heart failure. Comparative studies suggest that hawthorn is about as effective as a low dose of the conventional drug captopril, although whether it produces the same long-term benefits as captopril is unknown.[9]

DOSAGE

The standard dosage of hawthorn is 100 to 300 mg 3 times daily of an extract standardized to contain about 2 to 3% flavonoids or 18 to 20% procyanidins. Full effects appear to take several weeks or months to develop.

SAFETY ISSUES

Hawthorn appears to be safe. Germany's Commission E lists no known risks, contraindications, or drug interactions with hawthorn, and mice and rats have been given phenomenal doses without showing significant toxicity.[10] However, since hawthorn affects the heart, it shouldn't be combined with other heart drugs without a doctor's supervision. People with especially low blood pressure should also exercise caution.

Side effects are rare, mostly consisting of mild stomach upset and occasional allergic reactions (skin rash).

Safety in young children, pregnant or nursing women, or those with severe liver, heart, or kidney disease has not been established.

⚠ INTERACTIONS YOU SHOULD KNOW ABOUT

If you are taking any **heart medications,** it is possible that taking hawthorn could cause problems.

HE SHOU WU (*Polygonum multiflorum*)

Alternate Names   Fo Ti

Principal Proposed Uses   High Cholesterol, Insomnia, Constipation

The name of this herb literally means "Black-haired Mr. He," in reference to an ancient story of a Mr. He who restored his vitality, sexual potency, and youthful appearance by taking the herb now named after him. He shou wu is widely used in China for the traditional purpose of restoring black hair and other signs of youth.

More so than with most Chinese herbs, tradition supports taking He shou wu as a single herb, although it also figures as a component in many formulas. He shou wu is also called fo ti; pure unprocessed root is named white fo ti, while herb boiled in black-bean liquid according to a traditional process is called red fo ti. The two forms are believed to have somewhat different properties.

WHAT IS HE SHOU WU USED FOR TODAY?

Both animal and preliminary human studies performed in China suggest that He shou wu can reduce serum **cholesterol** (see page 88) and also improve symptoms of **insomnia** (see page 103).[1]

He shou wu is also said to be useful for **constipation** (see page 56); although if this is true, the effect is mild.

DOSAGE

He shou wu should be taken at a dosage of 9 to 15 g of raw herb per day, or according to the label for processed extracts. For most purposes, the processed or "red" fo ti is said to be superior. However, the raw herb is believed to be more effective for relieving constipation.

SAFETY ISSUES

Detailed modern safety studies have not been performed on this herb. Immediate side effects are infrequent, primarily limited to mild diarrhea and the rare allergic reaction. Safety for young children, pregnant or nursing women, or those with severe kidney or liver disease has not been established.

HISTIDINE

Supplement Forms/Alternate Names   L-Histidine

Principal Proposed Uses   There are no well-documented uses for histidine.

Other Proposed Uses   Rheumatoid Arthritis

Histidine is a semiessential amino acid, which means your body normally makes as much as it needs. Like most other amino acids, histidine is used to make proteins and enzymes. The body also uses histidine to make histamine, the culprit behind the swelling and itching you feel in an allergic reaction.

It appears that people with rheumatoid arthritis may have low levels of histidine in their blood. This has led to some speculation that histidine supplements might be a good treatment for this kind of arthritis, but so far no studies have confirmed this.

SOURCES

Although histidine is not required in the diet, histidine deficiencies can occur during periods of very rapid growth. Dairy products, meat, poultry, fish, and other protein-rich foods are good sources of histidine.

THERAPEUTIC DOSAGES

A typical therapeutic dosage of histidine is 4 to 5 g daily.

THERAPEUTIC USES

Although individuals with **rheumatoid arthritis** (see page 157) appear to have reduced levels of histidine in the blood,[1,2] this by itself doesn't prove that taking histidine will help. One study designed to evaluate this question directly found no significant benefit.[3]

SAFETY ISSUES

As a necessary nutrient, histidine is believed to be safe. However, maximum safe dosages of histidine have not been determined for young children, pregnant or nursing women, or those with severe liver or kidney disease. As with other supplements taken in large doses, it is important to purchase a quality product, as contaminants present even in very small percentages could conceivably add up and become toxic.

HMB *(Hydroxymethyl Butyrate)*

Supplement Forms/Alternate Names   Beta-Hydroxy Beta-Methylbutyric Acid

Principal Proposed Uses   Muscle Building for Strength Athletes and Bodybuilders

Technically "beta-hydroxy beta-methylbutyric acid," HMB is a chemical that occurs naturally in the body when the amino acid leucine breaks down.

Leucine is found in particularly high concentrations in muscles. During athletic training, damage to the muscles leads to the breakdown of leucine as well as increased HMB levels. Evidence suggests that taking HMB supplements might signal the body to slow down the destruction of muscle tissue.[1] However, while promising, the research record at present is contradictory and marked by an absence of large studies.

SOURCES

HMB is not an essential nutrient, so there is no established requirement. HMB is found in small amounts in citrus fruit and catfish. To get a therapeutic dosage, however, you need to take a supplement in powder or pill form.

THERAPEUTIC DOSAGES

A typical therapeutic dosage of HMB is 3 g daily.

Be careful not to confuse HMB with gamma hydroxybutyrate (GHB), a similar supplement. GHB can cause severe sedation, especially when combined with other sedating substances, such as alcohol or antianxiety drugs.

THERAPEUTIC USES

According to most but not all of the small double-blind trials performed thus far, HMB may improve response to weight training.[2–8] HMB might help prevent muscle damage during prolonged exercise.[9]

WHAT IS THE SCIENTIFIC EVIDENCE FOR HMB (HYDROXYMETHYL BUTYRATE)?

Muscle Building

Studies on chick and rat muscles suggest that HMB reduces the amount of muscle protein that breaks down during exercise.[10]

In a controlled study, 41 male volunteers aged 19 to 29 were given either 0, 1.5, or 3 g of HMB daily for 3 weeks.[11] The participants also lifted weights 3 days a week for 90 minutes. The results suggested that HMB can enhance strength and muscle mass in direct proportion to intake.

In another controlled study reported in the same article, 32 male volunteers took either 3 g of HMB daily or placebo, and then lifted weights for 2 or 3 hours daily, 6 days a week for 7 weeks. The HMB group saw a significantly greater increase in its bench-press strength than the placebo group. However, there was no significant difference in body weight or fat mass by the end of the study.

Another double-blind placebo-controlled trial of 39 men and 36 women found that over 4 weeks HMB supplementation improved response to weight training.[12]

Two placebo-controlled studies in women found that 3 g of HMB had no effect on lean body mass and strength in sedentary women, but it did provide an additional benefit when combined with weight training.[13]

However, two double-blind placebo-controlled studies, each lasting 28 days, failed to detect any effect on body composition or strength.[14] The first enrolled 52 college football players during off-season training, and the other followed 40 athletes engaged in weight training.

HMB

Visit Us at TNP.com

Although HMB at a dose of 3 or 6 g daily produced no effect different from placebo, creatine plus HMB did produce some improvements (see the full chapter on **sports performance** for more information). Marginal results were seen in another double-blind trial.[15]

All of these studies were small, and therefore, their results are not reliable. Larger studies will be necessary to truly establish whether HMB is helpful for power athletes working to enhance strength and muscle mass.

SAFETY ISSUES

HMB seems to be safe when taken at standard doses.[16,17] However, full safety studies have not been performed, so HMB should not be used by young children, pregnant or nursing women, or those with severe liver or kidney disease, except on the advice of a physician.

As with all supplements taken in very large doses, it is important to purchase a quality product, as an impurity present even in very small percentages could add up to a real problem.

HOPS (*Humulus lupulus*)

Principal Proposed Uses   Anxiety, Insomnia, Digestive Problems

Hops (the fruiting bodies of the hop plant) are most famous as the source of beer's bitter flavor, but they have a long history of use in herbal medicine as well. In Greece and Rome, hops were used as a remedy for poor digestion and intestinal disturbances. The Chinese used the herb for these purposes as well as to treat leprosy and tuberculosis.

As cultivation of hops for beer spread through Europe, it gradually became obvious that workers in hop fields tended to fall asleep on the job, more so than could be explained by the tedium of the work. This observation led to enthusiasm for using hops as a sedative. However, subsequent investigation suggests that much of the sedative effect seen in hop fields is due to an oil that evaporates quickly in storage.

Despite the absence of this oil, dried hop preparations do appear to be somewhat calming. While the exact reason is not clear, it seems that a sedating substance known as methylbutenol develops in the dried herb over a period of time.[1] It may also be manufactured in the body from other constituents of dried hops.

WHAT ARE HOPS USED FOR TODAY?

Germany's Commission E authorizes the use of hops for "discomfort due to restlessness or anxiety and sleep disturbances." Because its sedative effect is mild at most, the herb is often combined with other treatments for **anxiety** (see page 11) and **insomnia** (see page 103).

Like other bitter plants, hops are also used to improve appetite and digestion.

Scientists have had difficulty demonstrating that hops cause sedation.[2]

DOSAGE

The standard dosage of hops is 0.5 g taken 1 to 3 times daily.

SAFETY ISSUES

Hops are believed to be nontoxic. However, as with all herbs, some people are allergic to them. Interestingly, some species of dogs, greyhounds in particular, appear to be sensitive to hops with reports of deaths occurring.[3] The mechanism of this toxicity is not yet known. Those taken with the popular hobby of brewing beer at home are advised to keep pets away from the relatively large quantity of hops used in this process.

One animal study suggests that hops might increase the effect of sedative drugs,[4] so do not take hops with other medications for insomnia or anxiety except under a physician's supervision.

⚠ INTERACTIONS YOU SHOULD KNOW ABOUT

If you are taking **sedative drugs,** do not take hops except under a physician's supervision.

HORSE CHESTNUT (*Aesculus hippocastanum*)

Alternate or Related Names   Spanish Chestnut, Buckeye, Common Horse Chestnut, Conqueror Tree

Principal Proposed Uses
  Vein Problems: Varicose Veins, Phlebitis, Hemorrhoids

Other Proposed Uses   Easy Bruising, Swelling from Sprains and Other Injuries

The horse chestnut tree is widely cultivated for its bright white, yellow, or red flower clusters. Closely related to the Ohio buckeye, this tree produces large seeds known as horse chestnuts. A superstition in many parts of Europe suggests that carrying these seeds in your pocket will ward off rheumatism. More serious medical uses date back to nineteenth-century France, where extracts were used to treat hemorrhoids.

WHAT IS HORSE CHESTNUT USED FOR TODAY?

Serious German research of this herb began in the 1960s and ultimately led to the approval of a horse chestnut extract for vein diseases of the legs. Horse chestnut is the third most common single herb product sold in Germany, after ginkgo and St. John's wort. In Japan, an injectable form of horse chestnut is widely used to reduce inflammation after surgery or injury; however, it is not available in the United States.

The active ingredients in horse chestnut appear to be a group of chemicals called saponins, of which escin is considered the most important. Like **OPCs** (see page 373) and **bilberry** (see page 220), escin has the capacity to reduce swelling and inflammation, probably by slowing down the rate at which fluid leaks from irritated capillaries.[1] It's not exactly clear how escin works, but theories include "sealing" leaking capillaries, improving the elastic strength of veins, preventing the release of enzymes (known as glycosaminoglycan hydrolases) that break down collagen and open holes in capillary walls, and blocking other physiological events that lead to vein damage.[2,3]

Horse chestnut is most often used as a treatment for venous insufficiency. This is a condition associated with **varicose veins** (see page 184), when the blood pools in the veins of the leg and causes aching, swelling, and a sense of heaviness. While horse chestnut appears to reduce these symptoms, it is not believed to improve visible varicose veins very much.

Because **hemorrhoids** (see page 85) are actually a form of varicose veins, horse chestnut is often recommended for them as well.

Based on its known effects on veins, horse chestnut is also sometimes used along with conventional treatment in cases where the veins of the lower legs become seriously inflamed (**phlebitis**; see page 143). However, this condition is potentially dangerous and requires a doctor's supervision.

Just like OPCs, extracts of horse chestnut are sometimes recommended to help reduce swelling after sprains, other athletic injuries, and **surgery** (see page 173). Again, this use is based on the known effects of horse chestnut on blood vessels, and there is some evidence that it may be effective.[4]

Finally, one preliminary study suggests that a gel made from horse chestnut might be helpful for **bruises** (see page 74).[5]

WHAT IS THE SCIENTIFIC EVIDENCE FOR HORSE CHESTNUT?

More than 800 individuals have been involved in double-blind placebo-controlled studies of horse chestnut for treating venous insufficiency.[6–14]

One of the largest of these trials followed 212 people over a period of 40 days.[15] It was what is called a crossover study because the participants initially received horse chestnut or placebo, and then were crossed over to the other treatment (without their knowledge) after 20 days. The results showed that horse chestnut produced significant improvement in leg edema, pain, and sensation of heaviness.

However, the design of this study was not quite up to modern standards. A better-designed double-blind study of 74 individuals also found benefit.[16]

Good results were also seen in a partially double-blind placebo-controlled study, which compared the effectiveness of horse chestnut to that of compression stockings, a standard treatment.[17] This study followed 240 people over a course of 12 weeks. Compression stockings worked faster at reducing swelling, but by the end of the study the results were equivalent, and both treatments were better than placebo.

An extract of horse chestnut called escin may also help with bruising. One double-blind study of 70 people found that about 10 g of 2% escin gel, applied externally to bruises in a single dose 5 minutes after they were induced, reduced bruise tenderness.[18]

DOSAGE

The most common dosage of horse chestnut is 300 mg twice daily, standardized to contain 50 mg escin per dose, for a total daily dose of 100 mg escin. After good results have been achieved, the dosage can be reduced by about half for maintenance.

Horse chestnut preparations should certify that a toxic constituent called esculin has been removed (see Safety Issues). Also, a delayed-release formulation must be used to prevent gastrointestinal upset.

SAFETY ISSUES

Whole horse chestnut is classified as an unsafe herb by the FDA. Eating the nuts or drinking a tea made from the leaves can cause horse chestnut poisoning, the symptoms of which include nausea, vomiting, diarrhea, salivation, headache, breakdown of red blood cells, convulsions, and circulatory and respiratory failure possibly leading to death.[19] However, manufacturers of the typical European standardized extract formulations remove the most toxic constituent (esculin) and standardize the quantity of escin. To prevent stomach irritation caused by another ingredient of horse chestnut, the extract is supplied in a controlled-release product, which reduces the incidence of irritation to below 1%, even at higher doses.[20]

Properly prepared horse chestnut products appear to be quite safe.[21] After decades of wide usage in Germany, there have been no reports of serious harmful effects, and even mild reported reactions have been few in number.

In animal studies, horse chestnut and its principal ingredient escin have been found to be very safe, producing no measurable effects when taken at dosages seven times higher than normal. Dogs and rats have been treated for 34 weeks with this herb without harmful effects.[22] Studies in pregnant rats and rabbits found no injury to embryos at doses up to 10 times the human dose, and only questionable effects at 30 times the dose.

However, individuals with severe kidney problems should avoid horse chestnut.[23,24,25] In addition, injectable forms of horse chestnut can be toxic to the liver.[26]

Horse chestnut should not be combined with anticoagulant or "blood-thinning" drugs, as it may amplify their effect.[27,28] The safety of horse chestnut in young children and pregnant or nursing women has not been established. However, 13 pregnant women were given horse chestnut in a controlled study without noticeable harm.[29]

⚠ INTERACTIONS YOU SHOULD KNOW ABOUT

If you are taking **aspirin, Trental (pentoxifylline),** or **anticoagulant drugs** such as **Coumadin (warfarin)** or **heparin,** do not use horse chestnut except under medical supervision.

HORSETAIL (*Equisetum arvense*)

Alternate or Related Names   Bottle-Brush, Corn Horsetail, Dutch Rushes, Field Horsetail, Horse Willow

Principal Proposed Uses   Brittle Nails, Osteoporosis, Rheumatoid Arthritis

Horsetail is a living fossil, the sole descendent of primitive plants that served as dinosaur snacks 100 million years ago. The herb is unique for its high concentration of silicon, as well as for its ability to dissolve gold and other minerals into itself. Because of its silicon content, horsetail is abrasive enough to be used for polishing.

Medicinally, horsetail has been used for treating urinary disorders, **wounds** (see page 123), gonorrhea, **nosebleeds** (see page 129), digestive disorders, **gout** (see page 84), and many other conditions.[1]

WHAT IS HORSETAIL USED FOR TODAY?

Silicon plays a role in bone health,[2] and for this reason, horsetail has been recommended to keep bones and **nails** (see page 31) strong. The famous German herbalist Rudolf Weiss also suggests that horsetail can relieve symptoms of **rheumatoid arthritis** (see page 151).[3] However, there is no real scientific evidence for any of these uses.

DOSAGE

The standard dosage of horsetail is 1 g in capsule or tea form up to 3 times daily, as needed. Medicinal horsetail should *not* be confused with its highly toxic relative, the marsh horsetail (*Equisetum palustre*).

SAFETY ISSUES

Noticeable side effects from standard dosages of horsetail tea are rare. However, horsetail contains an enzyme that damages vitamin B_1 (thiamin) and has caused severe illness and even death in livestock that consumed too much of it.[4] In Canada, horsetail products are required to undergo heating or other forms of processing to inactivate this harmful constituent.

Also, perhaps because horsetail contains low levels of nicotine, children have been known to become seriously ill from using the branches as blow guns.[5] This plant can also concentrate toxic metals present in its environment.

For all of the above reasons, horsetail is not recommended for young children, pregnant or nursing women, or those with severe kidney or liver disease.

Horsetail may also cause loss of potassium, which may be dangerous for those taking drugs in the digitalis category.[6,7]

⚠ INTERACTIONS YOU SHOULD KNOW ABOUT

If you are taking **drugs in the digitalis category,** use horsetail only under medical supervision.

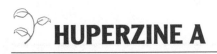

HUPERZINE A

Principal Proposed Uses   Alzheimer's Disease, Other Forms of Dementia, Ordinary Age-Related Memory Loss

Huperzine A is an extremely potent chemical derived from a particular type of club moss (*Huperzia serrata* [Thumb] Trev.). Like caffeine and cocaine, huperzine A is a medicinally active, plant-derived chemical that belongs to the class known as alkaloids. It was first isolated in 1948 by Chinese scientists.[1] This substance is really more a drug than an herb, but it is sold over the counter as a dietary supplement for memory loss and mental impairment.

WHAT IS THE SCIENTIFIC EVIDENCE FOR HUPERZINE A?

Many experiments have found that huperzine A can improve memory skills in aged animals as well as in younger animals whose memories have been deliberately impaired.[2–17]

All clinical trials of huperzine to date were performed in China and reported in Chinese.

A double-blind placebo-controlled study evaluated 103 people with Alzheimer's disease who received either huperzine A or a placebo twice daily for 8 weeks.[18] About 60% of the treated participants showed improvements in memory, thinking, and behavioral functions compared to 36% of the placebo-treated group, and the difference was significant.

Benefits were also seen in an earlier double-blind trial using injected huperzine in 160 individuals with dementia or other memory disorders.[19]

However, another double-blind trial of 60 individuals with Alzheimer's disease found no significant difference in symptoms between the treated and the placebo groups.[20]

Huperzine is also reportedly helpful for improving memory in healthy individuals. A double-blind trial of 34 matching pairs of junior middle school students reported improvements in memory in the treated group.[21]

Huperzine A inhibits the enzyme acetylcholinesterase. This enzyme breaks down acetylcholine, which seems to play an important role in mental function. When the enzyme that breaks it down is inhibited, acetylcholine levels in the brain tend to rise. Drugs that inhibit acetylcholinesterase (such as tacrine and donepezil) seem to improve memory and mental functioning in people with Alzheimer's and other severe conditions. The research on huperzine A indicates that it works in much the same way.

The chemical action of huperzine A is very precise and specific. It "fits" into a niche on the enzyme where acetylcholine is supposed to attach.[22,23] Because huperzine A is in the way, the enzyme can't grab and destroy acetylcholine. This mechanism has been demonstrated by considerable scientific work, including sophisticated computer modeling of the shape of the molecule.[24]

Although it originally comes from a plant, huperzine A is highly purified in a laboratory and is just a single chemical. It is just not much like an herb. Herbs contain hundreds or thousands of chemicals. In this way, huperzine A resembles drugs such as digoxin, codeine, Sudafed, and vincristine (a chemotherapy drug), which are also highly purified chemicals taken from plants. If we wish to call huperzine A a natural treatment, we need to call these (and dozens of other standard drugs) natural as well.

Visit Us at TNP.com

Hydroxycitric Acid

DOSAGE

Huperzine A is a highly potent compound with a recommended dose of only 100 to 200 mcg twice a day for age-related memory loss. We recommend using it only under a doctor's supervision.

SAFETY ISSUES

Perhaps because it works so specifically, huperzine A appears to have few side effects. However, children, pregnant or nursing women, or those with high blood pressure or severe liver or kidney disease should not take huperzine A except on a doctor's recommendation. We also don't know whether huperzine A interacts adversely with any drugs.

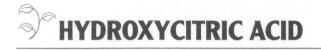

HYDROXYCITRIC ACID

Supplement Forms/Alternate Names   Hydroxycitrate, HCA, Malabar Tamarind, *Garcinia cambogia*, Gorikapuli

Principal Proposed Uses   There are no well-documented uses for hydroxycitric acid.

Other Proposed Uses   Weight Loss

Hydroxycitric acid (HCA), a derivative of citric acid, is found primarily in a small, sweet, purple fruit called the Malabar tamarind or, as it is most commonly called, *Garcinia cambogia*. Test-tube and animal research suggests that HCA may be helpful in weight loss because of its effects on metabolism. However, a recent, well-designed study found it ineffective.

SOURCES

HCA is not an essential nutrient. The Malabar tamarind is the only practical source of this supplement.

THERAPEUTIC DOSAGES

A typical dosage of HCA is 250 to 1,000 mg 3 times daily. Supplements are available in many forms, including tablets, capsules, powders, and even snack bars. Products are often labeled *Garcinia cambogia* and standardized to contain a fixed percentage of HCA.

THERAPEUTIC USES

According to animal studies, HCA can suppress appetite and thereby encourage **weight loss** (see page 192).[1–5] It is thought to work by interfering with the body's ability to produce and store fat.[6–9] However, the largest and best-designed human trial found no benefit.[10] Another small, placebo-controlled study found no effect on metabolism.[11]

WHAT IS THE SCIENTIFIC EVIDENCE FOR HYDROXYCITRIC ACID?

A 12-week double-blind placebo-controlled trial of 135 overweight individuals, who were given either placebo or 500 mg of HCA (as *Garcinia cambogia* extract standardized to contain 50% HCA) 3 times daily, found no effect on body weight or fat mass.[12] Another study tested HCA to see if it could cause weight loss by affecting metabolism, but no effects on metabolism were found.[13]

SAFETY ISSUES

The Malabar tamarind (from which HCA is extracted) is a traditional food and flavoring in Southeast Asia. No serious side effects have been reported from animal or human studies involving either fruit extracts or the concentrated chemical. However, formal safety studies have not been performed, and therefore, its safety remains unknown.

INDIGO (*Indigofera tinctoria, Indigofera oblongifolia*)

Principal Proposed Uses   There are no well-documented uses for indigo.

Other Proposed Uses   Liver Protection, Antiseptic

The leaflets and branches of the indigo plant yield an exquisite blue dye; people around the globe have used it to color textiles and clothing for centuries. Before the development of synthetic blue dyes, indigo was cultivated for this pigment rather than for medicinal use.

In the traditional medicine of India and China, indigo was used in the treatment of conditions we would now call epilepsy, bronchitis, liver disease, and psychiatric illness.[1] However, there is no real scientific evidence for any of these uses.

Warning: Several species of indigo are poisonous. See Safety Issues for more information.

WHAT IS INDIGO USED FOR TODAY?

Based on its traditional use for liver problems, researchers have investigated whether indigo might protect the liver against chemically induced injury. Animal studies do suggest that extracts of the indigo species *Indigofera tinctoria* protect the liver from damage by toxic chemicals.[2,3] No human trials, however, have been performed to examine indigo's effects on the liver.

The species *Indigofera oblongifolia* has been tested for its antibacterial and antifungal activity.[4] In a test tube trial, this plant showed significant activity against certain types of bacteria and fungi. This research is still in its preliminary stages, so it is too early to tell whether *Indigofera oblongifolia* will prove useful for the treatment of any infectious diseases.

Note: A different plant called wild indigo (*Baptisia tinctoria*), in combination with **echinacea** (see page 273) and white cedar, has been studied as a possible immune stimulant.[5] However, wild indigo is not part of the *Indigofera* family of plants and is not discussed here.

DOSAGE

No standard dosage of indigo has been established.

SAFETY ISSUES

The indigo species *Indigofera tinctoria* has a history of use in traditional medical systems, and is regarded by herbalists as safe, other than the occasional allergic reactions that have been reported.[6] However, comprehensive safety tests have not been performed. For this reason, indigo should not be used by pregnant or nursing women, young children, or individuals with severe liver or kidney disease. Safety in other individuals is unknown.

The species *Indigofera spicata* (formerly *Indigofera endecaphylla*), however, is poisonous: it has killed cattle and other animals[7,8] and has caused birth defects in rats.[9] Other indigo species have also been found to be lethal.[10,11] For this reason, it is important to avoid ingesting indigo internally unless you are absolutely certain that it has been harvested and processed by expert, reliable individuals.

INOSINE

Principal Proposed Uses　　There are no well-documented uses for inosine.

Other Proposed Uses　　Performance Enhancement, Heart Disease, Tourette's Syndrome

Inosine is an important chemical found throughout the body. It plays many roles, one of which is helping to make ATP (adenosine triphosphate), the body's main form of usable energy. Based primarily on this fact, inosine supplements have been proposed as an energy-booster for athletes, as well as a treatment for various heart conditions.

SOURCES

Inosine is not an essential nutrient. However, brewer's yeast and organ meats, such as liver and kidney, contain considerable amounts. Inosine is also available in purified form.

THERAPEUTIC DOSAGES

When used as a sports supplement, a typical dosage of inosine is 5 to 6 g daily (see Safety Issues).

THERAPEUTIC USES

Inosine has been proposed as a treatment for various forms of heart disease, from inflammation of the heart lining to irregular heartbeat and heart attacks. However, the evidence that it works is highly preliminary.[1]

Inosine is better known as a **performance enhancer** (see page 158) for athletes, although most of the available evidence suggests that it *doesn't* work for this purpose.[2–6]

Inosine has also been suggested as a possible treatment for Tourette's syndrome, a neurological disorder.[7]

SAFETY ISSUES

Although no side effects have been reported with the use of inosine, long-term use should be avoided. A very preliminary double-blind crossover study that enrolled 7 participants suggests that high doses of inosine (5,000 to 10,000 mg per day for 5 to 10 days) may increase the risk of uric acid–related problems, such as gout or kidney stones.[8]

The safety of inosine for young children, pregnant or nursing women, or those with serious liver or kidney disease has not been established.

As with all supplements taken in multigram doses, it is important to purchase a reputable product, because a contaminant present even in small percentages could add up to a real problem.

INOSITOL

Supplement Forms/Alternate Names   Vitamin B_8

Principal Proposed Uses   Depression, Panic Disorder

Other Proposed Uses   Alzheimer's Disease, Obsessive-Compulsive Disorder, Attention Deficit Disorder, Diabetic Neuropathy, Bipolar Disorder

Inositol, unofficially referred to as "vitamin B_8," is present in all animal tissues, with the highest levels in the heart and brain. It is part of the membranes (outer linings) of all cells, and plays a role in helping the liver process fats as well as contributing to the function of muscles and nerves.

Inositol may also be involved in depression. People who are depressed have much lower-than-normal levels of inositol in their spinal fluid. In addition, inositol participates in the action of *serotonin,* a neurotransmitter known to be a factor in depression. (Neurotransmitters are chemicals that transmit messages between nerve cells.) For this reason, inositol has been proposed as a treatment for depression, and preliminary evidence suggests that it may be helpful.

Inositol has also been tried for other psychological and nerve-related conditions.

SOURCES

Inositol is not known to be an essential nutrient. However, nuts, seeds, beans, whole grains, cantaloupe, and citrus fruits supply a substance called phytic acid, which releases inositol when acted on by bacteria in the digestive tract. The typical American diet provides an estimated 1,000 mg daily.

THERAPEUTIC DOSAGES

Experimentally, inositol dosages of up to 18 g daily have been tried for various conditions.

THERAPEUTIC USES

Preliminary double-blind studies suggest that high-dose inositol may be useful for **depression** (see page 59),[1,2,3] panic disorder,[4] **Alzheimer's disease** (see page 5),[5] obsessive-compulsive disorder,[6] and **attention deficit disorder** (see page 22).[7]

Inositol is also sometimes proposed as a treatment for complications of **diabetes** (see page 65), specifically diabetic neuropathy, but there have been no double-blind placebo-controlled studies, and two uncontrolled studies had mixed results.[8,9]

Finally, inositol has been recommended for **bipolar disorder** (see page 27) although there is no scientific evidence to support this use (see also Safety Issues below).

WHAT IS THE SCIENTIFIC EVIDENCE FOR INOSITOL?

Depression

Small double-blind studies have found inositol helpful for depression.[10,11] In one such trial, 28 depressed individuals were given a daily dose of 12 g of inositol for 4 weeks.[12] By the fourth week, the group receiving inositol showed significant improvement compared to the placebo group. However, by itself this study was too small to prove anything.

Panic Disorder

People with panic disorder frequently develop panic attacks, often with no warning. The racing heartbeat, chest pressure, sweating, and other physical symptoms can be so intense that they are mistaken for a heart attack. A small double-blind study (21 participants) found that people given 12 g of inositol daily had fewer, and less severe, panic attacks as compared to the placebo group.[13] Again, this study was too small to prove anything.

SAFETY ISSUES

No serious ill effects have been reported for inositol, even with a therapeutic dosage that equals about 18 times the average dietary intake. However, no long-term safety studies have been performed.

Although inositol has sometimes been recommended for bipolar disorder, there is evidence to suggest inositol may trigger manic episodes in people with this condition.[14] If you have bipolar disorder you should not take inositol unless under a doctor's supervision.

Safety has not been established in young children, women who are pregnant or nursing, and those with severe liver and kidney disease. As with all supplements used in multigram doses, it is important to purchase a reputable product, because a contaminant present even in small percentages could add up to a real problem.

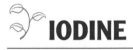

IODINE

Supplement Forms/Alternate Names   Iodide, Elemental Iodine

Principal Proposed Uses   Correcting Nutritional Deficiency

Other Proposed Uses   Cyclic Mastalgia

Your thyroid gland, located just above the middle of your collarbone, needs iodine to make thyroid hormone, which maintains normal metabolism in all cells of the body. Principally found in sea water, dietary iodine can be scarce in many inland areas, and deficiencies were common before iodine was added to table salt. Iodine deficiency causes enlargement of the thyroid, a condition known as goiter. However, if you are not deficient in iodine, taking extra iodine will not help your thyroid work better, and it might even cause problems.

For reasons that are not clear, supplementary iodine might also be helpful for cyclic mastalgia.

REQUIREMENTS/SOURCES

The official U.S. recommendations for daily intake of iodine are as follows:

- Infants 0–6 months, 40 mcg
    7–12 months, 50 mcg
- Children 1–3 years, 70 mcg
    4–6 years, 90 mcg
    7–10 years, 120 mcg
- Adults (and children 11 years and older), 150 mcg
- Pregnant women, 175 mcg
- Nursing women, 200 mcg

Iodine deficiency is rare in developed countries today because of the use of iodized salt.

Seafood and **kelp** (see page 340) contain very high levels of iodine, as do salty processed foods that use iodized salt.

Most iodine is in the form of iodide, but a few studies suggest that a special form of iodine called *molecular iodine* may be better than iodide (see What Is the Scientific Evidence for Iodine?).

THERAPEUTIC DOSAGES

A typical therapeutic dosage of iodide or iodine is 200 mcg daily.

THERAPEUTIC USES

Iodine supplements have been proposed as a treatment for **cyclic mastalgia** (breast pain and lumpiness that usually cycles in relation to the menstrual period, also called cyclic mastitis or fibrocystic breast disease; see page 58).[1]

WHAT IS THE SCIENTIFIC EVIDENCE FOR IODINE?

Cyclic Mastalgia (Cyclic Mastitis, Fibrocystic Breast Disease)

Three clinical studies indicate that supplements providing iodine may be helpful in treating cyclic mastalgia.[2] These studies suggest that either iodide or iodine (the

Iodine

Visit Us at TNP.com

pure molecular form) might be useful. In the one placebo-controlled trial among this group, a study that enrolled 56 individuals, molecular iodine was found
superior to placebo in relieving pain and reducing the
number of cysts.

Another of these studies compared molecular iodine
to iodide. Molecular iodine was no more effective than
iodide, but was deemed superior because it induced
fewer side effects and did not affect the thyroid.

SAFETY ISSUES

When taken at the recommended dosage, iodine and iodide appear to be safe nutritional supplements. However, excessive doses of iodide can actually cause thyroid
problems! There is also a speculative link between excessive iodide intake and thyroid cancer. For these reasons,
iodide intake above about 200 mcg daily is not recommended.

IPRIFLAVONE

Principal Proposed Uses   Preventing and Treating Osteoporosis

Other Proposed Uses   Reducing the Pain of Osteoporotic Fractures, Bodybuilding

Isoflavones (see page 335) are water-soluble chemicals found in many plants. Ipriflavone is a semisynthetic version of an isoflavone found in **soy** (see
page 411).

Soy isoflavones have effects in the body somewhat
similar to those of estrogen. This should be beneficial,
but it is possible that soy could present some of the risks
of estrogen as well. In 1969, a research project was initi-
ated to manufacture a type of isoflavone that would possess the bone-stimulating effects of estrogen without any
estrogen-like activity elsewhere in the body. Such a
product would help prevent osteoporosis but cause no
other health risks.

Ipriflavone was the result. After 7 successful years of
experiments with animals, human research was started
in 1981. Today, ipriflavone is available in over 22 countries and in most drugstores in the United States as a
nonprescription dietary supplement. It is an accepted
treatment for osteoporosis in Italy, Turkey, and Japan.

Like estrogen, ipriflavone appears to slow and perhaps slightly reverse bone breakdown. It also seems to
help reduce the pain of fractures caused by osteoporosis.
However, since it does not appear to have any estrogenic
effects anywhere else in the body, it shouldn't increase
the risk of breast or uterine cancer. On the other hand, it
won't reduce the hot flashes, night sweats, mood
changes, or vaginal dryness of menopause, nor prevent
heart disease. Ipriflavone is also touted as a bodybuilding
aid, but no real evidence supports this use.

SOURCES

Ipriflavone is not an essential nutrient and is not found
to any appreciable extent in food. It must be taken as a
supplement.

THERAPEUTIC DOSAGES

The proper dosage of ipriflavone is 200 mg 3 times daily,
or 300 mg twice daily.

THERAPEUTIC USES

Ipriflavone appears to be able to slow down and perhaps
slightly reverse **osteoporosis** (see page 136). It may be
helpful for this purpose in ordinary postmenopausal osteoporosis as well as osteoporosis caused by
medications.[1–17] Ipriflavone also seems to ease the pain
of fractures caused by osteoporosis.[18,19,20] There is no
real evidence that it is helpful for bodybuilding.

WHAT IS THE SCIENTIFIC EVIDENCE FOR IPRIFLAVONE?

Preventing and Treating Osteoporosis

Numerous double-blind placebo-controlled studies involving a total of over 1,000 participants have examined
the effects of ipriflavone on osteoporosis.[21–25] Overall, it
appears that ipriflavone can slow the progression of osteoporosis and perhaps reverse it to some extent. For example, a 2-year double-blind study followed 198
postmenopausal women who showed evidence of bone
loss.[26] At the end of the study, there was a gain in bone
density of 1% in the ipriflavone group and a loss of 0.7%
in the placebo group. These numbers may sound small,
but they can add up to a lot of bone over time.

Ipriflavone, like estrogen, probably works by fighting
bone breakdown.[27–30] However, there is some evidence
that it may also increase new bone formation, too.[31–33]

In Combination with Calcium

Taking calcium plus ipriflavone may also be an excellent idea. In one study, 60 women who had already been diagnosed with osteoporosis and had already suffered one spinal fracture were given either 1,000 mg of calcium or 1,000 mg of calcium with ipriflavone.[34] After 6 months, the ipriflavone group had an increase of bone density in the spine of 3.5%, compared to a net loss in the calcium-only group.

In Combination with Estrogen

Combining ipriflavone with estrogen may enhance anti-osteoporosis benefits.[35,36] However, we do not know for sure whether such combinations increase or reduce the other risks (or benefits) of estrogen. (See Safety Issues for more information.)

Preventing Side Effects of Medications

Ipriflavone may also be helpful for preventing osteoporosis in women who are taking Lupron or corticosteroids, medications that accelerate bone loss.[37,38]

Reducing Pain of Fractures Caused by Osteoporosis

For reasons that are not at all clear, ipriflavone appears to be able to reduce pain in osteoporosis-related fractures that have already occurred.[39,40,41]

SAFETY ISSUES

Nearly 3,000 people have used ipriflavone in clinical studies, with no more side effects than those taking placebo.[42] However, there are some potential risks. Because ipriflavone is metabolized by the kidneys, individuals with severe kidney disease should have their ipriflavone dosage monitored by a physician.[43]

Also, although ipriflavone itself does not affect tissues outside of bone, some evidence suggests that if it is combined with estrogen, estrogen's effects on the uterus are increased.[44,45] This might mean that risk of uterine cancer would be elevated over taking estrogen alone. It should be possible to overcome this risk, by taking progesterone along with estrogen, which is standard medical practice in any case. However, this finding does make one wonder whether ipriflavone-estrogen combinations raise the risk of breast cancer too, an estrogen side effect that has no easy solution. At present, there is no available information on this important subject.

Additionally, ipriflavone may interfere with certain drugs by affecting the way they are processed in the liver. For example, it may raise blood levels of the older asthma drug theophylline.[46,47,48] It could also raise levels of caffeine, meaning that if you drink coffee while taking ipriflavone you might stay up longer than you expect! Ipriflavone could also interact with tolbutamide (a drug for diabetes), phenytoin (used for epilepsy), and Coumadin (a blood thinner).[49] Such interactions are potentially dangerous, especially since phenytoin and warfarin cause osteoporosis, and some people might be tempted to try taking ipriflavone at the same time.

⚠ INTERACTIONS YOU SHOULD KNOW ABOUT

If you are taking

- **Theophylline, tolbutamide, Dilantin (phenytoin), Coumadin (warfarin),** or any other drug metabolized in the liver: Ipriflavone might change the levels of that drug in your body.
- **Estrogen:** Ipriflavone might help it strengthen your bones even more. However, it might also increase the risk of uterine cancer.

🌿 IRON

Supplement Forms/Alternate Names   Iron Sulfate, Chelated Iron

Principal Proposed Uses   Correction of Iron Deficiency, Performance Enhancement

Other Proposed Uses   Menorrhagia (Heavy Menstruation), Attention Deficit Disorder, Restless Legs Syndrome, HIV Support

---

The element iron is essential to human life. As part of hemoglobin, the oxygen-carrying protein found in red blood cells, iron plays an integral role in nourishing every cell in the body with oxygen. It also functions as a part of myoglobin, which helps muscle cells store oxygen.

Without iron, your body could not make ATP (adenosine triphosphate, the body's primary energy source), produce DNA, or carry out many other critical processes.

Iron deficiency can lead to anemia, learning disabilities, impaired immune function, fatigue, and depression.

However, you shouldn't take iron supplements unless lab tests show that you are genuinely deficient.

REQUIREMENTS/SOURCES

The official U.S. recommendations for daily intake of iron are as follows:

- Infants 0–6 months, 6 mg
- Children 7 months–10 years, 10 mg
- Males 11–18 years, 12 mg
      19 years and older, 10 mg
- Females 11–50 years, 15 mg
      51 years and older, 10 mg
- Menstruating women, 15 mg
- Pregnant women, 30 mg
- Nursing women, 15 mg

Iron deficiency is the most common nutrient deficiency in the world; worldwide, at least 700 million individuals have iron-deficiency anemia.[1] While iron deficiency is widespread in the developing world, it is also prevalent in developed countries. Groups at high risk are children, teenage girls, menstruating women, pregnant women, and the elderly.[2,3]

There are two major forms of iron: *heme* iron and *nonheme* iron. Heme iron is bound to the proteins hemoglobin or myoglobin, whereas nonheme iron is an inorganic compound. (In chemistry, "organic" has a very precise meaning that has nothing to do with farming. An organic compound contains carbon atoms. Thus "inorganic iron" is an iron compound containing no carbon.) Heme iron, obtained from red meats and fish, is easily absorbed by the body. Nonheme iron, derived from plants, is less easily absorbed.

Rich sources of heme iron include oysters, meat, poultry, and fish. The main sources of nonheme iron are dried fruits, molasses, whole grains, legumes, egg yolks, leafy green vegetables, nuts, seeds, and **kelp** (see page 340). Acidic foods, such as fruit preserves and tomatoes, are a good source of iron when they've been cooked in iron or stainless steel cookware (some of the iron leaches into the food).

Iron absorption may be affected by the following substances: antibiotics in the quinolone (Floxin, Cipro)[4–8] or tetracycline[9,10,11] families, levodopa,[12] methyldopa,[13,14] carbidopa,[15] penicillamine,[16] thyroid hormone,[17] captopril (and possibly other ACE inhibitors),[18] calcium,[19–22] soy,[23] zinc,[24] copper,[25] or manganese.[26] Conversely, iron may inhibit their absorption, too.

In addition, drugs in the H_2 blocker or proton pump inhibitor families may impair iron absorption.[27]

THERAPEUTIC DOSAGES

The typical short-term therapeutic dosage to correct iron deficiency is 100 to 200 mg daily. Once your body's iron stores reach normal levels, however, this dose should be reduced to the lowest level that can maintain iron balance.

THERAPEUTIC USES

The most obvious use of iron supplements is to treat iron deficiency. Severe iron deficiency causes anemia, which in turn causes many symptoms. Iron deficiency too slight to cause anemia appears to impair health as well. A double-blind trial suggests that women with mild iron deficiency might have difficulty increasing their physical fitness.[28] In addition, an observational study suggests that adolescent girls who are marginally iron deficient may experience reduced mental function.[29] However, don't take iron just because you feel tired. Make sure to get tested to see whether you are indeed deficient. With iron, more is definitely *not* better.

Heavy menstruation (menorrhagia) can certainly cause iron loss. However, for reasons that are not clear, iron supplementation can reportedly lighten heavy menstrual bleeding, but only if you are iron deficient to begin with.[30] Iron has also been tried as a treatment for **attention deficit disorder** (see page 22), but there is as yet no real evidence that it works.

Preliminary studies have linked low iron levels to **restless legs syndrome** (see page 150). In these studies supplemental iron decreased symptoms.[31,32,33] However, a double-blind study on subjects with normal iron levels showed no benefit in taking iron supplements.[34]

A study of 71 **HIV-positive** (see page 94) children noted a high rate of iron deficiency.[35] One observational study of 296 men with HIV infection linked high intake of iron to a decreased risk of AIDS 6 years later.[36]

WHAT IS THE SCIENTIFIC EVIDENCE FOR IRON?

Sports Performance

A double-blind placebo-controlled trial of 42 non-anemic women with evidence of slightly low iron reserves found that iron supplements significantly increased the benefits gained from exercise.[37] Participants were put on a daily aerobic training program for the latter 4 weeks of this 6-week trial. At the end of the trial, those receiving iron showed significantly greater gains in speed and endurance as compared to those given placebo.

Menorrhagia

One small double-blind study found good results using iron supplements to treat heavy menstruation. This study, which was performed in 1964, saw an improvement in 75% of the women who took iron (compared to 32.5% of those who took placebo). Women who began with higher iron levels did not respond to treatment.[38] This suggests once more that supplementing with iron is only a good idea if you are deficient in it.

SAFETY ISSUES

At the recommended dosage, iron is quite safe. Excessive dosages, however, can be toxic—damaging the intestines and liver, and possibly resulting in death. Iron poisoning in children is a surprisingly common problem, so make sure to keep your iron supplements out of their reach.

Mildly excessive levels of iron may be unhealthy for another reason: it acts as an oxidant (the opposite of an antioxidant), perhaps increasing the risk of cancer and heart disease. Elevated levels of iron may also play a role in brain injury caused by stroke.[39] In addition, excess iron appears to increase complications of pregnancy.[40]

Simultaneous use of iron and high-dose vitamin C can cause excessive iron absorption.[41–48]

⚠ INTERACTIONS YOU SHOULD KNOW ABOUT

If you are taking

- Antibiotics in the **tetracycline** or **quinolone** (**Floxin**, **Cipro**) families, **ACE inhibitors, levodopa, methyldopa, carbidopa, penicillamine, thyroid hormone, calcium**, **soy**, **zinc**, **copper**, or **manganese**: To avoid absorption problems, wait at least 2 hours following your dose of medication or supplement before taking iron.
- Drugs that reduce stomach acid such as **antacids, H₂ blockers** and **proton pump inhibitors**: You may need extra iron.
- High doses of **vitamin C**: You may absorb too much iron.

ISOFLAVONES

Supplement Forms/Alternate Names   Soy Isoflavones, Red Clover Isoflavones
Principal Proposed Uses   Menopausal Symptoms, High Cholesterol
Other Proposed Uses   Osteoporosis, Cancer Prevention

Isoflavones are water-soluble chemicals found in many plants. In this chapter, we will discuss a group of isoflavones that are phytoestrogens, meaning that they cause effects in the body somewhat similar to those of estrogen. The most investigated phytoestrogen isoflavones, **genistein** (see page 294) and daidzein, are found in **soy** products (see page 411) and the herb **red clover** (see page 397).

One of the ways these isoflavones appear to work is interesting. Although they are less powerful than the body's own estrogen, they latch on to the same places (receptor sites) on cells and don't allow actual estrogen to attach. In this way, when there is not enough estrogen in the body, isoflavones can partially make up for it; but when there is plenty of estrogen, they can partially block its influence. The net effect may be to reduce some of the risks of excess estrogen (breast and uterine cancer) while still providing some of estrogen's benefits (preventing osteoporosis). These isoflavones may work in other ways as well, such as by lowering the body's own level of estrogen.[1,2] However, there is some evidence that isoflavones isolated from soy are less effective alone than when taken as part of a high-soy diet.

SOURCES

Although isoflavones are not essential nutrients, they may help reduce the incidence of several diseases. Thus isoflavones may be useful for optimum health, even if they are not necessary for life like a classic vitamin.

Roasted soybeans have the highest isoflavone content: about 167 mg for a 3.5-ounce serving. Tempeh is next, with 60 mg, followed by soy flour with 44 mg. Processed soy products such as soy protein and soy milk contain about 20 mg per serving. The same isoflavones found in soy are also contained in certain red clover products; check the label to determine the content.

THERAPEUTIC DOSAGES

The optimum dosage of isoflavones obtained from food is not known.

We know that Japanese women eat up to 200 mg of isoflavones from soy daily, but we don't really know what amount of natural isoflavones is ideal. According to one study, 62 mg of isoflavones daily is sufficient to reduce cholesterol.[3] However, isolated isoflavones may not be as effective as more complete soy foods.[4]

THERAPEUTIC USES

Soy products are known to reduce **cholesterol** (see page 88), and soy isoflavones may be their active ingredient for this purpose according to some,[5,6] but not all, studies.[7,8] Soy isoflavones may also help prevent some forms of **cancer** (see page 32).[9–15]

Soy has also been found to reduce **menopausal symptoms** (see page 117).[16,17,18] However, isolated isoflavones extracted from red clover have not proved effective.[19,20]

Promising evidence suggests that soy or soy isoflavones may be helpful for preventing **osteoporosis** (see page 136).[21–29] However, there is much more evidence for the semisynthetic isoflavone **ipriflavone** (see page 332) for this purpose.

What *don't* soy isoflavones do? They don't seem to lower blood pressure.[30]

WHAT IS THE SCIENTIFIC EVIDENCE FOR ISOFLAVONES?

High Cholesterol

In 1995, a review of 38 controlled studies on soy and heart disease concluded that soy is definitely effective at reducing total cholesterol, LDL ("bad") cholesterol, and triglycerides.[31]

One double-blind study (not part of the review mentioned previously), which involved 66 older women, found improvements in HDL ("good") cholesterol as well.[32] The women were divided into three groups. The first group received 40 g of skim milk protein daily. The second group was given the same amount of soy protein, and the third received 40 g of soy protein with extra soy isoflavones. Compared with the skim milk (placebo) group, both soy groups showed significant improvements in both total cholesterol and HDL cholesterol.

Although there is some evidence that the isoflavones in soy are the active ingredient for lowering cholesterol,[33] other studies suggest that different components must be present for soy to work.[34,35]

Menopausal Symptoms ("Hot Flashes")

Soy protein, presumably due to its isoflavone content, seems to relieve "hot flashes," a common symptom of menopause.

A double-blind placebo-controlled study involving 104 women found that soy protein provided significant relief compared to placebo (milk protein). After 3 weeks, the women taking daily doses of 60 g of soy protein were having 26% fewer hot flashes.[36] By week 12, the reduc-

tion was 45%. Women taking placebo also experienced a big improvement by week 12 (30% fewer hot flashes), but soy gave significantly better results.

Similarly positive results were seen in a 6-week double-blind placebo-controlled trial of 39 women.[37]

However, isoflavones from red clover have not done well in studies on menopausal symptoms. A 28-week double-blind placebo-controlled crossover trial of 51 postmenopausal women found no reduction in hot flashes among those given 40 mg of red clover isoflavones daily.[38] No benefits were seen in another double-blind placebo-controlled trial, which involved 37 women also given isoflavones from red clover at a dose of either 40 mg or 160 mg daily.[39]

There are many potential explanations for this discrepancy. It may be that the exact mixture of isoflavones in red clover is significantly different from that which is found in soy. Another possibility is that, as with high cholesterol, soy constituents other than isoflavones play a role.

Osteoporosis

In one study that evaluated the benefits of soy isoflavones in osteoporosis, a total of 66 postmenopausal women took either placebo (soy protein with isoflavones removed) or soy protein containing 56 or 90 mg of soy isoflavones daily for 6 months.[40] The group that took the higher dosage of isoflavones showed significant gains in spinal bone density. There was little change in the placebo or low-dose isoflavone groups. This study suggests that soy isoflavones may be effective for osteoporosis.

Very nearly the same results were also seen in a similar study. This 24-week double-blind trial of 69 postmenopausal women found that isoflavone-rich soy products can significantly reduce bone loss from the spine.[41]

Similar benefits have been seen in animal studies.[42–48] However, a couple of animal studies and one human trial failed to find benefit.[49,50,51]

Estrogen and most other medications for osteoporosis work by fighting bone breakdown. Soy may work in the other way, by helping to increase new bone formation.[52,53]

SAFETY ISSUES

Studies in animals have found soy isoflavones essentially nontoxic.[54]

Nonetheless, because isoflavones work somewhat like estrogen, there are at least theoretical concerns that they may not be safe for women who have already had breast cancer. Furthermore, evidence from one highly preliminary study in humans found changes suggestive of increased breast cancer risk after women took a commercial soy protein product.[55] Preliminary studies and reports have raised concerns that intensive use of soy products by pregnant women could exert a hormonal effect that impacts unborn fetuses.[56,57]

Red clover isoflavones probably present similar risks.

However, while fears have been expressed by some experts that soy isoflavones might interfere with the action of oral contraceptives, one study of 40 women suggests that such concerns are groundless.[58] Another trial found that soy does not interfere with the action of estrogen-replacement therapy in menopausal women.[59]

Soy products may impair thyroid function or reduce absorption of thyroid medication, at least in children.[60,61,62] For this reason, individuals with impaired thyroid function should use soy with caution.

JUNIPER BERRY (*Juniperus communis*)

Alternate or Related Names   Juniper, Ginepro, Enebro

Principal Proposed Uses   Bladder Infection

In Dutch, juniper is called "geniver," from which came the name "gin." But juniper is not only good for making martinis. Its berries (actually not berries at all, but a portion of the cone) were used by the Zuni Indians to assist in childbirth, by British herbalists to treat congestive heart failure and stimulate menstruation, and by American nineteenth-century herbalists to treat congestive heart failure, gonorrhea, and urinary tract infections.

The explanation for some of these uses may be found in juniper's diuretic properties. Its volatile oils reportedly increase the rate of kidney filtration,[1] thereby perhaps helping to remove the accumulated fluid in congestive heart failure, and "wash out" the offending bacteria in urinary tract infections. However, there is no direct scientific evidence that juniper is effective for these purposes.

WHAT IS JUNIPER BERRY USED FOR TODAY?

Contemporary herbalists primarily use juniper as a component of herbal formulas designed to treat **bladder infections** (see page 28). A typical combination might include **uva ursi** (see page 427), **parsley** (see page 381), cleavers, and buchu. Such formulas are said to be most effective when taken at the first sign of symptoms and may not work well once the infection has really taken hold. Unfortunately, double-blind studies of juniper have not been performed.

Recently, gin-soaked raisins have been touted as an arthritis treatment. This is probably just a fad, but some weak evidence suggests that juniper may possess anti-inflammatory properties.[2] In the test tube, certain constituents of juniper have been found to inhibit the herpes virus.[3]

DOSAGE

You can make juniper tea by adding 1 cup of boiling water to 1 tablespoon of juniper berries, covering, and allowing the berries to steep for 20 minutes. The usual dosage is 1 cup twice a day. However, juniper is said to work better as a treatment for bladder infections when combined with other herbs. Combination products should be taken according to label instructions.

Warning: Bladder infections can go on to become kidney infections. For this reason, seek medical supervision if your symptoms don't resolve in a few days, or if you develop intense low back pain, fever, chills, or other signs of serious infection.

SAFETY ISSUES

Although juniper is regarded as safe and is widely used in foods, we don't recommend taking it during pregnancy. (We also recommend not drinking gin.) Remember, juniper was used historically to stimulate menstruation and childbirth. It has also been shown to cause miscarriages in rats.[4]

Juniper seldom causes any noticeable side effects. Prolonged use of juniper could possibly deplete the body of potassium, the way other diuretics do, but this hasn't been proven. Combining juniper with conventional diuretics, however, may cause excessive fluid loss.

Some texts warn that juniper oil may be a kidney irritant, but there is no real evidence that this is the case.[5] Nonetheless, people with serious kidney disease probably shouldn't take juniper. Safety for young children, nursing women, or those with severe liver disease has also not been established.

KAVA *(Piper methysticum)*

Alternate or Related Names   Kava Kava, Ava, Ava Pepper, Intoxicating Pepper, Kawa, Others

Principal Proposed Uses   Anxiety, Insomnia

Other Proposed Uses   Tension Headaches, Alcohol Withdrawal

Kava is a member of the pepper family that has long been cultivated by Pacific Islanders for use as a social and ceremonial drink. The first description of kava came to the West from Captain James Cook on his celebrated voyages through the South Seas. Cook reported that on occasions when village elders and chieftains gathered together for significant meetings, they would hold an elaborate kava ceremony at the beginning to break the ice (if there's any ice in the South Seas). Typically, each participant would drink two or three bowls of chewed-up kava mixed with coconut milk. Kava was also drunk in less formal social settings as a mild intoxicant.

When they learned about kava's effects, European scientists set to work trying to isolate its active ingredients. However, it wasn't until 1966 that substances named kavalactones were isolated and found to be effective sedatives. One of the most active of these is dihydrokavain, which has been found to produce a sedative, painkilling, and anticonvulsant effect.[1,2,3] Other named kavalactones include kavain, methysticin, and dihydromethysticin.

High dosages of kava extracts cause muscular relaxation, and at very high dosages paralysis without loss of consciousness develops.[4–7] Kava is also a local anesthetic, producing peculiar numbing sensations when held in the mouth.

The method of action of kava is not fully understood. Conventional tranquilizers in the Valium family interact with special binding sites in the brain called GABA receptors. Early studies of kava suggested that the herb does not affect these receptors.[8] However, more recent studies have found an interaction.[9,10] The early researchers may have missed the connection because kava appears to affect somewhat unusual parts of the brain.

WHAT IS KAVA USED FOR TODAY?

In the words of Germany's Commission E, kava is useful for relieving "states of nervous anxiety, tension, and agitation." While it is not considered powerful enough to treat severe **anxiety** or **panic attacks** (see page 11), kava is often used for milder symptoms. Its skeletal-muscle relaxing effects may make it particularly useful if you suffer from tension headaches. While prescription drugs for anxiety are generally more powerful, kava does not seem to impair mental functioning.[11,12]

The Commission E monograph recommends using kava for no more than 3 months, and accompanying its use with more curative treatments such as psychotherapy.

Warning: Various medical conditions, such as hyperthyroidism, can produce symptoms similar to anxiety. Medical evaluation is strongly recommended before self-treating with kava.

There is some evidence that kava can help **insomnia** (see page 103).[13,14] It has also been proposed as a treatment for tension headaches and as an aid to alcohol withdrawal.

WHAT IS THE SCIENTIFIC EVIDENCE FOR KAVA?

There have been five meaningful studies of kava, involving a total of about 400 participants. The best of these was a 6-month, double-blind study that tested kava's effectiveness in 100 people with various forms of anxiety.[15] Over the course of the trial, they were evaluated with a list of questions called the Hamilton Anxiety Scale (HAM-A). The HAM-A assigns a total score based on such symptoms as restlessness, nervousness, heart palpitations, stomach discomfort, dizziness, and chest pain. Lower scores indicate reduced anxiety. Participants who were given kava showed significantly improved scores beginning at 8 weeks and continuing throughout the duration of the treatment.

This study is notable for the long delay before kava was effective. Previous studies showed a good response in 1 week.[16,17,18] The reason for this discrepancy is unclear.

Besides these placebo-controlled studies, one 6-month, double-blind study compared kava against two standard anxiety drugs (oxazepam and bromazepam) in 174 people with anxiety symptoms.[19] Improvement in HAM-A scores was about the same in all groups. However, physicians who use kava state that prescription treatments are usually more powerful in real life. The HAM-A rating scale can only roughly document changes in mood and may not always be able to distinguish between excellent and modest improvement.

DOSAGE

Kava is usually sold in a standardized form where the total amount of kavalactones per pill is listed. For use as an antianxiety agent, the dose of kava should supply about 40 to 70 mg of kavalactones 3 times daily. The total daily dosage should not exceed 300 mg. People who use kava frequently report that effects begin to be obvious in a week or less, but that full benefits require 4 to 8 weeks to manifest.

The proper dosage for insomnia is 210 mg of kavalactones 1 hour before bedtime.

SAFETY ISSUES

When used appropriately, kava appears to be safe. Animal studies have shown that dosages of up to 4 times that of normal cause no problems at all, and 13 times the normal dosage causes only mild problems in rats.[20]

A study of 4,049 people who took a rather low dose of kava (70 mg of kavalactones daily) for 7 weeks found side effects in 1.5% of cases. These were mostly mild gastrointestinal complaints and allergic rashes.[21] A 4-week study of 3,029 individuals given 240 mg of kavalactones daily showed a 2.3% incidence of basically the same side effects.[22] However, long-term use (months to years) of kava in excess of 400 mg kavalactones per day can create a distinctive generalized dry, scaly rash called "kava dermopathy."[23] It disappears promptly when the kava use stops.

One case report suggests that a kava product might have caused liver inflammation in a 39-year-old woman.[24] However, because the product was not analyzed, it isn't clear whether kava itself or a contaminant was responsible; the authors also could not rule out other causes of liver inflammation.

Kava does not appear to produce mental cloudiness.[25,26] Nonetheless, we wouldn't recommend driving after using kava until you discover how strongly it affects you. It makes some people quite drowsy.

Contrary to many reports in the media, there is no evidence that kava actually improves mental function. Two studies are commonly cited as if to prove this, but actually there was only one study performed: It was described in two separate articles.[27,28] This tiny study found that kava does not impair mental function; however, it doesn't show that kava improves it. A slight improvement was seen on a couple of tests, but it was statistically insignificant (too small to mean anything).

High doses of kava are known to cause inebriation. For this reason, there is some concern that it could become an herb of abuse. There have been reports of young people trying to get high by taking products they thought contained kava. One of these products, fX, turned out to contain dangerous drugs but no kava at all. European physicians have not reported any problems with kava addiction.[29]

One study suggests that kava does not amplify the effects of alcohol.[30] However, there is a case report indicating that kava can increase the effects of other sedatives.[31] For this reason, kava should not be taken with alcohol, prescription tranquilizers or sedatives, or other depressant drugs. Kava should also not be used by individuals who have had dystonic reactions from antipsychotic drugs, or who have Parkinson's disease, due to the risk of increased problems with movement.[32]

The German Commission E monograph warns against the use of kava during pregnancy and nursing.

Safety in young children and those with severe liver or kidney disease has not been established.

TRANSITIONING FROM MEDICATIONS

If you're taking Xanax or other drugs in the benzodiazepine family, switching to kava will be very difficult. You must seek a doctor's supervision, because withdrawal symptoms can be severe and even life-threatening. Additionally, if you are taking Xanax on an "as needed" basis to stop acute panic attacks, kava cannot be expected to have the same rapidity of action.

It's easier to make the switch from milder antianxiety drugs, such as BuSpar, and antidepressants. Nonetheless, a doctor's supervision is still strongly advised.

⚠ INTERACTIONS YOU SHOULD KNOW ABOUT

If you are taking

- **Medications** for **insomnia** or **anxiety** such as **benzodiazepines:** Do not take kava in addition to them.
- **Antipsychotic drugs:** Kava might increase the risk of a particular side effect consisting of sudden abnormal movements, called a dystonic reaction.
- **Levodopa** for Parkinson's disease: Kava might reduce its effectiveness.

KELP

Supplement Forms/Alternate Names   Kombu, Brown Seaweed

Principal Proposed Uses   Vitamin and Mineral Supplement

Other Proposed Uses   Antiviral Agent, Cancer Prevention, Lowering Blood Pressure, Weight Loss

Kelp refers to several species of large, brown algae that can grow to enormous sizes far out in the depths of the ocean. Kelp is a type of seaweed, but not all seaweed is kelp: "seaweed" loosely describes any type of vegetation growing in the ocean, including many other types of algae and plants.

Kelp is a regular part of a normal human diet in many parts of the world, such as Japan, Alaska, and Hawaii. It is also incorporated into some vitamin and mineral supplements because of its nutrient value. Kelp is a good source of **folic acid** (a B vitamin; see page 288), as well as many other vitamins and minerals—especially **iodine** (see page 331); but iodine is also a potential source of side effects (see Safety Issues).

SOURCES

Supplements containing kelp can be purchased at most pharmacies and health food stores. Kelp used in food preparation is available at groceries that stock specialties for Asian cooking.

THERAPEUTIC DOSAGES

There is no appropriate "therapeutic" dosage of kelp, as it is not yet known whether kelp is truly therapeutic for any conditions. However, because of its high iodine content, it is important not to overdo your use of kelp. The iodine content in 17 different kelp supplements studied by one group of researchers varied from 45 to 57,000 mcg per tablet or capsule.[1] The recommended daily intake for iodine is 150 mcg per day for people over the age of 4, and taking a great deal more than this can cause thyroid problems (see Safety Issues).

THERAPEUTIC USES

Kelp is used primarily as a vitamin and mineral supplement.

The results of highly preliminary studies in test tubes and on animals have suggested other potential uses for kelp.

For example, there is some evidence that elements in kelp might help to prevent infection with several kinds of viruses, including **influenza** (see page 47),[2] **herpes simplex** (see page 86),[3] and **HIV** (see page 94).[4] Similarly, there is some evidence that kelp possesses anticancer effects [5–10] and may lower blood pressure.[11] But it would be premature to begin using kelp as a treatment for any of these health problems.

Additionally, kelp has been marketed as a weight-loss product, but scientific studies of its efficacy and safety for this purpose haven't been published.

Another unsubstantiated and misleading claim for kelp is that it can be used to treat all kinds of thyroid problems. It is true that if you are deficient in iodine, kelp is probably good for you, but it is unlikely to help your thyroid in any other circumstance. In fact, too much kelp can cause dysfunction of the thyroid in healthy people (see Safety Issues below).

SAFETY ISSUES

Taking excessive kelp can overload the body with iodine, and cause either hypo- or hyperthyroidism—conditions in which the thyroid gland either produces too little or too much thyroid hormone.[12–18] This is a potentially dangerous side effect, and is definitely cause for caution. Certainly, if your thyroid gland is already functioning incorrectly, you should avoid kelp except on a physician's advice.

In addition, published reports describe two cases of acne apparently caused or worsened by taking large doses of kelp.[19] This effect is also believed to be due to the large amounts of iodine in the supplement.

Finally, some kelp supplements have been found to contain levels of arsenic high enough to be toxic.[20,21] Seawater contains highly diluted arsenic, but kelp (like other ocean life) can concentrate arsenic in its tissues, and there are reports of two people with symptoms of arsenic poisoning who had been consuming kelp.

KUDZU (*Pueraria lobata*)

Principal Proposed Uses   There are no well-documented uses for kudzu.

Other Proposed Uses   Alcoholism, Cold with Pain in the Neck

Kudzu is cooked as food in China, and also is used as an herb in traditional Chinese medicine. However, in the United States, kudzu has become an invasive pest. It was deliberately planted earlier this century for use as animal fodder and to control soil erosion. It turned out to be incredibly prolific and soon spread throughout the South like an alien invader. The problem is that kudzu can grow a foot a day during the summer, and as much as 60 feet a year, giving it the folk name "mile-a-minute vine." It swallows telephone poles, chokes trees, and takes over yards. The only defense may be to find a use for it.

WHAT IS KUDZU USED FOR TODAY?

Besides cooking with it, feeding it to animals, and weaving baskets out of its rubbery vines, kudzu may also be useful in treating alcoholism. In Chinese folk medicine, a tea brewed from kudzu root is believed to be useful in "sobering up" a drunk. Taking the hint, a 1993 study evaluated the effects of kudzu in a species of hamsters known to enjoy drinking alcohol to intoxication.[1] Ordinarily, if given a choice, the Syrian golden hamster will prefer alcohol to water, but administration of kudzu reversed that preference.

This animal study led to widespread speculation that kudzu may be useful in the treatment of human alcoholism. However, a 1-month double-blind study of 38 individuals with alcoholism found no improvement in the participants given kudzu as compared to those given placebo.[2] These results significantly dimmed the excitement around using kudzu for this purpose. Perhaps it only works for hamsters.

In academic Chinese herbology (as opposed to Chinese folk medicine), kudzu is used for other purposes. One classic herbal formula containing kudzu is recommended for the treatment of **colds** (see page 47) accompanied by pain in the neck, and modern Chinese herbalists frequently use it for this purpose.

DOSAGE

The standard dosage of kudzu ranges from 0 to 15 g daily, in tea or tablets.

SAFETY ISSUES

Based on its extensive food use, kudzu is believed to be reasonably safe. However, safety in young children, pregnant or nursing women, or those with severe kidney or liver disease has not been established.

LADY'S SLIPPER ORCHID (*Cypripedium* species)

Alternate or Related Names   Nerve Root, American Valerian, Bleeding Heart, Moccasin Flower, Monkey Flower

Principal Proposed Uses   There are no well-documented uses for lady's slipper orchid.

Other Proposed Uses   Tension Relief, Muscle Relaxant, Pain Relief, Sleeping Aid

The common name "lady's slipper" refers to the distinctive shape of these beautiful orchids, members of the genus *Cypripedium* that are native to North America and Europe, as well as the *Paphiopedilum* species native to Southeast Asia. Other "slipper" orchid species are native to South America. Typically, the yellow lady's slipper *Cypripedium calceolus var. pubescens* (now called *Cypripedium parviflorum var. pubescens*) is used medicinally in Europe and North America. *Cypripedium montanum*, the rare mountain lady's slipper native to North America, is also wildcrafted (collected in the wild).

Many of the *Cypripedium* lady's slipper species are endangered and have proven very difficult to cultivate; even just collecting the flower alone may be enough to kill the plant, and transplantation from the wild is rarely successful. Alternatively, some herbalists recommend using the roots of another species called stream orchid or helleborine (*Epipactis helleborine*), which has the same purported effects, is more widespread, and is relatively easy to cultivate.[1]

Traditionally, lady's slipper root was classified as a "nervine," indicating its purported healing and calming effect on the nerves. This term, however, is no longer used in medicine today.

WHAT IS LADY'S SLIPPER ORCHID USED FOR TODAY?

Despite a complete absence of scientific evidence that it is effective, lady's slipper is sometimes used today either alone or as a component of formulas intended to produce relaxation and induce sleep.

Lady's slipper is also sometimes used topically as a poultice or plaster for muscular pain relief,[2] but again there is no evidence that it is effective.

DOSAGE

The optimum oral dosage of lady's slipper is not known. A typical recommendation for *Cyrpripedium* species is 3 to 9 g of root or 2 to 6 ml of a tincture of fresh or dried root.[3]

For muscle pain relief, a topical application of fresh or dried roots mashed into a poultice or plaster can be used.[4]

SAFETY ISSUES

The safety of any medicinal application of these orchid species has not been established. Contact with the small hairs on some species can cause skin irritation.

LAPACHO (*Tabebuia impestiginosa*)

Alternate or Related Names   Pau d'Arco, Taheebo

Principal Proposed Uses   Yeast Infection, Respiratory Infection, Bladder Infection

Other Proposed Uses   Diarrhea, Cancer?

The inner bark of the lapacho tree plays a central role in the herbal medicine of several South American indigenous peoples. They use it to treat cancer as well as a great variety of infectious diseases. There is intriguing, but far from conclusive, scientific evidence for some of these traditional uses. One of lapacho's major ingredients, lapachol, definitely possesses antitumor properties, and for a time was under active investigation as a possible chemotherapy drug. Unfortunately, when given in high enough dosages to kill cancer cells, lapachol causes numerous serious side effects. Another component, b-lapachone, continues to be investigated as an anticancer agent since it may have a better side-effect profile and acts similarly to a new class of prescription antitumor drugs.[1]

Herbalists believe that the whole herb can produce equivalent benefits with fewer side effects, but this claim has never been properly investigated.

Various ingredients in lapacho can also kill bacteria and fungi in the test tube.[2] However, it is not yet clear how well the herb works for this purpose when taken orally.

WHAT IS LAPACHO USED FOR TODAY?

Based on its traditional use and the fledgling scientific evidence, some herbalists recommend lapacho as a treatment for cancer. However, we do not endorse this usage.

There is no good evidence that lapacho is an effective cancer treatment, and cancer is clearly not a disease to trifle with! Furthermore, the mechanism by which lapacho possibly works may cause it to interfere with the action of prescription anticancer drugs. Definitely do not add it to a conventional chemotherapy regimen without consulting your physician.

Lapacho is also sometimes used to treat **candida** (see page 38) yeast infections, respiratory infections such as **colds** and **flus** (see page 47), infectious diarrhea, and **bladder infections** (see page 28).

Note: Do not count on lapacho to treat serious infections.

DOSAGE

Lapacho contains many components that don't dissolve in water, so making tea from the herb is not the best idea. It's better to take capsulized powdered bark, at a standard dosage of 300 mg 3 times daily. For the treatment of yeast and other infections, it is taken until symptoms resolve.

The inner bark of the lapacho tree is believed to be the most effective part of the plant. Unfortunately, inferior products containing only the outer bark and the wood are sometimes misrepresented as "genuine inner-bark lapacho."

SAFETY ISSUES

Full safety studies of lapacho have not been performed. When taken in normal dosages, it does not appear to cause any significant side effects.[3] However, because its constituent lapachol is somewhat toxic, the herb is not recommended for pregnant or nursing mothers. Safety in young children or those with severe liver or kidney disease has also not been established.

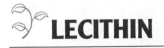

LECITHIN

Supplement Forms/Alternate Names   Egg Lecithin, Soy Lecithin, Phosphatidylcholine in Lecithin

Principal Proposed Uses   There are no well-documented uses for lecithin.

Other Proposed Uses   High Cholesterol, Liver Disease
Psychological and Neurological Disorders: Alzheimer's Disease, Bipolar Disorder, Tourette's Syndrome, Tardive Dyskinesia

---

For decades, lecithin has been a popular treatment for high cholesterol (although there is surprisingly little evidence that it works). More recently, lecithin has been proposed as a remedy for various psychological and neurological diseases, such as Tourette's syndrome, Alzheimer's disease, and bipolar disorder (also known as manic depression). Lecithin contains a substance called *phosphatidylcholine* (PC) that is presumed to be responsible for its medicinal effects. Phosphatidylcholine is a major part of the membranes surrounding our cells. However, when you consume phosphatidylcholine it is broken down into the nutrient *choline* rather than being carried directly to cell membranes. Choline acts like folate, TMG (trimethylglycine), and SAMe (S-adenosyl-methionine) to promote methylation (see the chapter on **TMG** for further discussion of this subject). It is also used to make *acetylcholine*, a nerve chemical essential for proper brain function. (For more information on the effects and possible benefits of **choline**, see the full chapter on that subject.)

SOURCES

Neither lecithin nor its ingredient phosphatidylcholine is an essential nutrient; however, choline has recently been recognized as essential. For use as a supplement or a food additive, lecithin is often manufactured from soy.

THERAPEUTIC DOSAGES

Ordinary lecithin contains about 10 to 20% phosphatidylcholine. However, European research has tended to use products concentrated to contain 90% phosphatidylcholine in lecithin, and the following dosages are based on that type of product. For psychological and neurological conditions, doses as high as 5 to 10 g taken 3 times daily have been used in studies. For liver disease, a typical dose is 350 to 500 mg taken 3 times daily; and for high cholesterol, 500 to 900 mg taken 3 times daily is common.

THERAPEUTIC USES

For a while, lecithin/phosphatidylcholine was one of the most commonly recommended natural treatments for high **cholesterol** (see page 88). This idea, however, appears to rest entirely on preliminary studies that lacked control groups.[1,2] A recent small double-blind study of 23 men with high blood cholesterol levels found that lecithin had *no* significant effects on blood levels of total cholesterol, HDL ("good") cholesterol, LDL ("bad") cholesterol, or lipoprotein(a) and triglycerides (two harmful fats found in the blood).[3]

In Europe, phosphatidylcholine is also used to treat liver diseases, such as alcoholic fatty liver, alcoholic hepatitis, **liver cirrhosis** (see page 112), and viral **hepatitis** (see page 189). While there is some evidence from animal and human studies that it may be helpful, other studies found no benefit.[4-13]

Finally, because phosphatidylcholine plays a role in nerve function, it has also been suggested as a treatment for various psychological and neurological disorders, such as **Alzheimer's disease** (see page 5), **bipolar disorder** (see page 27), Tourette's syndrome, and **tardive dyskinesia** (a late-developing side effect of drugs used for psychosis; see page 176). However, the evidence that it works is limited to small studies with somewhat conflicting results.[14-23]

Lecithin

Visit Us at TNP.com

SAFETY ISSUES

Lecithin is believed to be generally safe. However, some people taking high dosages (several grams daily) experience minor but annoying side effects, such as abdominal discomfort, diarrhea, and nausea. Maximum safe dosages for young children, pregnant or nursing women, or those with severe liver or kidney disease have not been determined.

LICORICE (Glycyrrhiza glabra)

Alternate or Related Names   Sweet Root, Sweet Wort

Principal Proposed Uses
Oral Uses (DGL form): Ulcers, Heartburn (Esophageal Reflux), Mouth Sores
Topical Uses (whole herb): Eczema, Psoriasis, Herpes
Oral Uses (whole herb): Cough, Asthma, Chronic Fatigue Syndrome

A member of the pea family, licorice root has been used since ancient times both as food and as medicine. In Chinese herbology, licorice is an ingredient in nearly all herbal formulas for the traditional purpose of "harmonizing" the separate herbs involved.

Licorice possesses a variety of active ingredients. The most analyzed is glycyrrhizin, which has been found to possess anti-inflammatory, cough-suppressant, antiviral, estrogen-like, and aldosterone-like activities.[1–7] The natural hormone aldosterone can cause fluid retention, increased blood pressure, and potassium loss. Glycyrrhizin can produce similar effects, which may cause a problem (see the discussion under Safety Issues). To avoid the aldosterone-like effects, manufacturers have found a way to remove glycyrrhizin from licorice, producing the much safer product deglycyrrhizinated licorice, or DGL. However, it is not clear that DGL provides all the same benefits as whole licorice.

WHAT IS LICORICE USED FOR TODAY?

Licorice appears to have a positive effect on the cells of the stomach, including increasing blood flow.[8,9] Licorice or DGL was once a standard European treatment for **ulcers** (see page 180).[10] Although it has been replaced by synthetic medications, there is a significant amount of evidence that DGL can be helpful. In particular, preliminary evidence suggests that DGL might help prevent ulcers caused by aspirin.[11] Licorice (primarily DGL) is also used to relieve the discomfort of **canker sores** (see page 40) and other mouth sores. Creams containing whole licorice (often combined with chamomile extract) are often used for **eczema** (see page 78), **psoriasis** (see page 148), and **herpes** (see page 86).

Whole licorice, not DGL, is used as an expectorant for respiratory problems such as coughs and **asthma** (see page 14).

Recently, licorice has been suggested as a treatment for **chronic fatigue syndrome** (CFS; see page 44), based on the observation that people with CFS appear to suffer from low levels of certain adrenal hormones. The glycyrrhizin portion of licorice may relieve symptoms by mimicking the effects of these hormones. However, this is a fairly dangerous approach to treatment that should be tried only under medical supervision.

Licorice has also been suggested as a treatment for numerous other conditions, including **hepatitis** (see page 189) and **menopausal symptoms** (see page 117), and for the prevention of **cancer** (see page 32), but there is as yet little evidence that it really works.

WHAT IS THE SCIENTIFIC EVIDENCE FOR LICORICE?

Several controlled, but not double-blind, studies suggest that regular use of DGL can heal ulcers as effectively as drugs in the Zantac family.[12,13,14] However, DGL must be taken continuously or the ulcer can be expected to return. Modern medical treatment tries to prevent the recurrence of ulcers permanently by eradicating the bacteria *Helicobacter pylori*. There is no evidence that DGL can do the same.

There is no solid evidence for the other proposed uses of licorice.

DOSAGE

For supportive treatment of ulcer pain along with conventional medical care, chew two to four 380-mg tablets of DGL before meals and at bedtime.

Sucking on these tablets can substantially relieve the discomfort of mouth sores, although some people find the taste unpleasant.

For respiratory problems, take 1 to 2 g of licorice root 3 times daily for no more than 1 week.

Licorice

For eczema, psoriasis, or herpes, apply licorice cream twice daily to the affected area.

When treating chronic fatigue syndrome, whole licorice must be taken at such a sufficiently high dosage that significant side effects are possible, and thus a physician's supervision is necessary.

SAFETY ISSUES

Due to its aldosterone-like effects, whole licorice can cause fluid retention, high blood pressure, and potassium loss when taken at dosages exceeding 3 g daily for more than 6 weeks. These effects can be especially dangerous if you take digitalis, or if you have high blood pressure, heart disease, diabetes, or kidney disease.

Licorice may also reduce testosterone levels in men.[15] For this reason, men with impotence, infertility, or decreased libido may wish to avoid this herb. Licorice may also increase both the positive and negative effects of treatment with corticosteroids, such as prednisone.[16,17,18]

DGL is believed to be safe, although extensive safety studies have not been performed. Side effects are rare.

Safety for either form of licorice in young children, pregnant or nursing women, or those with severe liver or kidney disease has not been established. According to one report, licorice possesses significant estrogenic activity and, as such, shouldn't be taken by women who have had breast cancer.[19]

⚠ INTERACTIONS YOU SHOULD KNOW ABOUT

If you are taking

- **Digitalis drugs:** Long-term use of licorice can be dangerous.
- **Thiazide** or **loop diuretics:** Use of licorice might lead to excessive potassium loss.[20]
- **Corticosteroid treatment:** Licorice could increase both its effects and its side effects. Do not take licorice internally if using corticosteroids.
- **Aspirin** or other **anti-inflammatory drugs:** Regular use of DGL might help lower the risk of ulcers.

LIGNANS

Principal Proposed Uses   There are no well-documented uses for lignans.

Other Proposed Uses   Breast Cancer Prevention, Colon Cancer Prevention, Other Cancer Prevention, Atherosclerosis Prevention, Elevated Cholesterol, Menopausal Symptoms, Kidney Disease

Lignans are naturally occurring chemicals widespread within the plant and animal kingdoms. Several lignans—with intimidating names such as secoisolariciresinol—are considered to be phytoestrogens, plant chemicals that mimic the hormone estrogen. These are especially abundant in **flaxseed** (see page 286). Bacteria in our intestines convert them into two other lignans, enterolactone and enterodiol, which also have estrogen-like effects. In this chapter, the term "lignans" refers to these two specific lignans as well as the phytoestrogen kind, but not to the wide variety of other lignans.

Lignans are being studied for possible use in cancer prevention, particularly breast cancer. Like other phytoestrogens, they hook onto the same spots on cells where estrogen attaches. If there is little estrogen in the body, after menopause for example, lignans may act like weak estrogen; but when natural estrogen is abundant in the body, lignans may instead reduce estrogen's effects by displacing it from cells. This displacement of the hormone may help prevent those cancers, such as breast cancer, that depend on estrogen to start and develop. In addition, at least one test tube study suggests that lignans may help prevent cancer in ways that are unrelated to estrogen.[1]

Very early evidence suggests that lignans may also be antioxidants, although the strength of their antioxidant activity is not yet clear.[2,3]

Besides their potential use in cancer, preliminary research suggests that lignans may have a role lowering cholesterol.[4,5] In addition, weak evidence suggests a possible role for lignans in preventing atherosclerosis,[6,7] treating menopausal symptoms,[8] and treating chronic kidney disease.[9,10]

SOURCES

The richest source of lignans is flaxseed (sometimes called linseed), containing more than 100 times the amount found in other foods![11] **Flaxseed oil** (see page

Lignans

285), however, does not contain appreciable amounts of lignans.[12] Other food sources are pumpkin seeds, whole grains, cranberries, and black or green tea.[13]

THERAPEUTIC DOSAGES

We don't yet know the dosages of flaxseed needed to prevent or treat disease. In some studies, participants took 5, 15, or even 38 g of ground flaxseed per day.

Flaxseed can be eaten raw, added to cereal, or baked into bread, muffins, pizza dough, or pancakes. Cooking flaxseed apparently does not decrease the amount of lignans absorbed by the body; however, it may damage another healthful flaxseed constituent, the essential fatty acid alpha-linolenic acid (ALA).

THERAPEUTIC USES

A number of preliminary human and animal studies suggest that lignans may be helpful in cancer treatment and prevention, particularly breast and colon cancer, as well reduction of cholesterol. In addition, highly preliminary research suggests that flaxseeds or lignans may help prevent atherosclerosis,[14,15] decrease menopausal symptoms[16] and improve kidney function in certain types of kidney disease.[17,18]

Warning: Flaxseed or other treatments for kidney disease should be taken only under a doctor's supervision, due to the serious nature of these disorders.

WHAT IS THE SCIENTIFIC EVIDENCE FOR LIGNANS?

Cancer Prevention/Treatment

The most promising use for lignans is in cancer prevention. Observational studies suggest that people who eat more lignan-containing foods have a lower incidence of breast and perhaps colon cancer;[19] however, other factors may have been responsible.

Animal studies offer support for a potential cancer-preventive or even cancer-treatment effect. Several studies showed that lignan-rich foods or lignans found in flax inhibited breast and colon cancer in animals[20,21,22] and reduced metastases from melanoma (a type of skin cancer) in mice.[23] Test tube studies found that flaxseed or one of its lignans inhibited the growth of human breast cancer cells[24] and that the lignans enterolactone and enterodiol inhibited the growth of human colon tumor cells.[25]

Although this preliminary research is promising, much more is needed before we can draw any conclusions. In many of these studies it isn't clear whether lignans are responsible for the benefit seen, as flaxseeds contain many other substances. Animal and human stud-

ies have begun to examine specific lignans, and results seem to confirm that at least some of the positive effects probably come from the lignans themselves;[26,27,28] still, until more and better designed trials are done, we will not know lignans' precise effects on the human body, or the precise dose needed to prevent cancer.

Cholesterol and Atherosclerosis

Preliminary research in rabbits and humans suggests that lignans may help protect against atherosclerosis, a condition in which fatty deposits line arteries. Lignans may directly provide such protection, or possibly indirectly by reducing the high cholesterol that is a risk factor for atherosclerosis.

Studies in rabbits found that both flaxseed and one of its lignans, secoisolariciresinol diglucoside, were able to decrease atherosclerosis;[29,30] the lignan also lowered the rabbits' cholesterol, but flaxseed by itself did not. In contrast, several human studies, two of them double-blind, found that flaxseed lowered cholesterol—both total cholesterol and low-density lipoproteins (LDL, or "bad") cholesterol.[31,32,33] However, it is entirely possible that other flaxseed components such as its fiber, oil, or proteins, rather than the lignans alone, contributed to the drop in cholesterol.[34,35] Again, more research is needed to determine whether lignans themselves play a role in reducing cholesterol and atherosclerosis.

SAFETY ISSUES

Flaxseed and its oil appear to be safe nutritional supplements when used as directed. Because of their potential effects on estrogen, however, avoid taking large amounts of either if you are pregnant or breast-feeding. One study found that pregnant rats who ate large amounts of flaxseed (5 or 10% of their diet), or a lignan present in flaxseed, gave birth to offspring with altered reproductive organs and functions, and that lignans were also transferred to the baby rats during nursing.[36] In humans, eating 25 g of flaxseed per day amounts to about 5% of the diet.[37]

There are no reports that lignans cause or worsen cancer when taken in usual amounts. However, a few sensitive test tube studies have found that cancer cells were stimulated by lignans[38]—in contrast to other studies in which lignans inhibited cancer cell growth.[39] Like estrogen, lignans' positive or negative effects on cancer cells may depend on dose, type of cancer cell, and levels of hormones in the body. If you have cancer, particularly breast cancer, talk with your doctor before consuming large amounts of flaxseed or lignans.

Finally, flaxseeds contain tiny amounts of cyanide-containing compounds, which can be a problem for livestock eating large amounts of flax.[40] Although normal cooking and baking of whole flaxseeds or flour eliminates any detectable amounts of cyanide,[41] it is at least theoretically possible that eating huge amounts of raw or unprocessed flaxseeds or flaxseed meal could pose a problem. However, most authorities are not concerned about this possibility.[42]

As with many substances, there have been reports of life-threatening allergic reactions to flaxseed.

LIPOIC ACID

Supplement Forms/Alternate Names   Alpha-Lipoic Acid, Thioctic Acid

Principal Proposed Uses   Diabetic Peripheral Neuropathy, Diabetic Autonomic Neuropathy

Other Proposed Uses   Diabetes (in General), Liver Disease, Cancer Prevention, Cataract Prevention, Heart Disease Prevention

Lipoic acid, also known as alpha-lipoic acid, is a sulfur-containing fatty acid that has recently become very popular as a dietary supplement. It is found inside every cell of the body, where it helps generate the energy that keeps us alive and functioning. Lipoic acid is a key part of the metabolic machinery that turns glucose (blood sugar) into energy for the body's needs.

Lipoic acid is an antioxidant, which means it neutralizes naturally occurring, but harmful, chemicals known as free radicals. Unlike other antioxidants, which work only in water or fatty tissues, lipoic acid is unusual in that it functions in both water and fat.[1,2] By comparison, vitamin E works only in fat and vitamin C works only in water. This gives lipoic acid an unusually broad spectrum of action.

Different antioxidants work together to keep free radicals under control (for more information, see the chapter on **vitamin E**). Antioxidants are a bit like kamikaze pilots, sacrificing themselves to knock out free radicals. One of the more interesting findings about lipoic acid is that it may help regenerate other antioxidants that have been used up. Some research also suggests that lipoic acid may do the work of other antioxidants in which the body is deficient.[3,4]

Thanks to its fat solubility, lipoic acid can get inside nerve cells, where it helps prevent free radical damage.

SOURCES

Because a healthy body makes enough lipoic acid to supply its energy requirements, there is no daily requirement for this supplement. However, several medical conditions appear to be accompanied by low levels of lipoic acid[5]—specifically, diabetes, liver cirrhosis, and heart disease—which suggests (but definitely does not prove) that supplementation would be helpful.

Liver and yeast contain some lipoic acid. Nonetheless, supplements are necessary to obtain therapeutic dosages.

THERAPEUTIC DOSAGES

The typical dosage of oral lipoic acid for treating complications of diabetes is 300 to 600 mg daily, although much higher doses have been tried in studies. Be patient, as the results take weeks to develop. For use as a general antioxidant, a lower dosage of 20 to 50 mg daily is commonly recommended.

THERAPEUTIC USES

Lipoic acid has been widely used for decades in Germany to treat diabetic peripheral neuropathy. This is a condition caused by **diabetes** (see page 65) in which nerves leading to the arms and legs become damaged, leading to numbness, pain, and other symptoms. However, the evidence that it works is largely limited to studies that used the intravenous form of this supplement.[6,7,8]

Lipoic acid has shown promise for another type of nerve damage caused by diabetes: autonomic neuropathy. This is a condition in which the nerves that control internal organs become damaged. When this occurs in the heart, the condition is called cardiac autonomic neuropathy, and it leads to irregularities of heart rhythm. There is some evidence that lipoic acid may be helpful for this condition.[9] When autonomic neuropathy occurs in the intestines, it causes extreme constipation. Based on its other effects, it appears possible that lipoic acid could help this condition as well, although there is no direct evidence to turn to.

Preliminary and sometimes contradictory evidence suggests that lipoic acid may improve other aspects of diabetes as well, including circulation in small blood vessels, metabolism of sugar and protein, and the body's response to insulin.[10–14] Lipoic acid has been proposed as a treatment for liver conditions as well as for preventing **cancer** (see page 32), **cataracts** (see page 42), and **heart disease** (see page 16). However, there is

Lipoic Acid

Visit Us at TNP.com

little to no real evidence that it is effective for these purposes.

One animal study suggests that lipoic acid might help prevent age-related hearing loss.[15]

WHAT IS THE SCIENTIFIC EVIDENCE FOR LIPOIC ACID?

Diabetic Peripheral Neuropathy

There is some evidence that intravenous lipoic acid can reduce symptoms of diabetic peripheral neuropathy, at least in the short term. Oral lipoic acid has not been well evaluated, and the best study of oral lipoic acid found it ineffective for long-term use.

A randomized, double-blind placebo-controlled study that enrolled 503 individuals with diabetic neuropathy found that intravenous lipoic acid helped reduce symptoms over a 3-week period, but long-term oral supplementation was not effective.[16]

A previous double-blind placebo-controlled study also found short-term benefit with intravenous lipoic acid.[17,18]

Warning: You should *never* attempt to take any drug or supplement intravenously except under the care of a doctor.

The positive evidence for oral lipoic acid is limited to open studies or to trials that were too small upon which to base conclusions.[19–23]

There is some preliminary evidence that lipoic acid may be more effective if it is combined with **GLA** (gamma-linolenic acid; see page 304), another supplement used for diabetic peripheral neuropathy.[24,25]

Diabetic Autonomic Neuropathy

Not only does diabetes damage the nerves in the arms and legs, but it can also affect deep nerves that control organs such as the heart and digestive tract. The DEKAN (Deutsche Kardiale Autonome Neuropathie) study followed 73 people with diabetes who had symptoms caused by nerve damage affecting the heart. Treatment with 800 mg daily of oral lipoic acid showed statistically significant improvement compared to placebo and caused no significant side effects.[26]

SAFETY ISSUES

Lipoic acid appears to have no significant side effects at dosages up to 1,800 mg daily.[27]

Safety for young children, women who are pregnant or nursing, or those with severe liver or kidney disease has not been established.

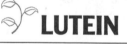

LUTEIN

Principal Proposed Uses   There are no well-documented uses for lutein.

Other Proposed Uses   Macular Degeneration, Cataracts, Atherosclerosis

Lutein, a chemical found in green vegetables, is a member of a family of substances known as *carotenoids*. Beta-carotene is the most famous nutrient in this class (for more information, see the chapter on **beta-carotene**). Like beta-carotene, lutein is an antioxidant that protects our cells against damage caused by dangerous, naturally occurring chemicals known as free radicals.

Recent evidence has found that lutein may play an important role in protecting our eyes and eyesight. It may work in two ways: by acting directly as a kind of natural sunblock, and also by neutralizing free radicals that can damage the eye.

SOURCES

Lutein is not an essential nutrient. However, it may be very important for optimal health. We're learning more all the time about nutrients like lutein that aren't re-

quired for life, but protect us in various ways. At present, an intake of about 6 mg daily of lutein is considered adequate.

Green vegetables are the best source of lutein, especially spinach, kale, collard greens, romaine lettuce, leeks, and peas. Unlike beta-carotene, lutein is *not* found in high concentrations in yellow and orange vegetables such as carrots.

THERAPEUTIC DOSAGES

We don't know how much lutein is necessary for a therapeutic effect, but estimates range from 5 to 30 mg daily.

THERAPEUTIC USES

Evidence suggests that people who eat foods containing lutein are less likely to develop **macular degeneration** (see page 115) or **cataracts** (see page 42), the two most common causes of vision loss in adults.[1–4] However, these were observational studies, in which people simply eat what they please and researchers follow them to see what illnesses they develop. Because lutein is found in vegetables that may also contain other helpful substances, we don't know for sure if it is the lutein itself that is providing the benefit. We really need studies in which some people are given pure lutein and others a placebo, but as yet they have not been performed.

However, there are reasons to believe that lutein may indeed play an important role in protecting the eyes. Lutein is the main pigment (coloring chemical) in the center of the retina, the region of maximum visual sensitivity known as the *macula*. Macular degeneration consists of injury to the macula, and leads to a severe loss in vision.

One of the main causes of macular degeneration appears to be sun damage to the sensitive tissue. Lutein appears to act as a natural eyeshade, protecting the retina against too much light.[5,6] This may explain why higher dietary intake of lutein appears to reduce the risk of this common cause of blindness in adults.

Besides protecting the macula, lutein may also shield the lens of the eye from light damage, slowing down the development of cataracts.

Furthermore, lutein fights free radicals. These chemicals can also damage the retina and the lens.

Note: Lutein may help prevent macular degeneration, but it has not been proven to treat the condition once it has developed. If you already have macular degeneration, medical supervision is essential.

Lutein might also help prevent **atherosclerosis** (see page 16).[7]

SAFETY ISSUES

Although lutein is a normal part of the diet, there has not been a formal evaluation of lutein's safety when taken as a concentrated supplement. Maximum safe dosages for young children, pregnant or nursing women, or those with severe liver or kidney disease have not been established.

LYCOPENE

Principal Proposed Uses Cancer Prevention

Other Proposed Uses Cataract Prevention, Macular Degeneration Prevention

Lycopene is a powerful antioxidant found in tomatoes, watermelon, guava, and pink grapefruit. Like the better-known supplement beta-carotene, lycopene belongs to the family of chemicals known as *carotenoids* (for more information about carotenoids, see the chapter on **beta-carotene**). As an antioxidant, it is about twice as powerful as beta-carotene.

There is some evidence that a diet high in lycopene may reduce the risk of cancer of the prostate as well as other cancers. Lycopene may also help prevent macular degeneration and cataracts.

SOURCES

Lycopene is not a necessary nutrient. However, like other substances found in fruits and vegetables, it may be very important for optimal health.

Tomatoes are the best source of lycopene. Happily, cooking doesn't destroy lycopene, so pizza sauce is just as good as a fresh tomato. In fact, some studies indicate that cooking tomatoes in oil may provide lycopene in a way that the body can use better,[1,2] although not all studies agree.[3] Lycopene is also found in watermelon, guava, and grapefruit.

THERAPEUTIC DOSAGES

The optimum dosage for lycopene has not been established. However, one study on lycopene and prostate cancer suggested that about 6.5 mg is an effective daily intake.[4]

THERAPEUTIC USES

Lycopene may help prevent **cancer** (see page 32), particularly cancer of the prostate, but also possibly cancer of the lung, colon, and breast.[5–11] However, the evidence we have for this idea comes from *observational* studies in which researchers analyze people's diets, rather than the more definitive *intervention* trials, in which people are actually given lycopene supplements. In observational trials, it is always possible that other unrecognized factors are at work.

Weak evidence also suggests that lycopene can reduce the risk of **cataracts** (see page 42) and **macular degeneration** (see page 115).[12]

Lycopene

Visit Us at TNP.com

WHAT IS THE SCIENTIFIC EVIDENCE FOR LYCOPENE?

Cancer Prevention

Although there are no double-blind studies on lycopene, the results of observational studies are impressive.

One study followed 47,894 men for 4 years.[13] Subjects who ate large amounts of tomatoes or tomato sauce (including that on pizza) had lower rates of prostate cancer. In an evaluation that compared these foods to others that were studied, lycopene appeared to be the common denominator.[14]

Some evidence suggests that lycopene may also help prevent lung, colon, and breast cancer as well.[15] In one study, elderly Americans who ate a diet high in tomatoes had 50% fewer cancers overall than those who did not.[16]

Animal studies have also found some cancer-preventative benefits with lycopene.[17,18]

However, other observational studies have not found lycopene to be the key cancer-fighting ingredient in fruits and vegetables.[19,20] What we really need are large double-blind studies in which people are given either pure lycopene supplements or placebo treatment. Unfortunately, none have yet been performed.

SAFETY ISSUES

Although lycopene is a normal part of the diet, there has not been a formal evaluation of lycopene's safety when it is taken as a concentrated supplement. Maximum safe dosages for young children, pregnant or nursing women, or those with severe liver or kidney disease have not been established.

LYSINE

Supplement Forms/Alternate Names   L-Lysine, Lysine Hydrochloride

Principal Proposed Uses   Herpes Simplex (Cold Sores, Genital Herpes)

Lysine is an essential amino acid, one that you need to get from food. Evidence suggests that supplemental lysine may be able to help prevent herpes infections (cold sores and genital herpes), especially when combined with certain dietary changes.

REQUIREMENTS/SOURCES

Most people need about 1 g of lysine per day. The requirement may be greater for athletes and people recovering from major injuries, especially burns. The richest sources of lysine are animal proteins such as meat and poultry, but it is also found in dairy products, eggs, and beans.

THERAPEUTIC DOSAGES

A typical therapeutic dosage of lysine for herpes is 1 g 3 times daily. You can take this as a regular part of your diet in hopes of preventing herpes flare-ups, or, perhaps, at the first sign of an attack. For best results, you should probably restrict your intake of foods that contain a lot of arginine (see Therapeutic Uses).

THERAPEUTIC USES

Some small studies suggest that regular use of lysine supplements can reduce the number of **herpes** (see page 86) flare-ups, although other studies have not found the same benefit.[1–6] Lysine has also been proposed as a treatment to take at the onset of a herpes attack, but at least one study has found it to be ineffective for this purpose.[7]

Both cold sores and genital herpes are caused by a virus called *herpes simplex*. After you are first infected, this virus hides in certain nerve cells, and reemerges under times of **stress** (see page 167). Test-tube research suggests that lysine fights this virus by blocking arginine, an amino acid the virus needs in order to replicate.[8]

For this reason, lysine may be most effective when used in conjunction with a low-arginine diet. Foods that you should avoid include chocolate, peanuts and other nuts, seeds, and, to a lesser extent, wheat. (See the chapter on **arginine** for more information about this amino acid.)

WHAT IS THE SCIENTIFIC EVIDENCE FOR LYSINE?

Herpes Simplex

Although the evidence is preliminary and somewhat contradictory, on balance it appears that regular use of lysine supplements might be able to reduce the number and intensity of herpes flare-ups.[9] However, a study evaluating lysine taken only at the onset of a herpes attack found no benefit.[10] (Consider using **melissa** for this latter purpose; see page 359.)

Lysine

One double-blind placebo-controlled study followed 52 participants with a history of herpes flare-ups.[11] While receiving 3 g of L-lysine every day for 6 months, the treatment group experienced an average of 2.4 fewer herpes flare-ups than the placebo group—a significant difference. The lysine group's flare-ups were also significantly less severe and healed faster.

Another double-blind placebo-controlled study on 41 subjects also found improvements in the frequency of attacks.[12] Interestingly, this study found that 1,250 mg of lysine daily worked, but 624 mg did not.

However, other studies, including one that enrolled 79 individuals, found no benefit.[13,14]

Although some are promising, none of these studies are large enough to give conclusive answers. At this point, more evidence is needed to determine whether lysine is an effective treatment for herpes simplex.

SAFETY ISSUES

Although lysine is an essential part of the diet, the safety of concentrated lysine supplements has not been well studied. In animal studies, high dosages have caused gallstones and elevated cholesterol levels,[15,16] so you may want to use caution when using lysine if you have either of these problems. Maximum safe dosages for young children, pregnant or nursing women, or those with severe liver or kidney disease have not been established.

⚠ INTERACTIONS YOU SHOULD KNOW ABOUT

If you are taking lysine to treat herpes, **arginine** might counteract the potential benefit.[17]

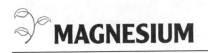

MAGNESIUM

Supplement Forms/Alternate Names   Magnesium Sulfate, Magnesium Gluconate, Magnesium Fumarate, Magnesium Citrate, Magnesium Malate, Magnesium Oxide, Magnesium Chloride

Principal Proposed Uses   Migraine Headaches, Noise-Related Hearing Loss, Kidney Stones, Hypertension (High Blood Pressure)

Other Proposed Uses   Atherosclerosis, Restless Legs Syndrome, PMS, Painful Menstruation (Dysmenorrhea), Diabetes, Osteoporosis, Low Blood Sugar, Glaucoma, Fibromyalgia, Fatigue, Low HDL ("Good") Cholesterol, Stroke, Autism
   Various Forms of Heart Disease: Mitral Valve Prolapse, Congestive Heart Failure
   Asthma

Magnesium is an essential nutrient mineral, meaning that your body needs it for healthy functioning. It is found in significant quantities throughout the body and used for numerous purposes, including muscle relaxation, blood clotting, and the manufacture of ATP (adenosine triphosphate, the body's main energy molecule).

It has been called "nature's calcium channel-blocker." The idea refers to magnesium's ability to block calcium from entering muscle and heart cells. A group of prescription heart medications work in a similar way, although much more powerfully. This may be the basis for magnesium's effects on migraine headaches and high blood pressure.

Magnesium is one of the few essential nutrients for which deficiencies are fairly common. For this reason, it is probably reasonable for most people to take magnesium on general principle, regardless of particular therapeutic use.

REQUIREMENTS/SOURCES

Requirements for magnesium increase as we grow and age. The official U.S. and Canadian recommendations for daily intake are as follows:

- Infants 0–6 months, 30 mg
   7–12 months, 75 mg
- Children 1–3 years, 80 mg
   4–8 years, 130 mg
- Males 9–13 years, 240 mg
   14–18 years, 410 mg
   19–30 years, 400 mg
   31 years and older, 420 mg
- Females 9–13 years, 240 mg
   14–18 years, 360 mg
   19–30 years, 310 mg
   31 years and older, 320 mg
- Pregnant women 18 years and younger, 400 mg
   19–30 years, 350 mg
   31–50 years, 360 mg

Magnesium

Visit Us at TNP.com

- Nursing women 18 years and younger, 360 mg
  19–30 years, 310 mg
  31–50 years, 320 mg

In the United States, the average dietary intake of magnesium is significantly lower than it should be.[1,2] Alcohol, surgery, diabetes, certain types of diuretics ("water pills"), estrogen and oral contraceptives, and zinc have been reported to reduce your body's level of magnesium or increase magnesium requirements.[3,4,5] If you are taking **potassium** (see page 390) or **manganese** (see page 354), you may need extra magnesium as well.[6,7]

While it is sometimes said that **calcium** (see page 234) interferes with magnesium absorption, it apparently has no significant effect on overall magnesium status.[8,9]

Estrogen (as in estrogen-replacement therapy and oral contraceptives) may decrease blood levels of magnesium by causing the mineral to move into body tissues and bone. For this reason, individuals who don't get enough dietary magnesium may need to take a magnesium supplement.

Kelp (see page 340) is very high in magnesium, as are wheat bran, wheat germ, almonds, and cashews. Other good sources include blackstrap molasses, brewer's yeast (not to be confused with nutritional yeast), buckwheat, and nuts and whole grains. You can also get appreciable amounts of magnesium from collard greens, dandelion greens, avocado, sweet corn, Cheddar cheese, sunflower seeds, shrimp, dried fruit (figs, apricots, and prunes), and many other common fruits and vegetables.

THERAPEUTIC DOSAGES

A typical supplemental dosage of magnesium ranges from the nutritional needs described above to as high as 600 mg daily. For premenstrual syndrome (PMS) and dysmenorrhea (painful menstruation), an alternative approach is to start taking 500 to 1,000 mg daily, beginning on day 15 of the menstrual cycle and continuing until menstruation begins.

Magnesium may interfere with the absorption of various other minerals. For this reason it's suggested that those taking magnesium should also take a multimineral supplement.

THERAPEUTIC USES

Several preliminary studies suggest that regular use of magnesium can help prevent **migraine headaches** (see page 120).[10,11,12]

Magnesium may also be useful for protecting the ears against hearing loss caused by exposure to loud noises,[13] reducing the incidence of **kidney stones** (see page 109),[14] and perhaps reducing **hypertension** (see page 98).[15,16,17] There is also some evidence that

magnesium may decrease the **atherosclerosis** (see page 16) risk caused by hydrogenated oils, margarine-like fats found in many "junk" foods.[18]

Preliminary double-blind trials suggest that magnesium may be useful for **dysmenorrhea** (menstrual cramps; see page 70)[19,20] and symptoms of **PMS** (premenstrual syndrome; see page 145), including menstrual migraines.[21,22] Open trials suggest that magnesium might decrease symptoms of **restless legs syndrome** (see page 150).[23,24] Although there is no direct evidence that magnesium helps people with **diabetes** (see page 65), such individuals are known to be deficient in magnesium,[25,26,27] and magnesium supplementation may be a good idea on general principle. (However, individuals with severe kidney disease should take magnesium supplements only on their physician's advice.)

Magnesium has also been suggested as a treatment for **osteoporosis** (see page 136), low blood sugar, glaucoma, **fibromyalgia** (see page 80), fatigue, stroke, low HDL ("good") cholesterol, **Alzheimer's disease** (see page 5), **angina** (see page 10), **attention deficit disorder** (see page 22), **periodontal disease** (see page 142), **rheumatoid arthritis** (see page 151), and various forms of heart disease including mitral valve prolapse and **congestive heart failure** (see page 54). However, there is little to no real evidence that it is effective for these purposes.

An interesting series of studies suggests (but certainly doesn't prove) that the combination of vitamin B_6 and magnesium can be helpful in **autism** (see page 23).[28–38]

Alternative medicine literature frequently mentions magnesium as a treatment for **asthma** (see page 14). However, this idea seems to be based entirely on the outdated practice of using intravenous magnesium as an emergency treatment for asthma. When you take something by mouth, it's a very different matter from having it injected into your veins. There is no real evidence that oral magnesium helps asthma, and even some evidence that it does not help.[39]

Warning: Do not self-inject magnesium! See your doctor for such treatment.

Finally, magnesium supplements have been suggested for reducing complications of pregnancy such as preeclampsia, but the results of large double-blind trials have been mixed.[40,41] It may be that magnesium is only helpful for this purpose in populations with particularly significant magnesium deficiency.

WHAT IS THE SCIENTIFIC EVIDENCE FOR MAGNESIUM?

Migraine Headaches

A recent double-blind study found that regular use of magnesium helps prevent migraine headaches. In this 12-week trial, 81 people with recurrent migraines were given either 600 mg of magnesium daily or placebo.[42] By the last 3 weeks of the study, the treated group's migraines had been reduced by 41.6%, compared to a reduction of 15.8% in the placebo group. The only side effects observed were diarrhea (in about one-fifth of the participants) and, less often, digestive irritation.

Similar results have been seen in other smaller double-blind studies.[43,44] One study found no benefit,[45] but it has been criticized on many significant points, including using an excessively strict definition of what constituted benefit.[46]

Noise-Related Hearing Loss

One double-blind placebo-controlled study on 300 military recruits suggests that 167 mg of magnesium daily can prevent hearing loss due to exposure to high-volume noise.[47]

Kidney Stones

Magnesium inhibits the growth of calcium oxalate stones in the test tube[48] and decreases stone formation in rats.[49] However, human studies have had mixed results. In one 2-year open study, 56 people taking magnesium hydroxide had fewer recurrences of kidney stones than 34 people not given magnesium.[50] In contrast, a double-blind (and, hence, more reliable) study of 124 individuals found that magnesium hydroxide was essentially no more effective than placebo.[51]

Hypertension (High Blood Pressure)

Magnesium works with calcium and potassium to regulate blood pressure. Several studies suggest that magnesium supplements can reduce blood pressure in people with hypertension,[52–55] although some have not.

Dysmenorrhea

A 6-month double-blind placebo-controlled study of 50 women with menstrual pain found that treatment with magnesium significantly improved symptoms.[56] The researchers reported evidence of reduced levels of prostaglandin F_2 alpha, a hormone-like substance involved in pain and inflammation.

Similarly positive results were seen in a double-blind placebo-controlled study of 21 women.[57]

PMS Symptoms

A double-blind placebo-controlled study of 32 women found that magnesium taken from day 15 of the menstrual cycle to the onset of menstrual flow could significantly improve premenstrual mood changes.[58]

Another small double-blind study (20 participants) found that magnesium supplementation can help prevent menstrual migraines.[59]

Preliminary evidence suggests that the combination of magnesium and **vitamin B_6** (see page 439) might be more effective than either treatment alone.[60]

Autism

Six double-blind placebo-controlled trials enrolling a total of about 150 children have evaluated the effects of vitamin B_6 and magnesium combination therapy for autism.[61–66] All of these studies found a significant improvement in autistic behaviors. However, the study design used in many of these trials was rather complicated and difficult to evaluate. For example, the largest trial (actually, a series of four closely intertwined trials) involved multiple groups of participants taking different treatments with inadequate time in between for the vitamins and minerals to wash out.[67] These studies were marked by other flaws as well; in addition, they were all performed by one research group.

For these reasons, until better-designed trials reported by independent laboratories are published, this therapy cannot be considered proven.

SAFETY ISSUES

In general, magnesium appears to be quite safe when taken at recommended dosages. The most common complaint is loose stools. However, people with severe kidney or heart disease should not take magnesium (or any other supplement) except on the advice of a physician. Maximum safe dosages have not been established for young children or women who are pregnant or nursing. There has been one case of death caused by excessive use of magnesium supplements in a developmentally and physically disabled child.[68]

Magnesium can interfere with the absorption of antibiotics in the tetracycline family.[69] Also, when combined with oral diabetes drugs in the sulfonylurea family (Tolinase, Micronase, Orinase, Glucotrol, Diabinese, DiaBeta), magnesium may cause blood sugar levels to fall more than expected.[70]

⚠ INTERACTIONS YOU SHOULD KNOW ABOUT

If you are taking

- **Potassium supplements, manganese, loop** and **thiazide diuretics, oral contraceptives, estrogen-replacement therapy:** You may need extra magnesium.
- **ACE inhibitors**, antibiotics in the **tetracycline** or **quinolone** (e.g., **Cipro**) families, **Dilantin (phenytoin), H_2 blockers** (e.g., **Zantac** or **Pepcid**), **Macrodantin,** or **zinc:** You should separate your magnesium dose from doses of these substances by at least 2 hours to avoid absorption problems.

- **Digoxin:** You may need extra magnesium, but magnesium can impair the absorption of digoxin. The solution: take them at least 2 hours apart.

- **Oral diabetes medications** in the sulfonylurea family: Work closely with your physician when taking magnesium to avoid hypoglycemia.
- **Amiloride:** Do not take magnesium supplements except on medical advice.[71]

MAITAKE (*Grifola frondose*)

Principal Proposed Uses   Adaptogen (Improve Resistance to Stress), Strengthen Immunity

Other Proposed Uses   Diabetes, Hypertension (High Blood Pressure), High Cholesterol

Maitake is a medicinal mushroom used in Japan as a general promoter of robust health. Like the similarly described reishi fungus (see the chapter on **reishi**), innumerable healing powers have been attributed to maitake, ranging from curing cancer to preventing heart disease. Unfortunately, there hasn't been enough reliable research yet to determine whether any of these ancient beliefs are really true.

ways, and one in particular, beta-D-glucan, has been studied for its potential benefit in treating cancer and AIDS.[1,2] Highly preliminary studies also suggest that maitake may be useful in treating **diabetes** (see page 65), **hypertension** (high blood pressure; see page 98), and high **cholesterol** (see page 88).[3,4] However, there is no real evidence as yet that maitake is effective for these or any other illnesses.

WHAT IS MAITAKE USED FOR TODAY?

Contemporary herbalists classify maitake as an adaptogen, a substance said to help the body adapt to **stress** (see page 167) and resist infection (see the chapter on **ginseng** for further explanation about adaptogens). However, as for other adaptogens, we lack definitive scientific evidence to show us that maitake really functions in this way.

Most investigation has focused on the polysaccharide constituents of maitake. This family of substances is known to affect the human immune system in complex

DOSAGE

Maitake is an edible mushroom that can be eaten as food or made into tea. A typical dosage of dried maitake in capsule or tablet form is 3 to 7 g daily.

SAFETY ISSUES

Maitake is widely believed to be safe, although formal safety studies have not been performed. Safety in young children, pregnant or nursing women, or those with severe liver or kidney disease has not been established.

MANGANESE

Supplement Forms/Alternate Names   Manganese Sulfate, Manganese Chloride, Manganese Picolinate, Manganese Gluconate

Principal Proposed Uses   Osteoporosis, Dysmenorrhea (Menstrual Pain)

Other Proposed Uses   Muscle Sprains/Strains, Rheumatoid Arthritis, Tardive Dyskinesia, Epilepsy, Diabetes

Our bodies contain only a very small amount of manganese, but this metal is important as a constituent of many key enzymes. The chemical structure of these enzymes is interesting: large protein molecules cluster around a tiny atom of metal.

Manganese plays a particularly important role as part of the natural antioxidant enzyme superoxide dismutase (SOD), which helps fight damaging free radicals. It also

helps energy metabolism, thyroid function, blood sugar control, and normal skeletal growth.

REQUIREMENTS/SOURCES

Manganese is thought to be an essential nutrient, but the precise daily requirement isn't known. The following daily amounts are considered safe and adequate:

- Infants 0–6 months, 0.3–0.6 mg
    7–12 months, 0.6–1 mg
- Children 1–3 years, 1–1.5 mg
    4–6 years, 1.5–2.0 mg
    7–10 years, 2.0–3.0 mg
- Adults (and children 11 years and older),
    2–5 mg

Antacids as well as calcium, iron, copper, magnesium, and zinc supplements can reduce the body's absorption of manganese.[1,2,3] The best sources of dietary manganese are whole grains, legumes, avocados, grape juice, chocolate, seaweed, egg yolks, nuts, seeds, boysenberries, blueberries, pineapples, spinach, collard greens, peas, and green vegetables.

THERAPEUTIC DOSAGES

A typical dosage used in studies on manganese is 3 to 6 mg daily. It is sometimes recommended at a much higher dose of 50 to 200 mg daily for 2 weeks following a muscle sprain or strain, but the safety of this dosage is not known.

THERAPEUTIC USES

Because manganese plays a role in bone metabolism, it has been suggested as a treatment for **osteoporosis** (see page 136), a condition in which bone mass deteriorates with age.[4] However, we have no direct evidence that manganese is helpful, except in combination with other minerals.

Manganese has also been suggested for **dysmenorrhea** (painful menstruation; see page 70),[5] muscle strains and sprains, **rheumatoid arthritis** (see page 151), and **tardive dyskinesia** (see page 176),[6] but the evidence that it works is very weak.

People with epilepsy have lower-than-normal levels of manganese in their blood.[7] This suggests (but doesn't prove) that manganese supplements might be helpful for epilepsy. Unfortunately, the studies that could prove or disprove this idea haven't been performed. A similar situation exists regarding **diabetes** (see page 65), where manganese deficiencies have been noted, but no trials

that used manganese supplements have been reported.[8,9]

WHAT IS THE SCIENTIFIC EVIDENCE FOR MANGANESE?

Osteoporosis

Although manganese is known to play a role in bone metabolism, there is no direct evidence that manganese supplements can help prevent osteoporosis. However, one double-blind placebo-controlled study suggests that a combination of minerals including manganese may be helpful.[10] Fifty-nine women took either placebo, calcium (1,000 mg daily), or calcium plus a daily mineral supplement consisting of 5 mg of manganese, 15 mg of zinc, and 2.5 mg of copper. After 2 years, the group receiving calcium plus minerals showed better bone density than the group receiving calcium alone. But this study doesn't tell us whether it was the manganese or the other minerals that made the difference.

Dysmenorrhea (Menstrual Pain)

One very small double-blind study suggested that 5.6 mg of manganese daily might ease menstrual discomfort.[11] In the same study, a lower dosage of 1 mg daily *wasn't* effective.

SAFETY ISSUES

Manganese appears to be safe when taken at the usual recommended dosage of 6 mg or less daily. However, the safety of higher doses is not known. Very high exposure to manganese (due either to environmental pollution or manganese mining) has resulted in a serious psychiatric disorder known as "manganese madness."

⚠ INTERACTIONS YOU SHOULD KNOW ABOUT

If you are taking

- **Iron, copper, zinc, magnesium,** or **calcium:** You may need extra manganese, and vice versa.
- **Antacids:** You may also need extra manganese.

MARSHMALLOW (*Althaea officinalis*)

Alternate or Related Names   Moorish Mallow, Cheeses, White Maoow, Althea, Mortification Root, Others
Principal Proposed Uses   Cough, Colds, Asthma, Sore Throat, Crohn's Disease, Ulcers, Diarrhea, Skin Inflammation

Marshmallow

Visit Us at TNP.com

The similarity in name between the herb marshmallow and the sweet treat is more than a coincidence, although the modern sugar puff ball no longer bears much relationship to the old-fashioned candy flavored with marshmallow herb.

Besides inspiring makers of campfire food, the marshmallow has also been used medicinally since ancient Greece. Hippocrates spoke of it as a treatment for bruises and blood loss, and subsequent Roman physicians recommended marshmallow for toothaches, insect bites, chilblains, and irritated skin. In medieval Europe, herbalists used marshmallow to soothe toothaches, coughs, sore throats, chapped skin, indigestion, and diarrhea.

WHAT IS MARSHMALLOW USED FOR TODAY?

Modern herbalists recommend marshmallow primarily for relieving digestive and respiratory problems, such as coughs, **colds** (see page 47), and **asthma** (see page 14). The herb contains very high levels of large sugar molecules called mucilage, which appear to exert a soothing effect on mucous membranes. While marshmallow is more a symptomatic treatment than a cure, its ability to soothe a raw throat can be very welcome. It is also some-

times recommended for **Crohn's disease** (see page 57) or **ulcers** (see page 180) to reduce discomfort. No double-blind studies have been reported at this time.

DOSAGE

Marshmallow can be made into a soothing tea by steeping roots overnight in water and diluting to taste. This tea can be drunk as desired for symptomatic relief. Alternatively, you can take marshmallow in capsules (5 to 6 g daily) or in tincture according to label directions.

Marshmallow ointments can be applied directly to soothe inflamed or irritated skin.

SAFETY ISSUES

Marshmallow is believed to be entirely safe. It is approved for use in foods, and its chemical makeup does not suggest any but benign effects.[1] However, detailed safety studies have not been performed. One study suggests that marshmallow can slightly lower blood sugar levels.[2] For this reason, people with diabetes should use caution when taking marshmallow. Safety in young children, pregnant or nursing women, or those with severe liver or kidney disease has not been established.

MEDIUM-CHAIN TRIGLYCERIDES (MCTS)

Principal Proposed Uses   Difficulty Digesting Fat (Especially in AIDS), Performance Enhancement

Other Proposed Uses   Weight Loss, Epilepsy

Medium-chain triglycerides (MCTs) are fats with an unusual chemical structure that allows the body to digest them easily. Most fats are broken down in the intestine and remade into a special form that can be transported in the blood. But MCTs are absorbed intact and taken to the liver, where they are used directly for energy. In this sense, they are processed very similarly to carbohydrates.

MCTs are different enough from other fats that they can be used as fat substitutes by people (especially those with AIDS) who need calories but are unable to absorb or metabolize normal fats.

MCTs are also popular among athletes as a proposed performance enhancer, although there is little evidence as yet that they really work.

SOURCES

There is no dietary requirement for MCTs. Coconut oil, palm oil, and butter contain up to 15% MCTs (plus a lot

of other fats). You can also buy MCTs as purified supplements.

THERAPEUTIC DOSAGES

MCTs can be eaten as salad oil or used in cooking. When taken as an athletic supplement, dosages in the neighborhood of 85 mg daily are common.

THERAPEUTIC USES

Preliminary evidence suggests that MCTs are a useful fat substitute for those who have trouble digesting fat. This includes people with serious diseases such as HIV or AIDS who need to find a way to gain weight.[1,2] It might also be helpful for those who have trouble digesting fatty foods because they lack the proper enzymes (pancreatic insufficiency).[3]

MCTs are also popular among athletes as a concentrated source of easily utilized energy.[4,5,6]

More controversially, MCTs have been used to promote ketosis, a fat-burning state that can cause weight loss,[7] and also improve certain symptoms of epilepsy. In ketosis, the body burns its stored fat for energy. It ordinarily occurs in starvation, but it can be produced on purpose by eating few or no carbohydrates and consuming protein and fat instead. However, intentional ketosis has potential health risks and it is controversial.

WHAT IS THE SCIENTIFIC EVIDENCE FOR MEDIUM-CHAIN TRIGLYCERIDES (MCTS)?

Fat Malabsorption

A double-blind placebo-controlled study on 24 men and women with AIDS suggests that MCTs can help improve AIDS-related fat malabsorption.[8] In this disorder, fat is not digested; it passes unchanged through the intestines, and the body is deprived of calories as well as fat-soluble vitamins.

The study subjects were split into two groups: One received a liquid diet containing normal fats, whereas the other group received mostly MCTs. After 12 days, the participants on the MCT formula showed significantly less fat in their stool and better fat absorption than the other group.

Another double-blind study found similar results in 24 men with AIDS-related fat malabsorption.[9]

The body depends on enzymes from the pancreas to digest fat. In one study, individuals with inadequate pancreatic function due to chronic pancreatitis appeared to be better able to absorb MCTs than ordinary fatty acids.[10] However, this didn't turn out to mean much on a practical basis, because without taking extra digestive enzymes they could only just barely absorb the MCTs; whereas, if they took digestive enzymes, they absorbed ordinary fats as well as MCTs without difficulty.

Athletic Performance

MCTs have been proposed as an "ergogenic aid," an energy-boosting supplement to enhance **athletic performance** (see page 158). During intense exercise, your body first burns up available energy from the blood (in the form of glucose) and then starts to use energy stored in the form of a larger carbohydrate called *glycogen*. When the glycogen is depleted, exhaustion begins to set in.

One solution to this is *carbo-loading*, the practice of taking large doses of carbohydrates prior to exercise in order to increase glycogen stores. Athletes can also sip carbohydrate-loaded drinks during exercise.

MCTs may provide an alternative. Like other fats, they provide more energy per ounce than carbohydrates; but unlike normal fats, this energy can be released rapidly.[11]

A very small study compared MCTs and carbohydrates as performance boosters for 6 trained cyclists. The athletes took a 4.3% MCT beverage, a 10% carbohydrate beverage, or a drink containing both 4.3% MCTs and 10% carbohydrate.[12] Researchers found a slight advantage to the combination drink. Another study on 12 cyclists also suggested that MCTs plus carbohydrates enhanced performance.[13] However, a recent small study found no benefit with MCTs, and the researchers felt that there was some impairment of performance due to a sensation of bloating.[14] Larger studies are necessary to discover whether MCTs are really as useful for athletes as some of its proponents claim.

SAFETY ISSUES

Studies in animals and humans tell us that MCTs are quite safe when consumed at a level of up to 50% of total dietary fat.[15] However, some people who consume MCTs, especially on an empty stomach, experience annoying (but not severe) abdominal cramps and bloating.

The maximum safe dosage of MCTs in young children, pregnant or nursing women, or people with serious kidney or liver disease has not been established.

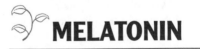

MELATONIN

Principal Proposed Uses
   Sleep Disorders: Insomnia, Jet Lag

Other Proposed Uses   Cancer (As an Addition to Conventional Therapy), Strengthening the Immune System, Preventing Heart Disease, Fighting Aging, Reducing Anxiety Before Surgery, Epilepsy in Children

Melatonin is a natural hormone that regulates sleep. During daylight, the pineal gland in the brain produces an important neurotransmitter called *serotonin*. (A neurotransmitter is a chemical that relays messages between nerve cells.) But at night, the pineal gland stops producing serotonin and instead makes melatonin. This melatonin release helps trigger sleep.

Melatonin

Visit Us at TNP.com

The production of melatonin varies according to the amount of light you're exposed to; for example, your body produces more melatonin in a completely dark room than in a dimly lit one.

Melatonin hit the news in 1995. Not only was it recommended as a treatment for insomnia and jet lag, but for various theoretical reasons it was also described as a "wonder hormone" that could fight cancer, boost the immune system, prevent heart disease, and generally make you live longer. But all we really know is that it helps people whose natural sleep cycle has been disturbed, such as travelers suffering from jet lag and night-shift workers.

Contrary to earlier reports, it does not appear that melatonin levels naturally decline with age.[1]

SOURCES

Melatonin is not a nutrient. However, travelers and workers on rotating or late shifts can experience sleep disturbances that seem to be caused by changing melatonin levels.

You can boost your melatonin production naturally by getting thicker blinds for the bedroom windows or wearing a night mask. You can also take melatonin tablets.

THERAPEUTIC DOSAGES

Melatonin is typically taken half an hour before bedtime for the first 4 days after traveling; however, the optimum dose is not clear.

Melatonin is available in two forms: quick-release and slow-release. There is some debate as to which one is better.

THERAPEUTIC USES

Reasonably good evidence tells us that melatonin can help people with jet lag or other similar sleep disturbances adjust to a new schedule,[2–6] although there have been negative studies as well.[7] Melatonin may also be helpful for shift workers[8,9] and those with general insomnia.[10–15]

Melatonin may also help individuals who have been using conventional sleeping pills and wish to quit.[16]

A recent preliminary study suggests that melatonin may be useful for epilepsy in children.[17]

Highly preliminary evidence suggests that melatonin may be useful for some forms of cancer when combined with conventional anticancer treatment.[18–21] The explanation for this possible effect is unknown, and it may not be true for certain forms of chemotherapy. It is strongly recommended that you consult with your oncologist if you wish to take melatonin during chemotherapy.

Based on fairly theoretical findings, it has been suggested that melatonin can boost the immune system, prevent heart disease, and help you live longer.[22–25]

One double-blind study found that melatonin was useful for reducing **anxiety** (see page 11) prior to surgery.[26]

WHAT IS THE SCIENTIFIC EVIDENCE FOR MELATONIN?

Sleep Disorders

There is good evidence that melatonin can help you fall asleep when your bedtime rhythm has been disturbed. For example, one double-blind placebo-controlled study enrolled 320 people and followed them for 4 days after plane travel. The participants were divided into four groups and given a daily dose of 5 mg of standard melatonin, 5 mg of slow-release melatonin, 0.5 mg of standard melatonin, or placebo.[27] The group that received 5 mg of standard melatonin slept better, took less time to fall asleep, and felt more energetic and awake during the day than the other three groups.

According to one review of the literature, melatonin treatment for jet lag is most effective for those who have crossed a significant number of time zones, perhaps eight.[28] One study on travelers found *no* benefit, but it may be that the change in time zones experienced by these travelers wasn't great enough to require melatonin.[29]

Good results were seen in a small double-blind trial of patients in a pulmonary intensive care unit.[30] It is famously difficult to sleep in an ICU, and the resulting sleep deprivation is not helpful for those recovering from disease or surgery. In this study of 8 hospitalized individuals, 3 mg of controlled-release melatonin "dramatically improved" sleep quality and duration.

A study of 19 individuals with schizophrenia who had disturbed sleep patterns found that 2 mg of controlled-release melatonin improved sleep.[31]

Mixed results have been seen in other studies involving night-shift workers and people with ordinary insomnia.[32–43]

Melatonin might be particularly helpful for individuals who rely on benzodiazepine drugs to sleep.[44] In addition, individuals trying to quit using sleeping pills may find melatonin helpful. A double-blind placebo-controlled study of 34 individuals who regularly used such medications found that melatonin at a dose of 2 mg nightly (controlled-release formulation) could help them discontinue the use of the drugs.[45]

Note: There can be risks in discontinuing benzodiazepine drugs. Consult your physician for advice.

Anxiety Prior to Surgery

Relaxing sedative medications are often used prior to surgery to help reduce the anxiety while waiting for surgery to begin. A double-blind placebo-controlled study of 75 women waiting for surgery compared melatonin against the standard drug midazolam.[46] Although midazolam was more effective, melatonin was definitely superior to placebo, and patients appeared to like each one equally. One advantage of melatonin was that it did not cause amnesia.

Cancer

Melatonin has been used with conventional anticancer therapy in more than a dozen clinical studies. Results have been surprisingly good, although this research must be considered preliminary. For example, a double-blind study on 30 people with advanced brain tumors suggested that melatonin might prolong life and also improve the quality of life.[47] Participants received standard radiation treatment with or without 20 mg daily of melatonin. After 1 year, 6 of 14 individuals in the melatonin group were still alive, compared with just 1 of 16 from the control group. The melatonin group also had fewer side effects due to the radiation treatment—a notable improvement in their quality of life.

Improvements in symptoms and a possible reduction of mortality were also seen in other studies.[48,49] Melatonin appears to work by increasing levels of the body's own tumor-fighting proteins, known as *cytokines*.[50]

SAFETY ISSUES

Melatonin is probably safe for occasional use, but its safety when used on a regular basis remains unknown. Keep in mind that melatonin is not truly a food supplement but a hormone.

As we know from other hormones used in medicine, such as estrogen and cortisone, harmful effects can take years to appear. Hormones are powerful substances that have many subtle effects in the body, and we're far from understanding them fully.

Because melatonin promotes sleep, you should not drive or operate machinery for several hours after taking it. In addition, melatonin may impair balance.[51] Also, based on theoretical ideas of how melatonin works, some authorities specifically recommend against using it in people with depression, schizophrenia, autoimmune diseases, and other serious illnesses. Maximum safe dosages for young children, pregnant or nursing women, or those with serious liver or kidney disease have not been established.

MELISSA (*Melissa officinalis*)

Alternate or Related Names   Lemon Balm, Balm, Sweet Mary, Honey Plant, Cure-All, Others

Principal Proposed Uses
   Topical Uses: Oral and Genital Herpes
   Oral Uses: Insomnia, Anxiety, Nervous Stomach

More well known in the United States as lemon balm, *Melissa officinalis* is a native of southern Europe, commonly planted in gardens to attract bees. Its leaves give off a delicate lemon odor when bruised.

Medical authorities of ancient Greece and Rome mentioned topical melissa as a treatment for wounds. The herb was later used orally as a treatment for influenza, insomnia, anxiety, depression, and nervous stomach.

WHAT IS MELISSA USED FOR TODAY?

Modern German researchers have focused on the ability of melissa creams and ointments to inhibit the **herpes** (see page 86) virus, as well as the stomach-calming and anti-insomnia benefits of the herb when taken by mouth.

Numerous test tube studies have found that extracts of melissa possess antiviral properties.[1,2,3] We don't really know how it works, but the predominant theory is that the herb blocks viruses from attaching to cells.[4]

Melissa cream is used at the first sign of genital or oral herpes. It appears to make flare-ups less intense and last

for a shorter period of time, but it doesn't completely eliminate them. There is no evidence that melissa reduces the chances that you can infect someone else. The cream is also applied on a daily basis to prevent flare-ups.

Oral melissa is also used for **insomnia** (see page 103), **anxiety** (see page 11), and nervous stomach.

WHAT IS THE SCIENTIFIC EVIDENCE FOR MELISSA?

Besides the clinical research described here, see also the description of how melissa cream is made (under Dosage). It, too, provides indirect evidence for melissa's antiviral effect.

Herpes

Early studies of melissa ointments showed a significant reduction in the duration and severity of herpes symptoms (both genital and oral) and, when the cream was used regularly, a marked reduction in the frequency of recurrences.[5] In one study, the melissa-treated participants recovered in 5 days, while participants receiving nonspecific creams required 10 days.[6] Researchers also described a "tremendous reduction" in the frequency of recurrence. However, because these studies weren't double-blind, the results can't be taken as reliable.

A subsequent double-blind study followed 116 individuals with oral or genital herpes at two dermatology centers.[7] Treated subjects showed a significantly better rate of recovery than those on placebo, according to physician and patient ratings.

A recent double-blind placebo-controlled study followed 66 individuals who were just starting to develop a cold sore (oral herpes).[8] Treatment with melissa cream produced significant benefits on day 2, reducing the intensity of discomfort, number of blisters, and the size of the lesion. The researchers specifically looked at day 2 because, according to them, that is when symptoms are most pronounced. Furthermore, long-term follow-up suggested that use of melissa can prolong the interval before the next herpes flare-up.

Insomnia

Melissa extracts have also been found to produce a sedative effect in mice.[9] Combined extracts of melissa and valerian have been studied as a treatment for insomnia. A 30-day double-blind placebo-controlled study of 98 individuals without insomnia found that a valerian–lemon balm combination improved sleep quality as compared to placebo.[10] Similarly, a double-blind crossover study of 20 people with insomnia compared the benefits of the sleeping drug Halcion (0.125 mg) against placebo and a combination of valerian and lemon balm, and found them equally effective.[11]

DOSAGE

For treatment of an active flare-up of herpes, the proper dosage is four thick applications daily of a standardized melissa (70:1) cream. The dosage may be reduced to twice daily for preventive purposes.

The best melissa extracts are standardized by their capacity to inhibit the growth of herpes virus in a petri dish.[12] To make sure the extract has been properly prepared, manufacturers place cells in such a growing medium, and then add herpes virus. Normally, the virus will gradually destroy all the cells. But when little disks containing melissa are added, cells in the immediate vicinity are protected. Although manufacturers use this method as a form of quality control, it also provides evidence that melissa really works.

When taken orally for its calming effect, the standard dosage of melissa is 1.5 to 4.5 g of dried herb daily.

SAFETY ISSUES

Topical melissa is not associated with any significant side effects, although allergic reactions are always possible. Oral melissa is on the FDA's GRAS (generally recognized as safe) list. There are no known drug interactions. However, there are theoretical concerns that if melissa is taken at the same time as standard sedative drugs, excessive sedation might occur.

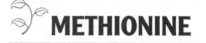

METHIONINE

Supplement Forms/Alternate Names　　L-Methionine

Principal Proposed Uses　　There are no well-documented uses for methionine.

Other Proposed Uses　　Urinary Tract Infections, "Liver Support," Parkinson's Disease

Methionine is an essential amino acid—one of the building blocks of proteins and peptides that your body cannot manufacture from other chemicals. The body uses methionine to manufacture **creatine** (see page 264) and uses the sulfur in methionine for normal metabolism and growth.

One preliminary study suggests that methionine can prevent bacteria from sticking to urinary tract cells,[1] which may make it useful for preventing bladder infections. (**Cranberry** juice is thought to help reduce the incidence of bladder infections in a similar fashion; see page 263.)

REQUIREMENTS/SOURCES

Depending on your body weight, you need between 800 and 1,000 mg of methionine daily for normal health. Deficiency is unlikely, because enough methionine is generally available from the diet.

Meat, fish, dairy products, and other high-protein foods are good sources of methionine.

THERAPEUTIC DOSAGES

A proper therapeutic dosage of methionine has not been determined. One study relating to urinary tract infections used a dosage of 500 mg 3 times daily.

THERAPEUTIC USES

Because it seems to discourage bacteria from sticking to the wall of the bladder, methionine has been suggested as a treatment for recurrent **bladder infections** (see page 28).[2] However, there is as yet little direct evidence that it works.

One study on rats suggests that methionine might protect the liver against acetaminophen (e.g., Tylenol) poisoning.[3] Based on this, it has been proposed as a generally helpful substance—what our great-grandparents might have called a "tonic"—for the liver. However, in this particular study the action of methionine was more to fight acetaminophen specifically than to protect the liver in general. There is much better evidence that the herb **milk thistle** (see page 361) is a general liver protectant.

Very preliminary evidence suggests methionine might be helpful in treating **Parkinson's disease** (see Safety Issues; see also page 140).[4,5]

WHAT IS THE SCIENTIFIC EVIDENCE FOR METHIONINE?

Bladder Infection

The clinical evidence for this use of methionine is based primarily on one study, a preliminary open trial that tested methionine against the standard treatment in 33 women with recurrent urinary tract infections. The dosage used in this study was 500 mg 3 times daily. Researchers found *no* infections in the methionine group during the 26-month study period.[6] Although methionine did not reduce the number of bacteria in the urinary tract, it appeared to lessen the bacteria's ability to latch on to cells.

SAFETY ISSUES

Methionine is thought to be generally safe. However, the maximum safe dosages for young children, pregnant or nursing women, or those with serious liver or kidney disease have not been established.

Like other amino acids, methionine may interfere with the absorption or action of the drug levodopa, which is used for Parkinson's disease.[7]

⚠ INTERACTIONS YOU SHOULD KNOW ABOUT

If you are taking

- **Methionine,** make sure to get enough folate, vitamin B_6, and vitamin B_{12}.[8]
- **Levodopa**, methionine might interfere with its action.

MILK THISTLE (*Silybum marianum*)

Alternate or Related Names   Marian Thistle, Mediterranean Milk Thistle, Mary Thistle

Principal Proposed Uses   Chronic Viral Hepatitis, Acute Viral Hepatitis, Alcoholic Liver Disease, Liver Cirrhosis, Mushroom Poisoning (Special Intravenous Form Only), Protection from Liver-Toxic Medications

The milk thistle plant commonly grows from 2 to 7 feet in height, with spiny leaves and reddish-purple, thistle-shaped flowers. It has also been called wild artichoke, holy thistle, and Mary thistle. Native to Europe, milk thistle has a long history of use as both a food and a medicine. At the turn of the twentieth century, English gardeners grew milk thistle to use its leaves like lettuce (after cutting off the spines), the stalks like asparagus, the roasted seeds like coffee, and the roots (soaked overnight) like oyster plant. The seeds and leaves of milk thistle were used for medicinal purposes as well, such as treating jaundice and increasing breast milk production.

German researchers in the 1960s were sufficiently impressed with the history and clinical effectiveness of milk thistle to begin examining it for active constituents. In 1986, Germany's Commission E approved an oral extract of milk thistle standardized to 70% crude silymarin content as a treatment for liver disease.

WHAT IS MILK THISTLE USED FOR TODAY?

Based on the extensive folk use of milk thistle in cases of jaundice, European medical researchers began to

Milk Thistle

Visit Us at TNP.com

investigate its medicinal effects. It is now widely used to treat alcoholic hepatitis, alcoholic fatty liver, **liver cirrhosis** (see page 112), liver poisoning, and **viral hepatitis** (see page 189), as well as to protect the liver from the effects of liver-toxic medications. Milk thistle is one of the few herbs that has no real equivalent in the world of conventional medicine.

According to reports and some research evidence that we'll review in the next section, treatment produces a modest improvement in symptoms of chronic liver disease, such as nausea, weakness, loss of appetite, fatigue, and pain. Liver enzymes as measured by blood tests frequently improve, and if a liver biopsy is performed, there may be improvements on the cellular level. Some studies have shown a reduction in death rate among those with serious liver disease.

The active ingredients in milk thistle appear to be four substances known collectively as silymarin, of which the most potent is named silibinin.[1] When injected intravenously, silibinin is one of the few known antidotes to poisoning by the deathcap mushroom, *Amanita phalloides.* Animal studies suggest that milk thistle extracts can also protect against many other poisonous substances, from toluene to the drug acetaminophen.[2–7] One animal study suggests that milk thistle can also protect against fetal damage caused by alcohol.[8]

Silymarin appears to function by displacing toxins trying to bind to the liver as well as by causing the liver to regenerate more quickly.[9] It may also scavenge free radicals and stabilize liver cell membranes.[10,11]

However, milk thistle is not effective in treating advanced liver cirrhosis, and only the intravenous form can counter mushroom poisoning.

In Europe, milk thistle is often added as extra protection when patients are given medications known to cause liver problems. However, milk thistle does not seem to prevent the liver inflammation caused by the anti-Alzheimer's drug Cognex (tacrine).[12]

Milk thistle is also used in a vague condition known as minor hepatic insufficiency, or "sluggish liver."[13] This term is mostly used by European physicians and American naturopathic practitioners—conventional physicians don't recognize it. Symptoms are supposed to include aching under the ribs, fatigue, unhealthy skin appearance, general malaise, constipation, premenstrual syndrome, chemical sensitivities, and allergies.

Milk thistle may also offer some protection to the kidney.[14]

Intriguing evidence suggests that milk thistle might help prevent breast **cancer** (see page 32).[15] Milk thistle is sometimes recommended for **gallstones** (see page 83) and **psoriasis** (see page 148), but there is little to no evidence as yet that it really works for these conditions.

WHAT IS THE SCIENTIFIC EVIDENCE FOR MILK THISTLE?

There is considerable evidence from studies in animals that milk thistle can protect the liver from numerous toxins. However, human studies of people suffering from various liver diseases have yielded mixed results.

Deathcap Poisoning

In *Amanita* mushroom poisoning, silibinin appears to dramatically reduce death rates, which are typically from 30 to 50%, down to less than 10%.[16] This mushroom destroys the liver if left untreated. In conditions like this one, it isn't ethical to perform double-blind studies. However, milk thistle seems to be so dramatically effective that its value is not disputed.

Chronic Viral Hepatitis

Preliminary double-blind studies of people with chronic viral hepatitis have found that milk thistle can produce significant improvement in symptoms such as fatigue, reduced appetite, and abdominal discomfort, as well as results on blood tests for liver inflammation.[17,18,19]

Acute Viral Hepatitis

While good results have been reported in one study of 57 people with acute viral hepatitis,[20] another study of 151 participants showed no benefit.[21]

Alcoholic Liver Disease

A double-blind placebo-controlled study performed in 1981 followed 106 Finnish soldiers with alcoholic liver disease over a period of 4 weeks.[22] The treated group showed a significant decrease in elevated liver enzymes and improvement in liver histology, as evaluated by biopsy in 29 subjects.

Two similar studies provided essentially equivalent results.[23,24] However, a 3-month randomized double-blind study of 116 people showed little to no additional benefit, perhaps because most participants reduced their alcohol consumption and almost half stopped drinking entirely.[25] Another study found no benefit in 72 patients followed for 15 months.[26]

Liver Cirrhosis

A double-blind placebo-controlled study followed 146 people with liver cirrhosis for 3 to 6 years. In the treated group, the 4-year survival rate was 58% as compared to only 38% in the placebo group.[27]

Another double-blind placebo-controlled trial, which followed 172 individuals with liver cirrhosis for 4 years, also found a significant reduction in mortality.[28]

However, a 2-year double-blind placebo-controlled study that followed 125 individuals with alcoholic cirrhosis found no reduction in mortality.[29] It may be that the study was not long enough to reproduce the benefits seen in the other studies.

Protection from Medications That Damage the Liver

Numerous medications can injure or inflame the liver. Preliminary evidence suggests that milk thistle might protect against liver toxicity caused by drugs such as acetaminophen, Dilantin (phenytoin), alcohol, and phenothiazines.[30,31] However, according to a 12-week double-blind study of 222 individuals, milk thistle does not seem to prevent the liver inflammation caused by the anti-Alzheimer's drug Cognex (tacrine).[32]

DOSAGE

The standard dosage of milk thistle is 200 mg 2 to 3 times a day of an extract standardized to contain 70% silymarin.

There is some evidence that silymarin bound to phosphatidylcholine may be better absorbed.[33,34] This form should be taken at a dosage of 100 to 200 mg twice a day.

Warning: Considering the severe nature of liver disease, a doctor's supervision is essential. Also, do not inject milk thistle preparations that are designed for oral use!

SAFETY ISSUES

Milk thistle is believed to possess very little toxicity. Animal studies have not shown any negative effects even when high doses were administered over a long period of time.[35]

A study of 2,637 participants reported in 1992 showed a low incidence of side effects, limited mainly to mild gastrointestinal disturbance.[36] However, on rare occasions severe abdominal discomfort may occur.[37]

On the basis of its extensive use as a food, milk thistle is believed to be safe for pregnant or nursing women, and researchers have enrolled pregnant women in studies.[38] However, safety in young children, pregnant or nursing women, and individuals with severe renal disease has not been formally established.

No drug interactions are known. However, one report has noted that silibinin (a constituent of silymarin) can inhibit a bacterial enzyme called beta-glucuronidase, which plays a role in the activity of certain drugs, such as oral contraceptives.[39] This could reduce their effectiveness.

⚠ INTERACTIONS YOU SHOULD KNOW ABOUT

If you are taking

- **Oral contraceptives:** Milk thistle may reduce their effectiveness.
- **Medications that could damage the liver:** Milk thistle might be protective for some such drugs.

MOTHERWORT (*Leonurus cardiaca, Leonurus artemisia*)

Alternate or Related Names   Lion's Tail, Lion's Ear, Throw-Wort

Principal Proposed Uses   Irregular or Rapid Heartbeat

Other Proposed Uses   Uterine Stimulant, Uterine Relaxant

As its Latin name *cardiaca* suggests, motherwort is primarily used to treat heart conditions. The ancient Greeks and Romans employed the motherwort species *cardiaca* to treat heart palpitations as well as depression, which they considered a problem of the heart. Centuries later, Europeans would believe motherwort helpful for "infirmities of the heart" but also considered the herb to have strengthening and stimulating effects on the uterus, using it to bring on a delayed menstrual period, as an aid during labor, and to relax a woman's womb after childbirth.

These uses of motherwort correspond well with those in traditional Chinese medicine, which employs the Asian variety, *Leonurus artemisia*, to treat menstrual disorders or to help a woman expel a dead fetus and placenta from her womb.[1] In eastern China, women still drink a syrup made from motherwort to promote the recovery of the uterus after childbirth; the herb has a strong bitter taste, so visitors to a recovering mother often bring along sugar as a gift.[2]

WHAT IS MOTHERWORT USED FOR TODAY?

Germany's Commission E has authorized motherwort for the treatment of heart disorders caused by anxiety and stress, as well as part of an overall treatment plan for an overactive thyroid (hyperthyroidism).[3] These two uses are linked by the fact that both stress and high levels of thyroid hormone can increase the heart rate.

As yet, there is no real evidence to support these applications; however, one test tube study found that motherwort slowed the contractions (beating) of normal rat heart cells and inhibited the ability of substances that speed up heart cell contractions to do so.[4]

Two test tube studies suggest that leonurine, a compound found in some species of motherwort, may affect the uterus.[5,6] One of these studies found that low concentrations of leonurine induced uterine contractions, but that higher concentrations inhibited contractions.[7] These opposing effects might explain how motherwort could induce both labor and menstruation, and could also relax the uterus after childbirth. However, until properly designed human studies are performed, we don't know for sure whether motherwort is actually safe or effective for these traditional uses.

One poorly designed study suggests that motherwort might improve blood circulation.[8] Another study of equally low quality suggests that motherwort might have some benefits for individuals who have had a stroke.[9]

One component of motherwort, ursolic acid, appears to possess antiviral and antitumor properties.[10,11] However, a highly preliminary animal study suggests that motherwort and/or various motherwort extracts can both inhibit or stimulate the growth of breast tumors.[12]

DOSAGE

The Commission E recommends a dose of 4.5 g of dried herb daily, or the equivalent.

Note: Irregular or rapid heartbeat can be a sign of serious medical illness. Do not self-treat these conditions with motherwort except under medical supervision. Also, do not combine motherwort with other heart medications, as they might interact unpredictably.

SAFETY ISSUES

The safety of motherwort has not been extensively studied; however, obvious side effects appear to be rare, except for occasional allergic reactions and gastrointestinal distress.

Because of the herb's traditional use for uterine stimulation and the corroborating results of some test tube studies,[13,14] motherwort should not be used by pregnant women until further scientific investigation has been performed.

In addition, preliminary animal evidence suggests that women with a history of breast cancer, or those at high risk for developing it, should avoid motherwort.[15]

Safety in young children, nursing women, or people with severe liver or kidney disease has not been established.

MSM (Methyl Sulfonyl Methane)

Supplement Forms/Alternate Names   Dimethyl Sulfone (DMSO2)

Principal Proposed Uses   Osteoarthritis

Other Proposed Uses   Rheumatoid Arthritis, Snoring, Cancer Prevention, Interstitial Cystitis, Scleroderma, Excess Stomach Acid, Allergies, Constipation

MSM (methyl sulfonyl methane) is a sulfur-containing compound normally found in many of the foods we eat. It is chemically related to DMSO (dimethyl sulfoxide), a popular (although unproven) treatment for arthritis. When DMSO is applied on the skin or taken orally, about 15% of it breaks down in the body to form MSM.[1] Some researchers have suggested that the resulting MSM could be responsible for DMSO's supposed benefits, although this has not been proven. MSM may be preferable, as it does not cause some of the unpleasant side effects associated with DMSO treatment, such as body odor and bad breath. Because it is a natural ingredient found in food, MSM might be safer as well.

REQUIREMENTS/SOURCES

There is no dietary requirement for MSM. However, it occurs naturally in cow's milk, meat, seafood, vegetables, fruits, and even coffee, tea, and chocolate. MSM supplements are sold in health food stores and some pharmacies. Although creams and lotions containing MSM are also available, it is hard to see the purpose of these topical products since MSM, unlike DMSO, is not absorbed through the skin.[2]

MSM is often combined with glucosamine in products sold for the treatment of osteoarthritis. However, there is no evidence that it provides any additional benefit to the much more well-established effects of glucosamine.

THERAPEUTIC DOSAGES

Dosages of oral MSM used for therapeutic purposes range from 250 mg to 2,250 mg daily.

THERAPEUTIC USES

MSM has been proposed as a treatment for most of the same conditions for which DMSO is popular. However, evidence that either of these treatments really work is highly preliminary at best.

According to one small double-blind trial, MSM may be helpful for **osteoarthritis** (see What Is the Scientific Evidence section for details; see also page 132).[3] Additionally, a study in mice found positive effects of MSM for rheumatoid arthritis.[4]

MSM is also proposed as a treatment for interstitial cystitis, an inflammation in the wall of the bladder that causes frequent and painful urination. When prescribed for this condition, MSM is often instilled directly into the bladder by an attending physician, although it is also sometimes taken orally. No clinical studies on this use have been performed: the only evidence for this treatment comes from case studies and anecdotal reports.[5] These, however, are far from conclusive, since this disease is known to respond very positively to placebo.[6] Properly-designed clinical trials are necessary to discover whether MSM really works for interstitial cystitis.

MSM is purported to be effective for snoring, based on an unpublished preliminary trial. Thirty-five individuals were given MSM, and for 28 of them, spouses reported "less noise."[7] Then, of the 28 whose snoring seemed quieter, 13 were given a new formula (without their knowledge), which didn't contain MSM. According to spouses' assessments, 11 of the 13 began snoring loudly again. Resuming use of the MSM appeared to reduce snoring volume once more. While these are promising results, the experimental design was substandard and the number of participants was very small. A better-designed study is necessary to determine whether MSM can truly help snoring.

Based on highly preliminary animal studies, MSM has been proposed to help prevent breast **cancer** (see page 32) and colon cancer.[8,9] MSM did not reduce the number of tumors found in the mice in these studies, but did appear to delay the onset of tumor development after exposure to a cancer-causing chemical.

Studies involving mice with an autoimmune disease predisposing them to develop tumors, as well as other symptoms, found that MSM exerted a protective effect.[10] The treated mice had significantly fewer tumors, fewer cases of anemia, and decreased development of antinuclear antibodies (a self-destructive type of cell typically seen in these mice). In addition, the life spans of the treated mice nearly doubled.

MSM has also been purported to be effective for **allergies** (including drug allergies; see page 2), scleroderma, **excess stomach acid** (see page 180), and **constipation** (see page 56), but there is little to no evidence to support these uses.

WHAT IS THE SCIENTIFIC EVIDENCE FOR MSM?

An unpublished and very small double-blind placebo-controlled trial of MSM treatment for osteoarthritis yielded positive results.[11] Sixteen people with x-ray evidence of osteoarthritis were randomly assigned to either 2,250 mg of MSM daily or placebo. Based on the participants' own assessments of their pain levels, those taking MSM experienced an 82% improvement by the end of 6 weeks, compared to an 18% improvement for those taking placebo.

SAFETY ISSUES

MSM is a natural component of the foods we normally eat and is not believed to be toxic. A laboratory study examining doses up to 8 g per kilogram of body weight per day (about 250 times the highest dose normally used by humans) reported that no toxic effects were seen.[12]

Maximum safe doses for young children, pregnant or nursing women, or people with liver or kidney disease are not known. Possible drug interactions are also not known.

MULLEIN (*Verbascum thapsus*)

Alternate or Related Names   Torch Weed, Aaron's Rod, Blanket-Leaf, Candlewick Plant, Flannelflower, Others
Principal Proposed Uses   Asthma, Colds, Cough, Sore Throat, Ear Infections

Mullein

Visit Us at TNP.com

Also called "grandmother's flannel" for its thick, soft leaves, mullein is a common wildflower that can grow almost anywhere. It reaches several feet tall and puts up a spike of densely packed tiny yellow flowers. Mullein has served many purposes over the centuries, from making candlewicks to casting out evil spirits, but as medicine it was primarily used to treat diarrhea, respiratory diseases, and hemorrhoids.

WHAT IS MULLEIN USED FOR TODAY?

Contemporary herbalists sometimes recommend hot mullein tea for **asthma** (see page 14), **colds** (see page 47), coughs, and sore throats. Mullein seldom produces dramatic effects, but its soothing qualities will be appreciated. You can also breathe the steam from a boiling pot of mullein tea.

Like marshmallow, mullein contains a high proportion of mucilage (large sugar molecules that appear to soothe mucous membranes). It also contains saponins that may help loosen mucus.[1] However, there has not been very much scientific investigation into this popular herb. Mullein is said to be most effective when combined with other herbs of similar qualities, such as **yerba santa** (see page 461), **marshmallow** (see page 355), cherry bark, and **elecampane** (see page 276).

Mullein is also often made into an oily eardrop solution to soothe the pain of **ear infections** (see page 73).

DOSAGE

To make mullein tea, add 1 to 2 teaspoons of dried leaves and flowers to 1 cup of boiling water and steep for 10 minutes. Make sure to strain the tea before drinking it because fuzzy bits of the herb can stick in your throat and cause an irritating tickle.

For painful ear infections, you can squeeze several drops of room-temperature mullein oil into the ear canal, so long as you are sure that the eardrum isn't punctured. But don't expect mullein oil to heal an ear infection: it only relieves the symptoms.

SAFETY ISSUES

Mullein leaves and flowers are on the FDA's GRAS (generally recognized as safe) list. Side effects are rare. Nonetheless, safety in young children, pregnant or nursing women, or those with severe liver or kidney disease has not been established.

N-ACETYL CYSTEINE (NAC)

Principal Proposed Uses   Chronic Bronchitis, Angina Pectoris (in Combination with Conventional Treatment)

Other Proposed Uses   Acute Respiratory Distress Syndrome, Kidney Protection, Colon Cancer Prevention, HIV Support, Chemotherapy Aid, Parkinson's Disease

N-acetyl cysteine (NAC) is a specially modified form of the dietary amino acid cysteine. NAC may help break up mucus, which is the basis for using it in respiratory conditions; however, this has been disputed. It also helps the body make the important antioxidant enzyme glutathione. However, the only well-documented uses of NAC are for conditions too serious for self-treatment.

SOURCES

There is no daily requirement for NAC, and it is not found in food.

THERAPEUTIC DOSAGES

Optimal levels of NAC have not been determined. The amount used in studies has varied from 250 to 1,500 mg daily.

THERAPEUTIC USES

Evidence suggests that regular use of NAC is helpful for individuals with **chronic bronchitis** (see page 45), a condition commonly associated with smoking and emphysema.[1–9]

Mixed evidence suggests that NAC may be helpful for people who take the drug nitroglycerin for **angina** (the chest pain associated with heart disease; see page 10).[10–15] However, severe headaches may develop as a side effect. NAC may also be helpful in a life-threatening condition called acute respiratory distress syndrome.[16] Very high dosages of NAC are used in hospitals as a conventional treatment for acetaminophen poisoning.

Note: Do not attempt to self-treat angina, acute respiratory distress syndrome, or acetaminophen poisoning!

Medical supervision is absolutely essential because of the very real risk of death in these conditions.

In order to get more information from certain types of x rays, radiologists often administer substances called "contrast agents." Unfortunately, contrast agents can damage the kidney. There is some evidence that NAC may help protect the kidney from such damage.[17]

Very preliminary evidence indicates that NAC may help prevent colon **cancer** (see page 32).[18]

NAC is often used by people with **HIV** (see page 94) in hopes of enhancing immune function. However, the evidence that it helps is somewhat conflicting.[19–22] It has also been suggested that the supplement NAC might help prevent side effects from the antibiotic TMP-SMX (trimethoprim-sulfamethoxazole), frequently taken long term by individuals with AIDS. However, two controlled studies found that NAC did not significantly decrease adverse reactions to TMP-SMX.[23,24]

NAC is also sometimes recommended for helping chemotherapy work better and reducing its side effects. It has also been suggested as a treatment for **Parkinson's disease** (see page 140). However, there is no solid scientific evidence that it is effective for these purposes, and one double-blind trial study found NAC ineffective for head and neck or lung cancer.[25]

WHAT IS THE SCIENTIFIC EVIDENCE FOR N-ACETYL CYSTEINE?

Chronic Bronchitis

Individuals who have smoked cigarettes for many years eventually develop deterioration in their lungs leading to various symptoms, including chronic production of thick mucus. This so-called chronic bronchitis tends to flare up periodically into severe acute attacks possibly requiring hospitalization.

Regular use of NAC may diminish the number of these attacks. A review and meta-analysis selected eight double-blind placebo-controlled trials of NAC for chronic bronchitis.[26–34] The results of these studies, involving a total of about 1,400 individuals, suggest that NAC taken daily at a dose of 400 to 1,200 mg can reduce the number of acute attacks of severe bronchitis. It is not clear how NAC works; the old concept that it acts by thinning mucus may not be correct.

Angina Pectoris

Angina pectoris is a squeezing feeling in the chest caused by inadequate blood supply to the heart. It can be a precursor of heart attacks. People with angina often use the drug nitroglycerin to relieve symptoms. One 4-month double-blind placebo-controlled study of 200 individuals with heart disease found that the combination of nitroglycerin and NAC significantly reduced the incidence of heart attacks and other severe heart problems.[35] NAC alone and nitroglycerin alone were not as effective. The only problem was that the combination of nitroglycerin and NAC caused severe headaches in many participants. This effect has been seen in other studies as well.[36]

NAC may also help in cases of nitroglycerin tolerance, a condition in which the drug becomes less effective over time. In a small double-blind study of 32 people with angina, tolerance developed in 15 of 16 individuals who took nitroglycerin only, but in just 5 of 16 individuals who took nitroglycerin plus 2 g of NAC daily.[37] However, other studies have found no benefit.[38]

Acute Respiratory Distress Syndrome

A double-blind placebo-controlled clinical trial compared the effectiveness of NAC, Procysteine (a synthetic cysteine building-block drug), and placebo in 46 people with a condition called acute respiratory distress syndrome.[39] This catastrophic lung condition can be caused when an unconscious person inhales his or her own vomit. Both NAC and Procysteine reduced the severity of the condition in some people (as compared with placebo). However, overall it did not reduce the number of deaths.

Colon Cancer Prevention

A preliminary double-blind placebo-controlled study of NAC enrolled 62 individuals, each of whom had had a polyp removed from the colon.[40] The abnormal growth of polyps is closely associated with the development of colon cancer. In this study, the potential anticancer benefits of NAC treatment were evaluated by taking a biopsy of the rectum. Individuals taking NAC at 800 mg daily for 12 weeks showed more normal cells in the biopsied tissue as compared to those in the placebo group.

HIV

Early human trials, including a double-blind study of 45 people, suggest that NAC may increase levels of CD4+ cells (a type of immune cell) in healthy people and slow CD4+ cell decline in people with HIV.[41,42] Another study of NAC combined with selenium had mixed results, affecting t-cell counts in some people but not others.[43] However, preliminary results of yet another study found that NAC had no effect on CD4+ counts or the amount of HIV virus in the blood.[44]

SAFETY ISSUES

NAC appears to be a very safe supplement when taken alone, although one study in rats suggests that 60 to 100 times the normal dose can cause liver injury.[45]

As mentioned earlier, the combination of nitroglycerin and NAC causes severe headaches. Safety in young children, women who are pregnant or nursing, and individuals with severe liver or kidney disease has not been established.

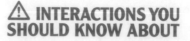

⚠ INTERACTIONS YOU SHOULD KNOW ABOUT

If you are taking **nitroglycerin,** NAC may cause severe headaches.

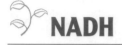

NADH

Supplement Forms/Alternate Names   Nicotinamide Adenine Dinucleotide

Principal Proposed Uses   There are no well-documented uses for NADH.

Other Proposed Uses   Alzheimer's Disease, Chronic Fatigue Syndrome, Depression, Parkinson's Disease, Performance Enhancement

NADH, short for *nicotinamide adenine dinucleotide,* is an important cofactor, or "assistant," that helps enzymes in the work they do throughout the body. NADH particularly plays a role in the production of energy. It also participates in the production of L-dopa, which the body turns into the important neurotransmitter dopamine.

Based on these basic biochemical facts, NADH has been suggested as a treatment for Alzheimer's disease, Parkinson's disease, chronic fatigue syndrome, and depression and as a sports supplement. However, there isn't enough scientific evidence to prove or disprove its usefulness for any of these conditions.

SOURCES

Healthy bodies make all the NADH they need, using **vitamin B₃** (also known as niacin, or nicotinamide; see page 437) as a starting point. The highest concentration of NADH in animals is found in muscle tissues, which means that meat might be a good source—were it not that most of the NADH in meat is destroyed during processing, cooking, and digestion. In reality, we don't get much NADH from our food.

THERAPEUTIC DOSAGES

The typical dosage for supplemental NADH ranges from 5 to 50 mg daily.

THERAPEUTIC USES

Supplemental NADH has been proposed as a treatment for **Alzheimer's disease** (see page 5), **chronic fatigue syndrome** (see page 44), **depression** (see page 59), and **Parkinson's disease** (see page 140). It has also been tried as an athletic **performance enhancer** (see page 158). However, although a few studies have been performed on these uses,[1–6] none were designed in such a way as to produce scientifically meaningful results.

SAFETY ISSUES

NADH appears to be quite safe when taken at a dosage of 5 mg daily or less. However, formal safety studies have not been completed, and safety in young children, pregnant or nursing women, or those with severe liver or kidney disease has not been established.

NEEM *(Azadirachta indica)*

Alternate or Related Names   Azedarach, Holy Tree, Nim

Principal Proposed Uses   Fevers, Respiratory Diseases, Skin Diseases, and Other Conditions Too Numerous to List

The neem tree has been called "the village pharmacy," because its bark, leaves, sap, fruit, seeds, and twigs have so many diverse uses in the traditional medicine of India. This member of the mahogany family has been used medicinally for at least 4,000 years, and is held in such esteem that Indian poets called it *Sarva Roga Nivarini: The One That Can Cure All Ailments*. Mohandas Gandhi encouraged scientific investigation of the neem tree as part of his program to revitalize Indian traditions, eventually leading to over 2,000 research papers and intense commercial interest.

At least 50 patents have been filed on neem, and neem-based products are licensed in the United States for control of insects in food and ornamental crops. However, the Indian government and many nongovernmental organizations have united to overthrow some patents of this type, which they regard as "folk-wisdom piracy." One fear is that if neem is patented, indigenous people who already use it will lose the right to continue to do so. Another point is the fundamental question: Who owns the genetic diversity of plants: the nations where the plants come from or the transnational corporations that pay for the research into those plants? Although this area of international law is rapidly evolving, a patent on the spice turmeric has already been overturned, and neem may follow soon.

At least 100 bioactive substances have been found in neem, including nimbidin, azadiracthins, and other triterpenoids and limonoids. Although the scientific evidence for all of neem's uses in health care remains preliminary, the intense interest in the plant will eventually lead to proper double-blind clinical trials.

WHAT IS NEEM USED FOR TODAY?

The uses of neem are remarkably diverse. In India, the sap is used for treating fevers, general debilitation, diges-

tive disturbances, and skin diseases; the bark gum for respiratory diseases and other infections; the leaves for digestive problems, intestinal parasites, and viral infections; the fruit for debilitation, malaria, skin diseases, and intestinal parasites; and the seed and kernel oil for **diabetes** (see page 65), fevers, fungal infections, bacterial infections, inflammatory diseases, fertility prevention, and as an insecticide.[1,2] Which, if any, of these uses will be verified when proper research is performed remains unclear.

DOSAGE

Because of the numerous parts of the neem tree used, and the many different ways these can be prepared, the only advice we can give at this time is to follow the directions on the label of the neem product you purchase.

SAFETY ISSUES

Based on its extensive traditional use, neem seems to be quite safe. This is particularly remarkable considering that the oil of neem is a powerful insecticide! However, there has not yet been a full scientific evaluation of the toxicity and side effects of neem and its many constituents.

A somewhat worrisome recent report suggests that neem might damage chromosomes.[3] Although this information is still highly preliminary, at the present time neem is not recommended for use by young children, pregnant or nursing women, or those with severe liver or kidney disease.

NETTLE (*Urtica dioica*)

Alternate or Related Names   Stinging Nettle

Principal Proposed Uses   Benign Prostatic Hyperplasia (Nettle Root), Allergies (Nettle Leaf)

Anyone who lives in a locale where nettle grows wild will eventually discover the powers of this dark green plant. Depending on the species, the fine hairs on its leaves and stem cause burning pain that lasts from hours to weeks. But this well-protected herb can also serve as medicine. Nettle juice was used in Hippocrates' time to treat bites and stings, and European herbalists recommended nettle tea for lung disorders. Nettle tea was used by Native Americans as an aid in pregnancy, childbirth, and nursing.

WHAT IS NETTLE USED FOR TODAY?

In Europe, nettle root is widely used for the treatment of **benign prostatic hyperplasia** (BPH; see page 24), or prostate enlargement. Like saw palmetto, pygeum, and beta-sitosterols, nettle appears to reduce obstruction to urinary flow and decrease the need for nighttime urination. However, the evidence is not as strong for nettle as it is for these other treatments.

Note: Before self-treating with nettle, be sure to get a proper medical evaluation to rule out prostate cancer.

Nettle leaf has recently become a popular treatment for **allergies** (hay fever; see page 2) based on one preliminary study at the National College of Naturopathic Medicine in Portland.

Nettle leaf is also highly nutritious, and in cooked form may be used as a general dietary supplement.

WHAT IS THE SCIENTIFIC EVIDENCE FOR NETTLE?

The evidence is much better for nettle root and prostatic enlargement than for nettle leaf and allergies.

Nettle Root

The use of nettle root for treating benign prostatic hyperplasia has not been as well studied as saw palmetto, but the evidence is at least moderately convincing.

Nettle root contains numerous biologically active chemicals that may influence the function of the prostate, interact with sex hormones, slow the growth of prostate cells, fight prostate **cancer** (see page 32), and reduce inflammation.[1–5]

Open studies involving a total of over 2,000 men with BPH have found significant improvements in prostate size, nighttime urination, urination frequency, urine flow, and residual urine.[6] However, open studies are not necessarily reliable in this case because up to 60% of men with BPH show good responses to placebo.

In a 4- to 6-week double-blind study of 67 men, treatment with nettle produced a 14% improvement in urine flow and a 53% decrease in residual urine.[7] Another double-blind study of 40 men found a significant decrease in frequency of urination after 6 months.[8] A double-blind study of 50 men over 9 weeks found a significant improvement in urination volume.[9]

Nettle Leaf

A preliminary double-blind placebo-controlled study following 69 individuals suggests that freeze-dried nettle leaf may at least slightly improve allergy symptoms.[10]

One small double-blind study suggests that direct application of stinging nettle leaf to a painful joint may improve symptoms.[11]

DOSAGE

According to Commission E, the proper dosage of nettle root is 4 to 6 g daily of the whole root, or a proportional dose of concentrated extract. There is some reason to believe that nettle root's effectiveness might be enhanced when it is combined with another herb used for prostate problems, **pygeum** (see page 395).[12,13]

For allergies, the proper dosage is 300 mg twice a day of freeze-dried nettle leaf.

SAFETY ISSUES

Because nettle leaf has a long history of food use, it is believed to be safe.

Nettle root does not have as extensive a history to go by. Although detailed safety studies have not been reported, no significant adverse effects have been noted in Germany where nettle root is widely used. In practice, it is nearly side-effect free. In one study of 4,087 people who took 600 to 1,200 mg of nettle root daily for 6 months, less than 1% reported mild gastrointestinal distress and only 0.19% experienced allergic reactions (skin rash).[14]

For theoretical reasons, there are some concerns that nettle may interact with diabetes, blood pressure, anti-inflammatory, and sedative medications, although there are no reports of any problems occurring in real life.

The safety of nettle root or leaf for pregnant or nursing mothers has not been established. However nettle leaf tea is a traditional drink for pregnant and nursing women.

⚠ INTERACTIONS YOU SHOULD KNOW ABOUT

If you are taking **anti-inflammatory, antihypertensive, sedative,** or **blood sugar–lowering medications,** nettle might conceivably interact with them, although it is unlikely.

Nettle

Visit Us at TNP.com

NONI (*Morinda citrifolia*)

Alternate or Related Names   Mengkudu

Principal Proposed Uses   There are no well-documented uses for noni.

Other Proposed Uses   Abrasions, Arthritis, Atherosclerosis, Bladder Infections, Boils, Bowel Disorders, Burns, Cancer, Chronic Fatigue Syndrome, Circulatory Weakness, Colds, Cold Sores, Congestion, Constipation, Diabetes, Drug Addiction, Eye Inflammations, Fever, Fractures, Gastric Ulcers, Gingivitis, Headaches, Heart Disease, Hypertension, Improved Digestion, Immune Weakness, Indigestion, Intestinal Parasites, Kidney Disease, Malaria, Menstrual Cramps, Menstrual Irregularities, Mouth Sores, Respiratory Disorders, Ringworm, Sinusitis, Skin Inflammation, Sprains, Stroke, Thrush, Wounds

Morinda citrifolia, also known as noni or Indian mulberry, is a small evergreen shrub or tree of the plant family Rubiaceae. Native to the Pacific islands, Polynesia, Asia, and Australia, it grows up to 10 feet high. The leaves are 8 or more inches long, dark green, oval shaped, and shiny, with deep veins. The flower heads are about an inch long and bear many small white flowers. These heads grow to become the mature fruit, 3 to 4 inches in diameter with a warty, pitted surface. Noni fruit starts out green, turns yellow with ripening, and has a foul odor, especially as it ripens to whiteness and falls to the ground.

Some cultures may eat noni fruit in times of scarcity (the unripened fruit is less noxious). Traditional Polynesian healers have apparently used the fruit for many purposes including bowel disorders (constipation and diarrhea), skin inflammation, infection, mouth sores, fever, contusions, and sprains—but it is said that only sick and desperate people will take it, due to its unpleasant odor and bitter taste. The primary indigenous use of this plant, however, appears to be of the leaves, as a topical treatment for wound healing.

In Chinese medicine, the root of *M. officinalis* is also a standard medication (known as bai ji tian or pa chi tien) used for the digestive system, kidneys, heart, and liver.

Other traditional uses for the plant include making a red dye from the bark and a yellow dye from the root.

WHAT IS NONI USED FOR TODAY?

Noni has been heavily promoted for an enormous range of uses, including abrasions, arthritis, atherosclerosis, bladder infections, boils, bowel disorders, burns, cancer, chronic fatigue syndrome, circulatory weakness, colds, cold sores, congestion, constipation, diabetes, drug addiction, eye inflammations, fever, fractures, gastric ulcers, gingivitis, headaches, heart disease, hypertension, improved digestion, immune weakness, indigestion, in-testinal parasites, kidney disease, malaria, menstrual cramps, menstrual irregularities, mouth sores, respiratory disorders, ringworm, sinusitis, skin inflammation, sprains, stroke, thrush, and wounds.[1] However, there is no real evidence that it is effective for any of these conditions.

Several animal studies have evaluated the effects of extracts derived from noni. The results suggest noni may have anti-cancer,[2,3,4] immune-enhancing,[5] and pain-relieving properties.[6] However, most of these studies used unrealistically high doses that would be difficult to get from taking the juice itself. There have been no human trials of noni.

DOSAGE

Commercial products that contain noni juice or a juice concentrate are widely available and heavily promoted. These preparations have either eliminated the odor or altered the taste to make it more palatable. Tablets and capsules of the fruit and of the whole plant are also available.

The usual recommendation is the equivalent of four ounces of noni juice one half-hour before breakfast. For liquid concentrates, the typical recommendation is 2 tablespoons daily, and for powdered extracts, 500 to 1,000 mg daily.

According to noni promoters, it should be taken on an empty stomach and not together with coffee, tobacco, or alcohol.[7] However, there is no scientific evidence for this recommendation.

SAFETY ISSUES

There are no known side effects of noni, but no safety studies have been performed. Due to the lack of evidence, use of noni by pregnant or nursing women or individuals with severe liver or kidney disease is not recommended.

OCTACOSANOL

Supplement Forms/Alternate Names   1-Octacosanol, N-Octacosanol, Octacosyl Alcohol, Policosanol, Wheat Germ Oil

Principal Proposed Uses   High Cholesterol

Other Proposed Uses   Performance Enhancement, Parkinson's Disease

Octacosanol is a naturally occurring waxy substance extracted from wheat germ oil; policosanol is a mixture of related substances that includes octacosanol, manufactured from sugar cane. Both are marketed as **performance-enhancing dietary supplements** (see page 158). They are said to increase muscle strength and endurance and improve reaction time and stamina, but there is no reliable scientific evidence as yet to support these claims. However, a substantial amount of research, most of it from Cuba, suggests that policosanol can help to lower elevated cholesterol levels.

REQUIREMENTS/SOURCES

Octacosanol and related substances are primarily produced from wheat germ oil; they are also found in vegetable oils, **alfalfa** (see page 202), and various animal products.[1,2]

THERAPEUTIC DOSAGES

Typical dosages of policosanol to lower elevated cholesterol levels range from 5 to 10 mg twice daily. Results may require 2 months to develop.[3,4]

THERAPEUTIC USES

Reasonably good evidence tells us that policosanol can significantly improve **cholesterol** (see page 88) levels.[5-14]

The only evidence for octacosanol as a performance enhancer comes from one small double-blind trial with marginal results.[15]

Marginal benefits were also seen in a very small double-blind trial of individuals with **Parkinson's disease** (see page 140).[16]

In a small double-blind trial, octacosanol failed to produce any benefits in amyotrophic lateral sclerosis.[17]

WHAT IS THE SCIENTIFIC EVIDENCE FOR OCTACOSANOL?

Elevated Cholesterol

Octacosanol appears to slow down cholesterol synthesis in the liver and also to increase liver reabsorption of LDL ("bad") cholesterol.[18,19]

Ten double-blind placebo-controlled studies, involving a total of more than 400 individuals and ranging in length from 6 weeks to 12 months, have found policosanol effective for improving cholesterol levels.[20-29] The results suggest that policosanol treatment can reduce total cholesterol and LDL ("bad") cholesterol by about 20%. Some studies found improvements in HDL ("good") cholesterol, but most did not. Interestingly, nine out of ten of these studies enrolled only individuals whose cholesterol levels had not previously improved with diet alone.

In one of the best of these double-blind studies, 74 men and women with elevated cholesterol were given policosanol or placebo for a total of 12 months.[30] The results in the treated group showed improvements in total cholesterol by 17%, LDL cholesterol by 26%, and HDL cholesterol by 14%, a significantly better result than was seen in the placebo group.

One study found policosanol to be safe and effective for reducing cholesterol levels in individuals with type 2 (adult-onset) diabetes.[31] However, individuals with any form of diabetes should seek medical advice before taking policosanol.

SAFETY ISSUES

Policosanol appears to be safe at the maximum recommended dose. A few side effects were observed in clinical trials using octacosanol or policosanol. These effects were short-term and mild, and mainly included nervousness, headache, diarrhea, and insomnia.[32]

No toxic signs were observed in animals given very high doses of policosanol (as much as 620 times the maximum recommended dose).[33-36]

Policosanol has been found not to interact with three types of medications used for high blood pressure: calcium-channel antagonists, diuretics, and beta-blockers.[37] Octacosanol might interact unfavorably with the medication levodopa, used for Parkinson's disease. There is no evidence to date that octacosanol or policosanol interacts with any other medications. However, for theoretical reasons, these supplements should not be combined with standard cholesterol-lowering medications except on the advice of a physician.

The maximum safe dosages for young children or pregnant or nursing women have not been established.

Octacosanol

Visit Us at TNP.com

OPCs (Oligomeric Proanthocyanidins)

Supplement Forms/Alternate Names   Procyanidolic Oligomers (PCOs), Grape Seed Extract, Pine Bark Extract

Principal Proposed Uses
Strengthening Blood Vessels/Reducing Inflammation: Varicose Veins, Hemorrhoids, Edema (Swelling) Following Injury, Edema (Swelling) Following Surgery, Easy Bruising

Other Proposed Uses   Aging Skin, Cancer Prevention, Diabetic Neuropathy, Diabetic Retinopathy, Atherosclerosis Prevention, Macular Degeneration, Allergies, Impaired Night Vision, Liver Cirrhosis

One of the bestselling herbal products of the early 1990s was an extract of the bark of French maritime pine. This substance consists of a family of chemicals known scientifically as oligomeric proanthocyanidin complexes (OPCs) or procyanidolic oligomers (PCOs). Similar substances are also found in grape seed.

The modern use of OPCs is closely linked to an event in 1534, when a French explorer and his crew were trapped by ice in the Saint Lawrence River. Many of the men were saved from scurvy by a Native American who suggested they make tea from the needles and bark of a local pine tree. Over 400 years later, Jacques Masquelier of the University of Bordeaux came across this story and decided to investigate the constituents of pine trees. In 1951, he extracted OPCs from the bark of the maritime pine and found that they could duplicate many of the functions of vitamin C. Later, he found an even better source of OPCs in grape seed, which is their major source in France today.

Like the anthocyanosides found in **bilberry** (to which they are closely related; see page 220), OPCs appear to stabilize the walls of blood vessels, reduce inflammation, and generally support tissues containing collagen and elastin.[1–4] OPCs are also strong antioxidants. Vitamin E defends against fat-soluble oxidants and vitamin C neutralizes water-soluble ones, but OPCs are active against both types.[5,6,7]

Evidence suggests that OPCs can reduce the discomfort and swelling of varicose veins and decrease the edema (swelling) that often follows injury or surgery. On the basis of much weaker evidence, OPCs are also popular for preventing heart disease, revitalizing aging skin, and reducing the tendency toward easy bruising.

SOURCES

Like other flavonoids, OPCs aren't necessary for life, although they may prove to be important for optimal health.

OPCs aren't a single chemical, but a group of closely related compounds. Several food sources contain similar chemicals: red wine, cranberries, blueberries, bilberries, tea (green and black), black currant, onions, legumes, parsley, and the herb hawthorn. However, most OPC supplements are made from either grape seed or the bark of the maritime pine. Grape seed is the preferred source in France, where this supplement was originally popularized, and is a more economical source than pine bark.

THERAPEUTIC DOSAGES

For use as a general antioxidant—much as you might use **vitamin E** or **vitamin C** (see the chapters on vitamins E and C)—50 mg of OPCs daily are sufficient. A higher dosage of 150 to 300 mg daily is generally used for treating specific diseases such as varicose veins. Grape seed OPCs are just as good and much less expensive than the maritime pine source.

THERAPEUTIC USES

The best-documented use of OPCs is to treat venous insufficiency, a condition closely related to **varicose veins** (see page 184). It refers to the situation when blood pools in the legs, causing aching, pain, heaviness, swelling, fatigue, and unsightly visible veins. Fairly good preliminary evidence suggests that OPCs can relieve the pain and swelling of venous insufficiency.[8–11] OPCs probably cannot make visible varicose veins disappear, but regular use might help prevent new ones from developing. Other approaches to varicose veins include **horse chestnut** (see page 325), **gotu kola** (see page 315), and **bromelain** (see page 229). On the basis of their evidence for varicose veins, OPCs are often recommended as a treatment for hemorrhoids as well.

There is also some evidence that OPCs can be useful for the swelling that often follows **injuries** (see page 101) or **surgery** (see page 173).[12,13,14] OPCs appear to speed the disappearance of swelling, presumably by strengthening damaged blood and lymph vessels that are leaking fluid.

For similar reasons, OPCs may also be helpful for people who bruise easily due to fragile blood vessels.[15,16] **Note:** Keep in mind that there may be medical causes for **easy bruising** (see page 74) that require more specific treatment.

OPCs in cream form are a popular treatment for aging skin, on the theory that by repairing elastin and collagen they will return skin to a more youthful appearance. However, there is no solid evidence as yet that they are effective for this purpose.

On the basis of preliminary evidence, regular use of OPCs has been proposed as a measure to prevent **cancer** (see page 32), diabetic neuropathy and diabetic retinopathy (side effects of **diabetes**; see page 65), **heart disease** (see page 16), **macular degeneration** (the major cause of age-related blindness; see page 115), as well as a treatment for **allergies** (hay fever; see page 2), **impaired night vision** (see page 128), and **liver cirrhosis** (see page 112). However, much more research needs to be performed to discover whether these potential benefits are real.

WHAT IS THE SCIENTIFIC EVIDENCE FOR OPCs?

Considerable evidence tells us that OPCs protect and strengthen collagen and elastin—proteins found in cartilage, tendons, blood vessels, and muscle.[17–22] There is also no question that OPCs are strong antioxidants, more powerful than either vitamin E or vitamin C by some measures.[23] The medicinal effects of OPCs are believed to be due to some combination of these properties.

Venous Insufficiency (Varicose Veins)

There is fairly good preliminary evidence for the use of OPCs to treat people with symptoms of venous insufficiency.

A double-blind placebo-controlled study of 71 subjects found that grape seed OPCs, taken at a dose of 100 mg 3 times daily, significantly improved major symptoms, including heaviness, swelling, and leg discomfort.[24] Over a period of 1 month, 75% of the participants treated with OPCs improved substantially. This result doesn't seem quite so impressive when you note that significant improvement was also seen in 41% of the placebo group; nonetheless, OPCs still did significantly better than placebo.

A 2-month double-blind placebo-controlled trial of 40 individuals with chronic venous insufficiency found that 100 mg 3 times daily of pine bark OPCs significantly reduced edema, pain, and the sensation of leg heaviness.[25]

A placebo-controlled study (blinding not stated) that enrolled 364 individuals with varicose veins found that treatment with OPCs produced statistically significant improvements as compared to baseline.[26] There was a lesser response in the placebo group, but whether this difference was statistically significant was not stated.

Finally, a double-blind study of 50 people with varicose veins of the legs found that doses of 150 mg per day of OPCs were more effective in reducing symptoms and signs than another natural treatment: the bioflavonoid diosmin, widely used in Europe for this condition.[27]

Edema After Surgery or Injury

Breast cancer surgery often leads to swelling of the arm. A double-blind placebo-controlled study of 63 post-operative breast cancer patients found that 600 mg of OPCs daily for 6 months reduced edema, pain, and peculiar sensations known as paresthesias.[28] Also, in a double-blind placebo-controlled study of 32 "face-lift" patients who were followed for 10 days, edema disappeared much faster in the treated group.[29]

Another 10-day double-blind placebo-controlled study enrolling 50 participants found that OPCs improved the rate at which edema disappeared following sports injuries.[30]

Night Vision

One interesting 6-week controlled (but not blinded) study evaluated the ability of grape seed OPCs to improve night vision in normal subjects.[31,32] In this trial of 100 healthy volunteers, those who received 200 mg per day of OPCs showed improvements in night vision and glare recovery as compared to untreated subjects.

Atherosclerosis

Although there are no reliable human studies, animal evidence suggests that OPCs can slow or reverse atherosclerosis.[33–36] This suggests (but definitely does not prove) that OPCs might be helpful for preventing heart disease.

SAFETY ISSUES

OPCs have been extensively tested for safety and are generally considered to be essentially nontoxic.[37] Side effects are rare, but when they do occur they are limited to occasional allergic reactions and mild digestive distress. However, maximum safe dosages for young children, pregnant or nursing women, or those with severe liver or kidney disease have not been established.

OPCs may have some anticoagulant properties when taken in high doses, and should be used only under medical supervision by individuals on blood-thinner drugs, such as Coumadin (warfarin) and heparin.

⚠ INTERACTIONS YOU SHOULD KNOW ABOUT

If you are taking **Coumadin (warfarin), heparin, Trental (pentoxifylline),** or **aspirin,** high doses of OPCs might cause a risk of excessive bleeding.

OREGON GRAPE (*Mahonia aquifolium, Berberis aquifolium*)

Alternate or Related Names   Mountain Grape, Holly-Leaved Berberis

Principal Proposed Uses   Psoriasis

Other Proposed Uses   Fungal Infections, Eczema, Acne

The roots and bark of the shrub *Mahonia aquifolium* (also called Oregon grape) have traditionally been used both orally and topically to treat skin problems. They were also used for other conditions such as gastritis, fever, hemorrhage, jaundice, gall bladder disease, and cancer. In addition, *Mahonia* was used as a bitter tonic to improve appetite.

There is considerable inconsistency about the correct name of this plant. According to some experts, *M. aquifolium* is identical to *Berberis aquifolium*, but others point to small distinctions. *Berberis vulgaris*, commonly called barberry, is a close relative of these herbs, but is not identical.

WHAT IS OREGON GRAPE USED FOR TODAY?

Mahonia is primarily used today as a topical treatment for **psoriasis** (see page 148). Preliminary evidence suggests that it may help reduce symptoms, although it does not seem to be as effective as standard medications.[1,2,3]

Mahonia has been proposed as a treatment for other skin diseases, such as fungal infections, **eczema** (see page 78), and **acne** (see page 2).[4,5,6] However, the evidence is extremely preliminary, and human trials must be conducted before we will know whether the herb is really effective for any of these conditions.

Many studies have been performed on purified berberine, a major chemical constituent of *Mahonia* and other herbs such as goldenseal, but it is not clear whether their results apply to the whole herb. In addition, impossibly high dosages of herb would be required to duplicate the amount of berberine used in many of these studies (for more information, see the chapter on **goldenseal**).

WHAT IS THE SCIENTIFIC EVIDENCE FOR OREGON GRAPE?

A double-blind placebo-controlled study involving 82 people with psoriasis tested the effectiveness of topical application of *Mahonia*.[7] Participants used a placebo ointment on one side of their bodies and *Mahonia* on the other. According to the participants' assessments, the *Mahonia* ointment produced significantly better results.

However, the physicians did not observe significant differences between the two. One possible design flaw was that the treatment salve was darker in color than the placebo, possibly allowing participants to guess which was which.

Another study found that dithranol, a conventional drug used to treat psoriasis symptoms, was more effective than *Mahonia*.[8] Regrettably, the authors fail to state whether this study was double-blind. Forty-nine participants applied one treatment to their left side and the other to their right for 4 weeks. Skin biopsies were then analyzed and compared with samples taken at the beginning of the study. The physicians evaluating changes in skin tissue were unaware which treatments had been used on the samples. Greater improvements were seen in the dithranol group.

A large open study in which 443 participants with psoriasis used *Mahonia* topically for 12 weeks found the herb to be helpful for 73.7% of the group.[9] Without a placebo group, it's not possible to know whether *Mahonia* was truly responsible for the improvement seen, but the trial does help to establish the herb's safety and tolerability (see Safety Issues below).

Laboratory research suggests *Mahonia* has some effects at the cellular level that might be helpful in psoriasis, such as slowing the rate of abnormal cell growth and reducing inflammation.[10,11]

DOSAGE

Topical ointments or creams containing 10% *Mahonia* extract are generally applied 3 times daily to the affected areas.

SAFETY ISSUES

Mahonia appears to be safe when used as directed. In the large open study described above, only 5 of the 443 participants reported side effects of burning, redness, and itching.[12]

However, because *Mahonia* contains berberine, which has been reported to cause uterine contractions and to increase levels of bilirubin, oral consumption of *Mahonia* should be avoided by pregnant women.[13,14] Safety in young children, nursing women, or people with severe liver or kidney disease has not been established.

Ornithine Alpha-Ketoglutarate

ORNITHINE ALPHA-KETOGLUTARATE

Principal Proposed Uses   Recovery From Severe Injury
Other Proposed Uses   Performance Enhancement

Ornithine alpha-ketoglutarate (OKG) is manufactured from two amino acids, ornithine and glutamine. OKG is not found in food, although its two building blocks are.

There is some evidence that ornithine may aid in the treatment of individuals recovering from severe physical injury. OKG has also been suggested as an aid to athletes in training.

SOURCES

The amino acids that make up OKG are found in high-protein foods such as meat, fish, and dairy, but OKG itself is not found in foods. Supplements are available in tablet or pill form.

THERAPEUTIC DOSAGES

Athletes have taken up to 35 g daily of OKG.

THERAPEUTIC USES

Ornithine may have a role in the treatment of individuals recovering from severe physical trauma.

When the body experiences severe trauma—such as **injury** (see page 101), **surgery** (see page 173), or **burns** (see page 123)—it goes into what is called a *catabolic*

state. In this condition, the body goes through a period in which it tends to tear itself down rather than build itself up. This is seen in an overall loss of protein and a poor ability to heal.

The opposite of a catabolic state is an *anabolic state,* in which the body tends to build itself up. Ornithine supplementation may help the body make the switch. In a double-blind placebo-controlled trial of 60 individuals who had suffered extensive burns, treatment with ornithine improved protein balance and speeded up the healing process.[1]

Based on studies like these, OKG has become popular among athletes in the hope that, like anabolic steroids, it will increase their muscle development in training. However, there is practically no foundation for this belief, other than two rather theoretical studies in rats.[2,3]

SAFETY ISSUES

OKG appears to be safe. However, as with all supplements used in multigram doses, it is important to purchase a reputable product, because a contaminant present even in small percentages could add up to a real problem. The maximum safe dosages for young children, women who are pregnant or nursing, or those with serious liver or kidney disease have not been established.

OSHA (*Ligusticum porteri*)

Principal Proposed Uses   Cough, Respiratory Infections, Digestive Disorders

Native to high altitudes in the Southwest and Rocky Mountain states, the root of the osha plant is a traditional Native American remedy for respiratory infections and digestive problems. A related plant, *Ligusticum wallichii,* has a long history of use in Chinese medicine, and most of the scientific studies on osha were actually performed on this species.

WHAT IS OSHA USED FOR TODAY?

Osha is frequently recommended for use at the first sign of a respiratory infection. Like a sauna, it will typically

induce sweating, and according to folk wisdom this may help avert the development of a full-blown **cold** (see page 47). Osha is also taken during respiratory infections as a cough suppressant and expectorant, hence the common name "Colorado cough root."

Although there have not been any double-blind studies to verify these proposed uses, Chinese research suggests that *Ligusticum wallichii* can relax smooth muscle tissue (perhaps thereby moderating the cough reflex) and inhibit the growth of various bacteria.[1] Whether these findings apply to osha as well is unknown.

Like other bitter herbs, osha also tends to improve symptoms of indigestion and increase appetite.

DOSAGE

Osha products vary in their concentration and should be taken according to directions on the label.

SAFETY ISSUES

Osha is believed to be safe, although the scientific record is far from complete. Traditionally, it is not recommended for use in pregnancy. Safety in young children, nursing women, or those with severe liver or kidney disease has also not been established.

One potential risk with osha is contamination with hemlock parsley, a deadly plant with a similar appearance.[2]

OXERUTINS

Supplement Forms/Alternate Names   Hydroxyethylrutosides (HERs), Troxerutin

Principal Proposed Uses   Varicose Veins, Venous Insufficiency, Hemorrhoids

Other Proposed Uses   Lymphedema, Postsurgical Edema, Vertigo, Lower-Leg Edema in People with Diabetes

Oxerutins have been widely used in Europe since the mid-1960s, primarily as a treatment for varicose veins, but this supplement remains hard to find in North America. Oxerutins are not a single substance, but a group of chemicals derived from a naturally occurring bioflavonoid called rutin. It is not clear whether this particular derivative of rutin is more effective than the many other bioflavonoid-based therapies believed to be effective for these conditions, but oxerutins are by far the best studied. Numerous experiments have found them to improve symptoms of varicose veins such as aching, swelling, and fatigue.

Oxerutins appear to strengthen the capillaries, tiny blood vessels that deliver oxygen and energy to every cell of the body. In people with **varicose veins** (see page 184), capillaries are under increased pressure, causing them to leak fluid and molecules of protein. The result is swelling (edema), pain, and fatigue in the lower legs. Oxerutins have been found to reduce these symptoms, probably by making the capillaries less permeable.

REQUIREMENTS/SOURCES

Although they are closely related to a natural flavonoid, oxerutins are not found in food. The only way to take them is in a supplement.

THERAPEUTIC DOSAGES

For varicose veins, oxerutins are usually taken in dosages ranging from 900 mg to 1,200 mg daily. A typical dosage is 1,000 mg daily, taken in two separate doses of 500 mg.

For treating lymphedema and postsurgical edema, a typical dosage is a good deal higher: 3,000 mg daily.

One particular oxerutin called troxerutin may be taken alone as a treatment for varicose veins, in similar dosages. There is no evidence as yet that rutin itself is effective.

THERAPEUTIC USES

"Varicose" means "enlarged" or "distended." A varicose vein is abnormally enlarged, allowing blood to pool and stagnate instead of moving it efficiently toward the heart. Surface veins of the leg are those most vulnerable to becoming varicose. **Venous insufficiency** (see page 184) is a closely related condition affecting larger veins deep within the leg. In either case, blood pools within the vein and exerts pressure against the vein walls and capillaries, resulting in pain, aching, swelling, and feelings of heaviness and fatigue. In addition, varicose veins present a cosmetic problem: bulging, often ropy, blue or purple lines visible on the skin of the lower legs.

Strong evidence shows that oxerutins can be helpful for these conditions, improving aching, swelling, and fatigue in the legs.[1-15]

Mixed evidence suggests that oxerutins might also be helpful for the leg ulcers that can develop in venous insufficiency.[16,17,18] There is no evidence as yet that oxerutins can improve the cosmetic appearance of varicose veins.

Oxerutins have also been found safe and effective for treating varicose veins when they occur during pregnancy.[19,20]

Hemorrhoids (see page 85) are a special type of varicose vein, and oxerutins may be helpful for treating them as well, although there have been some negative studies.[21,22]

Oxerutins

Some evidence suggests that oxerutins may be helpful for lymphedema (chronic arm swelling caused by damage to the lymph drainage system) following **surgery** (see page 173) for breast cancer,[23,24,25] as well as for **edema** (see page 173) in the immediate postsurgical period.[26]

One small double-blind study suggests oxerutins may be helpful for reducing **vertigo** (see page 188) and other symptoms of Meniere's disease.[27]

Preliminary evidence suggests that oxerutins might also be helpful for reducing foot and ankle swelling in people with diabetes.[28] In these trials, oxerutin therapy did not affect blood sugar control.

WHAT IS THE SCIENTIFIC EVIDENCE FOR OXERUTINS?

Varicose Veins/Venous Insufficiency

At least 17 double-blind placebo-controlled studies, enrolling a total of more than 2,000 participants, have examined oxerutins' effectiveness for treating varicose veins and venous insufficiency. All but one found oxerutins significantly more effective than placebo, giving substantial relief from swelling, aching, leg pains, and other uncomfortable symptoms, while causing no significant side effects. Together, this research makes a strong case for the use of oxerutins in these conditions.

For example, one large placebo-controlled double-blind study published in 1983 enrolled 660 people with symptoms of venous insufficiency.[29] Three out of four participants were randomly assigned to receive oxerutins (1,000 mg daily) while one out of four was given placebo. After 4 weeks of treatment, those who took oxerutins reported less heaviness, aching, cramps, and "restless leg" or "pins and needles" symptoms than those who took placebo. According to the researchers' calculations, oxerutins had produced significantly better results than placebo. This report has been criticized, however, for omitting key information (such as whether or not any participants also wore support stockings) and for failing to present data in a usable form.

A more recent, better-designed study supported these positive findings.[30] This 12-week double-blind placebo-controlled study enrolled 133 women with moderate chronic venous insufficiency. Half received 1,000 mg oxerutins daily, and the rest took a matching placebo. All participants were also fitted with standard compression stockings, and wore them for the duration of the study. The researchers measured subjective symptoms such as aches and pains, as well as objective measures of edema in the leg.

Those who took oxerutins had significantly less lower-leg edema than the placebo group. Furthermore, these results lasted through a 6-week follow-up period, even though participants were no longer taking oxerutins.

Compression stockings, on the other hand, produced no lasting benefit after participants stopped wearing them. They gave symptomatic relief while they were worn, but they didn't improve capillary circulation in a lasting way, as oxerutins apparently did.

Regarding aching, sensations of heaviness, and other uncomfortable symptoms, however, there was little difference between the two groups. The authors theorized that the compression stockings gave both groups so much symptomatic relief that it was difficult to demonstrate a separate subjective benefit of oxerutin therapy.

Several other double-blind placebo-controlled studies have also found benefits with oxerutins for varicose veins and venous insufficiency.[31–40]

As mentioned above, there is some evidence that troxerutin—one of the compounds in the standardized mixture sold as oxerutins—may be effective when taken alone. One study found it more effective than placebo,[41] but another (very small) study found it less effective than the standard oxerutin mixture.[42]

Pregnant women are at especially high risk for varicose veins and venous insufficiency. A 1975 study examined 69 pregnant women with varicose leg veins, and found that oxerutins (900 mg daily) were significantly more effective than placebo against pain as well as swelling.[43] A more recent study also found positive results,[44] but because it was neither placebo-controlled nor double-blind its results mean little.

Skin ulcers sometimes form on the legs of people with varicose veins or venous insufficiency, when capillary circulation has become too impaired to keep the skin healthy. A French study published in 1987 found that oxerutins combined with compression stockings were significantly more helpful for leg ulcers than the stockings alone.[45] Other positive results have been reported as well.[46]

However, some experiments found oxerutins to have no benefit in treating or preventing leg ulcers.[47,48] Until more research is done, the most we can say is that oxerutins *might* be helpful for leg ulcers—especially if combined with compression stockings.

Hemorrhoids

Some evidence suggests that oxerutins might be helpful for hemorrhoids as well. A double-blind study enrolling 97 pregnant women found oxerutins (1,000 mg daily) significantly better than placebo in reducing the pain, bleeding, and inflammation of hemorrhoids.[49]

Lymphedema

Women who have undergone surgery for breast cancer may experience a lasting and troublesome side effect: swelling in the arm caused by damage to the lymph system. Along with the veins, the lymph system is responsible for returning fluid to the heart, but when the system is damaged, fluid can accumulate. Three double-blind placebo-controlled studies enrolling more than 100 people total have examined the effectiveness of oxerutins in this condition.[50,51,52]

In one trial, oxerutins worked significantly better than placebo at reducing swelling, discomfort, immobility, and other measures of lymphedema over a 6-month treatment period, with better results appearing each month[53]—suggesting that, for women with this condition, the full effect of oxerutins might take months to realize.

Two smaller studies also found oxerutins to be more effective than placebo, but the researchers were not sure that the improvement was large enough to make a real difference.[54,55]

In all of these studies, the dosage used was 3 g daily—about 3 times the typical dosage for venous insufficiency.

Post-Surgical Edema

Swelling often occurs in the recovery period following surgery. In one double-blind trial, researchers gave oxerutins or placebo for 5 days to 40 people recovering from minor surgery or other minor injuries, and found it significantly helpful in reducing swelling and discomfort.[56]

SAFETY ISSUES

Oxerutins appear to be safe and well tolerated. In most studies, oxerutins have produced no more side effects than placebo. For example, in a study of 104 elderly people with venous insufficiency, 26 participants taking oxerutins reported adverse events, compared with 25 in the placebo group.[57] The most commonly observed side effects were gastrointestinal symptoms, headaches, and dizziness.[58]

Oxerutins have been given to pregnant women in some studies, with no apparent harmful effects. However, their safety for pregnant or nursing women cannot be regarded as absolutely proven. In addition, the safety of oxerutins has not been established for people with severe liver or kidney disease.

PABA (Para-Aminobenzoic Acid)

Principal Proposed Uses   There are no well-documented uses for PABA.

Other Proposed Uses   Scleroderma, Peyronie's Disease, Male Infertility, Vitiligo

Para-aminobenzoic acid (PABA) is best known as the active ingredient in sunblock. This use of PABA is not really medicinal: like a pair of sunglasses, PABA physically blocks ultraviolet rays when it is applied to the skin.

There are, however, some proposed medicinal uses of oral PABA supplements. PABA is sometimes suggested as a treatment for various diseases of the skin and connective tissue, as well as for male infertility. However, most of the clinical data on PABA comes from very old studies, some from the early 1940s.

SOURCES

PABA is not believed to be an essential nutrient. Nonetheless, it is found in foods, mainly in grains and meat. Small amounts of PABA are usually present in B vitamin supplements as well as in some multiple vitamins.

THERAPEUTIC DOSAGES

A typical therapeutic dosage of PABA is 300 to 400 mg daily. Some studies have used much higher dosages. However, serious side effects have been found in dosages above 8 g daily (see Safety Issues). You probably shouldn't take more than 400 mg daily except on medical advice.

THERAPEUTIC USES

PABA has been suggested as a treatment for scleroderma, a disease that creates fibrous tissue in the skin and internal organs.[1,2] However, a small double-blind study found it ineffective.[3]

PABA has also been suggested for other diseases in which abnormal fibrous tissue is involved, such as Peyronie's disease, a condition in which the penis becomes bent owing to the accumulation of such tissue.[4,5,6] However, no double-blind studies have yet been performed.

Based on one small World War II–era study, PABA has been suggested for treating **male infertility** (see page 116) as well as vitiligo, a condition in which patches of skin lose their pigment, resulting in pale blotches. However, this study didn't have a control group, so its results aren't meaningful.[7] Ironically, a recent study suggests that high dosages of PABA can *cause* vitiligo (see Safety Issues).

SAFETY ISSUES

PABA is probably safe when taken at a dosage up to 400 mg daily. Possible side effects at this dosage are minor, including skin rash and loss of appetite.[8]

Higher doses are a different story, however. There has been one reported case of severe liver toxicity in a woman taking 12 g daily of PABA.[9] Fortunately, her liver recovered completely after she discontinued her use of this supplement. Also, a recent study suggests that 8 g daily of PABA can cause vitiligo, the patchy skin disease described previously.[10]

Clearly, there are questions that need to be answered about the safety of high-dose PABA therapy. You shouldn't take more than 400 mg daily except under medical supervision.

PABA can interfere with certain medications, including sulfa antibiotics.[11,12]

Safety in young children, pregnant or nursing women, or those with serious liver or kidney disease has not been determined.

⚠ INTERACTIONS YOU SHOULD KNOW ABOUT

If you are taking **sulfa antibiotics** such as **Bactrim** or **Septra,** do not take PABA supplements except on medical advice.

PANTOTHENIC ACID AND PANTETHINE

Principal Proposed Uses   High Triglycerides/High Cholesterol

Other Proposed Uses   Rheumatoid Arthritis, Performance Enhancement, Stress

Note: Pantothenic acid is often sold as calcium pantothenate. Pantethine, a special form of pantothenic acid, appears to have some unique properties. Regular pantothenic acid cannot be used as a substitute for pantethine.

The body uses pantothenic acid (better known as vitamin B_5) to make proteins as well as other important chemicals needed to metabolize fats and carbohydrates. Pantothenic acid is also used in the manufacture of hormones, red blood cells, and *acetylcholine,* an important neurotransmitter (signal carrier between nerve cells). As a supplement, pantothenic acid has been proposed as a treatment for rheumatoid arthritis, an athletic performance enhancer, and an "antistress" nutrient.

In the body, pantothenic acid is converted to a related chemical known as pantethine. For reasons that are not clear, pantethine supplements (but not pantothenic acid supplements) appear to reduce levels of both triglycerides and cholesterol in the blood.

The supplement niacin, also called **vitamin B_3** (see page 437), is generally more effective at lowering cholesterol than pantethine and far cheaper as well. However, whereas niacin can inflame the liver, pantethine has not been associated with this side effect.

REQUIREMENTS/SOURCES

The word *pantothenic* comes from the Greek word meaning "everywhere," and pantothenic acid is indeed found in a wide range of foods. For this reason, pantothenic acid deficiency is rare. The official U.S. and Canadian recommendations for daily intake of pantothenic acid are as follows:

- Infants 0–5 months, 1.7 mg
    6–11 months, 1.8 mg
- Children 1–3 years, 2 mg
    4–8 years, 3 mg
    9–13 years, 4 mg
- Males and females 14 years and older, 4 mg
- Pregnant women, 6 mg
- Nursing women, 7 mg

Brewer's yeast, torula (nutritional) yeast, and calf liver are excellent sources of pantothenic acid. Peanuts, mushrooms, soybeans, split peas, pecans, oatmeal, buckwheat, sunflower seeds, lentils, rye flour, cashews, and other whole grains and nuts are good sources as well, as are red chili peppers and avocados. Pantethine is not found in foods in appreciable amounts.

THERAPEUTIC DOSAGES

For lowering cholesterol and triglycerides, the typical recommended dosage of pantethine is 300 mg 3 times daily. Dosages of pantothenic acid as high as 660 mg 3 times daily are sometimes recommended for people with arthritis.

THERAPEUTIC USES

Quite a few small studies suggest that pantethine may lower blood levels of triglycerides and, to a lesser extent,

cholesterol (see page 88).[1,2,3] In general, elevated cholesterol is more harmful than elevated triglycerides. However, some people have only modestly elevated cholesterol but very high triglycerides, so pantethine may be especially useful for them. It also may be helpful for people with diabetes who need to lower their triglyceride and/or cholesterol levels.[4–7]

Pantothenic acid has been proposed as a treatment for **rheumatoid arthritis** (see page 151), but the evidence for this use is quite weak.[8,9]

Pantothenic acid is also recommended as an athletic **performance enhancer** (see page 158), but there is no good evidence at all that it works. It is also sometimes referred to as an antistress nutrient because it plays a role in the function of the adrenal glands, but whether it really helps the body withstand stress is not known.

WHAT IS THE SCIENTIFIC EVIDENCE FOR PANTOTHENIC ACID AND PANTETHINE?

High Triglycerides/High Cholesterol

Several small studies suggest (but do not prove) that pantethine can reduce total blood triglycerides and perhaps cholesterol as well.[10,11,12] For example, a double-blind placebo-controlled study followed 29 people with high cholesterol and triglycerides for 8 weeks.[13] The dosage used was 300 mg 3 times daily, for a total daily dose of 900 mg. In this study, subjects taking pantethine experienced a 30% reduction in blood triglycerides, a 13.5% reduction in LDL ("bad") cholesterol, and a 10% rise in HDL ("good") cholesterol. However, for reasons that are unclear, some studies have found no benefit.[14,15]

Several open studies have specifically studied the use of pantethine to improve cholesterol and triglyceride levels in people with diabetes and found it effective.[16–19]

These findings are supported by experiments in rabbits, which show that pantethine may prevent the buildup of plaque in major arteries.[20] We don't know how pantethine works in the body.

Rheumatoid Arthritis

There is weak evidence for using pantothenic acid to treat rheumatoid arthritis. One observational study found 66 people with rheumatoid arthritis had less pantothenic acid in their blood than 29 healthy people. The more severe the arthritis, the lower the blood levels of pantothenic acid were.[21] However, this result doesn't prove that pantothenic acid supplements can effectively reduce any of the symptoms of rheumatoid arthritis.

To follow up on this finding, researchers then conducted a small placebo-controlled trial involving 18 subjects to see whether pantothenic acid would help. This study found that 2 g daily of pantothenic acid (in the form of calcium pantothenate) reduced morning stiffness, pain, and disability significantly better than placebo.[22] However, a study this small doesn't mean much on its own. More research is needed.

SAFETY ISSUES

No significant side effects have been reported for pantothenic acid or pantethine, used by themselves or with other medications. However, maximum safe dosages for young children, pregnant or nursing women, or people with serious liver or kidney disease have not been established.

PARSLEY (*Petroselinum crispum, Petroselinum hartense, Petroselinum sativum*)

Alternate or Related Names   Hamburg Parsley, Persely, Petersylinge, Rock Parsley

Principal Proposed Uses   There are no well-documented uses for parsley.

Other Proposed Uses   Flatulence, Indigestion/Colic, Amenorrhea, Abortifacant, Topical Antibiotic

Parsley is a culinary herb used in many types of cooking and as a nearly universal adornment to restaurant food. Originally a native plant of the Mediterranean region, parsley is grown today throughout the world. It is a nutritious food, providing dietary **calcium** (see page 234), **iron** (see page 333), carotenes, **ascorbic acid** (see page 444), and **vitamin A** (see page 432).[1]

Parsley's traditional use for inducing menstruation may be explained by evidence that apiol and myristicin, two substances contained in parsley, stimulate contractions of the uterus.[2,3] Indeed, extracted apiol has been tried for the purpose of causing abortions (see Safety Issues below).

A tea made from the "fruits" or seeds of parsley is also a traditional remedy for **colic** (see page 53), indigestion, and intestinal gas.[4,5]

Parsley

Visit Us at TNP.com

WHAT IS PARSLEY USED FOR TODAY?

Germany's Commission E suggests the use of parsley leaf or root to relieve irritation of the urinary tract and to aid in passing **kidney stones** (see page 109).[6] Although there is no evidence that parsley is helpful for these conditions, two of its constituents, apiol and myristicin, are believed to be diuretics;[7,8,9] because diuretics would increase the flow of urine, this might help the body to wash out bacteria as well as stones. However, no studies have as yet evaluated whether parsley is actually beneficial for either health problem.

A test tube study evaluated parsley extract as a topical antibiotic, finding that the extract had a weak effect against *Staphylococcus* bacteria.[10] However, it did not appear to be strong enough to be practically useful for this purpose.

DOSAGE

The usual dose of parsley leaf or root is 6 g of dried plant per day, consumed in 3 doses of 2 g, each steeped in 150 ml of water. Extract of parsley leaf and root are made at a ratio of 1 g of plant to 1 ml of liquid, and used at a dose of 2 ml 3 times daily. Tea made from parsley seeds is used at a lower dosage of 2 to 3 g per day, using 1 g of seed per cup of tea.[11,12]

SAFETY ISSUES

As a widely eaten food, parsley is generally regarded as safe. However, excessive quantities of parsley should be avoided during pregnancy, based on the evidence mentioned earlier that myristicin and apiol can stimulate the uterus.[13,14] Myristicin may also cross the placenta and increase the heart rate of the fetus.[15]

Parsley is known as a plant that can cause **photosensitivity** (see page 144), which is an increased tendency to **sunburn** (see page 171); this result, however, occurs from prolonged physical contact with the leaves, not from oral consumption of parsley.[16–19]

Maximum safe intake of parsley in young children, pregnant or nursing women, or people with severe liver or kidney disease has not been established.

PASSIONFLOWER (*Passiflora incarnata*)

Alternate or Related Names   Granadilla, Maypop, Passion Vine

Principal Proposed Uses   Anxiety, Insomnia, Nervous Stomach

The passionflower vine is a native of the Western hemisphere, named for symbolic connections drawn between its appearance and the crucifixion of Jesus. Native North Americans used passionflower primarily as a mild sedative. It quickly caught on as a folk remedy in Europe and was thereafter adopted by professional herbalists as a sedative and digestive aid.

WHAT IS PASSIONFLOWER USED FOR TODAY?

In 1985, Germany's Commission E officially approved passionflower as a treatment for "nervous unrest." The herb is considered to be a mildly effective treatment for **anxiety** (see page 11) and **insomnia** (see page 103), less potent than **kava** (see page 338) and **valerian** (see page 428), but nonetheless useful. Like **melissa** (lemon balm; see page 359), **chamomile** (see page 244), and **valerian** (see page 428), it is also used for nervous stomach.

Animal studies suggest that passionflower extracts can reduce agitation and prolong sleep.[1] There have been no controlled double-blind studies of passionflower in humans, except in combination with other herbs.[2]

Several constituents of passionflower have been credited with causing its sedative effect. However, none has been proven effective. At the current state of knowledge, the best we can say is that we don't yet know how the herb works.

DOSAGE

The proper dosage of passionflower is 1 cup 3 times daily of a tea made by steeping 1 teaspoon of dried leaves for 10 to 15 minutes. Passionflower tinctures and powdered extracts should be taken according to the label instructions.

SAFETY ISSUES

Passionflower is on the FDA's GRAS (generally recognized as safe) list.

The alkaloids harman and harmaline found in passionflower have been found to act somewhat like the drugs known as MAO inhibitors and also to stimulate the uterus,[3,4] but whether whole passionflower has these effects remains unknown. Passionflower might increase the action of sedative medications.[5,6,7] Finally, there are five case reports from Norway of individuals becoming temporarily mentally impaired from a combination herbal product containing passionflower.[8] It is not clear whether the other ingredients may have played a role.

Safety has not been established for pregnant or nursing mothers, very young children, or those with severe liver or kidney disease.

⚠ INTERACTIONS YOU SHOULD KNOW ABOUT

If you are taking **sedative medications,** passionflower might exaggerate their effect.

PC-SPES (*Isatis indigotica Fort, Glycyrrhiza glabra L, Panax pseudo-ginseng Wall, Ganoderma lucidium Karst, Scutellaria baicalensis Georgi, Dendranthema morifolium Tzvel, Robdosia rubescens, and Serenoa repens*)

Principal Proposed Uses   Prostate Cancer

PC-SPES is a formulation of eight herbs: seven are plants and one is a fungus. The name is derived from the common abbreviation for prostate cancer (PC) and the Latin word *spes* meaning hope. (Do not confuse it with a related herbal combination product simply called SPES, also under development as a possible cancer treatment.)

Since its commercial launch in 1996, PC-SPES has received increasing interest from the general public and prostate cancer researchers. Its constituents are believed to possess various pharmacological activities including immune stimulation, antitumor, antiviral, and anti-inflammatory properties. Seven of the herbs have long histories of use in traditional Chinese medicine; one of these, **saw palmetto** (see page 406), is widely recognized as an effective medical treatment for benign prostate enlargement.

Although no double-blind trials of PC-SPES have been reported, preliminary evidence suggests that it has significant effects on prostate cancer cells, perhaps due in part to its estrogen-like action.

WHAT IS PC-SPES USED FOR TODAY?

The only proposed use of PC-SPES is the treatment of prostate cancer. The formulation has been tried at various stages of the disease, and preliminary research indicates that it has real potential, particularly for treating prostate cancer that is no longer responsive to hormone therapies. Benefits have been reported in the two main types of prostate cancer: hormone-sensitive and hormone-insensitive cancer. Due to the absence of double-

blind trials, however, we cannot state at this time that PC-SPES is definitely effective.

Warning: Do not attempt to self-treat prostate cancer. Medical or surgical treatment may be life saving. PC-SPES has not been proven as effective as standard care.

WHAT IS THE SCIENTIFIC EVIDENCE FOR PC-SPES?

Test tube studies of cancer cells have found that PC-SPES decreases cell growth, promotes tumor cell death, and reduces PSA (prostate-specific antigen) levels in both hormone-sensitive and hormone-insensitive prostate cancers.[1–4]

In a rat study, PC-SPES treatment reduced the occurrence of prostate cancer tumors, inhibited their growth, and slowed the rate of cancer spread (metastasis) to the lungs.[5]

In one uncontrolled human study, PC-SPES produced a significant decrease in PSA levels for most of the 33 volunteers tested.[6]

An uncontrolled study of eight individuals with hormone-sensitive prostate cancer showed that PC-SPES decreased blood levels not only of PSA, but also of testosterone;[7] this finding indicates significant hormonal activity, which encourages future research but also raises safety concerns (see Safety Issues).

Another uncontrolled clinical trial followed 16 people with hormone-insensitive prostate cancer for a period of 5 months.[8] The results showed decreased PSA levels and also a reduction in pain and use of medication to control pain. However, because this was not a double-blind study, it is quite possible that the reported pain reduction was due to a placebo effect.

The most extensive study reported to date is an ongoing clinical trial involving 60 people, half with hormone-insensitive and half with hormone-sensitive prostate cancer.[9] A preliminary presentation of this work at a scientific conference in 1999 indicated that all of the participants with hormone-sensitive PC and over half of those with hormone-insensitive PC showed significantly decreased PSA levels.[10] Additionally, benefits were seen in individuals for whom conventional chemotherapy had ceased to work.

Tests in yeast cells and mice have shown that PC-SPES has strong estrogenic properties.[11] Because estrogen itself is sometimes used to treat prostate cancer, this estrogenic action is thought to play a significant role in the effects of PC-SPES.

DOSAGE

The standard dosage of PC-SPES is 6 to 9 capsules (320 mg each) per day, taken on an empty stomach at least 2 hours before or after meals.

SAFETY ISSUES

Note: The safety of this product has not been established. Use of PC-SPES is intended for adult men only: it should not be taken by women or children.

Side effects of PC-SPES resemble those of estrogen when taken by men for the treatment of prostate cancer;[12] it may cause breast or nipple tenderness or swelling, loss of body hair, hot flashes, and loss of libido. Some individuals have also reported leg cramps, nausea and vomiting, and blood clots in the legs.[13] Low-dose aspirin or anticoagulant medication may be useful for those at particular risk for blood clots.[14] Side effects of PC-SPES increase with dosage.

Researchers are concerned that these estrogenic effects could interfere with standard hormonal therapy for prostate cancer,[15] and also caution that the observed estrogenic effects could cause birth defects—however, as PC-SPES is only intended for men, this should not be an important issue for prospective users.

The formulation contains licorice, an herb with many known potential side effects that could occur with continued use of PC-SPES. See the chapter on **licorice** for more detail.

⚠ INTERACTIONS YOU SHOULD KNOW ABOUT

If you are taking **hormone treatments for prostate cancer**, PC-SPES might interfere with its effectiveness or increase its side effects.

PEPPERMINT *(Mentha piperita)*

Alternate or Related Names   Brandy Mint, Lamb Mint

Principal Proposed Uses   Irritable Bowel Syndrome, Colds, Cough, Dyspepsia, Gallstones, "Candida"

Peppermint is a relative of numerous wild mint plants, deliberately bred in the late 1600s in England to become the delightful tasting plant so well known today. It is widely used as a beverage tea and as a flavoring or scent in a wide variety of products.

Peppermint tea also has a long history of medicinal use, primarily as a digestive aid and for the symptomatic treatment of cough, colds, and fever. Peppermint oil is used for chest congestion (Vicks VapoRub), as a local anesthetic (Solarcaine, Ben-Gay), and most recently in the treatment of irritable bowel disease, also known as spastic colon.

WHAT IS PEPPERMINT USED FOR TODAY?

Germany's Commission E authorizes the use of peppermint oil for treating colicky pain in the digestive tract, specifically **irritable bowel syndrome** (see page 108), as well as for relieving mucus congestion of the lungs and sinuses caused by **colds and flus** (see page 47).

Peppermint is a carminative (gas-relieving) herb that has traditionally been used to relieve excessive gas. Preliminary evidence suggests peppermint oil, in combination with other essential oils such as caraway, may be helpful for the treatment of **dyspepsia** (minor indigestion; see page 71).

There is also some evidence that it might be helpful for **gallstones** (see page 83).[1] Peppermint is sometimes recommended for the treatment of **candida** (see page 38) yeast infections, but there is as yet no real evidence that it works.

WHAT IS THE SCIENTIFIC EVIDENCE FOR PEPPERMINT?

Irritable Bowel Syndrome

The scientific record for peppermint oil in treating irritable bowel syndrome is contradictory.

Menthol is the primary ingredient in peppermint oil. Studies have found that it relaxes the muscles of the small intestine in dilutions as low as 1:20,000 and counters the effect of other drugs that cause intestinal spasm.[2,3,4]

Three preliminary double-blind studies, involving a total of 146 individuals with irritable bowel syndrome, found that peppermint can provide significant relief from crampy abdominal pain.[5,6,7] However, other studies, involving a total of more than 90 people, have found no significant improvement in symptoms.[8,9,10]

The most probable reason for these contradictory results is that peppermint oil is not terrifically effective. Also, the placebo effect is fairly strong in irritable bowel syndrome, making it hard to detect small improvements due to the actual effects of a medicine.

Dyspepsia

Peppermint oil is often used in combination with other essential oils to treat dyspepsia; however the evidence that it works is preliminary as of yet.

A double-blind placebo-controlled study including 39 individuals found that an enteric-coated peppermint-caraway oil combination taken 3 times daily for 4 weeks significantly reduced dyspepsia pain as compared to placebo.[11] Of the treatment group, 63.2% was pain free after 4 weeks, compared to 25% of the placebo group.

Results from a double-blind comparative study including 118 individuals suggest that the combination of peppermint and caraway oil is comparably effective to the no-longer-available drug cisapride.[12] After 4 weeks, the herbal combination reduced dyspepsia pain by 69.7%, whereas the conventional treatment reduced pain by 70.2%.

A preparation of peppermint, caraway, fennel, and wormwood oils was compared to metoclopramide in another double-blind study enrolling 60 individuals.[13] After 7 days, 43.3% of the treatment group was pain free compared to 13.3% of the metoclopramide group.

DOSAGE

The proper dosage of peppermint oil when treating irritable bowel syndrome is 0.2 to 0.4 ml 3 times a day of an enteric-coated capsule. The capsule has to be enteric-coated to prevent stomach distress.

SAFETY ISSUES

At the normal dosage, enteric-coated peppermint oil is believed to be reasonably safe in healthy adults.[14,15]

However, if you take too much, peppermint oil can be toxic, causing kidney failure and even death. Excessive intake of peppermint oil can also cause nausea, loss of appetite, heart problems, loss of balance, and other nervous system problems.

Safety in young children, pregnant or nursing women, or those with severe liver or kidney disease has not been established. In particular, peppermint can cause jaundice in newborn babies, so don't try to use it for colic.

A total of at least 200 people have participated in studies of peppermint oil, without any significant problems other than the usual occasional mild gastrointestinal distress or allergic reactions.[16]

PHENYLALANINE

Supplement Forms/Alternate Names L-Phenylalanine, D-Phenylalanine, DL-Phenylalanine

Principal Proposed Uses Depression

Other Proposed Uses
  Chronic Pain: Rheumatoid Arthritis, Muscle Pain, Osteoarthritis
  Vitiligo, Multiple Sclerosis, Parkinson's Disease, Attention Deficit Disorder

Phenylalanine occurs in two chemical forms: *L-phenylalanine*, a natural amino acid found in proteins; and its mirror image, *D-phenylalanine*, a form synthesized in a laboratory. Some research has involved the L-form, others the D-form, and still others a combination of the two known as DL-phenylalanine.

In the body, phenylalanine is converted into another amino acid called **tyrosine** (see page 426). Tyrosine in turn is converted into L-dopa, norepinephrine, and

Phenylalanine

Visit Us at TNP.com

epinephrine, three key neurotransmitters (chemicals that transmit signals between nerve cells). Because some antidepressants work by raising levels of norepinephrine, various forms of phenylalanine have been tried as a possible treatment for depression.

D-phenylalanine (but not L-phenylalanine) has been proposed to treat chronic pain. It blocks *enkephalinase*, an enzyme that may act to increase pain levels in the body. Phenylalanine (various forms) has also been suggested as a treatment for vitiligo, a disease characterized by abnormal white blotches of skin due to loss of pigmentation.

REQUIREMENTS/SOURCES

L-phenylalanine is an essential amino acid, meaning that we need it for life and our bodies can't manufacture it from other chemicals. It is found in protein-rich foods such as meat, fish, poultry, eggs, dairy products, and beans. Provided you eat enough protein, you are likely to get enough L-phenylalanine for your nutritional needs. There is no nutritional need for D-phenylalanine.

THERAPEUTIC DOSAGES

When used as a treatment for depression, L-phenylalanine is typically started at a dosage of 500 mg daily, and then gradually increased to 3 to 4 g daily.[1] However, side effects may develop at dosages above 1,500 mg daily (see Safety Issues).

D- or DL-phenylalanine may be used for depression as well, but the typical dosage is much lower: 100 to 400 mg daily.[2]

For the treatment of chronic pain, usual recommended dosages of D-phenylalanine are as high as 2,500 mg daily.

It is best not to take your phenylalanine supplement at the same time as a high-protein meal, as it may not be absorbed well.

THERAPEUTIC USES

Preliminary studies suggest that both the L- and D-forms of phenylalanine may be helpful for **depression** (see page 59).[3,4]

Weak evidence suggests that D-phenylalanine may be useful for chronic pain,[5] such as **rheumatoid arthritis** (see page 151), muscle pain, and **osteoarthritis** (see page 132), but this conclusion has been contested.[6,7,8]

Preliminary uncontrolled and double-blind studies found that the combination of phenylalanine and ultraviolet radiation might be helpful for **vitiligo** (see page 191).[9–11]

Weak evidence suggests that phenylalanine may be helpful for **multiple sclerosis** (see page 124) when combined with transcutaneous electrical nerve stimulation (TENS).[12]

Very preliminary evidence suggests phenylalanine may reduce symptoms of **Parkinson's disease** (see Safety Issues; see also page 140).[13]

Although it is sometimes proposed as a treatment for **attention deficit disorder** (see page 22), phenylalanine taken alone does not appear to be helpful.[14,15] Some proponents claim that it works better when combined with **tyrosine** (see page 426), **glutamine** (see page 310), and gamma-aminobutyric acid (GABA), but this has not been proven.

WHAT IS THE SCIENTIFIC EVIDENCE FOR PHENYLALANINE?

Depression

A pair of double-blind studies have found that D- or DL-phenylalanine is as effective as imipramine, a standard antidepressant drug, and that it may take effect much more quickly. The larger of the two studies compared the effectiveness of D-phenylalanine at 100 mg daily against the same daily dose of imipramine.[16] Sixty people with depression were randomly assigned to take either imipramine or D-phenylalanine for 30 days. The results in both groups were statistically equivalent, meaning that phenylalanine was about as effective as imipramine. D-phenylalanine worked more rapidly, however, producing significant improvement in only 15 days. Like most antidepressant drugs, imipramine requires several weeks to take effect.

The other double-blind study followed 27 individuals, half of whom received DL-phenylalanine (150 to 200 mg daily) and the other half imipramine (100 to 150 mg daily).[17] When they were reevaluated after 30 days, both groups had improved by a statistically equal amount. Very preliminary studies have also found benefits with L-phenylalanine.[18,19]

Unfortunately, there have been no good studies comparing any form of phenylalanine against placebo. This is too bad, since without such evidence we can't be sure that the supplement is actually effective.

Chronic Pain

The use of D-phenylalanine to treat pain is primarily based on a study involving 43 individuals with chronic pain, mostly due to arthritis.[20] However, this was not a double-blind study, and it suffered from other flaws as well.[21]

A small double-blind study reportedly found evidence for the effectiveness of D-phenylalanine in chronic pain,[22] but a careful look at the math involved undermined that conclusion.[23] Another small study found no benefits.[24]

Phenylalanine

SAFETY ISSUES

Although most people do not report side effects from any type of phenylalanine, daily doses near or above 1,500 mg of L-phenylalanine can reportedly cause anxiety, headache, and even mildly elevated blood pressure.[25]

The long-term safety of phenylalanine in any of its forms is not known. Both L- and D-phenylalanine must be avoided by those with the rare metabolic disease phenylketonuria (PKU).

The safety of high dosages of L-phenylalanine, or any dosage of D-phenylalanine, has not been established for young children, pregnant or nursing women, or those with severe liver or kidney disease.

There are some indications that the combined use of phenylalanine with antipsychotic drugs might increase the risk of developing the long-term side effect known as tardive dyskinesia, or worsen symptoms in those who already have it.[26,27,28]

Like other amino acids, phenylalanine may interfere with the absorption or action of the drug levodopa which is used for Parkinson's disease.[29]

⚠ INTERACTIONS YOU SHOULD KNOW ABOUT

If you are taking

- **Antipsychotic medications:** Do not use phenylalanine.
- **Levodopa:** Like other amino acids, phenylalanine might interfere with its action.

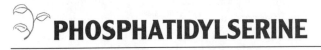

PHOSPHATIDYLSERINE

Principal Proposed Uses   Alzheimer's Disease, Age-Related Memory Loss

Other Proposed Uses   General Improvement of Mental Performance, Depression, Performance Enhancement

Phosphatidylserine, or PS for short, is a member of a class of chemical compounds known as *phospholipids*. PS is an essential component in all our cells; specifically, it is a major component of the cell membrane. The cell membrane is a kind of "skin" that surrounds living cells. Besides keeping cells intact, this membrane performs vital functions such as moving nutrients into cells and pumping waste products out of them. PS plays an important role in many of these functions.

Good evidence suggests that PS can help declining mental function and depression in the elderly, and it is widely used for this purpose in Italy, Scandinavia, and other parts of Europe. PS has also been marketed as a "brain booster" for people of all ages, said to sharpen memory and increase thinking ability.

Recently, PS has been marketed as a **sports supplement** (see page 158), said to help bodybuilders and power athletes develop larger and stronger muscles.

SOURCES

Your body makes all the PS it needs. However, the only way to get a therapeutic dosage of PS is to take a supplement.

PS was originally manufactured from the brains of cows, and all the studies described here used this form. However, because animal brain cells can harbor viruses, that form is no longer available, and most PS today is made from soybeans.

According to some experts, soy-based PS is just as effective as PS made from cows' brains.[1–5] However, not everyone agrees.[6]

Phosphatidylserine can also be manufactured from cabbage, but in one study the results with this form of the supplement were not impressive.[7]

THERAPEUTIC DOSAGES

For the purpose of improving mental function, PS is usually taken in dosages of 100 mg 2 to 3 times daily. After maximum effect is achieved, the dosage can sometimes be reduced to 100 mg daily without losing benefit. PS can be taken with or without meals.

When taking PS for sports purposes, athletes may use as much as 800 mg daily.

THERAPEUTIC USES

Impressive evidence from numerous double-blind studies suggests that PS is an effective treatment for **Alzheimer's disease** (see page 5) and other forms of age-related mental decline.[8–17]

PS is widely marketed as a treatment for ordinary age-related memory loss, and there is some evidence that it might work. Keep in mind that in studies of severe

Phosphatidylserine

Visit Us at TNP.com

mental decline, PS was equally effective whether the cause was Alzheimer's disease or something entirely unrelated (multiple small strokes). This certainly suggests that PS may have a positive impact on the brain that is not specific to any one condition. From this observation, it is not a great leap to suspect that it might make it useful for much less severe problems with memory and mental function, such as those that seem to occur in nearly all of us who are older than 40. Indeed, one double-blind study did find that phosphatidylserine could improve mental function in individuals with relatively mild age-related memory loss.[18]

PS may also be helpful for **depression** (see page 59).[19,20,21]

Recently, PS has become popular among athletes who hope it can help them build muscle more efficiently. This use is based on modest evidence that PS slows the release of cortisol following heavy exercise.[22,23,24] Cortisol is a hormone that causes muscle tissue to break down. For reasons that are unclear, the body produces increased levels of cortisol after heavy exercise. Strength athletes believe that this natural cortisol release works against their efforts to rapidly build muscle mass and hope that PS will help them advance more quickly. However, this idea has not been proven.

WHAT IS THE SCIENTIFIC EVIDENCE FOR PHOSPHATIDYLSERINE?

Alzheimer's Disease and Other Forms of Dementia

Overall, the evidence for PS in dementia is quite strong. Double-blind studies involving a total of over 1,000 people suggest that phosphatidylserine (at least the type from cow's brain) is an effective treatment for Alzheimer's disease and other forms of dementia.

The largest of these studies followed 494 elderly subjects in northeastern Italy over a course of 6 months.[25] All suffered from moderate to severe mental decline, as measured by standard tests. Treatment consisted of either 300 mg daily of PS or placebo. The group that took PS did significantly better in both behavior and mental function than the placebo group. Symptoms of depression also improved.

These results agree with those of numerous smaller double-blind studies involving a total of over 500 people with Alzheimer's and other types of age-related dementia.[26–33]

Ordinary Age-Related Memory Loss

There is some evidence that PS can also help people with ordinary age-related memory loss. In one double-blind study that enrolled 149 individuals with memory loss but not dementia, phosphatidylserine provided significant benefits as compared with placebo.[34] Individuals with the most severe memory loss showed the most improvement.

Athletic Performance

Weak evidence suggests that PS might decrease the release of the hormone cortisol after intense exercise.[35] Among its many effects, cortisol acts to break down muscle tissue—exactly the opposite of the effect desired by a strength athlete or bodybuilder. This double-blind placebo-controlled study on 11 intensely trained athletes found that 800 mg of PS taken daily reduced the cortisol rise by 20% as compared with placebo.[36] Another small study on 9 nonathletic males found that daily doses of 400 and 800 mg of PS reduced cortisol levels after exercise by 16% and 30%, respectively.[37] Another study found that phosphatidylserine could relieve some overtraining symptoms, including muscle soreness, possibly due to effects on cortisol.[38,39,40]

However, there is as yet no direct evidence to support the claims that PS actually helps athletes build muscles more quickly and with less training effort.

SAFETY ISSUES

Phosphatidylserine is generally regarded as safe when used at recommended dosages. Side effects are rare, and when they do occur they usually consist of nothing much worse than mild gastrointestinal distress.[41] However, the maximum safe dosages for young children, pregnant or nursing women, or those with severe liver or kidney disease have not been established.

PS is sometimes taken with **ginkgo** (see page 298) because they both appear to enhance mental function. However, some caution might be in order: Ginkgo is a "blood thinner," and PS might be one as well. Together, the two supplements might interfere with normal blood clotting enough to cause problems. Although this is still hypothetical, we do have reason to believe that PS can enhance the effect of heparin, a very strong prescription blood thinner.[42]

Keep in mind, too, that Alzheimer's disease and other types of severe age-related mental impairment are too serious to treat on your own with PS or any other supplement. In some cases, the symptoms of these diseases may be a sign of other serious conditions. If you suspect that you or a loved one may have a severe age-related mental impairment, see your doctor for diagnosis and treatment.

⚠ INTERACTIONS YOU SHOULD KNOW ABOUT

If you are taking

- **Prescription blood thinners,** such as **heparin** or

Coumadin (warfarin): Do not use phosphatidylserine except on a physician's advice.
- **Ginkgo:** Taking phosphatidylserine at the same time might conceivably "thin" the blood too much.

🌿 PHYLLANTHUS (*Phyllanthus amarus, Phyllanthus niruri, Phyllanthus urinaria*)

Principal Proposed Uses   Chronic Hepatitis B

Other Proposed Uses   Acute Hepatitis B

Tropical plants in the genus *Phyllanthus* have a long history of folk use for the treatment of hepatitis, kidney and bladder problems, intestinal parasites, and diabetes. The most studied species is *Phyllanthus amarus*, historically used for the treatment of jaundice. This traditional practice has led to scientific study of the herb in humans.

WHAT IS PHYLLANTHUS USED FOR TODAY?

Hepatitis B (see page 189) is a two-stage illness. Its has an acute phase which causes jaundice, severe fatigue, and other symptoms. These symptoms usually resolve in a month or so; however, the infection may become chronic. Long-term infection with hepatitis B can spread the disease to other people and can also lead to liver injury or liver cancer.

Promising results in animal and test tube trials have led to numerous double-blind studies evaluating *P. amarus* as a treatment for hepatitis B.

Most of the human studies have evaluated whether the herb can eradicate the hepatitis B virus from people in the chronic phase of the disease, but the results have not been promising. A study on *P. amarus* for the acute phase of hepatitis also had negative findings.

Test tube and animal research of other *Phyllanthus* species has revealed numerous active constituents of these plants as well. However, at present, properly designed double-blind human trials are lacking.[1]

WHAT IS THE SCIENTIFIC EVIDENCE FOR PHYLLANTHUS?

Despite numerous test tube and animal studies showing efficacy against the hepatitis B virus,[2] *P. amarus* has been found ineffective in all but one human trial.

One 30-day double-blind placebo-controlled trial of 60 individuals with chronic hepatitis B found that treatment with phyllanthus (200 mg 3 times daily) dramatically increased the odds of full recovery.[3] In the treated group, almost 60% were hepatitis B–negative at follow-up, as compared to only 4% in the placebo group.

However, the high drop-out rate in the placebo group significantly reduces the reliability of the results. Furthermore, follow-up studies attempting to reproduce these results have produced negative results.[4–11]

Another double-blind placebo-controlled trial enrolled 57 individuals with acute hepatitis B to see whether treatment with *P. amarus* (300 mg 3 times daily for 1 week) could improve speed of recovery.[12] The results showed no benefit. However, because acute hepatitis B usually lasts a month or more, the duration of treatment in this study was oddly short.

One study suggests that *P. urinaria*, a related species, might be more effective against hepatitis than other species of phyllanthus.[13] However, because this study was not placebo-controlled, its results can't be taken as more than highly preliminary.

DOSAGE

The usual dose of *P. amarus* used in studies is 600 to 900 mg daily.

SAFETY ISSUES

There are no indications that *P. amarus* is toxic when used at recommended doses, but comprehensive safety studies have not been performed.[14] In double-blind studies, significant side effects have not been reported. Safety in pregnant or nursing women, or individuals with severe liver or kidney disease, has not been established.

POTASSIUM

Supplement Forms/Alternate Names   Potassium Chloride, Potassium Bicarbonate, Chelated Potassium (Potassium Aspartate, Potassium Citrate)

Principal Proposed Uses   Hypertension (High Blood Pressure)

Potassium is a mineral found in many foods and supplements. But you will never see pure potassium in a health food store or pharmacy—it's a highly reactive metal that bursts into flame when exposed to water! The potassium you eat, or take as a supplement, is composed of potassium atoms bound to other nonmetallic substances—less exciting, perhaps, but chemically stable.

Potassium is one of the major electrolytes in your body, along with sodium and chloride. Potassium and sodium work together like a molecular seesaw: when the level of one goes up, the other goes down. All together, these three dissolved minerals play an intimate chemical role in every function of your body.

The most common use of potassium supplements is to make up for potassium depletion caused by diuretic drugs. These medications are often used to help regulate blood pressure, but by depleting the body of potassium they may inadvertently make blood pressure harder to control.

REQUIREMENTS/SOURCES

Potassium is an essential mineral that we get from many common foods. The minimum requirement of potassium for children ranges from 1,000 to 2,300 mg daily; adults should receive 1,600 to 2,000 mg daily.

True potassium deficiencies are rare except in cases of prolonged vomiting or diarrhea, or with the use of diuretic drugs.

However, in one sense potassium deficiency is common, at least when compared to the amount of sodium we receive in our diets. It is probably healthy to take in at least five times as much potassium as sodium (and perhaps 50 to 100 times as much). But the standard American diet contains twice as much sodium as potassium. Therefore, taking extra potassium may be a good idea in order to balance the sodium we consume to such excess.

Bananas, orange juice, potatoes, avocados, lima beans, cantaloupes, peaches, tomatoes, flounder, salmon, and cod all contain more than 300 mg of potassium per serving. Other good sources include chicken, meat, and various other fruits, vegetables, and fish.

Over-the-counter potassium supplements typically contain 99 mg of potassium per tablet. There is some evidence that, of the different forms of potassium supplements, potassium citrate may be most helpful for those with high blood pressure.[1]

Research indicates that it is important to get enough **magnesium** (see page 351), too, when you are taking potassium.[2,3,4] It might be wise to take extra **vitamin B$_{12}$** (see page 442) as well.[5]

THERAPEUTIC DOSAGES

When used by physicians, potassium is usually measured according to meqs (milliequivalents) rather than the more common mg (milligrams). A typical therapeutic dosage of potassium is between 10 and 20 meq (about 200 to 400 mg), taken 3 to 4 times daily.

THERAPEUTIC USES

Potassium appears to be helpful for **hypertension** (see page 98), especially among individuals who eat too much salt.[6,7]

WHAT IS THE SCIENTIFIC EVIDENCE FOR POTASSIUM?

High Blood Pressure

According to a review of 33 double-blind studies, potassium supplements can produce a slight but definite drop in blood pressure.[8] However, two large studies found *no* benefit.[9,10] The explanation is probably that potassium is only slightly helpful. When a treatment has only a small effect, it's not unusual for some studies to show no effect while others find a modest benefit. It's possible that potassium may only help people who are at least a bit deficient in this mineral.

Evidence suggests that potassium supplements may be most effective for people who eat too much salt.[11]

SAFETY ISSUES

As an essential nutrient, potassium is safe when taken at appropriate dosages. If you take a bit too much, your body will simply excrete it in the urine. However, people who have severe kidney disease cannot excrete potassium normally, and should consult a physician before taking a potassium supplement. Similarly, individuals taking potassium-sparing diuretics (such as spironolactone), ACE inhibitors (such as captopril),[12–16] or trimethoprim/sulfomethoxazole[17] should also not take potassium supplements except under doctor supervision.

Potassium pills can cause injury to the esophagus if they get stuck on the way down, so make sure to take them with plenty of water.

⚠ INTERACTIONS YOU SHOULD KNOW ABOUT

If you are taking

- **Loop diuretics** or **thiazide diuretics:** You may need more potassium.

- **ACE inhibitors** (e.g., **captopril**, **lisinopril**, **enalapril**), **potassium-sparing diuretics** (e.g., **triamterene** or **spironolactone**), or **trimethoprim/sulfamethoxazole:** You should not take potassium except on the advice of a physician.
- **Potassium:** You may need extra magnesium and vitamin B_{12}.

PREGNENOLONE

Principal Proposed Uses   There are no well-documented uses for pregnenolone.

Other Proposed Uses   Memory Enhancement, Age-Related Hormone Decline, Alzheimer's Disease, Menopausal Symptoms, Adrenal Disease, Parkinson's Disease, Osteoporosis, Fatigue, Stress, Depression, Rheumatoid Arthritis, Nerve Injury, Weight Loss

Pregnenolone has been called "the grandmother of all steroid hormones." The body manufactures it from cholesterol, and then uses it to make testosterone, cortisone, **progesterone** (see page 392), estrogen, **DHEA** (see page 268), **androstenedione** (see page 206), aldosterone, and all other hormones in the "steroid" family.

One reason given for using pregnenolone is that the level of many of these hormones declines with age. By taking pregnenolone supplements, proponents say, you can keep all your hormones at youthful levels. However, pregnenolone levels themselves don't decline with age,[1] and there is no indication that taking extra pregnenolone will increase the levels of any other hormones. Furthermore, even if it did, that doesn't mean using pregnenolone is a great idea.

Steroid hormones are powerful substances, and they can cause harm as well as benefit. Long-term use of cortisone causes severe osteoporosis; estrogen can increase the risk of cancer; and anabolic steroids (used by athletes) may cause liver problems and stress the heart. We really have very little idea what long-term consequences the use of pregnenolone might entail.

Actually, it is ironic that pregnenolone is legally classified as a "dietary supplement" at all. Pregnenolone is not a nutrient. It is a drug, just as estrogen, cortisone, and aldosterone are drugs. We recommend not using it until we know more about what it really does.

SOURCES

Pregnenolone is not normally obtained from foods. Your body manufactures it from cholesterol. Supplemental pregnenolone is made synthetically in a chemical laboratory from substances found in soybeans.

THERAPEUTIC DOSAGES

A typical recommended dosage of pregnenolone is 30 mg daily, but some studies have used as much as 700 mg.

THERAPEUTIC USES

If you browse the Internet or read health magazines, you'll find pregnenolone described as a treatment for an enormous list of health problems, including memory loss, **Alzheimer's disease** (see page 5), **menopausal symptoms** (see page 117), adrenal disease, **Parkinson's disease** (see page 140), **osteoporosis** (see page 136), fatigue, stress, **depression** (see page 59), **rheumatoid arthritis** (see page 151), and nerve injury. It is also supposed to help you lose **weight** (see page 192), improve your brain power, and make you feel young again. However, like so many overhyped new supplements, there is very little scientific evidence for any of these uses.

Studies involving rats suggest that pregnenolone may enhance memory,[2,3] but there have been no human studies.

SAFETY ISSUES

Pregnenolone is a powerful hormone, not a nutrient we would naturally get in our food. You should approach this supplement with caution, as if it were a drug—for all intents and purposes, it *is* a drug. It would be best to consult your doctor before taking it. Pregnenolone is definitely not recommended for children, pregnant or nursing women, or those with liver or kidney disease.

PROGESTERONE

Supplement Forms/Alternate Names   Natural Progesterone, Micronized Progesterone, Progesterone Cream

Principal Proposed Uses   Hot Flashes

Other Proposed Uses   Osteoporosis

Progesterone is one of the two primary female hormones. As the name implies, progesterone prepares ("pro") the womb for pregnancy (gestation). Progesterone works in tandem with **estrogen** (see page 278); indeed, if estrogen is taken as a medication without being balanced by progesterone (so called unopposed estrogen), there is an increased risk of uterine cancer.

However, progesterone is not well absorbed orally. For this reason, pharmaceutical manufacturers developed "progestins," substances similar to progesterone which are more easily absorbed. Most of the time, a woman prescribed "progesterone" is really being given a progestin. Two of the most commonly used progestins are medroxyprogesterone and norethindrone.

There may be benefits in using actual progesterone rather than progestins. Progesterone is fairly well absorbed through the skin; some alternative practitioners have, for years, promoted the use of progesterone creams. Such progesterone creams are typically, but misleadingly, said to contain "natural" progesterone. This is an oddly chosen term, as the progesterone in these creams is actually produced in a laboratory, just like other synthetic hormones. To avoid confusion in this chapter, we will call progesterone "true" progesterone, or just "progesterone."

Besides creams, a special form of true progesterone that can be absorbed orally, micronized progesterone, has recently become available as a prescription drug.

Progesterone cream appears to reduce menopausal symptoms. However, contrary to numerous misleading reports, it has not been found helpful for osteoporosis.

REQUIREMENTS/SOURCES

Progesterone is synthesized in the body and is not found in appreciable quantities in food. For use as a drug or "dietary supplement," progesterone is synthesized from chemicals found in **soy** (see page 411) or **Mexican yam** (see page 459).

Note: Contrary to widespread misrepresentation, Mexican yam by itself contains no progesterone, nor any substance that the body can turn into progesterone.

THERAPEUTIC DOSAGES

The usual dose of progesterone in cream form is 20 mg daily. Although this dose may decrease menopausal **hot flashes** (see page 117),[1] even 3 to 4 times that amount does not provide enough progesterone to protect the uterus from the effects of estrogen.[2,3] However, oral micronized progesterone taken at a dose of 200 to 400 mg daily should be approximately as effective as standard progestins.

THERAPEUTIC USES

Progesterone cream has been widely promoted as a treatment for **osteoporosis** (see page 136), primarily by one author.[4,5,6] However, the only meaningful study examining the issue found progesterone cream ineffective for this purpose.[7] In addition, oral micronized progesterone does not appear to add any additional bone-protective benefit in women taking estrogen.[8]

Like progestins, progesterone cream *has* been found effective in reducing **menopausal symptoms** (see page 117).[9]

Also like progestins, oral progesterone protects the uterus from the stimulating effects of unopposed estrogen. This use requires physician supervision. Progesterone cream is probably not effective for this purpose.

WHAT IS THE SCIENTIFIC EVIDENCE FOR PROGESTERONE?

Osteoporosis

Despite widespread reporting that true progesterone is effective against osteoporosis, the best evidence we have is that it does not offer any such benefit.

This notion began with test tube and other preliminary studies suggesting that progesterone or progestins can stimulate the activity of cells that build bone.[10,11] Subsequently, a poorly designed and uncontrolled study (really, a series of case histories from one physician's practice) purportedly demonstrated that progesterone cream can slow or even reverse osteoporosis.[12,13,14]

However, a 1-year double-blind trial of 102 women given either progesterone cream (providing 20 mg progesterone daily) or placebo cream, along with calcium and multivitamins, found no evidence of any improvements in bone density attributable to progesterone.[15]

Furthermore, in a 3-year study of 875 women, combination treatment with estrogen and oral progesterone was no more effective for osteoporosis than estrogen alone.[16]

Progesterone

Visit Us at TNP.com

Menopausal Symptoms

In the double-blind trial of 102 women described above, use of progesterone cream was, however, found to significantly reduce hot flashes and related symptoms.[17]

SAFETY ISSUES

Even though progesterone is sold as a dietary supplement, it is a hormone, not a food. We recommend that it *not* be used except under physician supervision.

Like progestins, progesterone causes side effects. In one study, oral micronized progesterone at a dose of 400 mg per day was associated with dizziness, abdominal cramping, headache, breast pain, muscle pain, irritability, nausea, fatigue, diarrhea, and viral infections.[18]

Finally, women taking progestins to protect the uterus from the effects of estrogen should not substitute progesterone cream, because it is not sufficiently potent.[19,20] Oral micronized progesterone, however, can be used for this purpose.

PROTEOLYTIC ENZYMES

Supplement Forms/Alternate Names   Bromelain, Papain, Trypsin, Chymotrypsin, Pancreatin, Digestive Enzymes

Principal Proposed Uses   Digestive Aid, Dyspepsia, Sports and Other Minor Injuries, Recovery from Surgery, Shingles (*Herpes zoster*)

Other Proposed Uses   Easy Bruising, Food Allergies, Rheumatoid Arthritis, Other Autoimmune Diseases

Proteolytic enzymes help you digest the proteins in food. Although your body produces these enzymes in the pancreas, certain foods also contain proteolytic enzymes.

Papaya and pineapple are two of the richest plant sources, as attested by their traditional use as natural "tenderizers" for meat. Papain and **bromelain** (see page 229) are the respective names for the proteolytic enzymes found in these fruits. The enzymes made in your body are called trypsin and chymotrypsin.

The primary use of proteolytic enzymes is as a digestive aid for people who have trouble digesting proteins. However, for reasons that are not clear, they also seem to help bruises and other **traumas** (see page 74) heal faster, which has made them popular in Europe as a treatment for sports injuries and as an aid in recovery from surgery. They may also help reduce the pain of shingles.

Many practitioners of alternative medicine believe that proteolytic enzymes can be helpful for a wide variety of other health conditions, including food allergies and autoimmune diseases. However, there is little to no scientific evidence as yet that they really work for these problems.

SOURCES

You don't need to get proteolytic enzymes from food, because the body manufactures them (primarily trypsin and chymotrypsin). However, deficiencies in proteolytic enzymes do occur, usually resulting from diseases of the pancreas. Symptoms include abdominal discomfort, gas, indigestion, poor absorption of nutrients, and passing undigested food in the stool.

For use as a supplement, trypsin and chymotrypsin are extracted from the pancreas of various animals. You can also purchase bromelain extracted from pineapple stems and papain made from papayas.

THERAPEUTIC DOSAGES

When you purchase an enzyme, the amount is expressed not only in grams or milligrams but also in *activity units* or *international units*. These terms refer to the enzyme's potency (i.e., its digestive power).

Recommended dosages of proteolytic enzymes vary with the form used. Due to the wide variation, we suggest following label instructions. Proteolytic enzymes can be broken down by stomach acid. To prevent this from happening, supplemental enzymes are often coated with a substance that doesn't dissolve until it reaches the intestine. Such a preparation is called "enteric coated."

THERAPEUTIC USES

The most obvious use of proteolytic enzymes is to assist digestion. However, a small double-blind placebo-controlled trial found no benefit from proteolytic enzymes as a treatment for **dyspepsia** (indigestion; see page 71).[1]

Proteolytic enzymes have been tried for a number of other conditions as well. Evidence suggests that they can

Proteolytic Enzymes

be absorbed whole[2] and may produce a variety of effects in the body.

For example, these enzymes might be able to improve the rate of healing of sports **injuries** (see page 101).[3–7] Proteolytic enzymes have also been evaluated as an aid to recovery from **surgery** (see page 173), with considerable success.[8–13] Similar reasoning has led to their use in treating **bruises** (see page 74).[14] Two double-blind studies suggest that proteolytic enzymes might be helpful for the treatment of the painful condition known as **shingles** (herpes zoster; see page 156).[15,16]

Proteolytic enzymes may also help reduce symptoms of **food allergies** (see page 82), presumably by digesting the food so well that there is less to be allergic to.

Proteolytic enzymes have also been proposed as a treatment for **rheumatoid arthritis** (see page 151) and other autoimmune diseases. According to a theory popular in alternative medicine circles, these diseases may be made worse by whole proteins from foods leaking into the blood and causing an immune reaction. Digestive enzymes may help foil this so-called "leaky gut" problem. (For another approach, see the chapter on **glutamine**.) However, there is no real evidence as yet to substantiate this use.

WHAT IS THE SCIENTIFIC EVIDENCE FOR PROTEOLYTIC ENZYMES?

Sports Injuries

A double-blind placebo-controlled study of 44 individuals with sports-related ankle injuries found that treatment with proteolytic enzymes resulted in faster healing and reduced the time away from training by about 50%.[17] Three other small double-blind studies, involving a total of about 80 athletes, found that treatment with proteolytic enzymes significantly speeded healing of bruises and other mild **athletic injuries** (see page 101) as compared to placebo.[18,19,20]

A double-blind placebo-controlled trial of 71 individuals with finger fractures found that treatment with proteolytic enzymes significantly improved recovery.[21]

Surgery

A double-blind placebo-controlled trial of 80 individuals undergoing knee surgery found that treatment with proteolytic enzymes after surgery significantly improved rate of recovery, as measured by mobility and **swelling** (see page 173).[22]

Another double-blind placebo-controlled trial evaluated the effects of proteolytic enzymes in 80 individuals undergoing oral surgery.[23] The results showed reduced pain, inflammation, and swelling in the treated group as compared to the placebo group.

Benefits were also seen in a controlled study of 53 individuals undergoing nasal surgery who were treated with bromelain.[24]

Bruises

In a controlled study, 74 boxers with **bruises** (see page 74) on their faces and upper bodies were given bromelain until all signs of bruising had disappeared;[25] another 72 boxers were given placebo. Fifty-eight of the group taking bromelain lost all signs of bruising within 4 days, compared to only 10 of the group taking placebo. Unfortunately, this study was apparently not double-blind, meaning that some of its results may have been due to the power of suggestion.

Other studies have found similar benefits.[26,27,28] However, not all studies have had positive results.[29,30]

Shingles (*Herpes zoster*)

Herpes zoster (shingles) is an acute, painful infection caused by the varicella-zoster virus, the organism that causes chickenpox. There is some evidence that proteolytic enzymes may be helpful for the initial attack of shingles, for reasons that aren't clear.

A double-blind study of 190 people with shingles compared proteolytic enzymes to the standard antiviral drug acyclovir.[31] Participants were treated for 14 days and their pain was assessed at intervals. Although both groups had similar pain relief, the enzyme-treated group experienced fewer side effects.

Similar results were seen in another double-blind study in which 90 individuals were given either an injection of acyclovir or enzymes, followed by a course of oral medication for 7 days.[32]

SAFETY ISSUES

Proteolytic enzymes are believed to be quite safe, although there are some concerns that they might further damage the exposed tissue in an ulcer (by partly digesting it).

One proteolytic enzyme, pancreatin, may interfere with folate absorption (see the chapter on **folate**).[33] In addition, the proteolytic enzyme papain might increase the blood-thinning effects of warfarin and possibly other anticoagulants.[34]

⚠ INTERACTIONS YOU SHOULD KNOW ABOUT

If you are taking

- The proteolytic enzyme **pancreatin:** You may need extra folate.
- **Warfarin:** You should not take the proteolytic enzyme papain unless under a doctor's supervision.

Visit Us at TNP.com

PYGEUM *(Pygeum africanus)*

Principal Proposed Uses   Benign Prostatic Hyperplasia (Prostate Enlargement)

Other Proposed Uses   Prostatitis (Prostate Infection), Impotence, Male Infertility

The pygeum tree is a tall evergreen native to central and southern Africa. Its bark has been used since ancient times to treat problems with urination.

WHAT IS PYGEUM USED FOR TODAY?

Today, pygeum is primarily used as a treatment for **benign prostatic hyperplasia** (BPH; see page 24), or prostate enlargement, a use that is supported by good scientific evidence. It is more popular in France and Italy than in Germany.

However, **saw palmetto** (see page 406) is probably the better treatment to use. The pygeum tree has been so devastated by collection for use in medicine that some regard it as a threatened species. Saw palmetto is cultivated rather than collected in the wild.

Pygeum is also sometimes used to treat prostatitis, as well as **impotence** (see page 100) and **male infertility** (see page 116);[1,2] however, there is little real evidence that it works.

Note: Before self-treating with pygeum, be sure to get a proper medical evaluation to rule out prostate cancer.

WHAT IS THE SCIENTIFIC EVIDENCE FOR PYGEUM?

At least 10 double-blind trials of pygeum have been performed, involving a total of over 600 people and ranging in length from 45 to 90 days.[3–7] Overall, the results make a reasonably strong case that pygeum can reduce symptoms such as nighttime urination, urinary frequency, and residual urine volume.

The best of these studies was conducted at 8 sites in Europe and included 263 men between 50 and 85 years of age.[8] Participants received 50 mg of a pygeum extract or placebo twice daily. The results showed significant improvements in residual urine volume, voided volume, urinary flow rate, nighttime urination, and daytime frequency.

We don't really know how pygeum works. Unlike the standard drug finasteride, it does not appear to work by affecting the conversion of testosterone to dihydrotestosterone.[9] Rather it is thought to reduce inflammation in the prostate, and also to inhibit prostate growth factors, substances implicated in inappropriate prostate enlargement.[10,11,12]

DOSAGE

The proper dosage of pygeum is 50 mg twice per day (occasionally 100 mg twice daily) of an extract standardized to contain 14% triterpenes and 0.5% n-docosanol. A dose of 100 mg once daily appears to be as effective as the most common dosage of 50 mg twice daily.[13]

There is some reason to believe that pygeum's effectiveness might be enhanced when it is combined with **nettle root** (see page 369).[14,15]

SAFETY ISSUES

Pygeum appears to be essentially nontoxic, both in the short and long term.[16] The most common side effect is mild gastrointestinal distress. However, safety in young children, pregnant or nursing women, or those with severe liver or kidney disease has not been established.

PYRUVATE

Supplement Forms/Alternate Names   Sodium Pyruvate, Calcium Pyruvate, Potassium Pyruvate, Magnesium Pyruvate, Dihydroxyacetone Pyruvate (DHAP)

Principal Proposed Uses   Weight Reduction

Other Proposed Uses   Performance Enhancement

Pyruvate

Visit Us at TNP.com

Pyruvate supplies the body with pyruvic acid, a natural compound that plays important roles in the manufacture and use of energy. Pyruvate supplements have become popular with bodybuilders and other athletes, based on claims that pyruvate can reduce body fat and enhance the ability to use energy efficiently. However, at the present time, there is only preliminary evidence that it really works.

SOURCES

Pyruvate is not an essential nutrient, since your body makes all it needs. But it can be found in food, with an average diet supplying anywhere from 100 mg to 2 g daily. Apples are the best source: a single apple contains about 450 mg of pyruvate. Beer and red wine contain about 75 mg per serving.

Therapeutic dosages are usually much higher than what you can get from food: you'd have to eat almost 70 apples a day to get the proper amount! To use pyruvate for therapeutic purposes, you must take a supplement.

Although most products on the market contain only (or almost only) pyruvate, some also contain small amounts of a related compound, dihydroxyacetone, which the body converts to pyruvate. The combination of the two products is known as DHAP.

THERAPEUTIC DOSAGES

A typical therapeutic dosage of pyruvate is 30 g daily.

THERAPEUTIC USES

Evidence from several small double-blind studies suggests that pyruvate may enhance **weight loss** (see page 192).[1–4] Preliminary evidence also suggests that pyruvate may slightly increase an athlete's capacity for endurance exercise.[5,6] Unfortunately, these studies were all too small for the results to mean very much.

WHAT IS THE SCIENTIFIC EVIDENCE FOR PYRUVATE?

Weight Reduction

In one double-blind placebo-controlled study, 34 people trying to lose weight were given either placebo or a dosage of pyruvate ranging from 22 to 44 g daily.[7] The treatment group lost significantly more weight.

Smaller studies have found similar benefits.[8,9,10]

SAFETY ISSUES

Both pyruvate and dihydroxyacetone appear to be quite safe, aside from mild side effects such as occasional stomach upset and diarrhea. However, maximum safe dosages for children, women who are pregnant or nursing, or those with liver or kidney disease have not been established.

Keep in mind that, because such enormous doses of pyruvate are used, if a contaminant were present even in very small percentages there could be harmful results. For this reason, you should make sure to use a high-quality product.

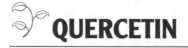

QUERCETIN

Supplement Forms/Alternate Names   Quercetin Chalcone

Principal Proposed Uses   There are no well-documented uses for quercetin.

Other Proposed Uses   Asthma, Allergies (Hay Fever), Eczema, Hives, Prostatitis (Chronic Pelvic Pain Syndrome), Heart Disease Prevention, Stroke Prevention, Cancer Prevention

You may have heard of the "French paradox." The French diet is very high in fat and cholesterol (just think of *pâté de fois gras* and croissants), yet France has one of the world's lowest rates of heart disease. One theory for this discrepancy is that another major player in the French diet—red wine—protects the arteries of the heart.

A natural antioxidant found in red wine, quercetin protects cells in the body from damage by free radicals (naturally occurring but harmful substances). Heart disease and high cholesterol are thought to be at least partly

caused by free radical damage to blood vessels, so it makes sense that quercetin might help protect against heart attacks and strokes. Quercetin belongs to a class of water-soluble plant coloring agents called *bioflavonoids*, a type of nutrient that we're learning more about all the time. Although they don't seem to be essential to life, it's likely that we need them for optimal health.

Another intriguing finding is that quercetin may help prevent immune cells from releasing *histamine,* the chemical that initiates the itching, sneezing, and swelling of an allergic reaction. Based on this very preliminary research, quercetin is often recommended as a treatment for allergies and asthma.

SOURCES

Quercetin is not an essential nutrient. It is found in red wine, grapefruit, onions, apples, black tea, and, in lesser amounts, in leafy green vegetables and beans. However, to get a therapeutic dosage, you'll have to take a supplement.

Quercetin supplements are available in pill and tablet form. One problem with them, however, is that they don't seem to be well absorbed by the body. A special form called quercetin chalcone appears to be better absorbed.

THERAPEUTIC DOSAGES

A typical dosage is 200 to 400 mg 3 times daily. Quercetin may be better absorbed if taken on an empty stomach.

THERAPEUTIC USES

The most popular use of quercetin is as a treatment for allergic conditions such as **asthma** (see page 14), **hay fever** (see page 2), **eczema** (see page 78), and **hives** (see page 181). This use is based on test-tube research showing that quercetin prevents certain immune cells from releasing histamine, the chemical that triggers an allergic reaction.[1,2] It also may block other substances involved with allergies.[3] But we have no evidence as yet that taking quercetin supplements will reduce your allergy symptoms.

Prostatitis is an inflammation or infection of the prostate gland. In some cases, no cause can be discovered. The condition causes chronic pain and difficulty with urination, and is sometimes called chronic pelvic pain syndrome. Conventional treatment for this condition is often unsatisfactory. According to a 1-month double-blind placebo-controlled trial of 30 men with chronic pelvic pain, quercetin at a dose of 500 mg twice daily might be helpful.[4]

Very preliminary evidence also suggests that quercetin might help prevent **heart disease** (see page 16) and strokes.[5–9]

Test-tube and animal research also suggests that quercetin might have anticancer properties.[10–14]

An animal study found that quercetin might protect rodents with diabetes from forming cataracts.[15] Another intriguing finding of test-tube research is that quercetin seems to prevent a wide range of viruses from infecting cells and reproducing once they are inside cells. One study found that quercetin produced this effect against herpes simplex, polio virus, flu virus, and respiratory viruses.[16,17] However, none of this research tells us whether humans taking quercetin supplements can hope for the same benefits. Much more research needs to be done on the use of quercetin for these conditions.

SAFETY ISSUES

Quercetin appears to be quite safe. However, at one point concerns were raised that it might cause cancer. Quercetin "fails" a standard laboratory test called the Ames test, which is designed to identify chemicals that might be carcinogenic. However, a bad showing on the Ames test does not definitely mean a chemical causes cancer. Other evidence suggests that quercetin does *not* cause cancer, and may in fact help prevent cancer.[18,19,20]

However, one highly preliminary study suggests that quercetin combined with other bioflavonoids in the diet of pregnant women might increase the risk of infant leukemia.[21]

Maximum safe dosages for young children, women who are pregnant or nursing, or those with serious liver or kidney disease have not been established.

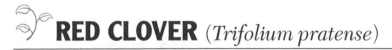

RED CLOVER (*Trifolium pratense*)

Alternate or Related Names   Purple Clover, Trefoil, Wild Clover

Principal Proposed Uses   Menopausal Symptoms

Other Proposed Uses   Acne, Eczema, Psoriasis, Cancer?

Red clover has been cultivated since ancient times, primarily to provide a favorite grazing food for animals. But, like many other herbs, red clover was also a valued medicine. Although it has been used for many purposes worldwide, the one condition most consistently associated with red clover is cancer. Chinese physicians and Russian folk healers also used it to treat respiratory problems.

In the nineteenth century, red clover became popular among herbalists as an "alterative" or "blood purifier."

Red Clover

Visit Us at TNP.com

This medical term, long since defunct, refers to an ancient belief that toxins in the blood are the root cause of many illnesses. Cancer, eczema, and the eruptions of venereal disease were all seen as manifestations of toxic buildup.

Red clover was considered one of the best herbs to "purify" the blood. For this reason, it is included in many of the famous treatments for cancer, including the Hoxsey cancer cure (see **burdock;** page 232) and Jason Winter's cancer-cure tea.

Recently, special red clover extracts high in substances called isoflavones have arrived on the market. For more information, see **isoflavones** (page 335).

WHAT IS RED CLOVER USED FOR TODAY?

Recently, red clover products have been marketed as a treatment for **menopausal symptoms** (see page 117). They contain high concentrations of four major isoflavones, substances similar but not identical to estrogen. However, a 28-week double-blind placebo-controlled crossover study of 51 postmenopausal women found no reduction in hot flashes among those given 40 mg of red clover isoflavones daily.[1] No benefits were seen in another double-blind placebo-controlled trial, which involved 37 women given isoflavones from red clover at a dose of either 40 or 160 mg daily.[2]

There is no evidence that red clover can help cancer. However, its usage in many parts of the world as a traditional cancer remedy has prompted scientists to take a close look at the herb. It turns out that the isoflavones in red clover may possess antitumor activity.[3,4] However, such preliminary research does not prove that red clover can treat cancer.

Red clover is sometimes recommended for the treatment of **acne** (see page 2), **eczema** (see page 78), **psoriasis** (see page 148), and other skin diseases.

DOSAGE

A typical dosage of red clover extract provides 40 to 160 mg of isoflavones daily.

SAFETY ISSUES

Red clover is on the FDA's GRAS (generally recognized as safe) list, and is included in many beverage teas. However, detailed safety studies have not been performed.

Because of its blood-thinning and estrogen-like constituents, red clover should not be used by pregnant or nursing women, or women who have had breast or uterine cancer. Safety in young children or those with severe liver or kidney disease has also not been established.

Based on their constituents, red clover extracts may conceivably interfere with hormone treatments and anticoagulant drugs.

For other potential risks due to the isoflavones in red clover (especially in concentrated isoflavone-rich extracts of red clover), see the chapter on isoflavones.

⚠ INTERACTIONS YOU SHOULD KNOW ABOUT

If you are taking hormones or **blood-thinning drugs** (such as **Coumadin [warfarin], heparin, Trental [pentoxifylline],** or even **aspirin**), red clover should be used only under a physician's supervision.

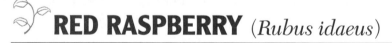

RED RASPBERRY (*Rubus idaeus*)

Alternate or Related Names   Raspberry

Principal Proposed Uses   Prevent Complications of Pregnancy

Herbalists have long believed that raspberry leaf tea taken regularly during pregnancy can prevent complications and make delivery easier. Raspberry has also been used to reduce excessive menstruation and relieve symptoms of diarrhea.

WHAT IS RED RASPBERRY USED FOR TODAY?

Red raspberry tea is still commonly recommended for pregnant women.

An interesting animal study suggests that red raspberry inhibits uterine contractions during pregnancy but not outside of pregnancy.[1] This naturally leads one to wonder whether raspberry leaf first stabilizes the uterus to prevent miscarriages and then somehow turns around and allows the uterus to relax for delivery. However, this is just speculation at the present time. If you take red raspberry during pregnancy, you are doing so based on long tradition, not on science.

Red Raspberry

Visit Us at TNP.com

DOSAGE

To make raspberry leaf tea, pour 1 cup of boiling water over 1 or 2 teaspoons of dried leaf, steep for 10 minutes, and then sweeten to taste. Unlike many medicinal herbs, raspberry leaf actually has a pleasant taste! During pregnancy, drink 2 to 3 cups daily.

SAFETY ISSUES

Strangely enough, the safety of red raspberry during pregnancy and nursing has not been established. Yet years of traditional use and the widespread availability of the beverage make it difficult to get very concerned. Safety in young children or those with severe liver or kidney disease has also not been established.

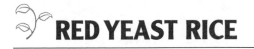

RED YEAST RICE

Supplement Forms/Alternate Names   *Monascus purpureus,* Hong Qu

Principal Proposed Uses   High Cholesterol

Red yeast rice is a traditional Chinese substance that is made by fermenting a type of yeast called *Monascus purpureus* over rice. This product (called Hong Qu) has been used in China since at least 800 A.D. as a food and also as a medicinal substance. Recently, it has been discovered that this ancient Chinese preparation contains at least 11 naturally occurring substances similar to prescription drugs in the "statin" family, such as Mevacor and Pravachol. These medications are highly effective at reducing cholesterol.

WHAT IS RED YEAST RICE USED FOR TODAY?

Presumably because it contains substances similar or identical to statin drugs, red yeast rice appears to be effective at lowering **cholesterol** (see page 88). However, because of potential risks, it should be used only under physician supervision.

WHAT IS THE SCIENTIFIC EVIDENCE FOR RED YEAST RICE?

A recent major U.S. study on red yeast rice was conducted at the UCLA School of Medicine.[1] This was a 12-week double-blind placebo-controlled trial involving 83 healthy participants (46 men and 37 women, aged 34 to 78 years) with high cholesterol levels. One group was given the recommended dose of red yeast rice, while the other group received a placebo. Both groups were instructed to consume a low-fat diet similar to the American Heart Association Step 1 diet.

The results showed that red yeast rice was significantly more effective than placebo. In the treated group, average total cholesterol (mg/dL) fell by about 18% by 8 weeks. During the same time period, LDL ("bad") cholesterol decreased by 22% and triglycerides by 11%. There was little to no improvement in the placebo group. HDL ("good") cholesterol did not change in either group during the study.

Similar or even better results have been seen in other U.S. and Chinese studies using various forms of red yeast rice.[2,3]

DOSAGE

Because red yeast rice products can vary widely in their strength, please refer to the labeling for appropriate dosage.

SAFETY ISSUES

While there have been no serious adverse reactions reported in the studies of red yeast rice, some minor side effects have been reported. In a large open trial in which 324 people received red yeast rice, heartburn (1.8%), bloating (0.9%), and dizziness (0.3%) were all mentioned.[4] Formal toxicity studies in rats and mice, giving doses up to 125 times the normal human dose for 3 months, showed no toxic effects, according to information provided by one of the manufacturers of red yeast rice.[5]

However, because red yeast rice contains ingredients similar to the statin drugs, there is a theoretical risk of the same side effects and risks that are seen with those drugs. These include elevated liver enzymes, damage to skeletal muscle, and increased risk of cancer.

Red yeast rice should not be combined with erythromycin, other statin drugs, the class of drugs called "fibrates," or high-dose niacin (for lowering cholesterol). Serious side effects have reportedly occurred when statin drugs were combined with these medications.

Additionally, like statin drugs, red yeast rice may deplete the body of a substance called coenzyme Q_{10} (CoQ_{10}).[6-9] Taking extra CoQ_{10} might be helpful.

Grapefruit juice can cause a significant and possibly dangerous increase in blood levels of statin drugs. For this reason, grapefruit juice should be avoided when taking red yeast rice.

This product should not be used by pregnant or nursing mothers, or those with severe liver or kidney disease except on a physician's advice.

⚠ INTERACTIONS YOU SHOULD KNOW ABOUT

If you are taking

- **Erythromycin,** cholesterol-lowering drugs in the **statin** or fibrate family, or high-dose **niacin:** Do not take red yeast rice.
- **Red yeast rice:** Do not drink grapefruit juice.
- **Red yeast rice:** You may need extra **CoQ_{10}**.

REISHI (*Ganoderma lucidum*)

Principal Proposed Uses   Adaptogen (Improve Resistance to Stress), Strengthen Immunity Against Colds and Other Infections, Improve Mental Function, Prevent Altitude Sickness

Other Proposed Uses   Asthma, Bronchitis, Viral Hepatitis, Cardiovascular Disease, Ulcers, Cancer?

The tree fungus known as reishi has a long history of use in China and Japan as a semi-magical healing herb. More revered than ginseng and, up until recently, more rare, many stories tell of people with severe illnesses journeying immense distances to find it. Presently, reishi is artificially cultivated and widely available in stores that sell herb products.

WHAT IS REISHI USED FOR TODAY?

Reishi is marketed as a cure-all, said to prevent and treat cancer, strengthen immunity against infection, restore normal immune function in autoimmune diseases (such as myasthenia gravis), improve symptoms of **asthma** (see page 14) and bronchitis, overcome **viral hepatitis** (see page 189), prevent and treat cardiovascular disease, improve mental function, heal **ulcers** (see page 180), and prevent **altitude sickness** (see page 4). However, there is no real evidence that reishi is effective for any of these conditions.

Contemporary herbalists regard it as an adaptogen, a substance believed to be capable of helping the body to resist **stress** (see page 167) of all kinds. (For more information on adaptogens, see the chapter on **ginseng**.) However, while there has been a great deal of basic scientific research into the chemical constituents of reishi, reliable double-blind studies are lacking.

DOSAGE

The proper dosage of reishi is 2 to 6 g per day of raw fungus, or an equivalent dosage of concentrated extract, taken with meals. Reishi is often combined with related fungi, such as shiitake, hoelen, or polyporus. Results may develop after about 1 to 2 weeks. It is often taken continually for its presumed overall health benefits.

SAFETY ISSUES

Reishi appears to be extremely safe. Occasional side effects include mild digestive upset, dry mouth, and skin rash. Reishi can "thin" the blood slightly, and therefore should not be combined with drugs such as Coumadin (warfarin) or heparin. Safety in young children, pregnant or nursing women, or those with severe liver or kidney disease has not been established.

⚠ INTERACTIONS YOU SHOULD KNOW ABOUT

If you are taking blood-thinning medications such as **Coumadin (warfarin)** or **heparin,** use reishi only under a doctor's supervision.

Reishi

RESVERATROL

Supplement Forms/Alternate Names   Grape Skin

Principal Proposed Uses   There are no well-documented uses for resveratrol.

Other Proposed Uses   Heart Disease, Cancer Prevention

You may have heard of the "French paradox." The national diet of France includes a lot of butter, cream, meat, and other high-fat, high-cholesterol foods suspected to be bad for the heart. Yet France has one of the world's *lowest* rates of heart disease. The leading theory attempting to explain this puzzle suggests that the French are somehow protected from cardiovascular disease because they drink red wine.

Resveratrol is an ingredient of red wine that may be at least partly responsible for this beneficial effect. (**Quercetin** is another such ingredient. See the chapter on quercetin.) Resveratrol is a *polyphenol,* a natural antioxidant that protects cells against dangerous, naturally occurring substances known as free radicals.

Test-tube and observational studies have linked resveratrol to reduced rates of heart disease and cancer. Unfortunately, there hasn't been any clinical research on human beings yet, but the attention resveratrol has been getting via news stories on the "French paradox" might lead to clinical studies in the near future.

SOURCES

Resveratrol is not an essential nutrient. It is found in red wine as well as in red grape skins and seeds and purple grape juice. Peanuts also contain a small amount of resveratrol. Resveratrol supplements are available as well.

THERAPEUTIC DOSAGES

Because there haven't been any clinical studies, the optimal therapeutic dosage hasn't been established for resveratrol. Based on animal studies, a reasonable therapeutic dosage of resveratrol might be about 500 mg daily.

THERAPEUTIC USES

Very preliminary evidence suggests that resveratrol may help prevent **heart disease** (see page 16),[1–4] although some studies have not been favorable.[5,6,7]

Test-tube studies also suggest that resveratrol might have a number of properties that might make it helpful for preventing **cancer** (see page 32).[8–13]

SAFETY ISSUES

Resveratrol appears to be quite safe according to the research done thus far, but full safety studies have not been performed. Maximum safe dosages for children, pregnant or nursing women, or those with severe liver or kidney disease have not been determined.

RIBOSE

Principal Proposed Uses   Coronary Artery Disease

Other Proposed Uses   Rare Enzyme Deficiencies, Performance Enhancement

Ribose is a carbohydrate vital for the body's manufacture of ATP, which is the major source of energy used by our cells.

Quite a few studies have been done on ribose, mostly relating to its potential usefulness for individuals with heart disease. When the heart is starved for oxygen, as can occur with a heart attack or angina, it loses much of its ATP, and its ATP levels remain low for several days, even after blood flow is resumed.[1] Scientists have found that supplying extra ribose in the blood helps restore the heart's normal ATP levels more quickly. This may there-fore mean that ribose supplements can improve heart functioning and increase exercise capacity, but these benefits have not yet been proven.

Ribose has also been tried for improving exercise capacity in individuals with certain enzyme deficiencies and other rare conditions that cause muscle pain during exertion. There is weak evidence that it may help people with some of these conditions—but not others—to exercise without pain.

Finally, ribose has recently been touted as an important new performance enhancer for athletes. However,

Ribose

Visit Us at TNP.com

there is as yet no evidence at all that it works in this capacity.

REQUIREMENTS/SOURCES

Ribose is not an essential nutrient. Although it is a common sugar present in the bodies of animals and plants, food sources don't supply recommended dosages.

THERAPEUTIC DOSAGES

The dose of ribose that will improve **sports performance** (see page 158) in ordinary athletes has not been determined. Typical doses recommended by sports supplement manufacturers are 1 to 10 g per day. Participants in a study of heart disease took 60 g of ribose in water (15 mg, 4 times a day) by mouth for 3 days.[2] In case reports, people with rare enzyme deficiencies reported benefit with oral doses of 3 to 4 g taken every 10 to 30 minutes during exercise, sometimes totaling 50 to 60 g per day.[3,4]

Warning: If you have either of these conditions, take ribose only under the supervision of a doctor.

Typically provided as a powder to be dissolved in water or in liquid form, ribose is also available commercially in capsules. The dissolved powder has a sweetish taste that some people find unpleasant.[5]

THERAPEUTIC USES

Ribose may be of benefit in improving exercise tolerance in people with severe coronary artery disease by helping the heart regenerate its ATP, but the evidence as yet is highly preliminary.[6]

Sports enthusiasts are more interested in ATP's effects on regular muscles than on the heart muscle. At least one animal study seems to show that skeletal muscle, like heart muscle, replenishes ATP more quickly when ribose is added to the blood,[7] but so far no research indicates improvement in sports performance.

In a few case reports, ribose has increased exercise ability in people with a rare condition involving deficiency of the enzyme myoadenylate deaminase (AMPD).[8,9] However, no double-blind studies of ribose in AMPD deficiency have been conducted. Small double-blind studies have found ribose to be ineffective for another rare enzyme deficiency called McArdle's disease and for Duchenne's muscular dystrophy.[10,11]

WHAT IS THE SCIENTIFIC EVIDENCE FOR RIBOSE?

Coronary Artery Disease

Individuals with sufficiently severe coronary artery disease suffer reduced blood flow to the heart (ischemia) with exercise, and experience angina pain. One small study examined whether giving ribose can improve exercise tolerance for people with coronary artery disease.[12] In the study, 20 men with severe coronary artery disease walked on a treadmill while researchers noted how long it took for signs of ischemia to develop. For the next 3 days, the men took either oral ribose (60 mg per day) or placebo, after which they repeated the treadmill test. Results of the final test showed that those taking ribose increased the time they were able to walk before developing EKG signs of ischemia, while those taking placebo had no such improvement. This preliminary study was too small to prove anything, but it certainly suggests that further investigation would be worthwhile.

SAFETY ISSUES

There are no reports of lasting or damaging side effects from ribose, but formal safety studies have not yet been conducted. Reported minor side effects include diarrhea, gastrointestinal discomfort, nausea, headache, and hypoglycemia.[13]

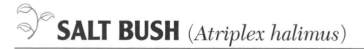

SALT BUSH (*Atriplex halimus*)

Principal Proposed Uses   Type 2 Diabetes (Non-Insulin-Dependent or Adult Onset Diabetes)

Salt bush is a shrub that grows throughout the Mediterranean region, in the Middle East, northern Africa, and southern Europe. As its name suggests, it is especially common in areas where the soil is saline. Salt bush is a nutritious plant, high in protein, **vitamins C** (see page 444), **A** (see page 432), and **D** (see page 449), and minerals such as **chromium** (see page 251). It is also fairly tasty—shepherds as well as their flocks enjoy eating salt bush.

WHAT IS SALT BUSH USED FOR TODAY?

Salt bush may prove useful in the treatment of type 2 (non-insulin-dependent or adult onset) **diabetes** (see page 65).

Salt Bush

Visit Us at TNP.com

This idea came to the attention of medical researchers in 1964, when they discovered that a rodent called the sand rat (*Psammomys obesus*) is highly susceptible to developing diabetes.[1] Yet wild sand rats, which regularly consume salt bush, never show any signs of diabetes—they tend to develop it in response to being fed regular laboratory food! As a result, scientists have explored the possibility that salt bush has an antidiabetic effect.

The results of animal studies suggest that salt bush does indeed have antidiabetic effects.[2,3,4] However, while these studies are certainly intriguing, human trials of salt bush are highly preliminary, and as yet we have no real evidence that it would be an effective treatment for human diabetes.[5,6]

Some animal researchers speculate that the effect of salt bush may be partly due to the chromium it contains.[7] Considerable evidence indicates that chromium supplementation can improve blood sugar control, especially in type 2 diabetes (see the **chromium** chapter for details). However, there may be other active ingredients in salt bush as well.

DOSAGE

No standard dosage of salt bush has been established.

Warning: Diabetes is a serious disease that should be treated only under medical supervision. Salt bush cannot be used as a substitute for insulin. Blood sugar levels should also be closely monitored. For more information, see Safety Issues.

SAFETY ISSUES

As a plant food commonly consumed by animals and humans, salt bush appears to be relatively safe. However, no comprehensive safety testing of salt bush has been performed. For this reason, it should not be used by young children, pregnant or nursing women, or people with severe liver or kidney disease.

Keep in mind that if salt bush is effective, the result might be excessive lowering of blood sugar levels. For this reason, people with diabetes who take salt bush should do so only under a physician's supervision.[8,9]

SAMe (S-Adenosylmethionine)

Supplement Forms/Alternate Names   SAM, Ademetionine

Principal Proposed Uses   Osteoarthritis, Depression

Other Proposed Uses   Liver Disease, Fibromyalgia, Parkinson's Disease, Protection Against Ulcers Caused by Alcohol

S-*adenosylmethionine* is quite a mouthful; the abbreviation *SAMe* (pronounced "sam-ee") is easier to say. Its chemical structure and name are derived from two materials you may have heard about already: methionine, a sulfur-containing amino acid; and adenosine triphosphate (ATP), the body's main energy molecule.

SAMe was discovered in Italy in 1952. It was first investigated as a treatment for depression, but along the way it was accidentally noted to improve arthritis symptoms—a kind of positive "side effect." SAMe is presently classed with **glucosamine** (see page 308) and **chondroitin** (see page 250) as a potential "chondroprotective" agent, one that can go beyond treating symptoms to actually slowing the progression of arthritis. However, this exciting possibility has not yet been proven.

Unfortunately, SAMe is an extraordinarily expensive supplement at present. Full dosages can easily cost more than $200 per month.

SOURCES

The body makes all the SAMe it needs, so there is no dietary requirement. However, deficiencies in **methionine** (see page 360), **folate** (see page 288), or **vitamin B$_{12}$** (see page 442) can reduce SAMe levels. SAMe is not found in appreciable quantities in foods, so it must be taken as a supplement. It's been suggested that the supplement **TMG** (see page 423) might indirectly increase SAMe levels and provide similar benefits, but this effect has not been proven.

THERAPEUTIC DOSAGES

A typical full dosage of SAMe is 400 mg taken 3 to 4 times per day. If this dosage works for you, take it for a few weeks and then try reducing the dosage. As little as 200 mg twice daily may suffice to keep you feeling better once the full dosage has "broken through" the symptoms.

However, some people develop mild stomach distress if they start full dosages of SAMe at once. To get around this, you may need to start low and work up to the full dosage gradually.

Recently, SAMe has come on the U.S. market at a recommended dosage of 200 mg twice daily. This dosage labeling makes SAMe appear more affordable (if you're

SAMe

Visit Us at TNP.com

only taking 400 mg per day, you'll spend only about a third of what you'd pay for the proper dosage), but it is unlikely that SAMe will actually work when taken at such a low dosage.

THERAPEUTIC USES

A substantial amount of evidence suggests that SAMe can be an effective treatment for **osteoarthritis** (see page 132), the "wear and tear" type of arthritis that many people develop as they get older.[1] However, the supplements glucosamine and chondroitin are much less expensive and just as well documented. (For more information on natural options for arthritis, see the chapters on **glucosamine** and **chondroitin**.)

Several small studies suggest that SAMe can be helpful for **depression** (see page 59).[2]

This supplement may also be helpful for certain liver conditions such as **liver cirrhosis** (see page 112), pregnancy-related jaundice, and Gilbert's syndrome.[3–10] Additionally, SAMe may help the painful muscle condition known as **fibromyalgia** (see page 80).[11,12]

SAMe might be helpful for individuals with **Parkinson's disease** (see page 140). It has been found to reduce the depression so commonly associated with the disease.[13] In addition, the drug levodopa, used for Parkinson's disease, depletes the body of SAMe.[14,15] This suggests that taking extra SAMe might be helpful. However, it is also possible that SAMe could interfere with the effect of levodopa, requiring an increase in dosage.

Preliminary evidence suggests that SAMe can protect the stomach against damage caused by alcohol.[16]

WHAT IS THE SCIENTIFIC EVIDENCE FOR SAME (S-ADENOSYLMETHIONINE)?

Although there have been many studies of SAMe, a substantial percentage of them involved intravenous use of the supplement instead of the oral form. Here we discuss only the evidence for SAMe when it is taken orally.

Osteoarthritis

A substantial body of scientific evidence supports the use of SAMe to treat osteoarthritis.[17] Double-blind studies involving a total of more than a thousand participants suggest that SAMe is about as effective as standard anti-inflammatory drugs. In addition, animal evidence suggests that SAMe may help protect cartilage from damage.[18,19]

For example, a double-blind placebo-controlled Italian study tracked 732 people taking SAMe, naproxen (a standard anti-inflammatory drug), or placebo.[20] After 4 weeks, participants taking SAMe or naproxen showed

about the same level of benefit as compared with those in the placebo group.

Another double-blind study compared SAMe with the anti-inflammatory drug piroxicam.[21] A total of 45 individuals were followed for 84 days. The two treatments proved equally effective. However, the SAMe-treated individuals maintained their improvement long after the treatment was stopped, whereas those on piroxicam quickly started to hurt again. Similarly long-lasting results have been seen with glucosamine and chondroitin. This pattern of response suggests that these treatments are somehow making a deeper impact on osteoarthritis than simply relieving symptoms. However, while we have direct evidence that glucosamine and chondroitin can slow the progression of osteoarthritis, we do not know for sure that SAMe offers the same benefit.

In other double-blind studies, oral SAMe has also shown equivalent benefits to various doses of indomethacin, ibuprofen, and naproxen.[22,23,24]

Depression

SAMe's antidepressant activity was first reported in 1976.[25] Since then, several small double-blind studies involving a total of more than 200 individuals have found oral SAMe to be an effective treatment for depression.[26–32] Some of these studies compared SAMe with placebo, while others used a control group given another antidepressant drug. Unfortunately, none of these trials enrolled more than 60 participants, and many of the studies suffered from significant design flaws. Solid evidence that SAMe is effective for depression will require a large (100 participants or more) double-blind placebo-controlled trial.

Liver Disease

A 2-year double-blind study of 117 individuals with alcoholic liver cirrhosis disease found that treatment with SAMe did not reduce mortality in the group as a whole.[33] Other studies showed benefits in a variety of other liver conditions, including liver toxicity caused by oral contraceptives, pregnancy-related jaundice, and Gilbert's syndrome.[34–40]

Fibromyalgia

Four double-blind trials have studied the use of SAMe for fibromyalgia,[41–44] three of them finding it to be helpful. Unfortunately, most of these studies gave SAMe either intravenously or as an injection into the muscles, sometimes in combination with oral doses. When you inject a medication, the effects can be quite different than when you take it orally. For that reason, these studies are of questionable relevance.

However, the one double-blind study that used only oral SAMe did find positive results.[45] In this trial, 44 people with fibromyalgia took 800 mg SAMe or placebo for 6 weeks. Compared to the group taking placebo, those taking SAMe had improvements in disease activity, pain at rest, fatigue, and morning stiffness, and in one measurement of mood. In other respects, such as the amount of tenderness in their tender points, the group taking SAMe did no better than those taking the placebo.

It isn't clear whether SAMe is helping fibromyalgia through its antidepressant effects, or by some other mechanism.

Parkinson's Disease

Evidence suggests that levodopa (the drug used to treat Parkinson's disease) can reduce brain levels of SAMe.[46,47,48] This depletion may contribute to the side effects of levodopa treatment, as well as the depression sometimes seen with Parkinson's disease. One study found that SAMe taken orally improved depression without changing the effectiveness of levodopa.[49] However, it is also possible that over time taking extra SAMe could interfere with levodopa's effectiveness (see Safety Issues).

SAFETY ISSUES

SAMe appears to be quite safe, according to both human and animal studies.[50–53] The most common side effect is mild digestive distress. However, SAMe does not actually damage the stomach.[54]

Like other substances with antidepressant activity, SAMe might trigger a manic episode in those with **bipolar disease** (manic-depressive illness; see page 27).[55–60]

Safety in young children, pregnant or nursing women, or those with severe liver or kidney disease has not been established.

SAMe might interfere with the action of the Parkinson's drug levodopa.[61] In addition, there may also be risks involved in combining SAMe with standard antidepressants.[62] For this reason, you shouldn't try either combination except under physician supervision.

⚠ INTERACTIONS YOU SHOULD KNOW ABOUT

If you are taking

- Standard antidepressants, including **MAO inhibitors**, **SSRIs**, and **tricyclics**: Do not take SAMe except on a physician's advice.
- **Levodopa** for Parkinson's disease: SAMe might help relieve the side effects of this drug. However, it might also reduce its effectiveness over time.

ᕘ SANDALWOOD (*Santalum album*)

Alternate or Related Names   Sanderswood, White Saunders, Yellow Saunders

Principal Proposed Uses   Bladder Infection

Other Proposed Uses   Herpes, Persistent Cough, Sore Throat, Bronchitis, Acne, Rashes, Dry Skin

---

Native to India, the sandalwood tree is used for many purposes—the wood for decorative carvings, the oil for fragrance in incense, perfumes, and soaps. Both its wood and oil have also been employed medicinally for a wide variety of conditions.

Unfortunately, harvesting of these trees is beginning to endanger the species. The Indian government has limited the amount of sandalwood that may be harvested each year, but has not restricted its export. Illegal harvesting of sandalwood has become very lucrative, as limits on legal harvesting have caused a price increase for sandalwood products.

In traditional Indian (Ayurvedic) medicine, sandalwood was used to treat gonorrhea and to decrease sex drive. Traditional Chinese medicine also lists sandalwood

as a treatment for gonorrhea, as well as for stomachache and vomiting. In Europe, sandalwood was used to treat fever and pain, as we use aspirin today. However, no clinical evidence exists to support any of these applications.

WHAT IS SANDALWOOD USED FOR TODAY?

Germany's Commission E has approved sandalwood for the treatment of bladder infections, not to be used alone, but along with other therapies.[1] Sandalwood is said to act as an antiseptic in the urinary system; if this is correct, it might help to rid the body of the bacteria that cause these infections,[2] but there is no evidence as yet to verify this belief.

In test tube studies, sandalwood was found to slow the growth of **herpes** (see page 86) virus.[3] An intriguing animal study found that components isolated from sandalwood caused responses similar to those seen with antipsychotic medications.[4] However, neither of these extremely preliminary investigations as yet provides evidence that can be applied to medicinal applications of sandalwood in humans.

Sandalwood is also advertised for other therapeutic uses, including bronchitis, sore throat, and persistent cough. External application of a sandalwood paste is sometimes suggested for **acne** (see page 2), skin rashes, or dry skin. None of these treatments, however, have been scientifically studied.

DOSAGE

For urinary tract infections, the Commission E suggests 1 to 1.5 g of essential oil or 10 to 20 g of ground sandalwood daily, not to be taken for more than 6 weeks except on the advice of a physician. If the essential oil of sandalwood is used, an enteric-coated capsule is recommended (such capsules delay the release of a substance until it has passed through the stomach into the intestine, helping to avoid an upset stomach).

SAFETY ISSUES

The safety of sandalwood has not been formally evaluated. For this reason, it should not be used by pregnant or nursing women, young children, or individuals with severe kidney or liver disease.

Reported side effects include nausea and itching.[5]

Sandalwood paste applied externally has been reported to cause skin irritation on rare occasions. There is also one case report of a man developing a skin rash after burning large quantities of sandalwood incense.[6,7,8]

SAW PALMETTO (*Serenoa repens* or *Sabal serrulata*)

Alternate or Related Names   Sabal, Shrub Palmetto

Principal Proposed Uses   Benign Prostatic Hyperplasia (Prostate Enlargement)

Other Proposed Uses   Prostatitis (Prostate Infection)

Saw palmetto is a native plant of North America, and although Europeans are its principal consumers, it is still primarily grown in the United States.

The saw palmetto tree grows only about 2 to 4 feet high, with fan-shaped serrated leaves and abundant berries. Native Americans used these berries for the treatment of various urinary problems in men, as well as for women with breast disorders. European and American physicians took up saw palmetto as a treatment for benign prostatic hyperplasia (BPH), but in the United States the herb ultimately fell out of favor, along with all other herbs.

European interest endured, and in the 1960s, French researchers discovered that by concentrating the oils of saw palmetto berry they could maximize the herb's effectiveness.

Saw palmetto contains many biologically active chemicals. Unfortunately, we don't know which ones are the most important. We also don't really know how saw palmetto works, although it appears to interact with various sex hormones.

WHAT IS SAW PALMETTO USED FOR TODAY?

Saw palmetto oil is an accepted medical treatment for **benign prostatic hyperplasia** (BPH; see page 24) in New Zealand, France, Germany, Austria, Italy, Spain, and other European countries. In some countries it is regarded as the "gold standard" against which new prostate drugs must prove themselves!

Typical symptoms of BPH include difficulty starting urination, weak urinary stream, frequent urination, dribbling after urination, and waking up several times at night to urinate. Research suggests that saw palmetto can markedly improve all these symptoms. Benefits require approximately 4 to 6 weeks of treatment to develop and endure for at least 3 years. It appears that about two thirds of men respond reasonably well.

Furthermore, while the prostate tends to continue to grow when left untreated,[1] saw palmetto causes a small but definite shrinkage.[2,3,4] In other words, it isn't just relieving symptoms, but may actually be retarding prostate enlargement. The drug Proscar does this too (and to even a greater extent than saw palmetto) but other standard medications for BPH have no effect on prostate size.

Research tells us that saw palmetto is equally effective to Proscar, but it has one great advantage: It leaves PSA (prostate-specific antigen) levels unchanged. Cancer raises PSA levels, and lab tests that measure PSA are used to screen for prostate cancer. Because Proscar lowers PSA measurements, its use may have the unintended effect of masking prostate cancer. Saw palmetto won't do this. On the other hand, Proscar has been shown to reduce the need for surgery, unlike saw palmetto or any of the other drugs used for BPH.

Note: Before self-treating with saw palmetto, be sure to get a proper medical evaluation to rule out prostate cancer.

Saw palmetto is also widely used to treat chronic prostatitis, but its effectiveness in this regard has not been documented.

WHAT IS THE SCIENTIFIC EVIDENCE FOR SAW PALMETTO?

The science for the effectiveness of saw palmetto in treating prostate enlargement is quite strong, although it could stand to improve.

At least seven double-blind studies involving a total of about 500 people have compared the benefits of saw palmetto against placebo over a period of 1 to 3 months.[5–11] In these studies, the herb significantly improved urinary flow rate and most other measures of prostate disease.[12] Only one study failed to find any benefit. This is fairly impressive, but it would be nice to have a long-term (6 months to 1 year) study of saw palmetto versus placebo.

A double-blind study followed 1,098 men who received either saw palmetto or the drug Proscar over a period of 6 months (unfortunately, there was no placebo group).[13] The treatments were equally effective, but while Proscar lowered PSA levels and caused a slight worsening of sexual function on average, saw palmetto caused no significant side effects.

A study involving 435 men found that the benefits of saw palmetto endure for at least 3 years.[14,15] However, there was no control group in this study, making the results unreliable.

Finally, a 6-month double-blind placebo-controlled trial of 44 men given a saw palmetto herbal blend (containing, in addition, nettle root and pumpkin seed oil) found shrinkage in prostate tissue.[16] No significant improvement in symptoms was seen, but the authors pointed out that the study size was too small to statistically detect such improvements if they did occur.

DOSAGE

The standard dosage of saw palmetto is 160 mg twice a day of an extract standardized to contain 85 to 95% fatty acids and sterols. A single daily dose of 320 mg seems to be just as effective.[17] However, taking more than this amount does not seem to produce better results.[18]

SAFETY ISSUES

Saw palmetto appears to be essentially nontoxic.[19] It is also nearly side-effect free. In a 3-year study only 34 of the 435 participants complained of side effects—primarily the usual mild gastrointestinal distress.[20] There are no known drug interactions.

Safety for those with severe kidney or liver disease has not been established.

SELENIUM

Supplement Forms/Alternate Names   Selenite, Selenomethionine, Selenized Yeast, Selenium Dioxide

Principal Proposed Uses   Cancer Prevention

Other Proposed Uses   Diabetic Neuropathy, HIV Support, Acne, AIDS, Asthma, Cataracts, Cervical Dysplasia, Heart Disease, Multiple Sclerosis, Rheumatoid Arthritis, Anxiety, Fibromyalgia, Gout, Male Infertility, Osteoarthritis, Psoriasis, Ulcers

Selenium is a trace mineral that our bodies use to produce *glutathione peroxidase,* an enzyme that serves as a natural antioxidant. Glutathione peroxidase works with vitamin E to protect cell membranes from damage caused by dangerous, naturally occurring substances known as free radicals.

You may have heard that China has very low rates of colon cancer, presumably because of the nation's lowfat diet. However, in some parts of China where the soil is depleted of selenium, the incidence of various types of cancer is much higher than in the rest of the country. This fact has given rise to a theory that selenium deficiency is a common cause of cancer, and that selenium supplements can reduce this risk.

As we will see, there is some evidence that selenium supplements may provide some protection against several types of cancer. This "chemopreventive" effect isn't fully understood. It might be due to the protective effects of the antioxidant glutathione peroxidase, but other explanations have also been suggested.[1,2]

REQUIREMENTS/SOURCES

The official U.S. and Canadian recommendations for daily intake of selenium are as follows:

- Infants 0–6 months, 15 mcg
    7–12 months, 20 mcg
- Children 1–3 years, 20 mcg
    4–8 years, 30 mcg
    9–13 years, 40 mcg
- Males and females 14 years and older, 55 mcg
- Pregnant women, 60 mcg
- Nursing women, 70 mcg

The "tolerable upper intake level" (UL) as determined by the U.S. government is 400 mcg per day.[3] The UL can be thought of as the highest daily intake over a prolonged time known to pose no risks to most members of a healthy population.

Selenium content of food varies depending on the selenium content of the soil in which it was grown. Studies suggest that many people in developed countries, including New Zealand, Belgium, and Scandinavia, do not get enough selenium in their diets.[4–7] In the United States, one recent study found relatively high soil selenium levels in South Dakota and Wyoming.[8] However most other studies of selenium content in the U.S. are outdated.[9–12]

Foods containing significant and reliable amounts of selenium include animal products like meat, seafood, and dairy foods, as well as whole grains and vegetables grown in selenium-rich soils. These include wheat germ, nuts (particularly Brazil nuts), oats, whole-wheat bread, bran, red Swiss chard, brown rice, turnips, garlic, barley, and orange juice.

However, even these foods won't give you an adequate intake if the soil they were grown in was poor in selenium. Unfortunately, most of us have no way of knowing what kind of soil our food was grown in, so supplements may be a good idea.

In addition, medications that reduce stomach acid such as proton pump inhibitors or H_2 blockers may impair absorption of selenium.[13]

The two general types of selenium supplements available to consumers are organic and inorganic. These terms have a very specific chemical meaning and have nothing to do with "organic" foods. In chemistry, organic means a substance's chemical structure includes carbon. Inorganic chemicals have no carbon atoms.

The inorganic form of selenium, selenite, is essentially selenium atoms bound to oxygen. Some research suggests that selenite is harder for the body to absorb than organic forms of selenium, such as selenomethionine (selenium bound to methionine, an essential amino acid) or high-selenium yeast (which contains selenomethionine).[14,15] However, other research on both animals and humans suggests that selenite supplements are almost as good as organic forms of selenium.[16,17]

THERAPEUTIC DOSAGES

In controlled trials of selenium, typical dosages were 100 to 200 mcg daily.

THERAPEUTIC USES

Evidence indicates that supplemental selenium may help prevent **cancer** (see page 32).[18–23] One study suggests that selenium might help diabetic neuropathy.[24]

Selenium is required for a well-functioning immune system.[25] Based on this, selenium has been suggested as a treatment for people with **HIV** (see page 94). However, the studies done so far have had mixed results.[26–33]

Based on what science knows about antioxidants in general, selenium has been proposed as a preventive measure or treatment for **acne** (see page 2), AIDS, **asthma** (see page 14), **cataracts** (see page 42), **cervical dysplasia** (see page 43), **heart disease** (see page 16), and **multiple sclerosis** (see page 124). In addition, low selenium levels have been associated with increased likelihood of developing certain kinds of rheumatoid arthritis.[34] However, there is some evidence that selenium supplements don't help rheumatoid arthritis once it has developed.[35]

Selenium has also been recommended for many other conditions, including **anxiety** (see page 11), **fibromyalgia** (see page 80), **gout** (see page 84), **male infertility** (see page 116), **osteoarthritis** (see page 132), **psoriasis** (see page 148), and **ulcers** (see page 180), but there is no real evidence as yet that it really works.

WHAT IS THE SCIENTIFIC EVIDENCE FOR SELENIUM?

Cancer Prevention

A large body of evidence has found that increased intake of selenium is tied to a reduced risk of cancer. The most important blind study on selenium and cancer was a double-blind intervention trial conducted by researchers at the University of Arizona Cancer Center. In this trial, which began in 1983, 1,312 individuals were divided into two groups. One group received 200 mcg of yeast-based selenium daily; the other received placebo.[36] The researchers were trying to determine whether selenium could lower the incidence of skin cancers.

Although they found no benefit for skin cancer, they saw dramatic declines in the incidence of several other cancers in the selenium group. For ethical reasons, researchers felt compelled to stop the study after several years and allow all participants to take selenium.

When all the results were tabulated, it became clear that the selenium-treated group developed almost 66% fewer prostate cancers, 50% fewer colorectal cancers, and about 40% fewer lung cancers as compared with the placebo group. (All these results were statistically significant.) Selenium-treated subjects also experienced a statistically significant (17%) decrease in overall mortality, a greater than 50% decrease in lung cancer deaths, and nearly a 50% decrease in total cancer deaths. While this evidence is very promising, it has one major flaw. The laws of statistics tell us that when researchers start to deviate from the question their research was designed to answer, the results may not be trustworthy. For this reason, more double-blind trials need to be done to truly confirm that selenium can help prevent these types of cancer.

Other evidence for the possible anticancer benefits of selenium comes from large-scale Chinese studies showing that giving selenium supplements to people who live in selenium-deficient areas reduces the incidence of cancer.[37]

Also, observational studies have indicated that cancer deaths rise when dietary intake of selenium is low.[38,39]

The results of animal studies corroborate these results. One recent animal study examined whether two experimental organic forms of selenium would protect laboratory rats against chemically induced cancer of the tongue.[40] Rats were given one of three treatments: 5 parts per million of selenium in their drinking water, 15 parts per million of selenium, or placebo. The study was blinded so that the researchers wouldn't know until later which rats received which treatment. Whereas 47% of the rats in the placebo group developed tongue tumors, none of the rats that were given the higher selenium dosage developed tumors.

Another study examined whether selenium supplements could stop the spread (metastasis) of cancer in mice. In this study, a modest dosage of supplemental selenium reduced metastasis by 57%.[41] Even more significant was the decrease in the number of tumors that had spread to the lungs: mice in the control group had an average of 53 tumors *each*, whereas mice fed supplemental selenium had an average of *one* lung tumor.

SAFETY ISSUES

Selenium is safe when taken at the recommended dosages. However, very high selenium dosages, above 850 mcg daily, are known to cause selenium toxicity. Signs of selenium toxicity include depression, nervousness, emotional instability, nausea, vomiting, and in some cases loss of hair and fingernails.

⚠ INTERACTIONS YOU SHOULD KNOW ABOUT

If you are taking medications that reduce stomach acid, such as **H₂ blockers** or **proton pump inhibitors,** you may need extra selenium.

❧ SITOSTEROLS

Principal Proposed Uses   Benign Prostatic Hyperplasia (Prostate Enlargement)

Other Proposed Uses   General Health Benefits

Numerous plants contain cholesterol-like compounds called sitosterols and their close relatives sitosterolins. Of these, beta-sitosterol and beta-sitosterolin are considered the most important therapeutically. These substances bind to prostate tissue and affect the metabolism of prostaglandins, substances found in the body that affect pain and inflammation.[1] However, it is not clear whether this is the correct explanation of how sitosterols work for benign prostatic hyperplasia (prostate enlargement) or merely an interesting finding.

WHAT ARE SITOSTEROLS USED FOR TODAY?

For some reason, there seem to be more useful herbal treatments for **benign prostatic hyperplasia** (BPH; see page 24) than any other disease (except perhaps varicose veins!). Sitosterols join **saw palmetto** (see page 406), **nettle** (see page 369), and **pygeum** (see page 395) as a documented treatment for BPH.

Based on preliminary evidence, it has been suggested that sitosterols may also offer general health benefits, in particular strengthening the immune system.[2] One study suggests that a sitosterol mixture can help prevent the immune weakness that typically occurs after marathon running.[3] Sitosterols may eventually take their place alongside flavonoids and carotenes as beneficial substances found in food that aren't essential for life but may enhance overall health. However, more research needs to be done.

WHAT IS THE SCIENTIFIC EVIDENCE FOR SITOSTEROLS?

A review of the literature, published in 1999, found a total of four randomized, double-blind placebo-controlled studies on sitosterol mixtures (primarily beta-sitosterol, with other sitosterols and sitosterolins as well) for BPH, enrolling a total of 519 men.[4] All these studies found significant benefits in both perceived symptoms and objective measurements, such as urine flow rate.

The largest study followed 200 men with BPH for a period of 6 months.[5] After the trial was completed, many of the participants were followed for an additional year, during which the benefits continued.[6]

DOSAGE

The daily dosage of beta sitosterol is 60 to 135 mg. Effects usually take 4 weeks to develop.

SAFETY ISSUES

Although detailed safety studies have not been performed, sitosterols are believed to be safe. No significant side effects or drug interactions have been reported.[7]

SKULLCAP (*Scutellaria lateriflora*)

Alternate or Related Names   Blue Pimpernel, Helmet Flower, Hoodwort, Mad-Dog Weed, Madweed, Others
Principal Proposed Uses   Anxiety, Insomnia, Drug and Alcohol Withdrawal

Native Americans as well as traditional European herbalists used skullcap to induce sleep, relieve nervousness, and moderate the symptoms of epilepsy, rabies, and other diseases related to the nervous system. In other words, skullcap was believed to function as an herbal sedative.

A relative of skullcap, *Scutellaria baicalensis,* is a common Chinese herb. However, the root instead of the above-ground plant is used, and overall effects appear to be far different. The discussion below addresses European skullcap *(Scutellaria lateriflora)* only.

WHAT IS SKULLCAP USED FOR TODAY?

Skullcap is still popular as a sedative. Unfortunately, there has been virtually no scientific investigation of how well the herb really works. In practice, skullcap seems to produce a mild calming effect, generally not as strong as that of the herb **kava** (see page 338), but enough to be helpful at times. It appears to take the edge off mild **anxiety** (see page 11) and to make falling asleep easier for those troubled by **insomnia** (see page 103). Skullcap is also sometimes used to ease drug or alcohol withdrawal.

DOSAGE

When taken by itself, the usual dosage of skullcap is approximately 1 to 2 g, 3 times a day. However, skullcap is more often taken in combination with other sedative herbs such as **valerian** (see page 428), **passionflower** (see page 382), **hops** (see page 324), and **melissa** (see page 359), also called lemon balm. When using an herbal combination, follow the label instructions for dosage. Skullcap is usually not taken long term.

SAFETY ISSUES

Not much is known about the safety of skullcap. However, if you take too much, it can cause confusion and stupor.[1] There have been reports of liver damage following consumption of products labeled skullcap; however, since skullcap has been known to be adulterated with germander, an herb toxic to the liver, it may not have been the skullcap that was at fault.[2,3] Safety in young children, pregnant or nursing women, or those with severe liver or kidney disease has not been established.

Skullcap

SLIPPERY ELM (*Ulmus rubra, Ulmus fulva*)

Alternate or Related Names   Red Elm, Sweet Elm

Principal Proposed Uses   Cough, Irritable Bowel Syndrome, Irritated Digestion, Hemorrhoids

The dried inner bark of the slippery-elm tree was a favorite of many Native American tribes, and was subsequently adopted by European colonists. Like **marshmallow** (see page 355) and **mullein** (see page 365), slippery elm was used as a treatment for sore throat, coughs, dryness of the lungs, **wounds** (see page 123), skin inflammations, and irritations of the digestive tract.[1] It was also made into a kind of porridge to be taken by weaned infants and during convalescence from illness: various heroes of the Civil War are said to have credited slippery elm with their recovery from war wounds.

WHAT IS SLIPPERY ELM USED FOR TODAY?

Slippery elm has not been scientifically studied to any significant extent. It's primarily used today as a cough lozenge, widely available in pharmacies. Based on its soothing properties, slippery elm is also sometimes rec-ommended for treating **irritable bowel syndrome** (see page 108), inflammatory bowel disease (see the chapters on **Crohn's disease** and **ulcerative colitis**), gastritis, esophageal reflux (heartburn), and **hemorrhoids** (see page 85).

DOSAGE

Suck cough lozenges as needed. For digestive disorders, make a porridge of slippery elm sweetened with honey and eat as desired, or take 500 to 1,000 mg of capsulized powder 3 times daily.

SAFETY ISSUES

Other than occasional allergic reactions, slippery elm has not been associated with any toxicity. However, its safety has never been formally studied. Safety in young children, pregnant or nursing women, or those with severe liver or kidney disease has not been established.

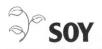 SOY

Supplement Forms/Alternate Names   Soy Protein Extract, Hydrolyzed Soy Protein, Soy Protein

Principal Proposed Uses   High Cholesterol

Other Proposed Uses   Menopausal Symptoms, Cancer Prevention, Osteoporosis

The soybean has been prized for centuries in Asia as a nutritious, high-protein food with myriad uses, and today it's popular in the United States not only in Asian food but also as a cholesterol-free meat and dairy substitute in traditional American foods. Soy burgers, soy yogurt, tofu hot dogs, and tofu cheese can be found in a growing number of grocery stores alongside the traditional white blocks of tofu.

Soy appears to reduce blood cholesterol levels, and the U.S. Food and Drug Administration has authorized allowing foods containing soy to carry a "heart-healthy" label.

Soybeans contain chemicals that are similar to estrogen, called isoflavones. These are widely thought to be the active ingredients in soy (although this may not be correct). They are described in more detail in the chapter on **isoflavones** (page 335).

SOURCES

If you like Japanese, Chinese, Thai, or Vietnamese food, it's easy to get a healthy dose of soy. Tofu is one of the world's most versatile foods. It can be stir-fried, steamed, or added to soup. You can also mash a cake of tofu and use it in place of ricotta cheese in your lasagna. If you don't like tofu, there are many other soy products to try: plain soybeans, soy cheese, soy burgers, soy milk, or tempeh. Or you can use a soy supplement instead.

THERAPEUTIC DOSAGES

The FDA suggests a daily intake of 25 g of soy protein to reduce cholesterol. This amount is typically found in about 2½ cups of soy milk or ½ pound of tofu. Evidence suggests that substituting as little as 20 g per day of soy protein for animal protein can significantly improve cholesterol levels.[1] Other studies have used dosages of up to 40 g daily.

THERAPEUTIC USES

According to the combined evidence of 38 controlled studies, soy can reduce blood **cholesterol** (see page 88) levels and improve the ratio of LDL ("bad") versus HDL ("good") cholesterol.[2] At an average dosage of 47 g daily, total cholesterol falls by about 9%, LDL cholesterol by 13%, and triglycerides by 10%. Soy's effects on HDL cholesterol itself are less impressive.

Soy also seems to reduce the common **menopausal symptom** (see page 117) known as "hot flashes."[3,4] Unlike estrogen, soy appears to reduce the risk of uterine cancer.[5] Its effect on breast cancer is not as well established, but there are reasons to believe that soy can help reduce breast **cancer** (see page 32) risk as well.[6,7,8] Although we don't know for sure, soy may do this by reducing levels of estrogen in the blood.[9,10] Soy may also help prevent prostate and colon cancer.[11,12,13] In addition, soy might help prevent **osteoporosis** (see page 136).[14–22]

WHAT IS THE SCIENTIFIC EVIDENCE FOR SOY?

High Cholesterol

In 1995, a review of 38 controlled studies on soy and heart disease concluded that soy is effective at reducing total cholesterol, LDL cholesterol, and triglycerides.[23] A double-blind study (not part of the review mentioned previously), which involved 66 older women, found improvements in HDL cholesterol as well.[24] The women were divided into three groups. The first group received 40 g of skim milk protein daily. The second group was given the same amount of soy protein, and the third received 40 g of soy protein with extra soy isoflavones. Compared with the skim milk (placebo) group, both soy groups showed significant improvements in both total cholesterol and HDL cholesterol.

Isoflavones in soy may be the active cholesterol-lowering ingredient,[25] although some studies disagree with this assertion.[26,27]

One indisputable benefit from eating soy is that, unlike animal sources of protein, it contains no saturated fat. However, soy appears to produce benefits above and beyond substituting for less healthful forms of protein.[28]

Menopausal Symptoms ("Hot Flashes")

Soy seems to relieve "hot flashes," a common symptom of menopause.

In one double-blind placebo-controlled study involving 104 women found that soy provided significant relief

compared to placebo (milk protein). After 3 weeks, the women taking daily doses of 60 g of soy protein were having 26% fewer hot flashes.[29] By week 12, the reduction was 45%. Women taking placebo also experienced a big improvement by week 12 (30% fewer hot flashes), but soy gave significantly better results.

Similarly positive results were seen in a 6-week double-blind placebo-controlled trial of 39 women.[30]

It is generally thought that the isoflavones in soy are responsible for these effects.[31] However, similar isoflavones from red clover have not been found effective;[32,33] for this reason, along with the results of studies involving soy and cholesterol, a rising current of thought suggests that there may be other important but unrecognized factors in soy.

Osteoporosis

In one study that evaluated the benefits of soy in osteoporosis, a total of 66 postmenopausal women took either placebo (soy protein with isoflavones removed) or soy protein with 56 or 90 mg of isoflavones daily for 6 months.[34] The group that took the higher dosage of isoflavones showed significant gains in spinal bone density. There was little change in the placebo or low-dose isoflavone groups. This study suggests that the soy isoflavones in soy protein may be effective for osteoporosis.

Very nearly the same results were also seen in a similar study. This 24-week double-blind study of 69 postmenopausal women found that soy can significantly reduce bone loss from the spine.[35]

Similar benefits have been seen in animal studies.[36–42] However, a couple of animal studies and one human trial failed to find benefit.[43,44,45]

Estrogen and most other medications for osteoporosis work by fighting bone breakdown. Soy may also work in the other way, by helping to increase new bone formation.[46,47]

SAFETY ISSUES

Studies in animals have found soy isoflavones essentially nontoxic.[48]

However, the isoflavones in soy could conceivably have some potentially harmful hormonal effects in certain specific situations. There is some evidence that although soy generally seems to reduce the risk of breast cancer, it also may cause some influences in the opposite direction.[49] For this and other reasons, we don't know if high doses of soy are safe for women who have already had breast cancer (for more information, see the chapter on **isoflavones**). There are also concerns that intensive use of soy products by pregnant women could exert a hormonal effect that impacts unborn fetuses.[50,51] Finally, fears have been expressed by some experts that soy might interfere with the action of oral contraceptives.

However, one study of 40 women suggests that such concerns are groundless.[52] Another trial found that soy does not interfere with the action of estrogen-replacement therapy in menopausal women.[53]

Soy may impair thyroid function or reduce absorption of thyroid medication, at least in children.[54,55,56] For this reason, individuals with impaired thyroid function should use soy with caution.

Soy also may reduce the absorption of the nutrients zinc, iron, and calcium.[57–61] To avoid absorption problems, you should probably take these vitamins at least 2 hours apart from eating soy.

⚠ INTERACTIONS YOU SHOULD KNOW ABOUT

If you are taking

- **Zinc, iron,** or **calcium** supplements: It may be best to eat soy at a different time of day to avoid absorption problems.
- **Thyroid hormone**: You should consult your physician before increasing your intake of soy products.

SPIRULINA

Supplement Forms/Alternate Names   Blue-Green Algae

Principal Proposed Uses   Nutritional Support

Other Proposed Uses   Weight Loss, High Cholesterol, Cancer Prevention, HIV Infection, Herpes Infection, Weak Immunity, Allergies, Liver Protection, Fibromyalgia

The supplement called spirulina consists of one or more members of a family of blue-green algae. The name was inspired by the spiral shapes in which these plants array themselves as they grow.[1]

Spirulina grows in the wild in salty lakes in Mexico and on the African continent. It reproduces quickly, and because the individual plants tend to stick together, it is easy to harvest. Records of the Spanish conquistadores suggest that the Aztecs used spirulina as a food source; we also know that the Kanembu people of Central Africa harvested it from what is now called Lake Chad.

Spirulina is currently cultivated and processed on an industrial scale in several countries, for sale in the health food market. African, Asian, and South American villagers also grow it in smaller amounts for local consumption, counting on spirulina's high protein and nutrient content to fight malnutrition. In countries where better diets are the norm, spirulina is used mainly as a dietary supplement for those seeking optimum wellness.

This plant contains high levels of various B vitamins, **beta-carotene** (see page 217), other carotenoids, and minerals, including **calcium** (see page 234), **iron** (see page 333), **magnesium** (see page 351), **manganese** (see page 354), **potassium** (see page 390), and **zinc** (see page 463). It is also a source of **gamma-linolenic acid** (GLA; see page 304). Spirulina is also a rich source of protein—dried spirulina contains up to 70% protein by weight.[2] Spirulina also contains **vitamin B$_{12}$** (see page 442), a nutrient otherwise found almost exclusively in animal foods. Unfortunately, the B$_{12}$ in spirulina is not absorbable.[3]

REQUIREMENTS/SOURCES

Unless you live within 35 degrees of the equator, on the shores of an alkaline lake, you will have difficulty finding spirulina anywhere but in a health food store. Most carry a number of brands of spirulina that has been dried and processed into powder or tablets.

THERAPEUTIC DOSAGES

Researchers studying spirulina's effects on health have used a variety of doses, ranging from 1 to 8.4 g daily; 50 g daily is generally regarded as the maximum safe dose (see Safety Issues).

THERAPEUTIC USES

There is no question that spirulina is a nutritious food, but it isn't cheap.[4] Protein can be obtained more cheaply from legumes, nuts, grains, and animal foods, iron from dark greens, prunes, and meat, and carotenes and vitamins from standard fruits and vegetables. However, spirulina contains these nutrients in a highly concentrated form, making it useful as a kind of natural vitamin pill.

Spirulina might have other specific therapeutic uses beyond general nutritional support, but the evidence supporting these recommendations is highly preliminary at best.

For example, manufacturers of spirulina supplements sometimes claim that the plant can reduce appetite,

Spirulina

Visit Us at TNP.com

thereby helping overweight individuals control their food intake. However, one small double-blind study of spirulina for **weight loss** (see page 192) failed to find a significant difference between spirulina and placebo treatment.[5]

Evidence from animal studies and one small controlled (but not blinded) study in humans suggests that spirulina might help lower cholesterol.[6,7,8] However, in the absence of double-blind placebo-controlled trials, it is too early to say that spirulina can be used for this purpose.

Preliminary evidence suggests that spirulina, like other nutritious plant foods, may help prevent **cancer** (see page 32).[9,10,11]

Test tube and animal studies suggest that spirulina might have some activity against the HIV virus, but much more research needs to be done before we could say that spirulina is helpful against **HIV infection** (see page 94).[12,13]

Highly preliminary evidence suggests that spirulina may activate the immune system,[14,15,16] counter allergic reactions,[17,18] help protect the liver from toxic chemicals,[19,20] and reduce **fibromyalgia** (see page 80) symptoms.[21]

WHAT IS THE SCIENTIFIC EVIDENCE FOR SPIRULINA?

A double-blind placebo-controlled trial investigated the possible weight loss effects of spirulina.[22] However, while individuals taking 8.4 g of spirulina daily lost weight, the difference between the spirulina group and the placebo group was not statistically significant. Larger and longer studies are needed to establish whether spirulina is indeed an effective treatment for obesity.

SAFETY ISSUES

Spirulina itself appears to be nontoxic.[23] A study in rats showed that high spirulina intake caused no weight reduction or toxicity symptoms in rats, nor did spirulina affect the rats' ability to reproduce normally.[24]

Nevertheless, there are areas of potential concern for consumers.

When spirulina is grown with the use of fermented animal waste fertilizers, contamination with dangerous bacteria could occur.[25] There are also concerns that spirulina might concentrate radioactive ions found in its environment.[26]

Probably of most concern is spirulina's ability to absorb and concentrate heavy metals such as lead and mercury if they are present in its environment. One study of spirulinas grown in a number of locations found them to contain an unacceptably high content of these toxic metals.[27] However, a second study on this topic claims that the first used an unreliable method of analyzing heavy metal content,[28] and concludes that a person would have to eat more than 77 g daily of the most heavily contaminated spirulina to reach unsafe mercury and lead consumption levels.

These researchers, however, go on to suggest that it is not prudent to eat more than 50 g of spirulina daily. The reason they give is that the plant contains a high concentration of nucleic acids, substances related to DNA. When these are metabolized, they create uric acid, which could cause **gout** (see page 84) or **kidney stones** (see page 109). This is of special concern to those who have already had uric acid stones or attacks of gout.

Maximum safe doses of spirulina in pregnant and nursing women, young children, and individuals with kidney or liver disease have not been determined.

ST. JOHN'S WORT (*Hypericum perforatum*)

Alternate or Related Names   Hardhay, Amber, Goatweed, Klamath Weed, Tipton Weed, Others

Principal Proposed Uses   Mild to Moderate Depression

Other Proposed Uses
   Depression-Associated Symptoms: Anxiety, Insomnia
   PMS, Menopause, Seasonal Affective Disorder (SAD)

Probably Ineffective Uses   Viral Diseases

St. John's wort is a common perennial herb of many branches and bright yellow flowers that grows wild in much of the world. Its name derives from the herb's tendency to flower around the feast of St. John. (A "wort" is simply a plant in Old English.) The species name *perfo-* *ratum* derives from the watermarking of translucent dots that can be seen when the leaf is held up to the sun.

St. John's wort has a long history of use in treating emotional disorders. During the Middle Ages, St. John's wort was popular for "casting out demons," conceivably an archaic description of curing mental illness. In the 1800s, the herb was classified as a "nervine," or a treatment for "nervous disorders." It began to be considered a treatment for depression in the early 1900s, and when pharmaceutical antidepressants were invented, German researchers began to look for similar properties in St. John's wort.

Today, St. John's wort is one of the best-documented herbal treatments, with a scientific record approaching that of many prescription drugs. Indeed, this herb *is* a prescription antidepressant in Germany, covered by the national health-care system, and is prescribed more frequently for depression than any synthetic drug. Evidence suggests that for mild to moderate depression, it is at least as effective as standard drugs, with fewer and less severe side effects.

The active components in St. John's wort are found in the buds, flowers, and newest leaves. Extracts are usually standardized to the substance hypericin, which has led to the widespread misconception that hypericin is the active ingredient. However, there is no evidence that hypericin itself is an antidepressant. Recent attention has focused on another ingredient of St. John's wort named hyperforin as the potential active ingredient.

Hyperforin was first identified as a constituent of *Hypericum perforatum* in 1971 by Russian researchers, but it was incorrectly believed to be too unstable to play a major role in the herb's action.[1] However, recent evidence has corrected this view. It now appears that standard St. John's wort extract contains about 1 to 6% hyperforin.[2]

We don't really know how St. John's wort works. Early research suggested that St. John's wort works like the oldest class of antidepressants, the MAO inhibitors.[3] However, later research essentially discredited this idea.[4,5] More recent research suggests that St. John's wort may inhibit the reuptake of serotonin, norepinephrine, and dopamine.[6,7]

Evidence from animal and human studies suggests that hyperforin is the ingredient in St. John's wort that raises these neurotransmitters.[8,9,10] Nonetheless, there may be other active ingredients in St. John's wort also at work.[11,12] In fact, two double-blind trials using a form of St. John's wort with low hyperforin content found it effective.[13,14]

St. John's wort appears to be reasonably safe when taken alone. However, there is good reason to believe that it may interfere with the effectiveness of numerous medications, including treatments for HIV infection. (See Safety Issues for details.)

WHAT IS ST. JOHN'S WORT USED FOR TODAY?

St. John's wort is primarily used to treat mild to moderate **depression** (see page 59). Typical symptoms include depressed mood, lack of energy, sleep problems, anxiety, appetite disturbance, difficulty concentrating, and poor stress tolerance. Irritability can also be a sign of depression.

Research suggests that St. John's wort is effective in about 55% of cases. As with other antidepressants, the full effect takes approximately 4 to 6 weeks to develop.

Warning: St. John's wort should never be relied on for the treatment of severe depression. If you or a loved one are feeling suicidal, unable to cope with daily life, paralyzed by anxiety, incapable of getting out of bed, unable to sleep, or uninterested in eating, see a physician at once. Drug therapy may save your life.

Furthermore, various systemic diseases may masquerade as depression, such as hypothyroidism, chronic hepatitis, and anemia. Make sure to find out whether you have an undiagnosed medical illness before treating yourself with St. John's wort.

Like other antidepressants, St. John's wort is also used in the treatment of chronic **insomnia** (see page 103) and **anxiety** (see page 11) when they are related to depression. It may be effective in relieving seasonal affective disorder (SAD) as well.

Early reports suggested that St. John's wort or synthetic hypericin might be useful against viruses such as **HIV** (see page 94), but these haven't panned out.[15] There is some evidence that the presumed active ingredient in St. John's wort, hyperforin, may be able to fight certain bacteria, including some that are resistant to antibiotics.[16] However, this evidence is far too preliminary to count St. John's wort as an effective antibiotic.

Highly preliminary evidence suggests that St. John's wort might be helpful for **PMS**[17] (see page 145) and **menopause** (see page 117).[18]

WHAT IS THE SCIENTIFIC EVIDENCE FOR ST. JOHN'S WORT?

Taken as a whole, the available research makes a convincing case that the herb is an effective antidepressant. There have been two main kinds of studies: those that compared St. John's wort to placebo, and others that compared it to prescription antidepressants.

St. John's Wort Versus Placebo

Probably the best-designed St.-John's-wort-versus-placebo study was reported in 1993 by the German physician K. D. Hansgen and his colleagues.[19] In this 4-week trial, 72 moderately depressed individuals were randomly assigned to receive either placebo or 300 mg 3 times per day of an extract of St. John's wort standardized to contain 0.3% hypericin.

Participants were evaluated using a set of questions called the Hamilton Depression Index (HAM-D). This scale rates the extent of depression, with higher numbers indicating more serious symptoms. Over 80% of the par-

St. John's Wort

Visit Us at TNP.com

ticipants taking St. John's wort improved significantly based on this index, while only 26% of the placebo group responded. Later, 36 additional people were added to the trial, with essentially identical results.

A recent double-blind study examined the effectiveness of a new kind of St. John's wort extract standardized to its content of hyperforin rather than to hypericin.[20] It followed 147 people with mild to moderate depression for a period of 42 days. Participants were given either a placebo or one of two forms of St. John's wort: a low-hyperforin product (0.5%) or a high-hyperforin product (5%).

The results showed that the St. John's wort containing 5% hyperforin was successful in controlling depression symptoms in about 50% of cases, a better result than placebo. Although identical to the high-hyperforin product in every respect other than hyperforin content, the low-hyperforin product did not do any better than the placebo. This study provides strong evidence that hyperforin is at least one of the active ingredients in St. John's wort.

However, another St. John's wort product with very low levels of hyperforin was also found effective in a double-blind placebo-controlled trial of 159 individuals with mild to moderate depression.[21]

There have been over 13 other double-blind placebo-controlled studies as well.[22] A review that evaluated most of the published studies up through 1994 found that nine of them were performed according to adequate scientific standards, involving a total of over 600 participants.[23] Adding in the hyperforin study just mentioned, the combined results make a compelling case for St. John's wort as an effective antidepressant.

This body of research has been criticized by some authorities who point out that none of the studies exceeded 8 weeks in length. However, as it states in the *Physician's Desk Reference*, Prozac was approved on the basis of studies no longer than 6 weeks. It isn't fair to apply a higher standard to herbs than to drugs.

St. John's Wort Versus Medications

A 6-week double-blind trial of 240 individuals with mild to moderate depression compared St. John's wort (250 mg twice daily of a 4–7:1 alcohol extract) to fluoxetine (Prozac) at the standard dose of 20 mg daily.[24] The results showed that St. John's wort was somewhat *more* effective, and caused far fewer and less severe side effects.

Another double-blind study of 149 seniors with mild to moderate depression found that St. John's wort extract at a dose of 800 mg daily was as effective as a standard dose of the drug fluoxetine (Prozac).[25] In addition, a double-blind study that enrolled 30 individuals found equivalent benefits comparing St. John's wort and sertraline (Zoloft).[26]

An 8-week study of 263 individuals with moderate depression compared the effectiveness of a slightly high dose of St. John's wort (350 mg 3 times daily of an extract standardized to contain 2 to 3% hyperforin) against placebo and the somewhat outdated, but nonetheless effective, antidepressant imipramine.[27] The results showed that imipramine and St. John's wort were equally effective, and both were more effective than placebo.

However, according to a double-blind study of 209 people, St. John's wort, even in double the usual dose, is not as effective as imipramine for severe depression.[28]

Ten other trials of individuals with mild to moderate depression have compared St. John's wort against old-fashioned but tried-and-true antidepressants including imipramine, maprotiline, and amitriptyline.[29,30,31] However, these studies used very low doses of the standard drug, and therefore proved little.

Depression-Related Symptoms

In many of the studies described above, anxiety and insomnia associated with depression were noted to improve with St. John's wort treatment.

Seasonal Affective Disorder

One small controlled study found St. John's wort to be effective in the treatment of seasonal affective disorder (SAD), a form of depression that occurs primarily during the winter.[32]

DOSAGE

The standard dosage of St. John's wort is 300 mg 3 times a day of an extract standardized to contain 0.3% hypericin. A few new products on the market are standardized to hyperforin content (usually 2 to 3%) instead of hypericin. These are taken at the same dosage. Some people take 500 mg twice a day, or 600 mg in the morning and 300 mg in the evening.

Yet another form of St. John's wort has also passed double-blind studies. This form contains little hyperforin, and is taken at a dose of 250 mg twice daily.[33,34]

If the herb bothers your stomach, take it with food.

Remember that the full effect takes 4 weeks to develop. Don't give up too soon!

SAFETY ISSUES

St. John's wort is essentially side-effect free. Strangely, this good news has an unfortunate consequence: Some people who try St. John's wort decide that it must not be very powerful since it doesn't make them feel ill, and quit. Be patient! When St. John's wort works, it is very smooth.

In a study designed to look for side effects, 3,250 people took St. John's wort for 4 weeks.[35] Overall, about 2.4% experienced side effects. The most common were mild stomach discomfort (0.6%), allergic reactions—

primarily rash—(0.5%), tiredness (0.4%), and restlessness (0.3%).

In the extensive German experience with St. John's wort as a treatment for depression, there have been no published reports of serious adverse consequences from taking the herb alone.[36] Animal studies involving enormous doses of St. John's wort extracts for 26 weeks have not shown any serious effects.[37]

Cows and sheep grazing on St. John's wort have sometimes developed severe and even fatal sensitivity to the sun. However, this has never occurred in humans taking St. John's wort at normal dosages.[38] In one study, highly sun-sensitive people were given twice the normal dose of the herb.[39] The results showed a mild but measurable increase in reaction to ultraviolet radiation. The moral of the story is, if you are especially sensitive to the sun, don't exceed the recommended dose of St. John's wort, and continue to take your usual precautions against burning. Nonetheless, there might be problems if you combine St. John's wort with other medications that cause increased sun sensitivity, such as sulfa drugs and the anti-inflammatory medication Feldene (piroxicam). In addition, the medications Prilosec (omeprazole) and Prevacid (lansoprazole) may increase the tendency of St. John's wort to cause photosensitivity.[40]

A recent report also suggests that regular use of St. John's wort might also increase the risk of cataracts.[41] While this is preliminary information, it may make sense to wear sunglasses when outdoors if you are taking this herb on a long-term basis.

One study raised questions about possible antifertility effects of St. John's wort. When high concentrations of St. John's wort were placed in a test tube with hamster sperm and ova, the sperm were damaged and less able to penetrate the ova.[42] However, since it is unlikely that this much St. John's wort can actually come in contact with sperm and ova when they are in the body rather than in a test tube, these results may not be meaningful in real life.

Older reports suggested that St. John's wort works like the class of drugs known as MAO inhibitors.[43] This led to a number of warnings, including avoiding cheese and decongestants while taking St. John's wort. However, St. John's wort is no longer believed to act like an MAO inhibitor, and these warnings are now thought to be groundless.[44,45]

Herbal experts have warned for some time that combining St. John's wort with drugs in the Prozac family (SSRIs) might raise serotonin too much and cause a number of serious problems. Recently, case reports of such events have begun to trickle in.[46,47] This is a potentially serious risk. Do not combine St. John's wort with prescription antidepressants except on the specific advice of a physician. Since some antidepressants, such as Prozac, linger in the blood for quite some time, you also need to exercise caution when switching from a drug to St. John's wort. (See Transitioning from Medications to St. John's Wort.)

The antimigraine drug sumatriptan (Imitrex) and the pain-killing drug tramadol also raise serotonin levels and might interact similarly with St. John's wort.[48,49]

Perhaps the biggest concern with St. John's wort is the possibility that it may decrease the effectiveness of various medications, including protease inhibitors (for HIV infection), cyclosporine (for organ transplants), digoxin (for heart disease), warfarin (a blood thinner), chemotherapy drugs, oral contraceptives, olanzapine or clozapine (for schizophrenia), and theophylline (for asthma).[50–58] Furthermore, if you are taking St. John's wort and one of these medications at the same time and then stop taking the herb, blood levels of the drug may rise. This rise in drug level could be dangerous in certain circumstances.

These interactions could lead to catastrophic consequences. Indeed, St. John's wort appears to have caused two cases of heart transplant rejection by interfering with the action of cyclosporine. Also, many people with HIV take St. John's wort in the false belief that the herb will fight the AIDS virus. The unintended result may be to reduce the potency of standard AIDS drugs. In addition, the herb might decrease the effectiveness of oral contraceptives, presenting a risk of pregnancy.[59]

The bottom line: We recommend that individuals taking any critical medication should avoid using St. John's wort until more is known.

It is probably advisable on general principles to discontinue all herbs and supplements prior to surgery and anesthesia, due to the possibility of unpredictable interactions. However, there does not appear to be any specific foundation to publicized claims that St. John's wort interacts with anesthetic drugs.

Safety in young children, pregnant or nursing women, or those with severe liver or kidney disease has not been established.

TRANSITIONING FROM MEDICATIONS TO ST. JOHN'S WORT

If you are taking a prescription drug for mild to moderate depression, switching to St. John's wort may be a reasonable idea if you would prefer taking an herb. To avoid overlapping treatments, the safest approach is to stop taking the drug and allow it to wash out of your system before starting St. John's wort. Consult with your doctor on how much time is necessary.

However, if you are taking medication for severe depression, switching over to St. John's wort is *not* a good idea. The herb probably won't work well enough, and you may sink into a dangerous depression.

⚠ INTERACTIONS YOU SHOULD KNOW ABOUT

If you are taking

- **Antidepressant drugs,** including **MAO inhibitors, SSRIs,** and **tricyclics;** or possibly the drugs **tramadol** or **sumatriptan (Imitrex):** Do not take St. John's wort at the same time. Actually, you need to let the medication flush out of your system for a while (perhaps weeks, depending on the drug) before you start the herb.

- **Digoxin, cyclosporine, protease inhibitors** (for HIV infection), **oral contraceptives, amitriptyline, Coumadin (warfarin), theophylline, chemotherapy drugs, newer antipsychotic medications** (such as **olanzapine and clozapine**) or, indeed, any critical medication: St. John's wort might cause the drug to be less effective.
- **Medications** that cause sun sensitivity such as **sulfa drugs** and the anti-inflammatory medication **Feldene (piroxicam),** as well as **Prilosec (omeprazole)** or **Prevacid (lansoprazole):** Keep in mind that St. John's wort might have an additive effect.

🌿 STANOLS

Supplement Forms/Alternate Names   Phytostanols, Sitostanol, Campestanol, Stigmastanol, 5-Alpha-Stanols, Stanol Esters

Principal Proposed Uses   Lowering Cholesterol

Stanols are substances that occur naturally in various plants. Their cholesterol-lowering effects were first observed in animals in the 1950s. Since then, a substantial amount of research suggests that plant stanols (modified into stanol esters) can help to lower cholesterol in individuals with normal or mildly to moderately elevated cholesterol levels. Stanols are available in margarine spreads, salad dressings, and dietary supplement tablets.

REQUIREMENTS/SOURCES

Stanols occur naturally in wood pulp, tall oil, and soybean oil. Stanols are also made commercially from related substances in plants called sterols, such as **beta-sitosterol** (see page 409).[1,2]

For incorporation into foods, stanols are processed with fatty acids from vegetable oils to form chemicals called stanol esters.[3] Plant stanol esters are found in margarine spreads and salad dressings, and are also available as dietary supplement tablets.

THERAPEUTIC DOSAGES

Typical dosages of stanol esters to lower cholesterol levels range from 3.4 to 5.1 g per day.[4] One manufacturer of a commercially prepared margarine spread recommends taking 3 teaspoons (1.5 g of sitostanol ester per teaspoon) per day. The suggested use varies depending on the product and the quantity of sitostanol ester per serving. It may take up to 3 months to show a substantial decrease in total cholesterol values.[5]

THERAPEUTIC USES

Reasonably good evidence tells us that stanol esters can significantly improve **cholesterol** (see page 88) levels.[6–18]

WHAT IS THE SCIENTIFIC EVIDENCE FOR STANOLS?

Plant stanol esters reduce serum cholesterol levels by inhibiting cholesterol absorption.[19] Because they are structurally similar to cholesterol, stanols can displace cholesterol from the "packages" that deliver cholesterol for absorption from the intestines to the bloodstream.[20] The displaced cholesterol is not absorbed and is excreted from the body; the stanols themselves are ultimately not absorbed either.

At least 13 double-blind placebo-controlled studies, ranging in length from 30 days to 12 months and involving a total of more than 935 individuals, have found stanols effective for improving cholesterol levels.[21–33] The combined results suggest that stanols can reduce total cholesterol and LDL ("bad") cholesterol by about 10 to 15%. Stanols did not have any significant effect on HDL ("good") cholesterol or triglycerides in most of these studies.[34]

In one of the best of the double-blind placebo-controlled studies, 153 individuals with mildly elevated cholesterol were given sitostanol esters in margarine (at 1.8 or 2.6 g of sitostanol per day), or margarine without sitostanol ester, for a total of 1 year.[35] The results in the treated group receiving 2.6 g per day showed improvements in total cholesterol by 10.2% and LDL cholesterol by 14.1%—significantly better than the results in the control group. Neither triglycerides nor HDL cholesterol levels were affected.

Two studies found stanols to be helpful for lowering cholesterol levels in individuals with type 2 (adult-onset) diabetes.[36,37] One of these studies examined two treatments: pravastatin (a cholesterol-lowering drug) versus pravastatin along with sitostanol. The combination treatment was more effective at lowering total cholesterol and LDL cholesterol levels than the drug treatment alone.[38] Additive benefits were also seen in a study of nondiabetics taking statin drugs who began taking stanols as well.[39]

SAFETY ISSUES

Stanols are considered safe because they are not absorbed.[40,41] No adverse effects have been reported in any of the studies on lowering cholesterol, with the exception of one study that reported mild gastrointestinal complaints in a few preschool children.[42] In addition, no toxic signs were observed in rats given stanol esters for 13 weeks at levels comparable to or exceeding those recommended for lowering cholesterol.[43]

Although concerns have been expressed that stanols might impair absorption of the fat-soluble **vitamins A** (see page 432), **D** (see page 449), and **E** (see page 451), this does not seem to occur at the dosages of stanols required to lower cholesterol.[44] Stanols might, however, interfere with absorption of alpha- and **beta-carotene** (see page 217),[45,46] although some studies have found no such effect.[47,48] Until more is learned, it may be reasonable for individuals using stanol products to make sure to consume carotenoid-rich vegetables (yellow/orange and dark green vegetables).[49]

STEVIA (*Stevia rebaudiana*)

Alternate or Related Names   Sweet Herb, Sweetleaf
Principal Proposed Uses   Sweetener

This member of the Aster family has a long history of native use in Paraguay as a sweetener for teas and foods. It contains a substance known as stevioside that is 100 to 300 times sweeter than sugar, but provides no calories.[1]

In the early 1970s, a consortium of Japanese food manufacturers developed stevia extracts for use as a zero-calorie sugar substitute. Subsequently, stevia extracts became a common ingredient in Asian soft drinks, desserts, chewing gum, and many other food products. Extensive Japanese research has found stevia to be extremely safe. However, there have not been enough U.S. studies for the FDA to approve stevia as a sugar substitute. Without identifying it as such, stevia is nonetheless widely used by savvy manufacturers to sweeten commercial beverage teas and other products.

WHAT IS STEVIA USED FOR TODAY?

Although some people have claimed that stevia can help regulate blood sugar, the evidence for such an effect is negligible. This dietary supplement is primarily useful as a sweetening agent.

DOSAGE

Stevia is sold as a powder to be added to foods as needed for appropriate sweetening effects. It tastes slightly bitter if placed directly in the mouth, but in liquids this is generally not noticeable, and most people find the taste delightfully unique.

SAFETY ISSUES

Neither animal tests nor the extensive Japanese experience with stevia have uncovered any significant adverse effects.[2,3] However, safety in young children, pregnant or nursing women, or those with severe liver or kidney disease has not been established.

Stevia

Visit Us at TNP.com

SUMA *(Pfaffia paniculata)*

Principal Proposed Uses   Adaptogen (Improve Resistance to Stress); Strengthen Immunity Against Colds, Flus, and Other Infections; Performance Enhancement

Other Proposed Uses   Chronic Fatigue Syndrome, Menopausal Symptoms, Ulcer Disease, Anxiety, Menstrual Problems, Impotence, Aphrodisiac

Suma is a large ground vine native to Central and South America. Sometimes called "Brazilian ginseng," native peoples have long used suma to promote robust health as well as to treat practically all illnesses. They called it *Para Toda,* which means "for all things."[1]

WHAT IS SUMA USED FOR TODAY?

Suma's ancient reputation has generated worldwide interest. However, there has been little formal scientific investigation at this time.

According to most contemporary herbalists, suma is best understood as an adaptogen, a substance that helps one adapt to **stress** (see page 167) and fight infection (see the chapter on **ginseng** for a more in-depth discussion about adaptogens). Along with other adaptogens, Russian Olympic athletes have used suma in the belief that it will enhance **sports performance** (see page 158). In the United States, suma is often recommended

as a general strengthener of the body, as well as for the treatment of chronic fatigue syndrome, **menopausal symptoms** (see page 117), **ulcers** (see page 180), **anxiety** (see page 11), menstrual problems, impotence, and low resistance to illness. The herb also enjoys a considerable reputation as an aphrodisiac.

DOSAGE

A typical dosage of suma is 500 mg twice daily. It is usually taken for an extended period of time.

SAFETY ISSUES

Suma has not been associated with any serious adverse reactions. However, comprehensive safety studies have not been undertaken. Safety in young children, pregnant or nursing women, or those with severe liver or kidney disease has not been established.

TAURINE

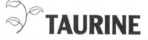

Supplement Forms/Alternate Names   L-Taurine

Principal Proposed Uses   Congestive Heart Failure, Viral Hepatitis

Other Proposed Uses   Alcoholism, Cataracts, Diabetes, Epilepsy, Gallbladder Disease, Hypertension (High Blood Pressure), Multiple Sclerosis, Psoriasis, Stroke

Taurine is an amino acid, one of the building blocks of proteins. Found in the nervous system and muscles, taurine is one of the most abundant amino acids in the body. It is thought to help regulate heartbeat, maintain cell membranes, and affect the release of neurotransmitters (chemicals that carry signals between nerve cells) in the brain.

Taurine's best-established use is to treat congestive heart failure (CHF), a condition in which the heart muscle progressively weakens. It may also be useful for hepatitis.

Warning: Please keep in mind that CHF is too serious for self-treatment. If you're interested in trying taurine or any other supplement for CHF, you should first consult your doctor.

SOURCES

There is no dietary requirement for taurine, since the body can make it out of **vitamin B$_6$** (see page 439) and the amino acids **methionine** (see page 360) and cysteine. Deficiencies occasionally occur in vegetarians, whose diets may not provide the building blocks for making taurine.

People with diabetes have lower-than-average blood levels of taurine, but whether this means they should take extra taurine is unclear.

Meat, poultry, eggs, dairy products, and fish are good sources of taurine. Legumes and nuts don't contain taurine, but they do contain methionine and cysteine.

THERAPEUTIC DOSAGES

A typical therapeutic dosage of taurine is 2 g 3 times daily.

THERAPEUTIC USES

Preliminary evidence suggests that taurine might be helpful in **congestive heart failure** (see page 54), a condition in which the heart has trouble pumping blood, which leads to fluid accumulating in the legs and lungs.[1]

There is also some evidence that taurine may be helpful for acute **viral hepatitis** (see page 189).[2]

Taurine has additionally been proposed as a treatment for numerous other conditions, including alcoholism, **cataracts** (see page 42), **diabetes** (see page 65), epilepsy, gallbladder disease, **hypertension** (see page 98), **multiple sclerosis** (see page 124), **psoriasis** (see page 148), and stroke, but the evidence for these uses is weak and, in some cases, contradictory.[3–7] Taurine is also sometimes combined in an "amino acid cocktail" with other amino acids for treatment of **attention deficit disorder** (see page 22), but there is no evidence as yet that it works for this purpose.

WHAT IS THE SCIENTIFIC EVIDENCE FOR TAURINE?

Congestive Heart Failure

Several studies (primarily by one research group) suggest that taurine may be useful for congestive heart failure (CHF). For example, in one double-blind trial, 58 people with CHF took either placebo or 2 g of taurine 3 times daily for 4 weeks.[8] Then the groups were switched. During taurine treatment, the study participants showed highly significant improvement in breathlessness, heart palpitations, fluid buildup, and heart x ray, as well as standard scales of heart failure severity.

Animal research as well as small blinded or open studies in humans have also found positive effects.[9–13] Interestingly, one very small study compared taurine with another supplement commonly used for congestive heart failure, **coenzyme Q$_{10}$** (see page 256). The results suggest that taurine is more effective.[14]

Viral Hepatitis

There are several viruses that can cause acute hepatitis, a disabling and sometimes dangerous infection of the liver. The most common are hepatitis A and B, although there are others (with such imaginative names as C and D).

One double-blind study suggests that taurine supplements might be useful for acute viral hepatitis. In this double-blind placebo-controlled study, 63 people with hepatitis were given either 12 g of taurine daily or placebo.[15] (The report does not state what type of viral hepatitis they had.) According to blood tests, the taurine group experienced significant improvements in liver function as compared to the placebo group.

Acute hepatitis can also develop into a long-lasting or permanent condition known as chronic hepatitis. One small double-blind study suggests that taurine does not help chronic hepatitis.[16] For this purpose, the herb **milk thistle** (see page 361) may be better.

SAFETY ISSUES

As an amino acid found in food, taurine is thought to be quite safe. However, maximum safe dosages of taurine supplements for children, pregnant or nursing women, or those with severe liver or kidney disease have not been determined.

As with any supplement taken in multigram doses, it is important to purchase a reputable product, because a contaminant present even in small percentages could add up to a real problem.

TEA TREE (*Melaleuca alternifolia*)

Principal Proposed Uses   Wound Healing, Athlete's Foot and Other Fungal Infections of the Skin, Acne, Vaginal Infections, Thrush (in HIV Infection), Periodontal Disease, Body Odor

Captain Cook named this tree, after finding that its aromatic, resinous leaves made a satisfying substitute for proper tea. One hundred and fifty years later, an Australian government chemist named A. R. Penfold studied tea tree leaves and discovered their strong antiseptic properties. Tea tree oil subsequently became a standard treatment in Australia for the prevention and treatment of wound infections. During World War II, the Australian government classified tea tree oil as an essential commodity and exempted producers from military service.

However, tea tree oil fell out of favor when antibiotics became widely available.

Thymus Extract

WHAT IS TEA TREE USED FOR TODAY?

There is little question that tea tree oil is an effective antiseptic, active against many bacteria and fungi, including some that are resistant to antibiotics.[1,2] It also possesses a penetrating quality that may make it particularly useful for treating infected wounds. However, it is probably not effective as an oral antibiotic.

Preliminary double-blind studies have found tea tree oil may be an effective treatment for **athlete's foot** (see page 21) and other fungal infections of the skin and nails.[3,4]

Like other topical antibiotics, tea tree oil may help control **acne** (see page 2) when applied to the skin directly.[5]

Preliminary studies also hint that it could be useful for treating **vaginal infections** (see page 182) caused by **candida** (see page 38) or other organisms.[6] Tea tree oil has been suggested as a treatment for thrush (oral *Candida* infection) in people with **HIV** (see page 94) infection.[7]

Australian dentists frequently use tea tree oil mouthwash prior to dental procedures and as a daily preventive against **periodontal disease** (see page 142).

Tea tree oil also appears to possess deodorant properties, probably through suppressing odor-causing bacteria.

WHAT IS THE SCIENTIFIC EVIDENCE FOR TEA TREE?

A double-blind placebo-controlled trial followed 104 individuals given either a 10% tea tree oil cream, the standard drug tolnaftate, or placebo.[8] The results showed that tea tree oil reduced the symptoms of athlete's foot more effectively than placebo, but less effectively than tolnaftate. Neither treatment cured the infection in 100% of the cases, but each treatment cured many cases.

Another double-blind study followed 112 people with fungal infections of the toenails, comparing 100% tea tree oil to a standard topical antifungal treatment, clotrimazole.[9] The results showed equivalent benefits; however, because topical clotrimazole is not regarded as a particularly effective treatment for this condition, the results mean little.

DOSAGE

Tea tree preparations contain various percentages of tea tree oil. For treating acne, the typical strength is 5 to 15%; for fungal infections, 70 to 100% is usually used; and for use as a vaginal douche (with medical supervision), 1 to 40% concentrations have been used. It is usually applied 2 to 3 times daily, until symptoms resolve. However, tea tree oil can be irritating to the skin, so start with low concentrations until you know your tolerance.

The best tea tree products contain oil from the *alternifolia* species of *Melaleuca* only, standardized to contain not more than 10% cineole (an irritant) and at least 30% terpinen-4-ol. Oil from a specially bred variant of tea tree may have increased activity against microorganisms, while irritating the skin less.[10]

SAFETY ISSUES

Like other essential oils, tea tree oil can be toxic if taken orally in excessive doses. Since the maximum safe dosage has not been determined, we recommend using it only topically, where it is believed to be quite safe. However, don't get it in your eye or it will sting badly.

In addition, an increasing number of cases of skin inflammation caused by allergy to tea tree oil have been reported.[11]

Safety in young children, pregnant or nursing women, or those with severe liver or kidney disease has not been established.

THYMUS EXTRACT

Supplement Forms/Alternate Names   Thymus Gland, Calf Thymus Extract, Thymic Extract, Thymomodulin

Principal Proposed Uses   There are no well-documented uses for thymus extract.

Other Proposed Uses   General Immune Support, Hepatitis, Food Allergies, Asthma, Cancer, Cold Sores, Dermatomyositis, Eczema, Genital Warts, Low White Blood Cell Count, Multiple Sclerosis, Psoriasis, Respiratory Infections, Rheumatoid Arthritis, Scleroderma, Shingles (*Herpes zoster*)

The thymus gland is found behind the sternum in the middle of the chest. Most active in unborn and very young children, it plays a significant role in the immune system. The theory behind the use of thymus extracts is that they might stimulate or normalize immunity. However, there is no real evidence as yet that any thymus extracts are effective, and they may present real health risks.

Visit Us at TNP.com

REQUIREMENTS/SOURCES

Thymus extract is produced primarily from the thymus gland of cows. This has led to concerns regarding "mad cow" disease. (See Safety Issues below.) Some studies have used chemically synthesized versions of chemicals found in thymus extract.

THERAPEUTIC DOSAGES

The dosage of thymus extract used in studies has varied widely, depending on the particular thymus product used.

THERAPEUTIC USES

Intensive athletic training can suppress immune function and lead to colds. However, a double-blind placebo-controlled trial failed to find any significant evidence of benefit with thymus extract.[1]

Highly preliminary evidence suggests that thymus extracts may be helpful for **food allergies**[2] (see page 82) and asthma;[3] it may do so not by boosting the immune system, but by calming it down and causing it to behave more normally.

Thymus extract has been tried as a treatment for **hepatitis B and C** (see page 189). However, the results of small double-blind trials have not been positive.[4–7]

Injectable forms of whole thymus extract or chemicals contained in it have been studied as a treatment for numerous conditions, including **cancer** (see page 32), cold sores, dermatomyositis, **eczema** (see page 78), genital warts, **hepatitis** (see page 189), **HIV infection** (see page 94), leukopenia (low white cell count), **multiple sclerosis** (see page 124), **psoriasis** (see page 148), **respiratory infections** (see page 47), **rheumatoid arthritis** (see page 151), scleroderma, and shingles (herpes zoster).[8–15] The results of these studies have been mixed. In any case, the results of trials involving injected thymus cannot be considered applicable to oral thymus products.

SAFETY ISSUES

Thymus extracts have not been definitely associated with any side effects. However, there are real concerns that any glandular extract might contain the virus causing "mad cow disease."[16] Keep in mind that there is no governmental regulation of thymus products sold as dietary supplements in the U.S. Even when a ban is placed on importation of cow glands from a country where mad cow disease has been found, the ban does not apply to dietary supplements! For this reason, we recommend that you do not use thymus products sold as dietary supplements.

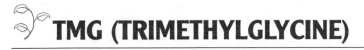

TMG (TRIMETHYLGLYCINE)

Supplement Forms/Alternate Names   Betaine (similar to betaine hydrochloride, but not identical)

Principal Proposed Uses   There are no documented uses for TMG.

Other Proposed Uses   Reducing Homocysteine Levels, Liver Protection, Substitute for SAMe, Performance Enhancement

TMG (trimethylglycine) has been available for decades. Recently, it has drawn attention as a possible treatment for elevated homocysteine levels.

Homocysteine is a naturally occurring chemical that may be as harmful to blood vessels as cholesterol. **Folate** (see page 288) and **vitamin B$_6$** (see page 439) destroy homocysteine by "methylating" it—attaching one carbon atom and three hydrogen atoms to it. This makes homocysteine harmless. Recent studies have found that vitamin B$_6$ and folate can help prevent heart disease, apparently by lowering homocysteine levels in the blood.

After this discovery, great interest developed in other substances that can methylate homocysteine. Chemicals of this type are called "methylating agents." **SAMe** (S-adenosylmethionine; see page 403) is one; TMG is

another. However, research into this subject is still in its infancy.

After TMG has done its work on homocysteine, it is turned into another substance, dimethylglycine (DMG). In Russia, DMG is used extensively as an athletic performance enhancer; however, TMG is cheaper and may have the same effects (if any).

SOURCES

TMG is not required in the diet because the body can manufacture it from other nutrients. Grains, nuts, seeds, and meats contain small amounts of TMG. However, most TMG in food is destroyed during cooking or processing, so food isn't a reliable way to get a therapeutic dosage.

Some manufacturers will tell you that DMG is identical to TMG, but this isn't true. DMG is not a methylating agent, so it can't have any effect on homocysteine.

THERAPEUTIC DOSAGES

There hasn't been enough research to establish the optimal therapeutic dosage of TMG. One manufacturer recommends using between 375 and 1,000 mg daily.

THERAPEUTIC USES

One small study suggests that TMG may lower homocysteine levels,[1] which might be helpful for those with **atherosclerosis** (see page 16).

TMG may also help protect the liver against the effects of alcohol, perhaps by stimulating the formation of SAMe.[2,3,4] Additionally, it may be useful for other purposes for which SAMe is used, although this has not been proven.

DMG (the substance TMG changes into in the body) has been extensively used as a **performance enhancer** (see page 158) by Russian athletes, and has recently become popular among American athletes. However, one small study suggests that it does not work.[5]

SAFETY ISSUES

TMG appears to be safe. However, the maximum safe dosages for young children, pregnant or nursing mothers, or those with severe liver or kidney disease have not been established.

TRIBULUS TERRESTRIS

Principal Proposed Uses   There are no well-documented uses for *Tribulus terrestris*.

Other Proposed Uses   Performance Enhancement, Sexual Dysfunction (in Men and Women)

Tribulus terrestris (commonly known as puncture vine) is a tropical plant with a long history of medicinal use. It has been tried for low libido in both men and women, **female infertility** (see page 79), and **impotence** (see page 100). In addition, it has been studied as a treatment for **heart disease** (see page 16).[1]

WHAT IS *TRIBULUS TERRESTRIS* USED FOR TODAY?

One theory regarding how tribulus might help with sexual problems regards a component from the plant, called protodioscin, which is converted in our bodies to the hormone dehydroepiandrosterone (DHEA; see page 268).[2] DHEA is used by the body as a building block for both testosterone and estrogen, as well as for other hormones.

This fact has led bodybuilders and strength athletes to try tribulus for increasing muscular development. So far, however, the scientific evidence does not support this use. This is not surprising, as DHEA itself has not been found effective as a **sports supplement** (see page 158) either.

One study compared the effects of tribulus (3.21 mg per kilogram of body weight—for example, 292 mg daily for a 200-lb man) against placebo on body composition and endurance among 15 men engaged in resistance training.[3] At the end of the 8-week study, the only significant difference between the treatment and placebo groups was that the placebo group showed greater gains in endurance.

There is no evidence as yet that tribulus is helpful for **impotence** (see page 100), low libido, or **sexual dysfunction in women** (see page 155). However, because DHEA may offer some benefits for sexual dysfunction, especially in older women, it is theoretically possible that tribulus could as well.

DOSAGE

Tribulus terrestris is usually taken at a dose ranging from about 85 to 250 mg three times daily with meals. Some tribulus products are standardized to provide 40% furostanol saponins.

SAFETY ISSUES

No significant adverse effects have been noted in any of the clinical trials or human research studies of tribulus. In animal studies, both short-term and long-term toxicity of the herb were found to be extremely low. However, tribulus is known to have a toxic effect on sheep.[4,5,6]

Note: Women who are pregnant or nursing should not use any tribulus product, as it might alter hormonal chemistry.

For additional possible safety concerns, see the chapter on DHEA.

Tribulus terrestris

Visit Us at TNP.com

TURMERIC *(Curcuma longa)*

Principal Proposed Uses   There are no well-documented uses for turmeric.

Other Proposed Uses   Arthritis, Gallstones, Dyspepsia, Cataracts, Chronic Anterior Uveitis, Dysmenorrhea

Turmeric is a widely used tropical herb in the ginger family. Its stalk is used both in food and medicine, yielding the familiar yellow ingredient that colors and adds flavor to curry. In the traditional Indian system of herbal medicine known as Ayurveda, turmeric is believed to strengthen the overall energy of the body, relieve gas, dispel worms, improve digestion, regulate menstruation, dissolve gallstones, and relieve arthritis, among other uses.

Modern interest in turmeric began in 1971 when Indian researchers found evidence that whole turmeric possesses anti-inflammatory properties. Much of this observed activity seems to be due to the presence of a constituent called curcumin.[1] Curcumin is also a powerful antioxidant.[2]

WHAT IS TURMERIC USED FOR TODAY?

Turmeric's antioxidant abilities make it a good food preservative, provided that the food is already yellow in color!

Based on its anti-inflammatory properties, curcumin is commonly recommended as a natural treatment for arthritis as well. However, the one small double-blind comparative study often cited as evidence for its effectiveness in **rheumatoid arthritis** (see page 151) actually provides no such evidence at all, because it lacked a placebo group.[3] Curcumin also has been suggested for **osteoarthritis** (see page 132).

Unlike standard anti-inflammatories, curcumin does not appear to cause stomach **ulcers** (see page 180) when taken in normal doses.[4] However, high doses might increase risk of ulcers.[5] Contrary to some reports, turmeric does not appear to be effective for treating ulcers.[6,7]

Curcumin appears to stimulate gallbladder contractions, which may explain its traditional use for **gallstones** (see page 83).[8] However, such contractions could cause pain or serious complications. For this reason, individuals with gallbladder disease should only use curcumin on the advice of a physician.

Because of its ability to stimulate the gall bladder, turmeric has also been suggested as a treatment for **dyspepsia** (see page 71) or indigestion.[9] In Europe, gallbladder dysfunction or a lack of bile is thought to be the main cause of dyspepsia, however there is no evidence that this is really the case.

There is some evidence that turmeric might be effective in its traditional role as an antiflatulent.[10,11]

Curcumin is also sometimes recommended for **cataracts** (see page 42), chronic anterior uveitis (an inflammation of the iris of the eye),[12] and **dysmenorrhea** (menstrual pain; see page 70), but there is as yet no real evidence that it works.

WHAT IS THE SCIENTIFIC EVIDENCE FOR TURMERIC?

Dyspepsia

A double-blind placebo-controlled study including 106 people compared the effects of 500 mg curcumin 4 times daily against placebo (as well as against a locally popular over-the-counter treatment). After 7 days, 87% percent of the curcumin group experienced full or partial symptom relief from dyspepsia as compared to 53% of the placebo group.[13]

DOSAGE

For medicinal purposes, turmeric is frequently taken in a form standardized to curcumin content, to provide 400 to 600 mg of curcumin 3 times daily.

Unfortunately, curcumin is not absorbed well by the body.[14] It is often sold in combination with **bromelain** (see page 229) for the supposed purpose of enhancing absorption. While there is no evidence or even sensible reason to believe that this strategy works, bromelain possesses some anti-inflammatory powers of its own that may add to those of curcumin.

SAFETY ISSUES

Turmeric is on the FDA's GRAS (generally recognized as safe) list, and curcumin, too, is believed to be extremely nontoxic.[15,16] Side effects are rare and are generally limited to the usual mild stomach distress. However, safety in young children, pregnant or nursing women, or those with severe liver or kidney disease has not been established. Due to curcumin's effects on the gallbladder, individuals with gallbladder disease should use curcumin only on the advice of a physician.

TYLOPHORA *(Tylophora indica, Tylophora asthmatica)*

Principal Proposed Uses   Asthma

Other Proposed Uses   Allergies, Bronchitis, Colds, Dysentery, Joint Pain

Tylophora indica is a climbing perennial plant indigenous to India, where it grows wild in the southern and eastern regions and has a long-standing reputation as a remedy for asthma (hence the name *T. asthmatica*).

The leaves and roots of tylophora have been included in the *Bengal Pharmacopoeia* since 1884. It is said to have laxative, expectorant, diaphoretic (sweating), and purgative (vomiting) properties. It has been used for the treatment of various respiratory problems besides asthma, including allergies, bronchitis and colds, as well as dysentery and joint pain.

WHAT IS TYLOPHORA USED FOR TODAY?

Based on its long-standing use as a folk remedy for **asthma** (see page 14), tylophora has been evaluated in several studies, but with mixed results.[1–8]

We don't know how tylophora might work in asthma, but it may have anti-inflammatory, antiallergic, adrenal gland–stimulating, and antispasmodic actions.[9–12]

WHAT IS THE SCIENTIFIC EVIDENCE FOR TYLOPHORA?

In a double-blind placebo-controlled crossover study of 195 individuals with asthma, participants showed significant improvement when given 40 mg of a tylophora alcohol extract daily for 6 days as compared to placebo. Surprisingly (so surprisingly, in fact, that it casts doubt on the study), the difference was even more marked months after use of the herb was stopped.[13] Similar long-lasting results were seen in a double-blind placebo-controlled study of 110 individuals with asthma.[14] However, the design of these studies was a bit convoluted,

and various pieces of information are missing from the reports, making it difficult to evaluate the validity of these trials.

Another double-blind study that enrolled 135 individuals and followed a more straightforward design found no benefit from tylophora in asthma.[15]

The bottom line: Although tylophora is promising, larger and better studies are necessary to discover whether tylophora is truly effective.

DOSAGE

The typical dosage of tylophora leaf in dried or capsule form is 200 mg twice daily or 400 mg total in 2 doses.

SAFETY ISSUES

In the second study mentioned above, tylophora caused nausea, vomiting, mouth soreness, and alterations in taste sensation in more than half of the participants. The other two studies found similar side effects, but far less frequently. The difference may have been because the second study had people chew the whole leaves from the plant, whereas other studies have used dried leaves or powdered extract in capsule form.

Preliminary studies on animals have found tylophora extracts to be toxic in extremely high doses; however, these extracts were safe in the far smaller doses needed to produce a therapeutic effect.[16]

Due to the lack of comprehensive safety studies on tylophora, the herb should not be used by children, pregnant or nursing women, or individuals with severe kidney or liver disease. Whether tylophora interacts with any drugs is unknown.

TYROSINE

Supplement Forms/Alternate Names   L-Tyrosine

Principal Proposed Uses   There are no well-documented uses for tyrosine.

Other Proposed Uses   Sleep Deprivation, Attention Deficit Disorder, Depression

Tyrosine is an amino acid found in meat proteins. Your body uses it as a starting material to make several neurotransmitters (chemicals that help the brain and nervous system function). Based on this fact, tyrosine has been proposed as a treatment for various conditions in which mental function is impaired or slowed down, such as sleep deprivation and depression. It has also been tried for attention deficit disorder (ADD).

SOURCES

Your body makes tyrosine from another common amino acid, **phenylalanine** (see page 385), so deficiencies are rare; however, they can occur in certain forms of severe kidney disease as well as in phenylketonuria (PKU), a metabolic disorder that requires complete avoidance of phenylalanine. (For more information, see the chapter on **phenylalanine**.)

Good sources of tyrosine include dairy products, meats, fish, and beans.

THERAPEUTIC DOSAGES

The typical recommended dosage of tyrosine is 7 to 30 g daily.

THERAPEUTIC USES

According to very preliminary evidence, tyrosine supplements may help fight fatigue and increase alertness in people who are deprived of sleep.[1]

Tyrosine may also provide some temporary benefit for **attention deficit disorder** (see page 22), but the benefits appear to wear off in a couple of weeks.[2,3,4] Tyrosine is said to work better for this purpose when it is combined in an "amino acid cocktail" along with gamma-aminobutyric acid (GABA), phenylalanine, and **gluta-**mine (see page 310); however, there is no scientific evidence to support this use.

Although one extremely tiny study found tyrosine helpful for **depression** (see page 59),[5] a recent larger study found it not effective.[6]

WHAT IS THE SCIENTIFIC EVIDENCE FOR TYROSINE?

Sleep Deprivation

A placebo-controlled study that enrolled 20 U.S. Marines suggests that tyrosine can improve alertness during periods of sleep deprivation. In this study, the participants were deprived of sleep for a night and then tested frequently for their alertness throughout the day as they worked. Compared to placebo, 10 to 15 g of tyrosine given twice daily seemed to provide a "pick-up" for about 2 hours.[7]

Depression

A study that enrolled nine individuals is widely quoted as evidence that tyrosine can help depression.[8] However, a recent double-blind placebo-controlled study of 65 people with depression found *no* benefit.[9]

SAFETY ISSUES

Tyrosine seems to be generally safe, though at high dosages some people have reported nausea, diarrhea, vomiting, or nervousness. As with any other supplement taken in multigram doses, it is important to use a high-quality product; even a very small percentage of contaminant in the product might add up to a dangerous amount.

Maximum safe dosages for young children, women who are pregnant or nursing, or those with severe liver or kidney disease have not been established.

UVA URSI *(Arctostaphylos uva-ursi)*

Alternate or Related Names   Arberry, Bearberry, Bear's Grape, Kinnikinnick, Mealberry, Others

Principal Proposed Uses   Treatment of Urinary Tract Infection (Not Recommended for Prevention of Urinary Tract Infection)

The uva ursi plant is a low-lying evergreen bush whose berries are a favorite of bears, hence the name "bearberry." However, it is the leaves that are used medicinally.

Uva ursi has a long history of use for treating urinary conditions in both America and Europe. Up until the development of sulfa antibiotics, its principal active compo-nent, arbutin, was frequently prescribed as a urinary antiseptic.

Although we don't know for sure how uva ursi works, it appears that the arbutin contained in uva ursi leaves is broken down in the intestine to another chemical, hydroquinone. This chemical is altered a bit by the liver

Uva Ursi

Visit Us at TNP.com

and then sent to the kidneys for excretion.[1] In the bladder, it acts as an antiseptic.

Uva ursi appears to be most effective in an alkaline urine, so taking vitamin C with uva ursi probably hampers its work.[2,3]

WHAT IS UVA URSI USED FOR TODAY?

The European Scientific Cooperative on Phytotherapy recommends uva ursi for "uncomplicated infections of the urinary tract such as cystitis when antibiotic treatment is not considered essential."[4] This herb is most useful for women who can tell when they are just starting to develop a bladder infection and can start treatment early. Once you have a severe **bladder infection** (see page 28), uva ursi probably won't work very well.

Warning: The herb is definitely not appropriate for kidney infections. If you develop symptoms such as high fever, chills, nausea, vomiting, diarrhea, or severe back pain, get medical assistance immediately.

Furthermore, because hydroquinone can be toxic (discussed under Safety Issues), it isn't a good idea to take uva ursi for a long period of time.

WHAT IS THE SCIENTIFIC EVIDENCE FOR UVA URSI?

The research foundation for uva ursi is surprisingly weak considering the popularity of this herb.[5]

Treatment

No double-blind studies have evaluated the clinical effectiveness of uva ursi. However, two studies have evaluated the antibacterial power of the urine of people given uva ursi, and have found activity against most major bacteria that infect the urinary tract.[6,7] This doesn't prove much, however.

Prevention

One double-blind study followed 57 women for 1 year. Half were given a standardized dose of uva ursi (in combination with dandelion leaf, intended to promote urine flow), while the others received placebo. Over the course of the study, none of the women taking the combination developed a bladder infection, while five of the untreated women did.[8] However, most experts do not believe that continuous treatment with uva ursi is a good idea (see Safety Issues).

DOSAGE

The dosage of uva ursi should be adjusted to provide 400 to 800 mg of arbutin daily.[9,10,11] This dosage should not be exceeded, and if the herb is not successful within a week you should definitely seek medical attention. No more than 2 weeks of treatment with uva ursi is recommended, and it should not be used more than five times a year.

Uva ursi should be taken with meals to minimize gastrointestinal upset. Because uva ursi is most effective in alkaline urine, it should not be combined with **vitamin C** (see page 444) or cranberry juice. You might try taking it along with calcium citrate to alkalinize the urine instead.

Uva ursi is also frequently sold in combination with other herbs traditionally thought to be helpful for bladder infections, including **dandelion** (see page 266), cleavers, **juniper berry** (see page 337), buchu, and parsley.

SAFETY ISSUES

Unfortunately, hydroquinone is a liver toxin, carcinogen, and irritant.[12–15] For this reason, uva ursi is not recommended for young children, pregnant or nursing women, or those with severe liver or kidney disease.

However, significant problems are rare among individuals using prepared uva ursi products in appropriate doses for a short period of time. Gastrointestinal distress (ranging from mild nausea and diarrhea to vomiting) can occur, especially with prolonged use.[16]

⚠ INTERACTIONS YOU SHOULD KNOW ABOUT

If you are taking **drugs** or **supplements that acidify the urine,** such as **cranberry juice,** uva ursi may not work very well.

🌿 VALERIAN (*Valeriana officinalis*)

Alternate or Related Names   All-Heal, Amantilla, Setwall, Setewale, Capon's Tail, Others

Principal Proposed Uses   Insomnia

Other Proposed Uses   Anxiety, Nervous Stomach

Over 200 plant species belong to the genus *Valeriana,* but the one most commonly used as an herb is *Valeriana officinalis.* The root is used for medicinal purposes.

Galen recommended valerian for insomnia in the second century A.D. From the sixteenth century onward, this herb became popular as a sedative in Europe (and later, the United States). Scientific studies on valerian in humans began in the 1970s, leading to its approval as a sleep aid by Germany's Commission E in 1985.

As for most herbs, we are not exactly sure which ingredients in valerian are most important.[1,2] Early research focused on a group of chemicals known as valepotriates, but they are no longer considered candidates. A constituent called valerenic acid is presently under study, but its role is far from clear.

Our understanding of how valerian functions is similarly incomplete. Several studies suggest that valerian affects GABA, a naturally occurring amino acid that appears to be related to the experience of anxiety.[3–6] Conventional tranquilizers in the Valium family are known to bind to GABA receptors in the brain, and valerian may work similarly. However, there are some significant flaws in these hypotheses, and the reality is that we don't really know how valerian works.[7,8]

WHAT IS VALERIAN USED FOR TODAY?

Valerian is commonly recommended as a mild treatment for occasional **insomnia** (see page 103). It appears to be somewhat more effective than herbs such as **hops** (see page 324), **skullcap** (see page 410), and **passionflower** (see page 382), but less effective than pharmaceutical sleeping pills such as Ambien.

Interestingly, a recent German herbal text suggests that valerian is most useful when taken over an extended period of time.[9] The authors suggest combining valerian extract with a comprehensive sleep-management program for people with chronic sleeping troubles.

Valerian is used to treat **anxiety** (see page 11) as well, although there is much more scientific evidence for the herb **kava** (see page 338).

Finally, valerian is sometimes suggested as a treatment for a nervous stomach; however, as of yet, there is no evidence for this use.

WHAT IS THE SCIENTIFIC EVIDENCE FOR VALERIAN?

The research basis for valerian is growing. The well-designed 28-day study described below still appears to be little known in the United States.

Insomnia

The best study to date of valerian's effectiveness in treating insomnia involved 121 people followed for 28 days.[10]

Half of the participants took 600 mg of an alcohol-based valerian extract 1 hour before bedtime, the other half placebo.

At first, placebo and valerian were running neck and neck. But by the end of the study, the participants treated with valerian were definitely sleeping better.

Although positive, these results are a bit confusing, because in another large study valerian was immediately more effective than placebo. This trial followed 128 subjects who had no sleeping problems.[11] On three consecutive nights they took either valerian or placebo. The results showed that on the nights they took valerian, participants fell asleep faster than when they were taking placebo. It is possible that different subspecies of valerian with differing medicinal effects have been used in the various trials.

Additional evidence for valerian's effectiveness comes from a double-blind placebo-controlled study of 78 elderly patients.[12] In this case, sleep improved by the end of the study, at 14 days.

Finally, the combination of valerian and **lemon balm** (see page 359) has been tried for insomnia. A 30-day double-blind placebo-controlled study of 98 individuals without insomnia found that a valerian–lemon balm combination improved sleep quality as compared to placebo.[13] Similarly, a double-blind crossover study of 20 people with insomnia compared the benefits of the sleeping drug Halcion (0.125 mg) against placebo and a combination of valerian and lemon balm, and found them equally effective.[14]

Anxiety

Forty-eight participants were placed under situations of "social stress" in a double-blind study of valerian.[15] Individuals in the treated group reported less anxiety.

Animal Studies

Both valerenic acid and whole valerian have been found to produce calm, sleepiness, and reduced activity in laboratory mice.[16–19] Both substances also help prevent seizures. Since most pharmaceutical tranquilizers also reduce seizures, the latter result can be taken as additional indirect evidence of valerian's tranquilizing powers.

Warning: Do not try to substitute valerian for your antiseizure medication. The herb is not powerful enough.

DOSAGE

For insomnia, the standard dosage of valerian is 2 to 3 g of dried herb, 270 to 450 mg of an aqueous valerian extract, or 600 mg of an ethanol extract, taken 30 to 60 minutes before bedtime.[20]

According to the study mentioned previously that used this dosage, valerian may require weeks to reach its

Valerian

Visit Us at TNP.com

Vanadium

full effects. The same amount, or a reduced dose, can be taken twice daily for anxiety.

Because of valerian's unpleasant odor, European manufacturers have created odorless valerian products. However, these are not yet widely available in the United States.

Valerian is not recommended for children under 3 years old.[21]

SAFETY ISSUES

Valerian is on the FDA's GRAS (generally recognized as safe) list, and is approved for use as a food. In animals, it takes enormous doses of valerian to produce any serious adverse effects.[22]

In a suicide attempt, one young woman took approximately 20 g of valerian (20 to 40 times the recommended dose). Only mild symptoms developed, including stomach cramps, fatigue, chest tightness, tremors and light-headedness. All of these resolved within 24 hours, after two treatments with activated charcoal.[23] Her lab tests—including tests of her liver function—remained normal. Keep in mind that this does not mean that you can safely exceed the recommended dose!

One report did find toxic results from herbal remedies containing valerian mixed with several other herbal ingredients, including skullcap. Four individuals who took these remedies later developed liver problems.[24] However, skullcap products are sometimes contaminated with the liver-toxic herb germander, and this could have been the explanation.

There have also been about 50 reported cases of overdose with a combination preparation called Sleep-Qik, containing valerian as well as conventional medications.[25,26] Researchers specifically looked for liver injury, but found no evidence that it occurred.

There are some safety concerns about valepotriates, constituents of valerian, because they can affect DNA and cause other toxic effects. However, valepotriates are not present to a significant extent in any commercial preparations.[27,28]

Although no animal studies or controlled human trials have found evidence that valerian ever causes withdrawal symptoms when stopped, one case report is sometimes cited in support of the possibility that this might occur.[29] It concerns a 58-year-old man who developed delirium and rapid heartbeat after surgery. According to the patient's family, he had been taking high doses of valerian root extract (about 2.5 to 10 g per day) for many years. His physicians decided that he was suffering from valerian withdrawal. However, considering the many other factors involved (such as multiple medications and general anesthesia), it isn't really possible to conclude that valerian caused his symptoms.

Except for the unpleasant odor, valerian generally causes no side effects.[30,31] A few people experience mild gastrointestinal distress, and there have been rare reports of people developing a paradoxical mild stimulant effect from valerian.

Valerian does not appear to impair driving ability or produce morning drowsiness when it is taken at night.[32–35] However, there does appear to be some impairment of attention for a couple of hours after taking valerian.[36] For this reason, it isn't a good idea to drive immediately after taking it.

There have been no reported drug interactions with valerian. A 1995 study found no interaction between alcohol and valerian as measured by concentration, attentiveness, reaction time, and driving performance.[37] However, valerian extracts may prolong drug-induced sleeping time in mice, rats, and rabbits.[38,39] Thus, it is possible that valerian could compound the effects of other central-nervous-system depressants.

Safety in young children, pregnant or nursing women, or those with severe liver or kidney disease has not been established.

⚠ INTERACTIONS YOU SHOULD KNOW ABOUT

If you are taking **medications for insomnia** or **anxiety** such as **benzodiazepines,** don't take valerian in addition to them.

🌿 VANADIUM

Supplement Forms/Alternate Names   Vanadyl Sulfate, Vanadate

Principal Proposed Uses   There are no well-documented uses for vanadium, and there are serious safety concerns regarding vanadium use.

Other Proposed Uses   Diabetes, Bodybuilding, Osteoporosis

Vanadium, a mineral, is named after the Scandinavian goddess of beauty, youth, and luster. Taking vanadium will not make you beautiful, youthful, and lustrous, but evidence from animal studies suggests it may be an essential micronutrient. That is, your body may need it, but in *very* low doses.

Based on promising animal studies, high doses of vanadium have been tested as an aid to controlling blood sugar levels in people with diabetes. Like **chromium** (see page 251), another trace mineral used in diabetes, vanadium has also been recommended as an aid in bodybuilding. However, animal studies suggest that taking high doses of vanadium can be harmful.

REQUIREMENTS/SOURCES

We don't know exactly how much vanadium people require, but estimates range from 10 to 30 mcg daily. (To realize how tiny this amount is, consider that it's about *one millionth* of the amount of calcium you need.) Human deficiencies have not been reported, but goats fed a low-vanadium diet have developed birth defects.[1]

Vanadium is found in very small amounts in a wide variety of foods, including breakfast cereals, canned fruit juices, wine, beer, buckwheat, parsley, soy, oats, olive oil, sunflower seeds, corn, green beans, peanut oil, carrots, cabbage, and garlic. The average daily American diet provides between 10 and 60 mcg of vanadium.[2]

THERAPEUTIC DOSAGES

In various studies, vanadium has been used at doses thousands of times higher than is present in the diet, as high as 125 mg per day. However, there are serious safety concerns about taking vanadium at such high doses (see Safety Issues). We do not recommend exceeding the nutritional dose of 10 to 30 mcg daily.

THERAPEUTIC USES

Vanadium has been proposed as a treatment for **diabetes** (see page 65), based on promising studies in animals and a few small human trials.[3,4]

Vanadium is also sometimes used by bodybuilders, but there is no evidence that it is effective.[5]

Because studies in mice have found that vanadium is deposited in bone,[6] some practitioners of nutritional medicine have suggested that it may be helpful for **osteoporosis** (see page 136). However, since many toxic metals also accumulate in the bones without strengthening them, this doesn't prove that vanadium is good for bones.

WHAT IS THE SCIENTIFIC EVIDENCE FOR VANADIUM?

Diabetes

Studies in rats with and without diabetes suggest that vanadium may have an insulin-like effect, reducing blood sugar levels.[7–17] Based on these findings, preliminary studies involving human subjects have been conducted, with promising results.[18–21] However, they were all too small to be taken as definitive proof. More research is needed to definitely establish whether vanadium is effective (not to mention safe) for the treatment of diabetes.

Bodybuilding

A double-blind placebo-controlled study involving 31 weight-trained athletes found *no* benefit at a dosage more than 1,000 times the nutritional dose.[22]

SAFETY ISSUES

Studies in humans and animals suggest that vanadium can cause toxic effects and might accumulate in the body if taken to excess.[23–26] Based on these results, high dosages of vanadium can't be considered safe for human use. If you wish to take it, stick to the 10 to 30 mcg a day mentioned earlier.

⚠ INTERACTIONS YOU SHOULD KNOW ABOUT

If you are taking **insulin** or **oral diabetes medications,** seek medical supervision before taking vanadium because you may need to reduce your dose of diabetes medication.

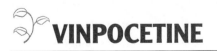

VINPOCETINE

Supplement Forms/Alternate Names   Periwinkle

Principal Proposed Uses   Alzheimer's Disease, Other Forms of Dementia, Ordinary Age-Related Memory Loss

Vinpocetine

Visit Us at TNP.com

Vinpocetine is a chemical derived from vincamine, a constituent found in the leaves of common periwinkle (*Vinca minor* L.) as well as the seeds of various African plants. It is used as a treatment for memory loss and mental impairment.

Developed in Hungary over 20 years ago, vinpocetine is sold in Europe as a drug under the name Cavinton. In the United States it is available as a "dietary supplement," although the substance probably doesn't fit that category by any rational definition. Vinpocetine doesn't exist to any significant extent in nature. Producing it requires significant chemical work performed in the laboratory.

WHAT IS THE SCIENTIFIC EVIDENCE FOR VINPOCETINE?

A significant level of evidence supports the idea that vinpocetine can enhance memory and mental function, especially in those with Alzheimer's disease and related conditions. It may also be helpful for those with ordinary age-related memory loss, although this has not been proven.

One 3-month double-blind placebo-controlled study followed 84 individuals with age-related mental impairment.[1] According to several standard rating scales, the severity of the illness improved by a statistically significant margin in the treatment group as compared to the placebo group. Similarly positive results have been seen in many other studies,[2] although at least one study did not find benefit.[3]

We don't know how vinpocetine works, although there are numerous theories. There is some evidence that vinpocetine can safeguard brain cells against damage caused by lack of oxygen.[4] However, whether this effect really has anything to do with its effects on mental function remains unclear.

DOSAGE

Vinpocetine is available in 10-mg capsules, usually taken 3 times per day. This supplement is probably best taken with meals, as it is better absorbed that way.[5] We recommend that it be used only on physician advice.

SAFETY ISSUES

No serious side effects have been reported in any of the clinical trials. However, there are some concerns that vinpocetine might impair the effectiveness of Coumadin (warfarin).[6]

Safety in pregnant or nursing women, young children, or those with severe liver or kidney disease has not been established.

⚠ INTERACTIONS YOU SHOULD KNOW ABOUT

If you are taking **Coumadin (warfarin),** vinpocetine might decrease its effectiveness.

🌿 VITAMIN A

Supplement Forms/Alternate Names   Retinol

Principal Proposed Uses   Viral Infections in Children in Developing Countries

Other Proposed Uses   Diabetes
Skin Disorders: Acne, Psoriasis
Menorrhagia (Heavy Menstruation), HIV Support, Down's Syndrome, Ear Infections, Eating Disorders, Glaucoma, Gout, Impaired Night Vision, Kidney Stones, Lupus, Multiple Sclerosis, Ulcerative Colitis, Ulcers, Crohn's Disease

Note: Beta-carotene is sometimes used interchangeably with vitamin A, because the body can turn beta-carotene into vitamin A.

Vitamin A is a fat-soluble antioxidant that protects your cells against damaging free radicals and plays other vital roles in the body. However, it is potentially more dangerous than most other vitamins because it can build up to toxic levels, causing liver damage and birth defects. Because of this risk, vitamin A supplements have few therapeutic uses.

In general, **beta-carotene** (see page 217) supplements taken at nutritional doses are a safer way to get

the vitamin A you need. Sometimes called "provitamin A," beta-carotene is transformed into vitamin A as your body needs it, and presents much less risk of toxicity.

REQUIREMENTS/SOURCES

Vitamin A is an essential nutrient—meaning you must get it in the diet. The official U.S. recommendations for vitamin A are expressed in micrograms (mcg) of retinol equivalents (RE). Supplement labels usually express vitamin A in international units (IU). The following list shows the official U.S. recommendations for daily intake of vitamin A in mcg and its equivalent in IU:

- Infants 0–12 months, 1,250 IU; 375 mcg (or retinol equivalent, RE)
- Children 1–3 years, 1,333 IU; 400 mcg
    4–6 years, 1,667 IU; 500 mcg
    7–10 years, 2,333 IU; 700 mcg
- Males 11 years and older, 3,333 IU; 1,000 mcg
- Females 11 years and older, 2,667 IU; 800 mcg
- Pregnant women, 2,667 IU; 800 mcg
- Nursing women, 4,000–4,333 IU; 1,200–1,300 mcg

These amounts can be obtained safely by taking beta-carotene instead of vitamin A. The proper dose may be calculated by keeping in mind that 1 IU of beta-carotene is equivalent to 1 IU of vitamin A; 1 mg of beta-carotene is equivalent to 500 mcg of vitamin A.

Warning: Pregnant women should not take vitamin A supplements. Instead they should take beta-carotene.

We get vitamin A from many foods, in the form of either vitamin A or beta-carotene. Liver and dairy products are excellent sources of vitamin A. Carrots, apricots, collard greens, kale, sweet potatoes, parsley, and spinach are good sources as well.

Deficiency in vitamin A is common in developing countries.[1] In the developed world, deficiency is relatively rare, except among teenagers and those in lower socioeconomic groups. Also, the older cholesterol-lowering drugs cholestyramine and colestipol can reduce vitamin A levels; however, the effect is slight and probably not significant.[2]

THERAPEUTIC DOSAGES

Doses of vitamin A above the basic nutritional requirement are not recommended.

THERAPEUTIC USES

There is some evidence that vitamin A supplements reduce deaths from measles and other causes among children in developing countries,[3] presumably because they correct a deficiency in the children's diets. This doesn't mean that vitamin A supplements above and beyond the basic nutritional requirement are a useful treatment for measles or any other childhood disease.

Vitamin A may be helpful for **diabetes** (see page 65). However, there are concerns that people with diabetes may be especially vulnerable to liver damage from excessive amounts of vitamin A (see Safety Issues). Therefore, if you have diabetes, you should take vitamin A only on the advice of a physician.

Vitamin A has been used in the past for a variety of skin diseases such as **acne** (see page 2) and **psoriasis** (see page 148), but since you need to use large amounts (which could cause toxicity) to achieve benefits, standard medications are safer. High-dose vitamin A may also be helpful for menorrhagia (heavy menstruation),[4] but again it is not safe.

Vitamin A deficiency may be linked to lower immune cell counts as well as higher death rates among people infected with **HIV** (see page 94).[5] A few preliminary studies have raised hopes that beta-carotene supplements (a source of vitamin A) might increase or preserve immune function or decrease symptoms among people with HIV.[6–9] However, not all studies have had positive results.[10,11]

In addition, vitamin A has been proposed as a treatment for a wide variety of other conditions, some of them quite serious, including AIDS, Down's syndrome, **ear infections** (see page 73), **eating disorders** (see page 77), glaucoma, **gout** (see page 84), impaired **night vision** (see page 128), **kidney stones** (see page 109), **lupus** (see page 114), **multiple sclerosis** (see page 124), **ulcerative colitis** (see page 179), and **ulcers** (see page 180). There is little to no evidence that it is effective for any of these conditions. One study suggests that vitamin A is not effective for **Crohn's disease** (see page 57).[12]

WHAT IS THE SCIENTIFIC EVIDENCE FOR VITAMIN A?

Viral Infections (in Children Living in Developing Countries)

Vitamin A has been tried as a treatment for various viral infections, including measles, respiratory syncytial virus (RSV, a common childhood viral disease of the respiratory tract), chicken pox, and AIDS.

Most of the research on vitamin A has concentrated on children in developing countries. A review article examining 12 studies suggested that vitamin A supplements can protect such children from dying, and should be used more widely.[13]

Success with measles led researchers to study its use in respiratory syncytial virus.[14,15] However, the results were not impressive.

Diabetes

According to many[16,17] but not all[18,19] studies, people with diabetes tend to be deficient in vitamin A.

An observational study suggests that vitamin A supplements may improve blood sugar control in people with diabetes.[20] However, due to safety concerns, they should not supplement with vitamin A except under medical supervision (see Safety Issues).

Vitamin A

Visit Us at TNP.com

Skin Disorders

Vitamin A has been tried for various skin disorders, including acne, psoriasis, rosacea, **seborrhea** (see page 154), and eczema.[21–24] However, the benefits have not been great, and generally vitamin A has to be taken in potentially toxic dosages to produce good effects.

Menorrhagia (Heavy Menstruation)

One study suggests that women with heavy menstrual bleeding can benefit from taking 25,000 IU daily of vitamin A.[25] But vitamin A cannot be recommended as an ongoing treatment for menorrhagia, since women who menstruate can become pregnant, and even low doses of supplemental vitamin A may cause birth defects.

HIV Support

One small double-blind study suggested that taking beta-carotene might raise white blood cell count in people with HIV.[26] However, two subsequent larger controlled trials found no significant differences between those taking beta-carotene or placebo in white blood cell count, CD4+ count, or other measures of immune function.[27,28]

Two observational studies lasting 6 to 8 years suggest that higher intakes of vitamin A or beta-carotene may be helpful, but they also found that caution is in order with regard to dosage.[29,30] This group of researchers generally linked higher intake of vitamin A or beta-carotene to lower risk of AIDS and lower death rates, with an important exception: people with the highest intake of either nutrient (more than 11,179 IU per day of beta-carotene; or more than 20,268 IU per day of vitamin A) did worse than those who took somewhat less.

Despite hopes that vitamin A given to pregnant, HIV-positive women might decrease the infection rate of their babies, two double-blind studies have found no significant differences between babies whose mothers took vitamin A compared to those whose mothers took placebo.[31,32] In any case, vitamin A is not considered safe in pregnancy; beta-carotene is preferred.

Crohn's Disease

According to a double-blind study of 86 people with Crohn's disease, vitamin A does *not* help prevent flare-ups.[33]

SAFETY ISSUES

Dosages of vitamin A above 50,000 IU per day taken for several years can cause liver injury, bone problems, fatigue, hair loss, headaches, and dry skin. If you already have liver disease, check with your doctor before taking vitamin A supplements, because even small doses may be harmful for you. Also, it is thought that people with diabetes may have trouble releasing vitamin A stored in the liver. This may mean that they are at greater risk for vitamin A toxicity. For different reasons, individuals who consume too much alcohol may also be at higher risk of vitamin A toxicity.[34] In addition, excessive intake of vitamin A may increase the risk of **osteoporosis** (see page 136).[35]

Women should avoid supplementing with vitamin A during pregnancy, because at toxic levels it may increase the risk of birth defects. Pregnant women taking valproic acid may be even more at risk of vitamin A toxicity.[36]

Vitamin A may also increase the anticoagulant effects of warfarin.[37] You should not take supplementary vitamin A unless under a physician's supervision.

Warning: Be sure to store vitamin A supplements where children cannot reach them!

⚠ INTERACTIONS YOU SHOULD KNOW ABOUT

If you are taking

- The older cholesterol-lowering drugs **cholestyramine** or **colestipol:** You may need more vitamin A (preferably as beta-carotene).
- **Isotretinoin (Accutane):** Don't take vitamin A as they might enhance each other's toxicity.
- **Valproic acid** or other **anticonvulsants:** Do not take vitamin A if you are pregnant unless on the advice of a physician.
- **Warfarin:** You should not take vitamin A unless under a doctor's supervision.

VITAMIN B₁

Supplement Forms/Alternate Names   Thiamin

Principal Proposed Uses   Congestive Heart Failure, Nutritional Support

Other Proposed Uses   HIV Support, Alzheimer's Disease, Epilepsy, Canker Sores, Fibromyalgia

Vitamin B_1, also called thiamin, was the first B vitamin ever discovered. Your body uses it to process fats, carbohydrates, and proteins. Every cell in your body needs thiamin to make adenosine triphosphate, or ATP, the body's main energy-carrying molecule. The heart, in particular, has considerable need for thiamin in order to keep up its constant work.

Severe deficiency results in beriberi, a disease common among sailors through the nineteenth century, but rare today. Beriberi is still seen, however, in developing countries as well as in alcoholics and people with diseases that significantly impair the body's ability to absorb vitamin B_1. Many of the principal symptoms of beriberi relate to impaired heart function.

REQUIREMENTS/SOURCES

Your need for vitamin B_1 varies with age. The official U.S. and Canadian recommendations for daily intake are as follows:

- Infants 0–5 months, 0.2 mg
    6–11 months, 0.3 mg
- Children 1–3 years, 0.5 mg
    4–8 years, 0.6 mg
    9–13 years, 0.9 mg
- Males 14 years and older, 1.2 mg
- Females 14–18 years, 1.0 mg
    19 years and older, 1.1 mg
- Pregnant women, 1.4 mg
- Nursing women, 1.5 mg

Alcoholism, congestive heart failure, Crohn's disease, anorexia, kidney dialysis, folate deficiency, and multiple sclerosis may all lead to a vitamin B_1 deficiency, and people with these conditions should consider taking B_1 supplements. Certain foods may impair your body's absorption of B_1 as well, including fish, shrimp, clams, mussels, and the herb horsetail.

Brewer's and nutritional yeast are the richest sources of B_1. Peas, beans, nuts, seeds, and whole grains also provide fairly good amounts.

THERAPEUTIC DOSAGES

Very high dosages of B_1—up to 8 g daily—have been recommended for a variety of conditions.

Since the B vitamins tend to work together, many nutritional experts recommend taking B_1 with other B vitamins in the form of a B-complex supplement.

THERAPEUTIC USES

Congestive heart failure (CHF; see page 54) is a condition in which the pumping ability of the heart declines, and fluid begins to accumulate in the lungs and legs. Standard treatment for CHF includes strong "water pills" called loop diuretics. These diuretics, however, deplete the body of B_1.[1] Since the heart depends on vitamin B_1 for its proper function, this is potentially quite worrisome. There is some evidence that supplementation with B_1 can improve symptoms.[2,3]

Individuals with alcoholism, **Crohn's disease** (see page 57), anorexia, or **multiple sclerosis** (see page 124) may also benefit from thiamin supplementation as part of general nutritional support.

An observational study found that **HIV-positive** (see page 94) men with the highest intakes of thiamin and other B vitamins had significantly longer survival rates, while a similar study found that those taking the most B_1 or niacin had a significantly lower rate of developing AIDS.[4,5]

In addition, weak and contradictory evidence suggests that vitamin B_1 may be helpful for **Alzheimer's disease** (see page 5).[6–10] Vitamin B_1 has also been proposed as a treatment for epilepsy, **canker sores** (see page 40), and **fibromyalgia** (see page 80), but the evidence for these uses is too preliminary to cite.

WHAT IS THE SCIENTIFIC EVIDENCE FOR VITAMIN B_1?

Congestive Heart Failure

Evidence suggests that individuals with congestive heart failure are commonly deficient in vitamin B_1, due to their use of loop diuretics.[11] A small double-blind study found that intravenous administration of thiamin could improve heart function in individuals with CHF.[12] Similar results were seen in an earlier uncontrolled study.[13]

SAFETY ISSUES

Vitamin B_1 appears to be quite safe even when taken in very high doses.

⚠ INTERACTIONS YOU SHOULD KNOW ABOUT

If you are taking **loop diuretics** (e.g., **furosemide [Lasix]**), you may need extra vitamin B_1.

Vitamin B_1

VITAMIN B₂

Supplement Forms/Alternate Names   Riboflavin, Riboflavin-5-Phosphate

Principal Proposed Uses   There are no well-documented uses for vitamin B₂.

Other Proposed Uses   Migraine Headaches, Cataracts, Sickle-Cell Anemia, HIV Support, Performance Enhancement

Vitamin B₂

Visit Us at TNP.com

Riboflavin, also known as vitamin B₂, is an essential nutrient required for life. This vitamin works with two enzymes critical to the body's production of adenosine triphosphate, or ATP, its main energy source. Vitamin B₂ is also used to process amino acids and fats, and to activate vitamin B₆ and folate.

Preliminary evidence suggests that riboflavin supplements may offer benefits for two illnesses: migraine headaches and cataracts.

REQUIREMENTS/SOURCES

The official U.S. and Canadian recommendations for daily intake of riboflavin are as follows:

- Infants 0–5 months, 0.3 mg
    - 6–11 months, 0.4 mg
- Children 1–3 years, 0.5 mg
    - 4–8 years, 0.6 mg
    - 9–13 years, 0.9 mg
- Males 14 years and older, 1.3 mg
- Females, 14–18 years, 1.0 mg
    - 19 years and older, 1.1 mg
- Pregnant women, 1.4 mg
- Nursing women, 1.6 mg

Riboflavin is found in organ meats (such as liver, kidney, and heart) and in many vegetables, nuts, legumes, and leafy greens. The richest sources are torula (nutritional) yeast, brewer's yeast, and calf liver. Almonds, wheat germ, wild rice, and mushrooms are good sources as well.

Although serious riboflavin deficiencies are rare, slightly low levels can occur in children, the elderly, and those in poverty.[1–4] In addition, use of oral contraceptives may reduce levels of riboflavin.[5,6,7]

THERAPEUTIC DOSAGES

For migraine headaches, the typical recommended dosage of riboflavin is much higher than nutritional needs: 400 mg daily. For cataract prevention, riboflavin may be taken at the nutritional dosages described. Since the B vitamins tend to work together, many nutritional experts recommend taking B₂ with other B vitamins, perhaps in the form of a B-complex supplement.

THERAPEUTIC USES

There are no well-documented uses of riboflavin. However, preliminary evidence suggests that riboflavin supplements taken at high dosages may reduce the frequency of **migraine headaches** (see page 120).[8]

One very large study suggests that riboflavin at nutritional doses may be helpful for **cataracts** (see page 42), but in this study it was combined with another B vitamin, niacin or **vitamin B₃** (see page 437), so it's hard to say which vitamin was responsible for the effect.[9]

Riboflavin has also been proposed as a treatment for sickle-cell anemia,[10] **HIV** (see page 94) infection,[11] and as a **performance enhancer** (see page 158) for athletes, but there is no real evidence that it is effective for these uses.

WHAT IS THE SCIENTIFIC EVIDENCE FOR VITAMIN B₂?

Migraine Headaches

According to a 3-month double-blind placebo-controlled study of 55 people with migraines, riboflavin can significantly reduce the frequency and duration of migraine attacks.[12] This study found that, when given at least 2 months to work, a daily dose of riboflavin (400 mg) can produce dramatic migraine relief. The majority of the participants experienced a greater than 50% decrease in the number of migraine attacks as well as the total days with headache pain. A larger and longer study is needed to follow up on these results.

Cataracts

Riboflavin supplements may help prevent cataracts, but the evidence isn't yet clear. In a large, double-blind placebo-controlled study, 3,249 people were given either placebo or one of four nutrient combinations (vitamin A/zinc, riboflavin/niacin, vitamin C/molybdenum, or selenium/beta-carotene/ vitamin E) for a period of 6 years.[13] Those receiving the niacin/riboflavin supplement showed a significant (44%) reduction in the incidence of cataracts. Strangely, there was a small, but statistically significantly *higher* incidence of a special type of cataract (called a subcapsular cataract) in the niacin/riboflavin group. However, it is unclear whether the effects seen in this group were due to niacin, riboflavin, or the combination of the two.

SAFETY ISSUES

Riboflavin seems to be an extremely safe supplement.

⚠ INTERACTIONS YOU SHOULD KNOW ABOUT

If you are taking **oral contraceptives,** you may need extra riboflavin.

VITAMIN B₃

Supplement Forms/Alternate Names   Niacin, Niacinamide, Nicotinamide, Inositol Hexaniacinate

Principal Proposed Uses   High Cholesterol/Triglycerides (Niacin), Diabetes Prevention and Treatment (Niacinamide), Intermittent Claudication (Inositol Hexaniacinate), Osteoarthritis (Niacinamide), Photosensitivity (Niacinamide), Raynaud's Phenomenon (Inositol Hexaniacinate)

Other Proposed Uses   Bursitis, Cataracts, HIV Support, Pregnancy Support, Tardive Dyskinesia

Vitamin B₃ is required for the proper function of more than 50 enzymes. Without it, your body would not be able to release energy or make fats from carbohydrates. Vitamin B₃ is also used to make sex hormones and other important chemical signal molecules.

Vitamin B₃ comes in two principal forms: niacin (nicotinic acid) and niacinamide (nicotinamide). When taken in low doses for nutritional purposes, they are essentially identical. However, each has its own particular effects when taken in high doses. High-dose niacin is principally used for lowering cholesterol. High-dose niacinamide may be helpful in preventing type 1 (childhood-onset) diabetes and reducing symptoms of osteoarthritis. However, there are concerns regarding liver inflammation when any form of niacin is taken at high dosages.

Additionally, good evidence suggests that a special form of niacin, *inositol hexaniacinate,* can improve walking distance in intermittent claudication. It may also reduce symptoms of Raynaud's phenomenon.

REQUIREMENTS/SOURCES

The official U.S. and Canadian recommendations for daily intake of niacin are as follows:

- Infants 0–5 months, 2 mg
    6–11 months, 3 mg
- Children 1–3 years, 6 mg
    4–8 years, 8 mg
    9–13 years, 12 mg
- Males 14 years and older, 16 mg
- Females 14 years and older, 14 mg
- Pregnant women, 18 mg
- Nursing women, 17 mg

Because the body can make niacin from the common amino acid tryptophan, niacin deficiencies are rare in developed countries. However, the antituberculosis drug isoniazid (INH) impairs the body's ability to produce niacin from tryptophan, and may create symptoms of niacin deficiency (see Interactions You Should Know About).[1,2]

Good food sources of niacin are seeds, yeast, bran, peanuts (especially with skins), wild rice, brown rice, whole wheat, barley, almonds, and peas. Tryptophan is found in protein foods (meat, poultry, dairy products, fish). Turkey and milk are particularly excellent sources of tryptophan.

THERAPEUTIC DOSAGES

When used as therapy for a specific disease, niacin, niacinamide, and inositol hexaniacinate are taken in dosages much higher than nutritional needs, about 1 to 4 g daily. Because of the risk of liver inflammation at these doses, medical supervision is essential.

For prevention of diabetes in children, the usual dosage of niacinamide is 25 mg per kilogram body weight per day. There are 2.2 pounds in a kilogram, so a 40-pound child would get about 450 mg daily.

Warning: Medical supervision is essential before giving your child long-term niacinamide treatment.

Many people experience an unpleasant flushing sensation and headache when they take niacin. These symptoms can usually be reduced by gradually increasing the dosage over several weeks or by using slow-release niacin. However, slow-release niacin appears to be more likely to cause liver inflammation than other forms. Inositol hexaniacinate may also cause less flushing than plain niacin, and if you take an aspirin along with niacin, the flushing reaction will usually decrease.

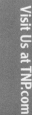

Vitamin B₃

Visit Us at TNP.com

THERAPEUTIC USES

There is no question that niacin (but not niacinamide) can significantly lower total **cholesterol** (see page 88) and LDL ("bad") cholesterol and raise HDL ("good") cholesterol.[3–8] However, unpleasant flushing reactions and the risk of liver inflammation have kept niacin from being widely used (see Safety Issues).

Intriguing evidence suggests that regular use of niacinamide (but not niacin) may help prevent **diabetes** (see page 65) in children at special risk of developing it.[9] Risk can be determined by measuring the ratio of antibodies to islet cells (ICA antibody test).

Niacinamide may improve blood sugar control in both children and adults who already have diabetes.[10,11]

According to several good-size double-blind studies, inositol hexaniacinate may be able to improve walking distance in **intermittent claudication** (severe leg cramps caused by hardening of the arteries; see page 106).[12] For other treatments that may help intermittent claudication, see the chapters on **carnitine** and **ginkgo**.

Preliminary evidence suggests that inositol hexaniacinate may be able to reduce symptoms of **Raynaud's phenomenon** (see page 149) as well.[13] This condition includes an extreme response to cold, usually most severely in the hands.

Preliminary evidence suggests that niacinamide may be able to reduce symptoms of **osteoarthritis** (see page 132).[14] Niacinamide may also reduce symptoms of polymorphous light eruption, a type of **photosensitivity** (see page 144).[15] Very weak evidence suggests one of the several forms of niacin may be helpful in bursitis,[16] **cataracts** (see page 42),[17] **HIV** (see page 94) infection,[18,19] pregnancy,[20] and **tardive dyskinesia** (see page 176).[21]

WHAT IS THE SCIENTIFIC EVIDENCE FOR VITAMIN B₃?

Niacin is one of the best researched of all the vitamins, and the evidence for using it to treat at least one condition—high cholesterol—is strong enough that it has become an accepted mainstream treatment.

High Cholesterol/Triglycerides

Niacin has been used since the 1950s to lower harmful blood lipids (cholesterol, triglycerides, and lipoproteins) and to raise levels of HDL cholesterol. According to numerous studies, niacin can lower total cholesterol and LDL cholesterol by 15 to 25%, lower triglycerides by 2 to 50%, and raise HDL cholesterol by about 15 to 25%.[22–25] A double-blind study of 140 individuals found extended-release niacin (2,000 mg per day) increased levels of HDL cholesterol from baseline twice as much

as did the cholesterol-lowering drug gemfibrozil (1,200 mg per day).[26] Furthermore, long-term use of niacin has been shown to significantly reduce death rates from cardiovascular disease.[27]

Preventing Diabetes

Exciting evidence from a huge study conducted in New Zealand suggests that niacinamide can prevent high-risk children from developing diabetes.[28] In this study, more than 20,000 children were screened for diabetes risk by measuring ICA antibodies. It turned out that 185 of these children had detectable levels. About 170 of these children were then given niacinamide for 7 years (not all parents agreed to give their children niacinamide or stay in the study for that long). About 10,000 other children were not screened, but they were followed to see whether they developed diabetes.

The results were very impressive. In the group in which children were screened and given niacinamide if they were positive for ICA antibodies, the incidence of diabetes was reduced by as much as 60%.

These findings suggest that niacinamide is a very effective treatment for preventing diabetes. (It also shows that tests for ICA antibodies can very accurately identify children at risk for diabetes.)

At present, an enormous-scale, long-term trial called the European Nicotinamide Diabetes Intervention Trial is being conducted to definitively determine whether regular use of niacinamide can prevent diabetes. Results from the German portion of the study have been released, and they are not positive.[29] However, until the entire study is complete, it is not possible to draw conclusions.

Treating Diabetes

If your child has just developed diabetes, niacinamide may prolong what is called the honeymoon period.[30] This is the interval in which the pancreas can still make some insulin, and insulin needs are low. By giving your child niacinamide, you may be able to buy some time to allow him or her to adjust to a life of insulin injections.

A recent study suggests that niacinamide may also improve blood sugar control in type 2 (adult-onset) diabetes, but it did not use a double-blind design.[31]

Intermittent Claudication

Double-blind studies involving a total of about 400 individuals have found that inositol hexaniacinate can improve walking distance for people with intermittent claudication.[32–35] For example, in one study, 100 individuals were given either placebo or 4 g of inositol hexaniacinate daily. Over a period of 3 months, walking distance improved significantly in the treated group.[36]

Osteoarthritis

There is some evidence that niacinamide may provide some benefits for those with osteoarthritis. In a double-blind study, 72 individuals with arthritis were given either 3,000 mg daily of niacinamide (in 5 equal doses) or placebo for 12 weeks.[37] The results showed that treated participants experienced a 29% improvement in symptoms, whereas those given placebo worsened by 10%. However, at this dose, liver inflammation is a concern that must be taken seriously.

Raynaud's Phenomenon

According to one small double-blind study, the inositol hexaniacinate form of niacin may be helpful for Raynaud's phenomenon.[38] The dosage used was 4 g daily, again a dosage high enough for liver inflammation to be a real possibility.

SAFETY ISSUES

When taken at a dosage of more than 100 mg daily, niacin frequently causes annoying skin flushing, especially in the face. This reaction may be accompanied by stomach distress, itching, and headache. In studies, as many as 43% of individuals taking niacin quit because of unpleasant side effects.[39]

A more dangerous effect of niacin is liver inflammation. Although most commonly seen with slow-release niacin, it can occur with any type of niacin when taken at a daily dose of more than 500 mg (usually 3 g or more). Regular blood tests to evaluate liver function are therefore mandatory when using high-dose niacin (or niaci-namide or inositol hexaniacinate). This side effect almost always goes away when niacin is stopped.

If you have liver disease, ulcers (presently or in the past), or gout, or drink too much alcohol,[40] do not take high-dose niacin except on medical advice.

Although there have been concerns that high-dose niacin in combination with statin drugs could cause muscle damage and kidney injury, recent studies suggest the risk may be slight, especially in those with normal kidney function.[41,42] Nonetheless, a doctor's supervision is recommended before trying this combination.

Another potential drug interaction involves the anticonvulsant drugs carbamazepine and primidone. Niacinamide might increase blood levels of these drugs, possibly requiring reduction in drug dosage.[43] Do not use this combination except under physician supervision.

Maximum safe dosages for young children and pregnant or nursing women have not been established.

⚠ INTERACTIONS YOU SHOULD KNOW ABOUT

If you are taking

- Cholesterol-lowering drugs in the **statin** family, or if you drink **alcohol** excessively: Do not take niacin except under physician supervision.
- The antituberculosis drug **isoniazid (INH):** You may need extra niacin.
- **Anticonvulsant drugs** such as **carbamazepine** or **primidone:** Do not take niacinamide except under physician supervision.

VITAMIN B₆

Supplement Forms/Alternate Names   Pyridoxine, Pyridoxine Hydrochloride, Pyridoxal-5-Phosphate

Principal Proposed Uses   Heart Disease Prevention, Morning Sickness in Pregnancy, PMS

Other Proposed Uses   MSG Sensitivity, Carpal Tunnel Syndrome, Diabetic Neuropathy, Kidney Stones, Depression, Asthma, HIV Support, Tardive Dyskinesia, Photosensitivity, Vertigo, Autism (B6 Combined with Magnesium), Seborrheic Dermatitis, Parkinson's Disease

Vitamin B₆ plays a major role in making proteins, hormones, and neurotransmitters (chemicals that carry signals between nerve cells). Because mild deficiency of vitamin B₆ is common, this is one vitamin that is probably worth taking as insurance.

There's good evidence that adequate intake of vitamin B₆ can help prevent heart disease and reduce the nausea of morning sickness. This vitamin is also widely recommended for premenstrual syndrome (PMS) and asthma, but there is little evidence that it is effective for either use. When combined with magnesium, vitamin B₆ may be helpful for autism.

Vitamin B₆

Visit Us at TNP.com

REQUIREMENTS/SOURCES

Vitamin B_6 requirements increase with age. The official U.S. and Canadian recommendations for daily intake are as follows:

- Infants 0–5 months, 0.1 mg
    6–11 months, 0.3 mg
- Children 1–3 years, 0.5 mg
    4–8 years, 0.6 mg
    9–13 years, 1.0 mg
- Males 14–50 years, 1.3 mg
    51 years and older, 1.7 mg
- Females 14–18 years, 1.2 mg
    19–50 years, 1.3 mg
    51 years and older, 1.5 mg
- Pregnant women, 1.9 mg
- Nursing women, 2.0 mg

Severe deficiencies of vitamin B_6 are rare, but mild deficiencies are extremely common. In a survey of 11,658 adults, 71% of men and 90% of women were found to have diets deficient in B_6.[1] Vitamin B_6 is the most commonly deficient water-soluble vitamin in the elderly,[2] and children, too, don't get enough.[3]

Dietary deficiency might be worsened by use of hydralazine (for high blood pressure),[4] penicillamine (used for rheumatoid arthritis and certain rare diseases),[5] theophylline (an older drug for asthma),[6–10] MAO inhibitors,[11] and the antituberculosis drug isoniazid (INH),[12–15] all of which are thought to interfere with B_6 to some degree. Good sources of B_6 include nutritional (torula) yeast, brewer's yeast, sunflower seeds, wheat germ, soybeans, walnuts, lentils, lima beans, buckwheat flour, bananas, and avocados.

THERAPEUTIC DOSAGES

When used therapeutically, B_6 is commonly recommended at a daily dose of 10 to 300 mg daily, much higher than the basic nutritional requirement. However, it's probably not wise to take more than 50 mg daily, except on a physician's advice (see Safety Issues).

Since the B vitamins tend to work together, many nutritional experts recommend taking B_6 with other B vitamins, perhaps in the form of a B-complex supplement.

THERAPEUTIC USES

There is impressive evidence that an intake of vitamin B_6 somewhat above the recommended daily intake levels (4.6 mg or more daily) can significantly reduce the risk of **heart disease** (see page 16).[16]

A large double-blind study suggests that a higher dose (30 mg daily) of vitamin B_6 can reduce the **nausea** (see page 126) of morning sickness.[17] (For another approach, see the chapter on **ginger**.)

Other common uses of B_6 are not very well established. For example, vitamin B_6 is widely recommended by conventional physicians as a treatment for **carpal tunnel syndrome** (see page 41). However, there is little to no evidence that it actually works.[18–21] Similarly, although B_6 is frequently suggested as a treatment for **PMS** (premenstrual syndrome; see page 145), there is some fairly good evidence that it doesn't work for this purpose.[22]

Some natural medicine authorities state that vitamin B_6 is a useful treatment for diabetic neuropathy. This idea is based on the fact that B_6 deficiency can cause neuropathy, and people with diabetes may be low in B_6. However, there is clinical evidence that B_6 supplements do *not* help diabetic neuropathy.[23,24,25]

Vitamin B_6 might help prevent calcium oxalate,[26] and a small uncontrolled study found that supplementation decreased oxalate excretion in people with a history of **kidney stones** (see page 109),[27,28] although not all studies agree.[29]

Very weak evidence suggests that B_6 may be helpful for **depression** (see page 59),[30] allergy to monosodium glutamate (MSG, a highly allergenic food additive used to enhance flavor), **asthma** (see page 14),[31,32] diabetes caused by pregnancy (gestational diabetes),[33] **HIV** (see page 94) infection,[34,35] **tardive dyskinesia** (see page 176),[36,37,38] **photosensitivity** (see page 144),[39] and **vertigo** (see page 188).[40] Vitamin B_6 also might help reduce nervous system side effects such as hand tremors associated with the use of the asthma drug theophylline.[41,42,43]

An interesting series of studies suggests (but certainly doesn't prove) that the combination of vitamin B_6 and magnesium can be helpful in **autism** (see page 23).[44–54] Finally, one preliminary study suggests topical vitamin B_6 may help with the skin disease **seborrheic dermatitis** (see page 154).[55]

Vitamin B_6 is sometimes suggested as a treatment for **Parkinson's disease** (see page 140); however, no real evidence as yet supports this use.

WHAT IS THE SCIENTIFIC EVIDENCE FOR VITAMIN B_6?

Prevention of Atherosclerosis/Heart Disease

According to data gathered in the Nurses' Health Study, one of the largest long-term medical studies ever performed, vitamin B_6 supplements can significantly reduce a woman's risk of developing heart disease.[56] A total of 80,000 women with no history of heart disease were studied for possible links between vitamin B_6, folate, and the development of heart disease. The results showed that increased intake of B_6 could significantly reduce the risk of heart disease. Folate was also effective. (For more information, see the chapter on **folate**.)

Vitamin B_6 reduces blood levels of *homocysteine,* a chemical that has been linked to hardening of the arteries and heart disease. At first, it was assumed that the benefits of vitamin B_6 were all due to reducing homocysteine. However, a subsequent study found *no* association between high homocysteine levels and the risk of heart disease.[57] Instead, researchers found a connection between heart disease and low levels of vitamin B_6. People with the highest vitamin B_6 levels were 28% less likely to develop heart disease than those with the lowest B_6 levels. This study has led to the hypothesis that it is vitamin B_6 itself that reduces heart disease risk, and the reduction of homocysteine seen at the same time is simply incidental. However, the matter remains controversial.

Vitamin B_6 may help the heart in several ways. Preliminary studies suggest that it can reduce the tendency of platelets in the blood to form clots,[58] and also lower blood pressure to some extent.[59]

Morning Sickness (Nausea and Vomiting in Pregnancy)

Vitamin B_6 supplements have been used for years by conventional physicians as a treatment for morning sickness. In 1995, a large double-blind study validated this use.[60] A total of 342 pregnant women were given placebo or 30 mg of vitamin B_6 daily. Subjects then graded their symptoms by noting the severity of their nausea and recording the number of vomiting episodes. The women in the B_6 group experienced significantly less nausea than those in the placebo group, suggesting that regular use of B_6 can be helpful for morning sickness. However, vomiting episodes were not significantly reduced.

Premenstrual Syndrome (PMS)

More than a dozen double-blind studies investigated the effectiveness of vitamin B_6 for premenstrual syndrome (PMS). Many of these studies reported positive results, but a careful review of the literature found serious flaws in nearly all of them, so the results can't be taken as reliable.[61]

A recent properly designed double-blind trial of 120 women found *no* benefit.[62] In this study, three prescription drugs were compared against vitamin B_6 (pyridoxine, at 300 mg daily) and placebo. All study participants received 3 months of treatment and 3 months of placebo. Vitamin B_6 proved to be no better than placebo.

However, preliminary evidence suggests that the combination of **magnesium** (see page 351) and B_6 might be more effective than either treatment alone.[63]

Autism

Six double-blind placebo-controlled trials enrolling a total of about 150 children have evaluated the effects of vitamin B_6 and magnesium combination therapy for autism.[64–69] All of these studies found a significant improvement in autistic behaviors. However, the study design used in many of these trials was rather complicated and difficult to evaluate. For example, the largest trial (actually, a series of four closely intertwined trials) involved multiple groups of participants taking different treatments with inadequate time in between for the vitamins and minerals to wash out.[70] These studies were marked by other flaws as well; in addition, they were all performed by one research group.

For these reasons, until better-designed trials reported by independent laboratories are published, this therapy cannot be considered proven.

Asthma

A double-blind study of 76 children with asthma found significant benefit from vitamin B_6 after the second month of usage.[71] Children in the vitamin B_6 group were able to reduce their doses of asthma medication (bronchodilators and steroids). However, a recent double-blind study of 31 adults who used either inhaled or oral steroids did *not* show any benefit.[72] The dosages of B_6 used in these studies were quite high, in the range of 200 to 300 mg daily. Because of the risk of nerve injury, it is not advisable to take this much B_6 without medical supervision (see Safety Issues).

SAFETY ISSUES

Vitamin B_6 appears to be completely safe for adults at dosages up to 50 mg daily. However, at higher dosages (especially above 2 g daily) there is a very real risk of nerve damage. Nerve-related symptoms have even been reported at doses as low as 200 mg.[73] (This is a bit ironic, given that B_6 deficiency *also* causes nerve problems.) In some cases, very high doses of vitamin B_6 can cause or worsen acne symptoms.[74,75]

In addition, doses of vitamin B_6 over 5 mg may interfere with the effects of the drug levodopa when it is taken alone.[76,77,78] However, levodopa/carbidopa combinations are immune to this effect.

Maximum safe dosages for children, pregnant or nursing women, or those with severe liver or kidney disease have not been established.

⚠ INTERACTIONS YOU SHOULD KNOW ABOUT

If you are taking

Vitamin B_6

Visit Us at TNP.com

- **Isoniazid (INH), penicillamine, hydralazine, theophylline,** or **MAO inhibitors:** You may need extra vitamin B_6, but take only nutritional doses. Higher doses of B_6 might interfere with the action of the drug.

- **Levodopa** (for Parkinson's disease): Do not take more than 5 mg of vitamin B_6 daily except on medical advice.

VITAMIN B_{12}

Supplement Forms/Alternate Names   Methylcobalamin, Cyanocobalamin, Hydrocobalamin, Cobalamin

Principal Proposed Uses   Pernicious Anemia, Correcting Absorption Problems Caused by Medications

Other Proposed Uses   Male Infertility, Asthma, HIV Support, Amyotrophic Lateral Sclerosis (Lou Gehrig's Disease), Diabetic Neuropathy, Multiple Sclerosis, Restless Legs Syndrome, Tinnitus, Alzheimer's Disease, Vitiligo, Depression, Osteoporosis, Periodontal Disease

Vitamin B_{12}, an essential nutrient, is also known as cobalamin. The "cobal" in the name refers to the metal cobalt contained in B_{12}. Vitamin B_{12} is required for the normal activity of nerve cells, and works with folate and vitamin B_6 to lower blood levels of *homocysteine*, a chemical in the blood that is thought to contribute to heart disease. (For more information about homocysteine and heart disease, see the chapters on **folate** and **vitamin B_6**.) B_{12} also plays a role in the body's manufacture of S-adenosylmethionine, or SAMe (see the chapter on **SAMe**).

Anemia is usually the first sign of B_{12} deficiency. Earlier in this century, doctors coined the name "pernicious anemia" for a stubborn anemia that didn't improve even when the patient was given iron supplements. Today we know that pernicious anemia is usually caused by a condition in which the stomach fails to excrete a special substance called intrinsic factor. The body needs the intrinsic factor for efficient absorption of vitamin B_{12}. In 1948, vitamin B_{12} was identified as the cure for pernicious anemia.

More recent evidence suggests that B_{12} supplements may improve sperm count and mobility, possibly enhancing fertility. Vitamin B_{12} has also been proposed as a treatment for numerous other conditions, but as yet there is no definitive evidence that it is effective.

REQUIREMENTS/SOURCES

Extraordinarily small amounts of vitamin B_{12} suffice for daily nutritional needs. The official U.S. and Canadian recommendations for daily intake are as follows:

- Infants 0–5 months, 0.4 mcg
  6–11 months, 0.5 mcg

- Children 1–3 years, 0.9 mcg
  4–8 years, 1.2 mcg
  9–13 years, 1.8 mcg
- Males and females 14 years and older, 2.4 mcg
- Pregnant women, 2.6 mcg
- Nursing women, 2.8 mcg

Vitamin B_{12} deficiency is rare in the young, but it's not unusual in older people: Probably 10 to 20% of the elderly are deficient in B_{12}.[1–4] This may be because older people have lower levels of stomach acid. The vitamin B_{12} in our food comes attached to proteins, and must be released by acid in the stomach in order to be absorbed. When stomach acid levels are low, we don't absorb as much vitamin B_{12} from our food. Fortunately, vitamin B_{12} supplements don't need acid for absorption. For this reason, people who take medications that greatly reduce stomach acid, such as Prilosec (omeprazole) or Zantac (ranitidine), should probably also take B_{12} supplements.[5–10]

Stomach surgery and other conditions affecting the digestive tract can also lead to B_{12} deficiency. Vitamin B_{12} absorption is also impaired by colchicine (for gout), metformin and phenformin (for diabetes), AZT (for AIDS), and nitrous oxide.[11–14]

Slow-release **potassium** (see page 390) supplements can also impair B_{12} absorption.[15]

Severe B_{12} deficiency can cause anemia and, potentially, nerve damage. The latter may become permanent if the deficiency is not corrected in time. Anemia usually develops first, leading to treatment before permanent nerve damage develops. However, folate supplements can get in the way of this "early warning system." This is why people are cautioned against taking high doses of folate without medical supervision. When taken at a dosage higher than 400 mcg daily, folate can prevent anemia caused by B_{12} deficiency, thereby allowing permanent nerve damage to develop without any warning. Therefore, you should not take folate at high dosages without first getting a blood test to evaluate your B_{12} levels.

Vitamin B_{12} is found in most animal foods. Beef, liver, clams, and lamb provide a whopping 80 to 100 mcg of B_{12} per 3.5-ounce serving, at least 40 times the dietary requirement. Sardines, chicken liver, beef kidney, and calf liver are also good sources, providing between 25 and 60 mcg per serving. Trout, salmon, tuna, eggs, whey, and many cheeses provide at least the recommended daily intake. Nondairy, or total, vegetarians can eventually become B_{12}-deficient, unless they take B_{12} supplements or eat B_{12}-enriched yeast.

Vitamin B_{12} is available in three forms: cyanocobalamin, hydrocobalamin, and methylcobalamin. The first is the most widely available and least expensive, but some experts think that the other two forms are preferable.

THERAPEUTIC DOSAGES

For correcting absorption problems caused by medications, taking vitamin B_{12} at the level of dietary requirements should suffice.

For other purposes, enormously higher daily doses—ranging from 100 to 2,000 mcg—are sometimes recommended.

Because the B vitamins tend to work together, many nutritional experts recommend taking B_{12} with other B vitamins in the form of a B-complex supplement.

THERAPEUTIC USES

It appears that individuals who take medications that dramatically lower stomach acid would profit by taking B_{12} supplements.[16–21]

For pernicious anemia, B_{12} injections are traditionally used but research has shown that oral B_{12} works just as well, provided you take enough of it (between 300 and 1,000 mcg daily).[22–25]

Preliminary evidence suggests that B_{12} supplements may improve sperm activity and sperm count and perhaps treat **male infertility** (see page 116).[26,27]

Vitamin B_{12} is widely recommended as a treatment for **asthma** (see page 14),[28] but there is little real evidence that it is effective. On the basis of weak and sometimes contradictory evidence, vitamin B_{12} has been suggested for **HIV** (see page 94),[29–33] **amyotrophic lateral sclerosis** (see page 9),[34] diabetic neuropathy,[35,36] **multiple sclerosis** (MS; see page 124),[37–41] **restless legs syndrome** (see page 150),[42,43] and **tinnitus** (see page 178).[44]

Although vitamin B_{12} has been proposed as a treatment for **Alzheimer's disease** (see page 5), this recommendation is based solely on the results of one small, poorly designed study.[45] More recent and better-designed studies found little to no benefit.[46,47]

Some evidence suggests that people with **vitiligo** (splotchy loss of skin pigmentation; see page 191) might be deficient in vitamin B_{12} and supplementation along with folate may be helpful.[48,49] However, the evidence is very weak and not all studies agree.[50] Vitamin B_{12} is also sometimes recommended for numerous other problems, including **depression** (see page 59), **osteoporosis** (see page 136), and **periodontal disease** (see page 142), but there is little to no evidence as yet that it really works.

WHAT IS THE SCIENTIFIC EVIDENCE FOR VITAMIN B_{12}?

Male Infertility

Vitamin B_{12} deficiencies in men can lead to reduced sperm counts and lowered sperm mobility. For this reason, B_{12} supplements have been tried for improving fertility in men with abnormal sperm production. In one double-blind study of 375 infertile men, supplementation with vitamin B_{12} produced no benefits on average in the group as a whole.[51] However, in a particular subgroup of men with sufficiently low sperm count and sperm motility, B_{12} appeared to be helpful. Such "dredging" of the data is suspect from a scientific point of view, however, and this study cannot be taken as proof of effectiveness.

SAFETY ISSUES

Vitamin B_{12} appears to be extremely safe. However, in some cases very high doses of vitamin B_{12} can cause or worsen acne symptoms.[52,53]

⚠ INTERACTIONS YOU SHOULD KNOW ABOUT

If you are taking

- Medications that reduce stomach acid such as **H₂ blockers** (e.g., **Zantac [ranitidine]**) and **proton pump inhibitors** (e.g., **Prilosec [omeprazole]**), **colchicine, metformin** and **phenformin, AZT,** or if you are exposed to **nitrous oxide** anesthesia: You may need extra B_{12}.
- **Potassium:** You may need extra B_{12}.

VITAMIN C

Supplement Forms/Alternate Names   Ascorbic Acid, Ascorbate

Principal Proposed Uses   Colds, Post-Exercise Colds, Cataracts, Macular Degeneration

Other Proposed Uses   Preeclampsia Prevention, RSD Prevention, Easy Bruising, Asthma, Hypertension, Muscle Soreness, Bedsores, Low Sperm Count, Autism, Minor Injuries, Sunburn Prevention, Photosensitivity, Acute Anterior Uveitis, Gallbladder Disease Prevention, Vascular Dementia Prevention, Bipolar Disorder, Bladder Infection, Diabetes, Hepatitis, Herpes, Insomnia, Menopausal Symptoms, Migraine Headaches, Nausea, Parkinson's Disease, Periodontal Disease, Restless Legs Syndrome, Rheumatoid Arthritis, Ulcers, Allergies, Cancer Prevention, Cancer Treatment, HIV Support, Heart Disease Prevention, Osteoarthritis, General Antioxidant

Although most animals can make vitamin C from scratch, humans have lost the ability over the course of evolution. We must get it from food, chiefly fresh fruits and vegetables. One of this vitamin's main functions is helping the body manufacture collagen, a key protein in our connective tissues, cartilage, and tendons.

From ancient times through the early nineteenth century, sailors and others deprived of fresh fruits and vegetables developed a disease called *scurvy*. Scurvy involves so-called scorbutic symptoms, which include non-healing wounds, bleeding gums, bruising, and overall weakness. Now we know that scurvy is nothing more than vitamin C deficiency.

Scurvy was successfully treated with citrus fruit during the mid-1700s. In 1928, when Albert Szent-Gyorgyi isolated the active ingredient, he called it the "anti-scorbutic principle," or ascorbic acid. This, of course, is vitamin C.

Vitamin C is a powerful antioxidant that protects against damaging natural substances called free radicals. It works in water, both inside and outside of cells. Vitamin C complements another antioxidant vitamin, **vitamin E** (see page 451), which works in lipid (fatty) parts of the body.

Vitamin C is the single most popular vitamin supplement in the United States, and perhaps the most controversial as well. In the 1960s, two-time Nobel Prize winner Dr. Linus Pauling claimed that vitamin C could effectively treat both cancer and the common cold. Research has been mixed on both counts, but that hasn't dampened enthusiasm for this essential nutrient. The vitamin C movement has led to hundreds of clinical studies testing the vitamin on dozens of illnesses.

REQUIREMENTS/SOURCES

Vitamin C is an essential nutrient that must be obtained from food or supplements—the body cannot manufacture it. The official U.S. and Canadian recommendations for daily intake are as follows:

- Infants 0–6 months, 40 mg
    7–12 months, 50 mg
- Children 1–3 years, 15 mg
    4–8 years, 25 mg
    9–13 years, 45 mg
- Males 14–18 years, 75 mg
    19 years and older, 90 mg
- Females 14–18 years, 65 mg
    19 years and older, 75 mg
- Pregnant women 85 mg (80 mg if under 19 years old)
- Nursing women 120 mg (115 mg if under 19 years old)

Note: Smoking significantly reduces levels of vitamin C in the body.[1] The recommended daily intake for smokers is 35 mg higher across all age groups.

Scurvy, the classic vitamin C deficiency disease, is now a rarity in the developed world, although a more subtle deficiency of vitamin C is fairly common.[2–6] According to one study, 40% of Americans do not get enough vitamin C.[7] Also, aspirin and possibly other anti-inflammatory drugs might lower body levels of vitamin C.[8,9,10] Finally, oral contraceptives might decrease blood levels of vitamin C.[11–15] Supplementation may be helpful if you are taking any of these medications.

Most of us think of orange juice as the quintessential source of vitamin C, but many vegetables are actually even richer sources. Red chili peppers, sweet peppers, kale, parsley, collard, and turnip greens are excellent sources, as are broccoli, brussels sprouts, watercress, cauliflower, cabbage, and strawberries. (Oranges and other citrus fruits are good sources, too.)

One great advantage of getting vitamin C from foods rather than from supplements is that you will get many other healthy nutrients at the same time, such as bioflavonoids and carotenes. However, vitamin C in food is partially destroyed by cooking and exposure to air, so for maximum nutritional benefit you might want to try freshly made salads rather than dishes that require a lot of cooking.

Vitamin C

Visit Us at TNP.com

Vitamin C supplements are available in two forms: ascorbic acid and ascorbate. The latter is less intensely sour.

THERAPEUTIC DOSAGES

Ever since Linus Pauling, proponents have recommended taking vitamin C in enormous doses, as high as 20,000 to 30,000 mg daily. However, some evidence suggests that there might not be any reason to take more than 200 mg of vitamin C daily (10 to 100 times less than the amount recommended by vitamin C proponents).[16] The reason is that if you consume more than 200 mg daily (researchers have tested up to 2,500 mg) your kidneys begin to excrete the excess at a steadily increasing rate, matching the increased dose. Your digestive tract also stops absorbing it well. The net effect is that no matter how much you take, your blood levels of vitamin C don't increase.

However, there are some flaws in this research. It is possible that vitamin C levels might rise in other tissues even if they remain constant in the blood. Furthermore, this study did not take into account the effects of taking vitamin C several times daily.

Many nutritional experts recommend a total of 500 mg of vitamin C daily. This dose is almost undoubtedly safe. Others recommend that you take as much vitamin C as you can, up to 30,000 mg daily, cutting back only when you start to develop stomach cramps and diarrhea. This recommendation is not so much based on any evidence that such huge doses of vitamin C are good for you, but primarily on a semireligious enthusiasm.

THERAPEUTIC USES

According to numerous double-blind studies, vitamin C supplements can reduce symptoms of **colds** (see page 47) and shorten the length of the illness.[17,18] In addition, vitamin C might help prevent post race colds in endurance athletes.[19,20]

A sizable double-blind study suggests that the use of vitamin C and vitamin E supplements can reduce the risk of developing preeclampsia, a complication of pregnancy.[21]

Observational studies (studies in which researchers observe the participants to try to identify lifestyle factors associated with better health) tell us that people who regularly use vitamin C supplements are less likely to develop either of two eye problems, **cataracts** (see page 42) and **macular degeneration** (see page 115).[22–27]

One double-blind study suggests that vitamin C at a dose of 500 mg daily may help prevent reflex sympathetic dystrophy (RSD), a little-understood condition that can follow injuries such as fractures.[28]

Another double-blind trial found that vitamin C supplements can decrease the tendency to **bruise** (see page 74) in individuals with marginal deficiency of the vitamin.[29]

Many studies have tried to evaluate whether vitamin C supplements can help **asthma** (see page 14), with mixed results.[30] The same may be said of using vitamin C to treat **hypertension** (see page 98).[31–36]

One double-blind trial compared vitamin C, vitamin E, and placebo for muscle soreness in 24 male volunteers.[37] Vitamin C was found to relieve muscle soreness, while vitamin E did not. However, larger trials are needed to resolve whether or not vitamin C is effective in preventing muscle soreness. (See the full chapter on **sports performance** for more information.)

Small double-blind studies suggest that vitamin C may be able to speed recovery from bedsores.[38] Vitamin C may improve sperm count and function;[39] however, a recent double-blind study of 31 individuals found no benefit.[40]

A 10-week double-blind placebo-controlled study of 18 **autistic** (see page 23) children found some evidence that vitamin C might be helpful for improving behavior.[41]

Preliminary evidence from a somewhat poorly reported double-blind trial of 40 college football players suggests that a combination of vitamin C and citrus bioflavonoids taken before practice can reduce the severity of athletic **injuries** (see page 101).[42]

Studies on laboratory animals found that topical vitamin C and vitamin E, alone or together, helped prevent burning on exposure to ultraviolet light.[43–46] One double-blind study of 10 people found that 2 g of vitamin C and 1,000 IU of vitamin E taken for 8 days resulted in a modest decrease of "sunburn" induced by ultraviolet light.[47] A 50-day placebo-controlled study of 40 people found that higher doses of these vitamins provided a sun-protection factor of about 2.[48] (Compare this to the sun protection factor of 15 or higher in many sunscreens.) However, so far, research hasn't found that these vitamins, taken separately, are any more helpful than placebo.[49,50] In addition, preliminary evidence from a small double-blind placebo-controlled trial suggests that a face cream containing vitamin C could improve the appearance of sun-damaged skin.[51]

There is also evidence that vitamin C in combination with vitamin E (and the standard drug treatment) may be helpful for acute anterior uveitis. This condition involves painful inflammation of the iris of the eye, with acute sensitivity to light, increased ocular pressure, and a loss of visual clarity; it most often occurs in conjunction with autoimmune diseases. While acute anterior uveitis usually responds to conventional treatment after 10 to 14 days, vision problems may persist. In one study, the use

Vitamin C

Visit Us at TNP.com

Vitamin C

of vitamin C at a dose of 500 mg twice daily and vitamin E (alpha-tocopherol) at 100 mg twice daily improved vision after 8 weeks as compared to placebo.[52] **Note:** Acute anterior uveitis is a potentially dangerous condition. Physician supervision is mandatory.

Weak evidence suggests that vitamin C supplements may reduce the risk of **gallbladder disease** (see page 83) in women[53] and help prevent **vascular dementia** (see page 5) but not Alzheimer's disease.[54]

A small double-blind placebo-controlled study including 20 **smokers** (see page 131) suggests that vitamin C supplements may improve arterial function, but the effects aren't long-lasting.[55]

In addition, vitamin C supplements have been recommended for **bipolar disorder** (see page 27), **bladder infections** (see page 28), **diabetes** (see page 65), **hepatitis** (see page 189), **herpes** (see page 86), **insomnia** (see page 103), **menopausal symptoms** (see page 117), **migraine headaches** (see page 120), **nausea** (see page 126), **Parkinson's disease** (see page 140), **periodontal disease** (see page 142), **restless legs syndrome** (see page 150), **rheumatoid arthritis** (see page 151), and **ulcers** (see page 180), but there is no solid scientific basis for any of these uses.

Vitamin C is often suggested as a treatment for **allergies** (see page 2), but the research results are very preliminary and somewhat contradictory.[56,57,58]

Dietary vitamin C appears to reduce the risk of **cancer** (see page 32) and **heart disease** (see page 16) and slow the progression of **osteoarthritis** (see page 132).[59,60] However, there is little evidence that vitamin C supplements provide the same benefits. As noted earlier, foods containing vitamin C also contain many other healthful ingredients (such as bioflavonoids and carotenes), so it's not clear that pills containing vitamin C alone work just as well.

Vitamin C has been proposed as a treatment for cancer, but this claim is very controversial, and there is as yet no scientifically meaningful evidence that it works.[61–64]

Massive doses of vitamin C have at times been popular among people with **HIV** (see page 94) infection based on highly preliminary evidence.[65,66] An observational study linked high doses of vitamin C with slower progression to AIDS.[67] However, a double-blind study of 49 people with HIV who took combined vitamins C and E or placebo for 3 months did not show any significant effects on the amount of HIV virus detected or the number of opportunistic infections.[68]

According to a double-blind placebo-controlled study of 141 women with **cervical dysplasia** (early cervical cancer; see page 43), vitamin C, taken at a dosage of 500 mg daily, does *not* help to reverse the dysplasia.[69]

Heated disagreement exists regarding whether it is safe or appropriate to combine vitamin C with standard chemotherapy drugs.[70,71] The reasoning behind this concern is that many chemotherapy drugs work in part by creating free radicals that destroy cancer cells. Antioxidants like vitamin C might interfere with this beneficial effect. Indeed, some cancer cells appear to accumulate vitamin C to protect themselves from injury! On the other hand, some evidence suggests that vitamin C may help reduce the side effects of certain chemotherapy drugs without decreasing their effectiveness.[72,73] Nonetheless, in view of the high stakes involved, we strongly recommend that you do not take any supplements while undergoing cancer chemotherapy except on the advice of a physician.

WHAT IS THE SCIENTIFIC EVIDENCE FOR VITAMIN C?

Colds

As the most famous of all natural treatments for colds, vitamin C has been subjected to irresponsible hype from both proponents and opponents. Enthusiasts claim that if you take vitamin C daily, you will never get sick, while critics of the treatment insist that vitamin C has no benefit at all.

However, a cool-headed evaluation of the research indicates something in between. Numerous studies have found that vitamin C supplements taken at a dose of 1,000 mg daily or more *can* significantly reduce symptoms of colds and help you get over a cold faster.[74,75,76] Benefits appear to be greater for children than for adults, and the exact amount of the benefit varies widely between studies.

In most of these studies, participants took vitamin C supplements on a daily basis throughout the period of the study.[77] However, a few studies evaluated the benefits of taking vitamin C only right at the onset of cold symptoms. This method, which is perhaps the most popular way of using vitamin C for colds, appears to be just as effective.

There is no real evidence that vitamin C supplements can prevent colds in general. However, there are two exceptions to this. One is the "post-marathon sniffle." Heavy endurance exercise temporarily weakens the immune system, leading to a high incidence of infection following marathons, triathlons, or similar forms of exercise. There is some evidence that vitamin C can prevent such colds[78,79] (see Post Exercise Colds below for more information). **Glutamine** (see page 310) might also be helpful for this purpose.

The other situation in which vitamin C may help prevent colds is when you are actually *deficient* in the vitamin. There is some evidence that making sure to get your dietary allowance might help keep you healthier.[80]

Post-Exercise Colds

According to a double-blind placebo-controlled study involving 92 runners, taking 600 mg of vitamin C for 21 days prior to a race made a significant difference in the incidence of sickness afterwards.[81] Within 2 weeks after the race, 68% of the runners taking placebo developed cold symptoms, versus only 33% of those taking the vitamin C supplement. As part of the same study, non-runners of similar age and gender to those running were also given vitamin C or placebo. Interestingly, for this group, the supplement had no apparent effect on the incidence of upper respiratory infections. Vitamin C seemed to be effective in this capacity only for those who exercised intensively!

Two other studies found that vitamin C could reduce the number of colds experienced by groups of people involved in rigorous exercise in extremely cold environments.[82] One study involved 139 children attending a skiing camp in the Swiss Alps, while the other enrolled 56 military men engaged in a training exercise in Northern Canada during the winter months. In both cases, the participants took either 1 g of vitamin C or placebo daily at the time their training program began. Cold symptoms were monitored for 1 to 2 weeks following training, and significant differences in favor of vitamin C were found.

However, one very large study of 674 marine recruits in basic training found no such benefit.[83] The results showed no difference in the number of colds between the treatment and placebo groups.

What's the explanation for this discrepancy? There are many possibilities. Perhaps basic training in the marines is significantly different from the other forms of exercise studied. Another point to consider is that the marines didn't start taking vitamin C right at the beginning of training, but waited 3 weeks. The study also lasted a bit longer than the positive studies mentioned above, continuing for 2 months; maybe vitamin C is more effective at preventing colds in the short term. Of course, another possibility is that it doesn't really work. More research is needed to know for sure.

Cataracts

Regular use of vitamin C may reduce the risk of cataracts, probably by fighting free radicals that damage the lens of the eye. In an observational study of 50,800 nurses followed for 8 years, it was found that people who used vitamin C supplements for more than 10 years had a 45% lower rate of cataract development.[84] Interestingly, diets high in vitamin C were *not* found to be protective—only supplemental vitamin C made a difference. This is the opposite of what has been found with vitamin C in the prevention of other diseases, such as cancer (see the section titled Cancer Prevention).

A more recent study of 247 women suggests that vitamin C supplements taken for more than 10 years reduce the incidence of cataracts by 77%.[85] In this study, no benefit was found for shorter-term vitamin C supplementation.

It has been suggested that vitamin C may be particularly useful against cataracts in people with diabetes, because of its influence on *sorbitol,* a sugar-like substance that tends to accumulate in the cells of diabetics. Excess sorbitol is believed to play a role in the development of diabetes-related cataracts, and vitamin C appears to help reduce sorbitol buildup.[86]

Macular Degeneration

After cataracts, injury to the macula (the most important part of the retina) is the second most common cause of vision loss in people 65 and older.

Observational studies involving a total of over 4,000 people suggest that regular use of vitamin C supplements may help prevent macular degeneration.[87,88] Vitamin C is thought to work by protecting the retina against damaging free radicals.

According to one study, a combination of many antioxidants including vitamin C might be able to halt macular degeneration that has already begun. In this 18-month double-blind trial, a daily supplement containing 750 mg of vitamin C, 200 IU of vitamin E, 50 mcg of selenium, and 20,000 IU of beta-carotene (along with other ingredients) actually stopped progression of macular degeneration.[89]

Warning: If you have macular degeneration, do not self-treat it without first seeing a physician. One particular type of macular degeneration must be treated with laser surgery.

Preeclampsia Prevention

Preeclampsia is a dangerous complication of pregnancy that involves high blood pressure, swelling of the whole body, and improper kidney function. A double-blind placebo-controlled study of 283 women at increased risk for preeclampsia found that supplementation with vitamin C (1,000 mg daily) and vitamin E (400 IU daily) significantly reduced the chances for developing this disease.[90]

While this research is promising, larger studies are necessary to confirm whether vitamins C and E will actually work. The authors of this study point out that similarly sized studies found benefits with other treatments, such as aspirin, that later proved to be ineffective when large-scale studies were performed. Furthermore, keep in mind that we don't know whether such high dosages of these vitamins are absolutely safe for pregnant women.

Cancer Prevention

While there is some evidence that dietary vitamin C from fruits and vegetables can reduce the risk of cancer, we don't know if vitamin C *supplements* are particularly helpful. This is a crucial distinction. When you get vitamin C from fruits and vegetables, you also receive myriad other substances such as bioflavonoids and carotenes

Vitamin C

Visit Us at TNP.com

that may provide health benefits. The studies involving vitamin C supplements and cancer prevention have not shown stellar results.

One study found that vitamin C supplementation at 500 mg or more daily was connected to a lower incidence of bladder cancer.[91] However, another study found *no* benefit.[92]

Supplemental vitamin C at 1,000 mg daily failed to prevent new colon cancers after one had developed.[93] In another large observational study, 500 mg or more of vitamin C daily over a period of 6 years provided *no* significant protection against breast cancer.[94] Another study found similar results.[95]

Cancer Treatment

Cancer treatment is one of the more controversial proposed uses of vitamin C. An early study tested vitamin C in 1,100 terminally ill cancer patients. One hundred patients received 10,000 mg daily of vitamin C, while 1,000 other patients (the control group) received no treatment. Those taking the vitamin survived more than 4 times longer on average (210 days) than those in the control group (50 days).[96] A large (1,826 subjects) follow-up study by the same researchers found a nearly doubled survival rate (343 days versus 180 days) in vitamin C–treated patients whose cancers were deemed "incurable," as compared to untreated controls.[97] However, these studies were poorly designed, and other generally better-constructed studies have found no benefit of vitamin C in cancer.[98,99] At the present time, vitamin C cannot be regarded as a proven treatment for cancer.

Heart Disease Prevention

As with cancer prevention, there is some evidence that eating vitamin C–rich foods can reduce your risk of heart disease. However, the evidence that vitamin C supplements taken by themselves are helpful for atherosclerosis is weak.[100,101,102] A combination of supplemental vitamins C and E may offer some heart-protective benefits, although the evidence for this comes only from observational studies.[103]

Reflex Sympathetic Dystrophy (RSD)

RSD is a set of symptoms that occasionally develops in the legs or arms after fractures and other injuries. The condition involves persistent pain, changes in skin temperature, redness, swelling, and difficulty in movement. Its cause is unknown, and it is very difficult, if not impossible, to treat, creating significant suffering and disability.

A double-blind study set out to find whether vitamin C could prevent RSD from developing in individuals who had sustained wrist fractures.[104] A total of 123 adults with wrist fractures were enrolled and followed for 1 year. All were given 500 mg of vitamin C or placebo daily for 50 days. The results showed significantly fewer cases of RSD in the treated group.

If these results hold up in larger studies, vitamin C treatment could become part of the standard treatment of fractures.

Easy Bruising

A 2-month double-blind study of 94 elderly people with marginal vitamin C deficiency found that vitamin C supplements decreased their tendency to bruise.[105]

Hypertension (High Blood Pressure)

According to a 30-day double-blind study of 39 individuals taking medications for hypertension, treatment with 500 mg of vitamin C daily can reduce blood pressure by about 10%.[106] Smaller benefits were seen in studies of individuals with normal blood pressure or borderline hypertension.[107,108]

However, in another study of 363 individuals given vitamin C (1,000 mg per day), vitamin E, beta-carotene, or placebo, no differences in blood pressure were seen among the groups.[109] Other studies have returned inconclusive results.[110,111]

The bottom line: Whether vitamin C truly affects blood pressure remains unclear.

SAFETY ISSUES

Vitamin C is indisputably safe at dosages up to 500 mg daily in adults, and is probably safe for most individuals at significantly higher doses. In recognition of this, the U.S. government has issued recommendations regarding "tolerable upper intake levels" (ULs) for vitamin C. The UL can be thought of as the highest daily intake over a prolonged time known to pose no risks to most members of a healthy population. The ULs for vitamin C are as follows:

- Children 1–3 years, 400 mg
    4–8 years, 650 mg
    9–13 years, 1,200 mg
- Males and females 14–18 years, 1,800 mg
    19 years and older, 2,000 mg
- Pregnant women 2,000 mg (1,800 mg if under 19 years old)
- Nursing women 2,000 mg (1,800 mg if under 19 years old)

However, the maximum safe dosages of vitamin C for those with severe liver or kidney disease have not been determined.

Even within the safe intake range for vitamin C, some individuals may develop diarrhea. This side effect will likely go away with continued use of vitamin C, but you might have to cut down your dosage for a while and then gradually build up again.

In addition, vitamin C supplements can cause **copper**[112–115] (see page 262) deficiency and excessive **iron**[116–123] (see page 333) absorption.

There is also reason for concern that long-term vitamin C treatment can cause **kidney stones** (see page 109).[124] However, in large-scale observational studies, individuals who consume large amounts of vitamin C have shown either no change or a decreased risk of kidney stone formation.[125,126,127] Still, there may be certain individuals who are particularly at risk for vitamin C–induced kidney stones.[128] People with a history of kidney stones and those with kidney failure who have a defect in vitamin C or oxalate metabolism should probably restrict vitamin C intake to approximately 100 mg daily. You should also avoid high-dose vitamin C if you have glucose-6-phosphate dehydrogenase deficiency, iron overload, or a history of intestinal surgery.

One study from the 1970s suggests that very high doses of vitamin C (3 g daily) might increase the levels of acetaminophen (e.g., Tylenol) in the body.[129] This could potentially put you at higher risk for acetaminophen toxicity. This interaction is probably relatively unimportant when acetaminophen is taken in single doses for pain and fever, or for a few days during a cold. However, if you use acetaminophen daily or have kidney or liver problems, simultaneous use of high-dose vitamin C is probably not advisable.

Finally, weak evidence suggests that vitamin C, when taken in high doses, might reduce the blood-thinning effects of Coumadin (warfarin) and heparin.[130–133]

⚠ INTERACTIONS YOU SHOULD KNOW ABOUT

If you are taking

- **Aspirin** other **anti-inflammatory drugs,** or **oral contraceptives:** You may need more vitamin C.
- **Acetaminophen (Tylenol):** The risk of liver damage from high doses of acetaminophen may be increased if you also take large doses of vitamin C.
- **Coumadin (warfarin)** or **heparin:** High-dose vitamin C might reduce their effectiveness.
- **Iron supplements:** High-dose vitamin C can cause you to absorb too much iron. This is especially a problem for people with diseases that cause them to store too much iron.
- High doses of **vitamin C:** Your ability to absorb copper may be impaired.

VITAMIN D

Supplement Forms/Alternate Names   Cholecalciferol (Vitamin D$_3$), Ergocalciferol (Vitamin D$_2$)

Principal Proposed Uses   Preventing and Treating Osteoporosis

Other Proposed Uses   Cancer Prevention, Polycystic Ovary Syndrome, Psoriasis

Vitamin D is both a vitamin and a hormone. It's a vitamin because your body cannot absorb calcium without it; it's a hormone because your body manufactures it in response to your skin's exposure to sunlight.

There are two major forms of vitamin D, and both have the word *calciferol* in their names. In Latin, calciferol means "calcium carrier." Vitamin D$_3$ (cholecalciferol) is made by the body and is found in some foods. Vitamin D$_2$ (ergocalciferol) is the form most often added to milk and other foods, and the form you're most likely to use as a supplement.

Strong evidence tells us that the combination of vitamin D and calcium supplements can be quite helpful for preventing and treating osteoporosis.

REQUIREMENTS/SOURCES

As with **vitamin A** (see page 432), dosages of vitamin D are often expressed in terms of international units (IU) rather than milligrams. The official U.S. and Canadian recommendations for daily intake of vitamin D are as follows:

- Infants 0–12 months, 200 IU (5 mcg) daily
- Males and females 1–50 years, 200 IU (5 mcg)
  - 51–70 years, 400 IU (10 mcg)
  - 71 years and older, 600 IU (15 mcg)
- Pregnant women, 200 IU (5 mcg)
- Nursing women, 200 IU (5 mcg)

A study of veiled Moslem women living in Denmark found that 600 IU of vitamin D daily was insufficient to raise vitamin D levels in the blood to normal levels.[1] The authors of this study recommend that sun-deprived individuals should receive 1,000 IU of vitamin D daily. Another researcher investigated the origin of current vitamin D recommendations and found them startlingly ungrounded in science.[2] He concluded that consideration be given to increasing current vitamin D intake recommendations by as much as a factor of 10. However, this idea has not been universally accepted, and other authorities feel that vitamin D toxicity is a real risk.[3]

There is very little vitamin D found naturally in the foods we eat (the best sources are coldwater fish). In many countries, vitamin D is added to milk and other foods like breakfast cereals and margarine, contributing to our daily intake.

By far the best source of vitamin D is sunlight. However, in view of current recommendations stressing sunblock and sun avoidance, we can't advise you to get your vitamin D this way. It is interesting to note that severe vitamin D deficiency was common in England in the 1800s due to coal smoke obscuring the sun. Cod liver oil, which is high in vitamin D, became popular as a supplement for children to help prevent rickets. (Rickets is a disease in which developing bones soften and curve because they aren't receiving enough calcium.) It is possible that recent emphasis on avoiding the sun will have some negative consequences. In addition, rickets has recently been observed among African American and Hispanic children with poor nutrition and little sunshine exposure.[4]

Vitamin D deficiency is known to occur in the elderly as well as in people who live in northern latitudes and don't drink vitamin D–enriched milk.[5,6,7] Women with significant osteoporosis are also often vitamin D deficient.[8] Additionally, phenytoin (Dilantin), primidone (Mysoline), and phenobarbital for seizures; corticosteroids; cimetidine (Tagamet) for ulcers; the blood-thinning drug heparin; and the antituberculosis drugs isoniazid (INH) and rifampin may interfere with vitamin D absorption or activity.[9–27]

THERAPEUTIC DOSAGES

For therapeutic purposes, vitamin D is taken at the nutritional doses described in Requirements/Sources (and sometimes in even higher amounts). If you wish to exceed nutritional levels of vitamin D intake, physician supervision is recommended (see Safety Issues).

THERAPEUTIC USES

Without question, if you are concerned about **osteoporosis** (see page 136), you should take **calcium** (see page 234) and vitamin D. The combination definitely helps prevent bone loss.[28,29] This is true even if you are taking estrogen or any other treatment for osteoporosis; after all, you can't build bone without calcium, and you can't properly absorb and utilize calcium without adequate intake of vitamin D. Other uses of vitamin D are less well documented. Some evidence suggests that vitamin D may help prevent **cancer** (see page 32) of the breast, colon, pancreas, and prostate, but the research on this question has yielded mixed results.[30–36]

One preliminary study suggests that supplementation with vitamin D and calcium may be helpful for women with polycystic ovary syndrome.[37]

Vitamin D is sometimes mentioned as a treatment for **psoriasis** (see page 148). However, this recommendation is based on Danish studies using calcipotriol, a variation of vitamin D_3 that is used externally (applied to the skin).[38] Calcipotriol does *not* affect your body's absorption of calcium, so it is a very different substance from the vitamin D you can purchase at a store.

WHAT IS THE SCIENTIFIC EVIDENCE FOR VITAMIN D?

Osteoporosis

Women with severe osteoporosis have low levels of vitamin D.[39] Supplementing with vitamin D alone may not be helpful,[40] but the combination of calcium and vitamin D can slow down or even reverse osteoporosis.

One double-blind study followed 249 women in Boston for 1 year; the location of this study is important because your body can't produce significant amounts of vitamin D from sunlight during the winter in Boston.[41] These were postmenopausal women with an average age of 61, none of whom were taking estrogen or other medications for bone loss. Half of the women received a calcium citrate malate supplement (400 mg daily) plus a vitamin D supplement (400 IU daily), while the other half received placebo. The women in this study who were taking the vitamin D and calcium experienced a net increase in spinal bone mass (0.85%), while the placebo group showed no net change—a significant difference.

Another double-blind placebo-controlled study enrolling 3,270 women (nearly all of whom had never been on estrogen-replacement therapy) found that higher dosages of vitamin D produced even better results. For a period of 1.5 years, participants received either placebo or 1,200 mg of calcium and 800 IU of vitamin D. At the end of the study period, the researchers found that the bone density in the hips of the women who had taken calcium and vitamin D had *increased* by 2.7%, while the hip bone density of the women who had taken placebo *decreased* by 4.6%. The calcium/vitamin D group also had 43% fewer hip fractures. A reduced fracture rate was also seen in another large, double-blind placebo-controlled study.[42]

There is also some good evidence that the use of calcium combined with vitamin D can help protect against the bone loss caused by corticosteroid drugs (such as prednisone). In a 2-year double-blind placebo-controlled study of 130 individuals, supplementation with 1,000 mg of calcium and 500 IU of vitamin D daily actually reversed steroid-induced bone loss, causing a net bone gain.[43]

SAFETY ISSUES

When taken at recommended dosages, vitamin D appears to be safe. However, when used at considerable excess, vitamin D can build up in the body and cause toxic symptoms. According to current recommendations, the maximum safe dosage of vitamin D, in the absence of sunlight or other sources, is 2,000 IU daily. However, the actual dosage at which intake becomes toxic is a matter of dispute.[44,45]

People with sarcoidosis or hyperparathyroidism should never take vitamin D without first consulting a physician.

Taking vitamin D and calcium supplements might interfere with some of the effects of calcium channel–blockers.[46] It is very important that you consult your physician before trying this combination.

The combination of calcium, vitamin D and thiazide diuretics can lead to excessive calcium levels in the body.[47,48,49] If you are taking thiazide diuretics, you should consult with a physician about the right doses of vitamin D and calcium for you.

⚠ INTERACTIONS YOU SHOULD KNOW ABOUT

If you are taking

- Antiseizure drugs (**phenobarbital, primidone [Mysoline], valproic acid [Depakene] or phenytoin [Dilantin]), corticosteroids, cimetidine (Tagamet), heparin, isoniazid (INH),** or **rifampin:** You may need extra vitamin D.
- **Calcium channel–blockers:** Do not take high-dose vitamin D (with calcium) except under physician supervision.
- **Thiazide diuretics:** Do not take calcium and vitamin D supplements unless under a doctor's supervision.

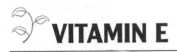

VITAMIN E

Supplement Forms/Alternate Names Alpha Tocopherol, D-Tocopherol, DL-Tocopherol, DL-Alpha-Tocopherol, Tocopheryl Succinate, Tocopheryl Acetate, D-Alpha-Tocopherol, D-Delta-Tocopherol, D-Beta-Tocopherol, D-Gamma-Tocopherol, Mixed Tocopherols

Principal Proposed Uses Cancer Prevention

Other Proposed Uses Heart Disease Prevention, Tardive Dyskinesia, Sunburn Prevention, Acute Anterior Uveitis, Preeclampsia Prevention, Impaired Immunity, Alzheimer's Disease, Rheumatoid Arthritis, Diabetic Neuropathy, Male Infertility, Cataracts, Diabetes, Macular Degeneration, Osteoarthritis, Restless Legs Syndrome, Vascular Dementia, PMS, Sports Performance, HIV Support, Cyclic Mastalgia, Parkinson's Disease, Asthma, Acne, Dupuytren's Contracture, Gout, Fibromyalgia, Psoriasis, Menopause, Intermittent Claudication, Hypertension, Nutritional Support for Smokers

Vitamin E is an antioxidant that fights damaging natural substances known as free radicals. It works in lipids (fats and oils), which makes it complementary to vitamin C, which fights free radicals dissolved in water.

There is evidence that vitamin E can prevent certain forms of cancer. Vitamin E has also shown considerable promise for preventing preeclampsia (a complication of pregnancy), treating tardive dyskinesia (a side effect of antipsychotic drugs), improving immunity, slowing the progression of Alzheimer's disease, and improving male fertility. However, contrary to earlier indications, vitamin E does not appear to prevent heart disease.

REQUIREMENTS/SOURCES

Vitamin E dosage recommendations are a bit complex, because the vitamin exists in many forms.

New vitamin E recommendations are in milligrams (mg) of alpha-tocopherol. Alpha-tocopherol can come from either natural vitamin E (called, somewhat incorrectly, d-alpha-tocopherol) or synthetic vitamin E (called, also somewhat incorrectly, dl-alpha-tocopherol). However much of the alpha-tocopherol in synthetic vitamin E is inactive. For this reason, you have to take about twice as much of it to get the same effect.[1,2,3]

Vitamin E

Visit Us at TNP.com

There are other forms of vitamin E as well, such as beta-, delta-, and gamma-tocopherols, all of which occur in food. It has been suggested that the best vitamin E supplement would be a mixture of all these.[4,5,6] However, other experts disagree and suggest that only alpha-tocopherol is important.[7,8,9]

To make matters even more confusing, vitamin E dosages are commonly listed on labels as international units (IU). Here's how you make the conversion. One IU natural vitamin E equals 0.67 mg alpha-tocopherol; one IU synthetic vitamin E equals 0.45 mg alpha-tocopherol. Therefore, to meet the new dietary recommendations for vitamin E (15 mg per day), you need to get either 22 IU natural vitamin E (22 IU × 0.67 = 15 mg) or 33 IU synthetic vitamin E (33 IU × 0.45 = 15 mg). The official U.S. and Canadian recommendations for daily intake of vitamin E are as follows:

- Infants 0–6 months, 4 mg
    7–12 months, 6 mg
- Children 1–3 years, 6 mg
    4–8 years, 7 mg
    9–13 years, 11 mg
- Males and females 14 years and older, 15 mg
- Pregnant women, 19 mg (15 mg if under 19 years old)
- Nursing women, 19 mg

In developed countries, dietary deficiency of vitamin E is relatively common.[10,11,12] In addition, bile acid sequestrants might inhibit absorption of vitamin E.[13]

The best food sources of vitamin E are polyunsaturated vegetable oils, seeds, nuts, and whole grains. To get a therapeutic dosage, though, you need to take a supplement.

THERAPEUTIC DOSAGES

The optimal therapeutic dosage of vitamin E has not been established. Most studies have used between 50 and 800 IU daily, and some have used even higher doses. This would correspond to about 50 to 800 mg of synthetic vitamin E (dl-alpha-tocopherol), or 25 to 400 mg of natural vitamin E (d-alpha- or mixed tocopherols).

Note: In general, IUs rather than mg are used in the following discussion, as that was the most commonly used measurement at the time the studies were performed.

If you wish to purchase natural vitamin E, look for a label that says "mixed tocopherols." However, some manufacturers use this term to mean the synthetic dl-alpha-tocopherol, so you need to read the contents closely. Natural tocopherols come as d-alpha-, d-gamma-, d-delta-, and d-beta-tocopherol.

THERAPEUTIC USES

Vitamin E appears to help prevent various forms of **cancer** (see page 32),[14–26] especially prostate cancer,[27] but more research is needed.

Vitamin E might be slightly helpful for **angina** (see page 10).[28] However, contrary to earlier indications, it does not seem to help prevent **heart disease** (see page 16).[29]

Tardive dyskinesia (see page 176) consists of involuntary movements of the face, arms, and head, usually caused by the long-term use of antipsychotic drugs. Vitamin E appears to reduce symptoms of this disorder.[30–34] However, not all studies agree.

When combined with vitamin C, vitamin E appears to help prevent **sunburn** (see page 171).[35–39] There is also evidence that vitamin E in combination with vitamin C (and the standard drug treatment) may be helpful for acute anterior uveitis. This condition involves painful inflammation of the iris of the eye, with acute sensitivity to light, increased ocular pressure, and a loss of visual clarity; it most often occurs in conjunction with autoimmune diseases. While acute anterior uveitis usually responds to conventional treatment after 10 to 14 days, vision problems may persist. In one study, the use of vitamin E (alpha-tocopherol) at 100 mg twice daily and vitamin C at a dose of 500 mg twice daily improved vision after 8 weeks as compared to placebo.[40] **Note:** Acute anterior uveitis is a potentially dangerous condition. Physician supervision is mandatory.

Intriguing evidence suggests that vitamin E may also prevent preeclampsia,[41] improve immunity,[42] slow the progression of **Alzheimer's disease** (see page 5),[43] reduce pain in **rheumatoid arthritis** (see page 151) and also possibly help prevent it,[44,45] improve symptoms of diabetic neuropathy,[46,47] and help protect people with diabetes from developing damage to their eyes and kidneys.[48] Vitamin E may also be helpful in treating **male infertility** (see page 116),[49] although a recent double-blind study of 31 individuals found no benefit.[50] Weaker evidence suggests that vitamin E can prevent **cataracts** (see page 42),[51–54] improve blood sugar control in people with type 2 **diabetes** (see page 65),[55,56,57] help prevent or treat **macular degeneration** (see page 115), slow the progression of **osteoarthritis** (see page 132),[58] control symptoms of **restless legs syndrome** (see page 150),[59] help prevent **vascular dementia** (see page 5),[60] and reduce symptoms of **PMS** (see page 145).[61,62]

There is also some evidence that vitamin E may be useful during weight training.[63] Heavy exercise produces free radicals that can disrupt the muscles and cause pain. Vitamin E appears to exert a protective effect in this regard.

Additionally, vitamin E might help reduce the lung-related side effects caused by the drug amiodarone (used to prevent abnormal heart rhythms).[64]

In one observational study, high intake of vitamin E was linked to decreased risk of progression to AIDS in **HIV** (see page 94) infected people.[65] However, a double-blind study of 49 people with HIV who took combined vitamins C and E or placebo for 3 months did not show any significant effects on the amount of HIV virus detected or the number of opportunistic infections.[66] It has been suggested that vitamin E may enhance the antiviral effects of AZT, but evidence for this is minimal.[67]

Vitamin E does *not* appear to be helpful for cyclic breast pain, sometimes called fibrocystic breast disease, cyclic mastitis, or **cyclic mastalgia** (see page 58).[68] In addition, despite some claims to the contrary, supplemental vitamin E does not seem to be helpful for treating **Parkinson's disease** (see page 140).[69,70,71] Vitamin E and other antioxidants are frequently recommended for **asthma** (see page 14), on the grounds that they may protect inflamed lung tissue, but there is no scientific evidence that they work. Similarly, although vitamin E has been suggested as a treatment for **acne** (see page 2), **Dupuytren's contracture** (see page 69), **gout** (see page 84), **fibromyalgia** (see page 80), and **psoriasis** (see page 148), there is no real supporting evidence for any of these uses.

Although vitamin E is often recommended for **menopausal** (see page 117) hot flashes, there is no real evidence that it is effective. One 9-week double-blind placebo-controlled trial followed 104 women with hot flashes associated with breast cancer treatment, but it found marginal benefits at best.[72]

A double-blind placebo-controlled trial of 1,484 individuals with **intermittent claudication** (see page 106) found no benefit from vitamin E (50 mg daily), beta-carotene (20 mg daily), or a combination of the two.[73]

Vitamin E has sometimes been suggested as a treatment for **hypertension** (see page 98), but there is some evidence that it does not work.[74]

Similarly, while vitamin E has been suggested as a treatment to prevent symptoms that can occur after endurance running, such as gastrointestinal bleeding, stomach cramps, nausea, or muscle injury, one double-blind trial found no significant benefit for any of these symptoms.[75]

Although vitamin E is sometimes recommended for **smokers** (see page 131) to help reduce their chances of getting lung cancer or heart disease, large double-blind trials found neither a beneficial nor a harmful effect.[76,77,78] However, vitamin E consumption might significantly reduce risk of prostate cancer in smokers.[79]

WHAT IS THE SCIENTIFIC EVIDENCE FOR VITAMIN E?

Cancer Prevention

In a double-blind trial that involved 29,133 smokers, those who were given 50 mg of synthetic vitamin E daily for 5 to 8 years showed a 32% reduction in the incidence of prostate cancer and a 41% drop in prostate cancer deaths.[80]

Surprisingly, results were seen soon after the beginning of supplementation. This was unexpected because prostate cancer grows very slowly. A cancer that shows up today actually started to develop many years ago. The fact that vitamin E almost immediately lowered the incidence of prostate cancer suggests that it somehow blocks the step at which a hidden prostate cancer makes the leap to being detectable.

Similarly promising results have been seen in stomach cancer; mouth, throat, and laryngeal cancer; and liver cancer.[81–84] However, vitamin E does not appear to be helpful against lung cancer, and the evidence regarding colon cancer is quite mixed.[85–93]

Heart Disease

The latest research findings appear to have turned the tables on our once high hopes for vitamin E. Now it looks increasingly unlikely that this antioxidant vitamin is a "magic bullet" that by itself can put a dent in heart disease.

The Heart Outcomes Prevention Evaluation (HOPE) trial found that natural vitamin E (d-alpha-tocopherol) at a dose of 400 IU daily did not reduce the number of heart attacks, strokes, or deaths from heart disease any more than placebo.[94] The details of this well-designed double-blind trial were published in the January 20, 2000, issue of *The New England Journal of Medicine*. The trial, lasting an average of 4.5 years, followed over 9,000 men and women who had existing heart disease or were at high risk for it.

We already knew that vitamin E supplements (50 IU synthetic) didn't work for heart disease in smokers,[95,96,97] but that could be readily explained away: Perhaps vitamin E, especially in that relatively small dose, could not overcome the damaging effects of smoking.

The Cambridge Heart Antioxidant Study (CHAOS) trial,[98] published in 1996, is what really had gotten our hopes up. In that trial, people with existing heart disease who took natural vitamin E (400 IU or 800 IU daily) had substantially fewer nonfatal heart attacks compared to the placebo group after about 1.5 years. Even so, and this may resonate with the latest findings, heart-related deaths were not reduced in the vitamin E group. Furthermore, it has been suggested that possible flaws in the design of this trial might make its findings questionable.

Large observational studies in both men and women found substantial benefits for vitamin E (100 IU).[99,100,101] One observational study of 11,178 people aged 67 to 105 years found good results from combining vitamins E and C.[102] Those who were taking vitamin E supplements at the beginning of the study had a 34% lower risk of death from heart disease than those who were not. Vitamin C supplements alone did not seem to make a difference, but the combination of vitamins E and C boosted the risk reduction to 53%. Long-term use of vitamin E granted an even stronger risk reduction of 63%. By their nature, though, observational studies cannot fully control for lifestyle factors, so it is possible that people taking vitamin E might also eat better and exercise more, which would influence the results.

So where does all this leave us? Experts uncomfortable with abandoning vitamin E have wondered whether it could be that vitamin E supplements exert a benefit in people who do not already have heart disease or are at low risk for it. Or, perhaps it takes vitamin E longer to exert a clinical benefit than the follow-up period of the studies. Realistically, though, there is no real evidence that this is true.

It might be that we just can't expect vitamin E—or perhaps any other single nutrient—to carry the full burden alone. The antioxidants are a package deal in nature. This group of nutrients, including vitamins E, A, C, selenium, and others, may work best as a team in nature's finely tuned botanical orchestra. The fact that lone vitamin E supplementation appears not to be the magic bullet we had hoped for hints that it might be better to take a balanced, comprehensive array of nutrients rather than depending on high doses of a few key nutrients to carry the load. We will be eagerly awaiting the outcome of ongoing trials of vitamin E combined with other antioxidants.

In addition, vitamin E itself is present in several forms in food, and some researchers believe that this mixture may work best and that perhaps taking too much of one form of vitamin E may blunt the effect of the others.[103]

Preeclampsia Prevention

Preeclampsia is a dangerous complication of pregnancy that involves high blood pressure, swelling of the whole body, and improper kidney function. A double-blind placebo-controlled study of 283 women at increased risk for preeclampsia found that supplementation with vitamin E (400 IU daily of natural vitamin E) and vitamin C (1,000 mg daily) significantly reduced the chances for developing this disease.[104]

While this research is promising, larger studies are necessary to confirm whether vitamins E and C will actually work. The authors of this study point out that studies of similar size found benefits with other treatments, such as aspirin, that later proved to be ineffective when large-scale studies were performed. Furthermore, keep in mind that we don't know whether such high dosages of these vitamins are absolutely safe for pregnant women.

Tardive Dyskinesia

Between 1987 and 1998, at least five double-blind studies were published which indicated that vitamin E was beneficial in treating TD.[105,106] Although most of these studies were small and lasted only 4 to 12 weeks, one 36-week study enrolled 40 individuals.[107] Three small double-blind studies reported that vitamin E was not helpful.[108,109] Nonetheless, a statistical analysis of the double-blind studies done before 1999 found good evidence that vitamin E was more effective than placebo.[110] Most studies found that vitamin E worked best for TD of more recent onset.[111]

However, in 1999, the picture on vitamin E changed with the publication of one more study—the largest and longest to date.[112] This double-blind study included 107 participants from nine different research sites who took 1,600 IU of vitamin E or placebo daily for at least 1 year. In contrast to most of the previous studies, this trial found that vitamin E was not effective in decreasing TD symptoms.

Why the discrepancy between this study and the earlier ones? The researchers, some of whom had worked on the earlier, positive studies of vitamin E, were at pains to develop an answer.[113,114] They proposed a number of possible explanations. One was that the earlier studies were too small or too short to be accurate, and that vitamin E really didn't help at all. Another was the most complicated: that vitamin E might help only a subgroup of people who had TD—those with milder TD symptoms of more recent onset—and that fewer of these people had participated in the latest study. They also pointed to changes in schizophrenia treatment since the last study was done, including the growing use of antipsychotic medications that do not cause TD.

The bottom line: The effectiveness of vitamin E for a given individual is simply not known. Given the lack of other good treatments for TD, and the general safety of the vitamin, it may be worth discussing with your physician.

Immunity

A recent double-blind study suggests that vitamin E may be able to strengthen immunity. In this study, 88 people over the age of 65 were given either placebo or vitamin E at 60 IU, 200 IU, or 800 IU dl-alpha-tocopherol daily.[115] The researchers then gave all participants immunizations against hepatitis B, tetanus, diphtheria, and pneumonia, and looked at subjects' immune response to these vaccinations. The researchers also used a skin test that evaluates the overall strength of the immune response.

The results were impressive. Vitamin E at all dosages significantly increased the strength of the immune response. However, a daily dosage of 200 IU produced the most marked benefits.

Alzheimer's Disease

Preliminary evidence suggests that high-dose vitamin E may slow the progression of Alzheimer's disease.[116] In a double-blind placebo-controlled study, 341 subjects received either 2,000 IU daily of vitamin E (dl-alpha-tocopherol), the antioxidant drug selegiline, or placebo. Those given vitamin E took nearly 200 days longer to reach a severe state of the disease than the placebo group. (Selegiline was even more effective.)

Warning: Such high dosages of vitamin E should not be taken except under a doctor's supervision (see Safety Issues).

Low Sperm Count/Infertility

In a double-blind placebo-controlled study of 110 men whose sperm showed subnormal activity, treatment with 100 IU of vitamin E daily resulted in improved sperm activity and higher actual fertility (measured in pregnancies).[117] However, a smaller double-blind trial found no benefit.[118]

SAFETY ISSUES

Vitamin E is generally regarded as safe when taken at the recommended therapeutic dosage of 400 to 800 IU daily. However, vitamin E does have a "blood-thinning" effect that could lead to problems in certain situations. In one study of 28,519 men, vitamin E supplementation at the low dose of about 50 IU synthetic vitamin E per day caused an increase in fatal hemorrhagic strokes, the kind of stroke caused by bleeding. (However, it reduced the risk of a more common type of stroke, and the two effects essentially canceled out.)[119] Based on its blood-thinning effects, there are concerns that vitamin E could cause problems if it is combined with medications that also thin the blood, such as Coumadin (warfarin), heparin, Trental (pentoxifylline), and aspirin. Theoretically, the net result could be to thin the blood *too* much, causing bleeding problems. A study that evaluated vitamin E plus aspirin did in fact find an additive effect.[120] In contrast, the results of a study on vitamin E and Coumadin found no evidence of interaction, but it would still not be advisable to combine these treatments except under a physician's supervision.[121]

There is also at least a remote possibility that vitamin E could also interact with herbs that possess a mild blood-thinning effect, such as **garlic** (see page 291) and **ginkgo** (see page 298). Individuals with bleeding disorders such as hemophilia, and those about to undergo surgery or labor and delivery should also approach vitamin E with caution.

In addition, vitamin E might enhance the body's sensitivity to its own insulin in individuals with adult-onset diabetes.[122,123] This could lead to risk of blood sugar levels falling too low. If you are taking oral hypoglycemic medications, do not take high-dose vitamin E without first consulting your physician.

Finally, considerable controversy exists regarding whether it is safe or appropriate to combine vitamin E with standard chemotherapy drugs.[124] The reasoning behind this concern is that many chemotherapy drugs work in part by creating free radicals that destroy cancer cells. Antioxidants like vitamin E might interfere with this beneficial effect. However, there is also some evidence that vitamin E might help protect against the side effects of certain chemotherapy drugs without interfering with their action.[125] Nonetheless, in view of the high stakes involved, we strongly recommend that you do not take any supplements while undergoing cancer chemotherapy, except on the advice of a physician.

⚠ INTERACTIONS YOU SHOULD KNOW ABOUT

If you are taking

- **Blood-thinning drugs**, such as **Coumadin (warfarin), heparin, Trental (pentoxifylline),** or **aspirin:** Seek medical advice before taking vitamin E.
- **Amiodarone**: Vitamin E may help protect you from lung-related side effects.
- **Phenothiazine drugs:** Vitamin E may help reduce side effects.
- **Chemotherapy drugs:** Seek medical advice before taking vitamin E.
- **Oral hypoglycemic medications:** High-dose vitamin E might cause your blood sugar levels to fall too low, requiring an adjustment in medication dosage.
- **Bile acid sequestrant drugs:** You may need more vitamin E.

Vitamin E

VITAMIN K

Supplement Forms/Alternate Names   Vitamin K_1 (Phylloquinone), Vitamin K_2 (Menaquinone), Vitamin K_3 (Menadione)
Principal Proposed Uses   Treating Medication-Induced Vitamin K Deficiency
Other Proposed Uses   Osteoporosis, Menorrhagia (Heavy Menstruation), Nausea

There's a good chance you haven't even heard of vitamin K. However, this obscure member of the vitamin clan is very important for good health. Without it, your blood wouldn't clot properly. There are three forms of vitamin K: K_1 (phylloquinone), found in plants; K_2 (menaquinone), produced by bacteria in your intestines; and K_3 (menadione), a synthetic form.

Vitamin K is used medically to reverse the effects of "blood-thinning" drugs such as warfarin (Coumadin). Growing evidence suggests that it may also be helpful for osteoporosis.

REQUIREMENTS/SOURCES

Vitamin K is an essential nutrient, but you need only a tiny amount of it. The official U.S. recommendation for daily intake is 1 mcg per kilogram body weight. This translates into the following:

- Infants 0–6 months, 5 mcg
  7–12 months, 10 mcg
- Children 1–3 years, 15 mcg
  4–6 years, 20 mcg
  7–10 years, 30 mcg
- Males 11–14 years, 45 mcg
  15–18 years, 65 mcg
  19–24 years, 70 mcg
  25 years and older, 80 mcg
- Females 11–14 years, 45 mcg
  15–18 years, 55 mcg
  19–24 years, 60 mcg
  25 years and older, 65 mcg
- Pregnant women, 65 mcg, preferably the K_1 variety (phylloquinone)
- Nursing women, 65 mcg, preferably the K_1 variety

However, a recent study suggests that a higher intake of vitamin K, in the range of 110 mcg daily, might be helpful for preventing osteoporosis.[1]

Vitamin K (in the form of K_1) is found in green leafy vegetables. Kale, green tea, and turnip greens are the best food sources, providing about 10 times the daily adult requirement in a single serving. Spinach, broccoli, lettuce, and cabbage are very rich sources as well, and you can get perfectly respectable amounts of vitamin K in such common foods as oats, green peas, whole wheat, and green beans, as well as watercress and asparagus.

Vitamin K (in the form of K_2) is also manufactured by bacteria in the intestines, and is a major source of vitamin K. Long-term use of antibiotics can cause a vitamin K deficiency by killing these bacteria. However, this effect seems to be significant only in people who are deficient in vitamin K to begin with.[2–5] Pregnant and postmenopausal women are also sometimes deficient in this vitamin.[6,7,8] In addition, children born to women taking anticonvulsants while pregnant may be significantly deficient in vitamin K, causing them to have bleeding problems and facial bone abnormalities.[9,10,11] Vitamin K supplementation during pregnancy may be helpful in these situations.

The blood-thinning drug warfarin (Coumadin) works by antagonizing the effects of vitamin K. Conversely, vitamin K supplements, or intake of foods containing high levels of vitamin K, block the action of this medication and can be used as an antidote.[12]

Cephalosporins and possibly other antibiotics may also interfere with vitamin K–dependent blood clotting.[13–16] However, this interaction seems to be significant only in people who have vitamin K–poor diets.

People with disorders of the digestive tract, such as chronic diarrhea, celiac sprue, **ulcerative colitis** (see page 179), or **Crohn's disease** (see page 57), may become deficient in vitamin K.[17–20] Alcoholism can also lead to vitamin K deficiency.[21]

THERAPEUTIC DOSAGES

For some purposes, vitamin K has been recommended at a daily dose of 150 to 500 mcg. Although such dosages are much higher than required for nutritional purposes, they are not out of the range of what can be reached through eating plenty of green leafy vegetables.

THERAPEUTIC USES

Evidence suggests (but does not prove) that vitamin K supplements may be helpful for preventing osteoporosis.[22–32]

Based on its ability to help blood clot normally, vitamin K has been proposed as a treatment for excessive menstrual bleeding.[33] However, the last actual study testing this idea was carried out more than 55 years ago.[34] Vitamin K has also been recommended for **nausea** (see page 126), although there is as yet little evidence that it really works.

WHAT IS THE SCIENTIFIC EVIDENCE FOR VITAMIN K?

Osteoporosis

Vitamin K plays a known biochemical role in the formation of new bone. This has led researchers to look for relationships between vitamin K intake and osteoporosis.

Research has found that people with osteoporosis have much lower blood levels of vitamin K than other people. For example, in a study of 71 postmenopausal women, participants with reduced bone mineral density showed lower serum vitamin K_1 levels than those with normal bone density.[35] Similar results have been seen in other studies.[36,37,38]

A recent report from 12,700 participants in the Nurse's Health Study found that higher dietary intake of vitamin K is associated with a significantly reduced risk of hip fracture.[39]

Interestingly, the most common source of vitamin K used by individuals in the study was iceberg lettuce, followed by broccoli, spinach, romaine lettuce, brussels sprouts, and dark greens. Women who ate lettuce each day had only 55% the risk of hip fracture as those who ate it only weekly. However, among women taking estrogen, no benefit was seen, probably because estrogen is so much more powerful.

Another observational study also found evidence that higher vitamin K intake is associated with a reduced incidence of hip fractures.[40]

Research also suggests that supplemental vitamin K can reduce the amount of **calcium** (see page 234) lost in the urine.[41,42,43] This is indirect evidence of a beneficial effect on bone.

Taken together, these findings suggest that vitamin K supplements might help prevent osteoporosis.

SAFETY ISSUES

Vitamin K is probably quite safe at the recommended therapeutic dosages, since those quantities are easily obtained from food.

Vitamin K directly counters the effects of the anticoagulant warfarin. If you are taking warfarin, you should not take vitamin K supplements or alter your dietary intake of vitamin K without doctor supervision.[44,45]

Newborns are commonly given vitamin K_1 injections to prevent bleeding problems. Although some have suggested that this practice may increase the risk of cancer,[46] enormous observational studies have found no such connection (one such trial involved more than a million participants).[47,48]

⚠ INTERACTIONS YOU SHOULD KNOW ABOUT

If you are taking

- **Warfarin (Coumadin):** Do not take vitamin K supplements or eat foods high in vitamin K except under the supervision of a physician. (You will need to have your medication dosage adjusted.)
- **Cephalosporins** or other **antibiotics:** You may need more vitamin K if you are already deficient in this nutrient.
- Anticonvulsants (such as **phenytoin [Dilantin], carbamazepine phenobarbital,** and **primidone [Mysoline]**) and are pregnant: You may need more vitamin K to protect your child.

🌿 WHITE WILLOW (*Salix alba*)

Alternate or Related Names   Willow, Salicin Willow, Withe Withy, Black Willow, Cartkins Willow, Others

Principal Proposed Uses
   Pain Relief: Osteoarthritis, Back Pain, Bursitis, Dysmenorrhea, Headaches, Rheumatoid Arthritis, Tendinitis

Willow bark has been used as a treatment for pain and fever in China since 500 B.C. In Europe, it was primarily used for altogether different purposes, such as stopping vomiting, removing warts, and suppressing sexual desire. However, in 1828, European chemists made a discovery that would bring some of these different uses together. They extracted the substance salicin from white willow, which was soon purified to salicylic acid. Salicylic acid is an effective treatment for pain and fever, but it is also sufficiently irritating to do a good job of burning off warts.

White Willow

Visit Us at TNP.com

Chemists later modified salicylic acid (this time from the herb meadowsweet) to create acetylsalicylic acid, or aspirin.

WHAT IS WILLOW USED FOR TODAY?

As interest in natural medicine has grown, many people have begun to turn back to white willow as an alternative to aspirin. One double-blind trial found it effective for back pain; it is also used for other painful conditions such as **osteoarthritis** (see page 132), bursitis, **dysmenorrhea** (see page 70), headaches, **rheumatoid arthritis** (see page 151), and tendinitis.

Aspirin and related anti-inflammatory drugs are notorious for irritating or damaging the stomach. However, when taken in standard doses, willow does not appear to produce this same side effect.[1,2] This may be partly due to the fact that most of the salicylic acid in white willow is present in chemical forms that are only converted to salicylic acid after absorption into the body.[3] In addition, evidence suggests that standard doses of willow bark are the equivalent of 1 baby aspirin daily rather than a full dose.[4]

This latter finding raises an interesting question: If willow provides only a small amount of salicylate, how can it work? It appears most likely that other ingredients must play a role as well, such as a substance called tremulacin.

WHAT IS THE SCIENTIFIC EVIDENCE FOR WILLOW?

In a 4-week double-blind placebo-controlled study of 210 individuals with back pain, two doses of willow bark extract were compared against placebo.[5] The higher-dose group received extract supplying 240 mg of salicin daily; in this group, 39% were pain free for at least 5 days of the last week of the study. In the lower-dose group (120 mg salicin daily), 21% became pain free. In contrast, only 6% of those given placebo became pain free. Stomach distress did not occur in this study. The only significant side effect seen was an allergic reaction in one participant given willow.

Benefits were also seen in an earlier, unpublished double-blind placebo-controlled trial of 78 individuals with osteoarthritis of the knee or hip.[6]

DOSAGE

Standardized willow bark extracts should provide 120 to 240 mg of salicin daily.

SAFETY ISSUES

Evidence suggests that willow, taken at standard doses, is the equivalent of 50 mg of aspirin, a very small dose.[7] Willow doesn't impair blood coagulation to the same extent as aspirin, and also doesn't appear to significantly irritate the stomach.[8]

Nonetheless, willow could still cause the side effects associated with aspirin such as stomach irritation and even bleeding ulcers if used over the long term. All the other risks of aspirin therapy apply as well. For example, white willow should not be given to children, due to the risk of Reye's syndrome. It should also not be used by people with aspirin allergies, bleeding disorders, ulcers, kidney disease, liver disease, or diabetes, and it may interact adversely with alcohol, "blood thinners," other anti-inflammatories, methotrexate, metoclopramide, phenytoin, probenecid, spironolactone, and valproate.

Safety in pregnant or nursing women, or those with severe liver or kidney disease has not been established.

⚠ INTERACTIONS YOU SHOULD KNOW ABOUT

If you are taking blood-thinning medications such as **Coumadin (warfarin), heparin, Trental (pentoxifylline),** or **aspirin; methotrexate; metoclopramide; Dilantin (phenytoin); sulfonamide drugs; spironolactone** and other **potassium-sparing diuretics;** or the antiseizure drug **valproic acid:** It may be wise to avoid combining white willow with these substances.

WILD CHERRY (*Prunus serotina*)

Alternate or Related Names   Wild Black Cherry, Virginian Prune, Black Choke, Choke Cherry, Rum Cherry

Principal Proposed Uses   Cough

The bark of the wild cherry tree is a traditional Native American remedy for two seemingly unrelated conditions: respiratory infections and anxiety. European settlers quickly adopted the herb for similar purposes.

WHAT IS WILD CHERRY USED FOR TODAY?

Over time, wild cherry has come to be used primarily as a component of cough syrups. It is tempting to connect the two traditional uses of wild cherry by imagining that it functions like codeine to affect both the mind and the cough reflex. However, this is just speculation, as there has been very little scientific evaluation of this herb.

DOSAGE

Syrups containing wild cherry should be taken as directed.

SAFETY ISSUES

Wild cherry is generally regarded as safe when used at recommended dosages. However, since it contains small amounts of cyanide, it should not be taken to excess. It is not recommended for use by young children, pregnant or nursing women, or those with severe liver or kidney disease.

WILD YAM (*Dioscorea species*)

Alternate or Related Names   Mexican Yam, China Root, Colic Root, Devil's Bones, Rheumatism Root, Others

Principal Proposed Uses   There are no well-documented uses for wild yam.

Incorrect Uses   Source of Women's Hormones

Various species of wild yam grow throughout North and Central America and Asia. Traditionally, this herb has been used as a treatment for indigestion, coughs, morning sickness, gallbladder pain, menstrual cramps, joint pain, and nerve pain.[1] The main use of wild yam in the United States today, however, is based on a fundamental misconception: that it contains women's hormones such as **progesterone** (see page 392) and **DHEA** (see page 268).

In reality, there is no progesterone, DHEA, or any other hormone in wild yam, nor are there any substances that the body can directly use to make such hormones.

To explain this widespread misunderstanding, we have to go back a number of years. When progesterone was first discovered, it was very expensive to produce. The first methods involved direct extraction of progesterone from cow ovaries, a process that required 50,000 cows to yield 20 mg of purified hormone![2] Other hormones such as estrogen and DHEA were also difficult to manufacture. Although doctors wanted to experiment with prescribing these treatments as medicine, until a simpler production method could be developed, it simply wasn't feasible.

The race to discover a more economical source of hormones was won by a scientist/businessman named Russell Marker. In the 1940s, he perfected a method of synthesizing progesterone from a constituent of wild yams called diosgenin. This process involves several chemical transformations carried out in the laboratory.

Marker focused his attention on two species of yam found in Mexico, *Dioscorea macrostachya* and *Dioscorea barabasco,* the latter of which is richer in diosgenin, while the former is much easier to harvest in the wild. He formed a manufacturing company in Mexico that produced progesterone and DHEA from these raw materials.

Unfortunately, corporate competition and difficult labor conditions eventually forced him to close his plant. But Marker's method of synthesizing progesterone continued to be used, bringing the price down drastically and helping to pave the way for the modern birth control pill. Progesterone continued to be manufactured from wild yam for decades, until a cheaper source of raw material was found in cultivated soybeans.

But neither soybeans nor wild yam contain progesterone. They only contain chemicals that chemists can use as a starting point to manufacture progesterone. Furthermore, the body almost certainly can't turn diosgenin into progesterone, because the synthetic steps used by chemists to do so don't even remotely resemble natural processes. Thus, any product that claims to contain "natural progesterone from wild yam" is misleading.

Nonetheless, some wild yam products do contain progesterone. Are we contradicting ourselves? Not at all: Manufacturers add synthetic progesterone to these creams. There may be a value to taking progesterone in cream form, but the Mexican yam part of the product is a red herring!

Wild Yam

Visit Us at TNP.com

YARROW (*Achillea millefolium*)

Alternate or Related Names   Band Man's Plaything, Bloodwort, Carpenter's Weed, Devil's Nettle, Soldier's Woundwort, Others

Principal Proposed Uses
Oral Uses: Respiratory Infections (Preventing)
Topical Uses: Bleeding

According to legend, the Greek general Achilles used yarrow to stop the bleeding of his soldiers' wounds during the Trojan War: hence the scientific name *Achillea* and the common names "soldier's wound-wort," "bloodwort," and *"herbe militaire."*

Yarrow has also been used traditionally as treatment for respiratory infections, menstrual pain, and digestive upsets.

WHAT IS YARROW USED FOR TODAY?

Like osha, yarrow tea is commonly taken at the first sign of a **cold** (see page 47) or flu to bring on sweating and, according to tradition, ward off infection. Crushed yarrow leaves and flower tops are also applied directly as first aid to stop **nosebleeds** (see page 129) and bleeding from **minor wounds** (see page 123). However, there has not been any formal scientific study of how well yarrow works.

DOSAGE

To make yarrow tea, steep 1 to 2 teaspoons of dried herb per cup of water. Combination products should be taken according to label instructions.

SAFETY ISSUES

No clear toxicity has been associated with yarrow.[1] The FDA has expressed concern about a toxic constituent of yarrow known as thujone and permits only thujone-free yarrow extracts for use in beverages. Nonetheless, the common spice sage contains more thujone than yarrow, and the FDA lists sage as generally recognized as safe.

Yarrow seldom produces any side effects other than the occasional allergic reaction. Nonetheless, safety in young children, pregnant or nursing women, or those with severe liver or kidney disease has not been established.

YELLOW DOCK

Alternate or Related Names   Curled Dock

Principal Proposed Uses   There are no well-documented uses for yellow dock.

Other Proposed Uses   Constipation, Diarrhea, Minor Skin Wounds, Hemorrhoids, Nasal and Lung Congestion

Yellow dock (*Rumex crispus*) is a perennial flowering herb, native to Europe, which grows throughout the United States. Its yellow roots were traditionally thought to have medicinal properties, and its sour-sweet leaves can be used (in moderation) as a salad green.

Historically, the plant has been used to treat a variety of problems, including constipation *and* diarrhea, as well as dermatitis and venereal diseases.[1] Powdered yellow dock root has also been used as a mouthwash or dentifrice.

WHAT IS YELLOW DOCK USED FOR TODAY?

Yellow dock root has no established medical uses. However, it contains chemicals called anthroquinones (also found in the more famous herbal laxative senna),[2] which stimulate bowel movements. For this reason, yellow dock is occasionally included in herbal laxative mixtures.

Like many other plants, yellow dock contains a substantial amount of tannins. These have astringent properties that may offer some benefit for treating minor skin **wounds** (see page 123) and **hemorrhoids** (see page 85). Yellow dock is also sometimes recommended for nasal and lung congestion.

DOSAGE

Typical doses of yellow dock root are 2 to 4 g of the dried root, 2 to 4 ml of the liquid extract, or 1 to 2 ml of the tincture.[3]

SAFETY ISSUES

Comprehensive safety studies of yellow dock have not been performed, and for this reason it should not be used by pregnant or nursing women, young children, or individuals with severe liver or kidney disease.

As with any stimulant laxative, yellow dock should not be used if there is an intestinal obstruction. Possible side effects of overuse include cramps, diarrhea, nausea, intestinal dependence on the laxative, and excessive loss of **potassium** (see page 390).[4]

In addition, yellow dock (like spinach) contains oxalic acid. Consuming excessive quantities of oxalic acid can cause severe toxic symptoms including vomiting and abdominal pain, and, in extreme cases, **kidney stones** (see page 109) or kidney failure. One case of fatal yellow dock poisoning has been documented.[5] The victim, who had diabetes, ingested one kilogram of the raw herb in a salad, and died of liver and kidney failure. The liver failure was not explained.

YERBA SANTA (*Eriodictyon californicum*)

Alternate or Related Names   Bear's Weed, Consumptive's Weed, Eriodictyon, Gum Bush, Holy Herb, Others

Principal Proposed Uses
Oral Uses: Respiratory Diseases (Asthma, Bronchitis, Etc.)
Topical Uses: Rash (Poison Ivy)

Yerba santa is a sticky-leafed evergreen that is native to the American Southwest. It was given its name ("holy weed") by Spanish priests impressed with its medicinal properties. The aromatic leaves were boiled to make a tea to treat coughs, colds, asthma, pleurisy, tuberculosis, and pneumonia, and a poultice of the leaves was applied to painful joints.

Unlike most medicinal herbs, yerba santa actually has a pleasant taste. It has been used as a general food flavoring and in cough syrups to disguise the bad taste of other ingredients.

WHAT IS YERBA SANTA USED FOR TODAY?

Some modern herbalists regard yerba santa as one of the most effective natural treatments for chronic respiratory problems such as bronchitis and **asthma** (see page 14). Unfortunately, scientific studies of this herb have not been carried out. About the most that can be said is that one of its constituents, eriodictyol, appears to be a mild expectorant.[1]

Yerba santa is occasionally used topically as a treatment for poison ivy.[2]

DOSAGE

Yerba santa tea may be made by adding 1 teaspoon of crushed leaves to a cup of boiling water and steeping for half an hour. However, because many of its resinous constituents do not dissolve in water, alcoholic tinctures of yerba santa may be more effective. Such tinctures should be taken according to the directions on the label. Drink 3 cups a day until symptoms subside.

Yerba santa is often combined with the herbs **osha** (see page 376) and grindelia.

SAFETY ISSUES

Yerba santa is on the FDA's GRAS (generally recognized as safe) list for use as a food flavoring. There have been no reports of significant side effects or adverse reactions,[3] except for the inevitable occasional allergic reaction. Nonetheless, safety in young children, pregnant or nursing women, or those with severe liver or kidney disease has not been established.

YOHIMBE (*Pausinystalia yohimbe*)

Principal Proposed Uses   Impotence (Not Recommended), Sexual Dysfunction in Women

The bark of the West African yohimbe tree is a traditional aphrodisiac and the source of yohimbine, a prescription drug for impotence.

Yohimbine (the drug) is only modestly effective at best, better than placebo but only successful in about 30 to 45% of the men who use it.[1] However, it seems to work even in men whose impotence is caused by a serious illness such as diabetes.

One small double-blind study on women found yohimbine combined with arginine to be somewhat effective for treating women with **sexual dysfunction** (see page 155).[2]

An open trial of yohimbine alone to treat sexual dysfunction induced by the antidepressant fluoxetine (Prozac) found improvement in eight out of nine people, two of whom were women.[3] However, in the absence of a placebo group, these results can't be taken as reliable; in addition, there are concerns about the safety of combining yohimbe with antidepressants.

We don't really know how yohimbine works, but recent thinking suggests that it operates by suppressing parts of the brain that keep sexual arousal under control.[4] In other words, it takes the brake off, which can be useful when the engine has lost some of its power.

WHAT IS YOHIMBE USED FOR TODAY?

Like the drug yohimbine, the bark of the yohimbe tree is widely used to treat impotence. Many herbalists report that the herb is more effective than the purified drug, perhaps due to the presence of other unidentified active ingredients. However, there have been no good studies to prove this.

Yohimbe is also sometimes recommended as an antidepressant. However, its effectiveness is unknown and there are much safer herbs for this purpose, such as **St. John's wort** (see page 414).

DOSAGE

Yohimbe bark is best taken in a form standardized to yohimbine content. Most people take a dose that supplies 15 to 30 mg of yohimbine daily. However, higher doses are not necessarily better, and some people respond optimally to 10 or even 5 mg daily. Furthermore, while some people appear to respond immediately to a single dose, for others it takes 2 to 3 weeks of treatment to provide significant benefits.

Because yohimbine is a somewhat dangerous substance (see Safety Issues), we recommend a physician's supervision when taking it.

SAFETY ISSUES

Yohimbe should not be used by pregnant or nursing women, or those with kidney, liver, or ulcer disease or high blood pressure. Dosages that provide more than 40 mg a day of yohimbine can cause a severe drop in blood pressure, abdominal pain, fatigue, hallucinations, and paralysis. (Interestingly, lower dosages can cause an increase in blood pressure.) Since 40 mg is not very far above the typical recommended dose, yohimbe has what is known as a *narrow therapeutic index*. This means that there is a relatively small dosing range, below which the herb doesn't work and above which it is toxic.

Even when taken in normal dosages, side effects of dizziness, anxiety, hyperstimulation, and nausea are not uncommon.

Yohimbe is not recommended for young children, pregnant or nursing women, or those with severe liver or kidney disease.

⚠ INTERACTIONS YOU SHOULD KNOW ABOUT

If you are taking **tricyclic antidepressants, phenothiazines, clonidine,** other drugs for lowering blood pressure, **central nervous system stimulants:** don't use yohimbine.[5–14]

🌿 YUCCA (*Yucca brevifolia* and other species)

Principal Proposed Uses   Rheumatoid Arthritis, Osteoarthritis

Various species of yucca plant were used as food by Native Americans and early California settlers. Yucca contains high levels of soapy compounds known as saponins that also made it a useful natural shampoo and soap.

WHAT IS YUCCA USED FOR TODAY?

When taken for a long period of time, yucca is said to reduce **osteoarthritis** (see page 132) and **rheumatoid arthritis** (see page 151) symptoms. However, the only

Yucca

Visit Us at TNP.com

scientific evidence for this claim comes from one preliminary study.[1]

Yucca extracts are also widely used to enhance the foaming effect of carbonated beverages.

DOSAGE

The standard dosage is 2 to 4 tablets of concentrated yucca saponins daily.

SAFETY ISSUES

Yucca is generally accepted as safe based on its long history of use as a food. However, it sometimes causes diarrhea if taken to excess. Safety in young children, pregnant or nursing women, or those with severe liver or kidney disease has not been established. According to one report, yucca possesses significant estrogenic activity and, as such, should not be taken by women who have had breast cancer.[2]

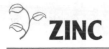 # ZINC

Supplement Forms/Alternate Names   Zinc Sulfate, Zinc Gluconate, Zinc Citrate, Zinc Picolinate, Chelated Zinc

Principal Proposed Uses   Colds, General Nutritional Supplementation, Pregnancy Support

Other Proposed Uses   Acne, Sickle-Cell Anemia, Ulcers, Rheumatoid Arthritis, HIV Support, Male Infertility, Anorexia Nervosa, Attention Deficit Disorder, Bladder Infection, Cataracts, Eczema, Macular Degeneration, Periodontal Disease, Psoriasis, and Many Others

Zinc is an important element that is found in every cell in the body. More than 300 enzymes in the body need zinc in order to function properly. Although the amount of zinc we need in our daily diet is tiny, it's very important that we get it. However, the evidence suggests that many of us do *not* get enough. Mild zinc deficiency seems to be fairly common.

Severe zinc deficiency can cause a major loss of immune function, and mild zinc deficiency might impair immunity slightly. For this reason, making sure to get enough zinc may help keep you from catching colds or other infections. But zinc may be helpful for colds in a completely different way, too, by directly killing viruses in the throat. When used in this way, it is taken in the form of lozenges every 2 hours from the first sign of cold symptoms. At press time, a large study reported that zinc nasal spray might be even more effective, shortening colds by almost 75%.

Intriguing evidence suggests that zinc supplements may have other specific benefits as well, including helping stomach ulcers heal, relieving symptoms of rheumatoid arthritis, slightly improving acne symptoms, increasing sperm count, and preventing "sickle-cell crisis" (a serious condition in people with sickle-cell anemia).

REQUIREMENTS/SOURCES

The official U.S. recommendations for daily intake of zinc are as follows:

- Infants 0–12 months, 5 mg
- Children 1–10 years, 10 mg
- Males 11 years and older, 15 mg
- Females 11 years and older, 12 mg
- Pregnant women, 15 mg
- Nursing women, 16–19 mg

However, the average diet in the developed world commonly provides insufficient zinc, especially in women, adolescents, infants, and the elderly.[1–5] Thus, it may be a wise idea to increase your intake of zinc on general principles.

Individuals with alcoholism, sickle-cell anemia, diabetes, or kidney disease are also at risk for zinc deficiency.

Various drugs may also inhibit zinc absorption, including AZT, captopril and possibly other ACE inhibitors, drugs which reduce stomach acid (including H_2 blockers and proton pump inhibitors), thiazide diuretics, and oral contraceptives.[6–12] Certain nutrients may have the same effect, such as calcium, soy, manganese, copper, and iron.[13–29] Contrary to previous reports, folate is not likely to significantly affect zinc absorption.[30]

Thiazide diuretics ("water pills") can cause excessive loss of zinc in the urine.[31,32]

Oysters are by far the best food source of zinc—a single serving will give you *10 times* the recommended daily intake! Seeds and nuts, peas, whole wheat, rye, and oats are not nearly as high in zinc, but you can get about 3 mg per serving of these foods.

Zinc can also be taken as a nutritional supplement, in one of many forms. Zinc citrate, zinc acetate, or zinc picolinate may be the best absorbed, although zinc sulfate is less expensive. When you purchase a supplement, you should be aware of the difference between the milligrams of actual zinc the product contains (so-called "elemental zinc") and the total milligrams of the zinc product. All figures given in this chapter refer to the amount of actual zinc to take.

THERAPEUTIC DOSAGES

For most purposes, zinc should simply be taken at the recommended daily requirements listed previously. For best absorption, zinc supplements should not be taken at the same time as high-fiber foods;[33,34] however, many high-fiber foods provide zinc in themselves.

When taking zinc long term it is advisable to take 1 to 3 mg of **copper** (see page 262) daily as well, because zinc supplements can cause copper deficiency.[35,36] Zinc may also interfere with **magnesium**[37] (see page 351) and **iron**[38] (see page 333) absorption.

For treatment of colds, much higher doses of zinc are used, although only for a short period of time. The usual dosage is 13 to 23 mg of zinc as zinc gluconate every 2 hours for a week or two (but no longer). The purpose is not to increase zinc levels in your body, but to kill viruses in the back of your throat. It appears that of the common forms of zinc, only zinc gluconate and zinc acetate have the required antiviral properties.[39,40] Also, some sweeteners and flavorings used in lozenges can block zinc's antiviral action. Dextrose, sucrose, mannitol, and sorbitol appear to be fine, but citric acid and tartaric acid are not. The information on glycine as a flavoring agent is a bit equivocal.

Long-term use of relatively high-dose zinc (90 mg daily or more) has been tried for various conditions such as acne, sickle-cell anemia, and rheumatoid arthritis, but medical supervision is essential because of the risk of toxicity (see Safety Issues).

THERAPEUTIC USES

Good evidence suggests that if you take zinc lozenges every 2 hours at the beginning of a **cold** (see page 47), you will recover much more quickly.[41] This approach involves using high doses of zinc for a short period. Long-term zinc supplementation at nutritional doses, which are much lower than what is used for colds, may also reduce the chance of getting sick, but probably only if you are deficient in zinc to begin with.[42,43]

Pregnant women should make sure to get enough zinc. One large double-blind study in zinc-deficient pregnant women found that a standard zinc supplement could significantly improve the birth weight and head size of their newborn children.[44] However, zinc supplements failed to make any difference in another large double-blind study of pregnant women that did not specifically select zinc-deficient women.[45]

Evidence also suggests that, when taken in fairly high dosages, zinc can reduce symptoms of **acne** (see page 2).[46]

Zinc may also help prevent the development of sickle-cell crisis in sickle-cell anemia[47] and speed the healing of stomach **ulcers** (see page 180).[48,49]

People with **rheumatoid arthritis** (see page 151) have been found to have lower-than-average blood levels of zinc. Although this doesn't necessarily mean that zinc supplements will reduce symptoms of rheumatoid arthritis, small studies suggest that they might help slightly.[50,51] However, others have shown no benefit at all.[52–55] It may be that zinc is only helpful for those who are zinc deficient in the first place.[56]

Some, but not all, studies have found that **HIV-positive** (see page 94) individuals tend to be deficient in zinc, with levels dropping lower in more severe disease.[57–62] Higher zinc levels have been linked to better immune function and higher CD4+ cell counts, whereas zinc deficiency has been linked to increased risk of dying from HIV.[63,64,65] One preliminary study among people taking AZT found that 30 days of zinc supplementation led to decreased rates of opportunistic infection over the following 2 years.[66] However, other research has linked higher zinc intake to more rapid development of AIDS.[67,68] The bottom line: if you have HIV, consult your physician before supplementing with zinc.

One small uncontrolled study found that zinc supplements increased sperm counts and improved **fertility** (see page 116) for men with low testosterone levels.[69] But no such effect was seen in men whose testosterone levels were normal to begin with.

Although the evidence that it works is not yet meaningful, zinc is sometimes recommended for the following conditions as well: **Alzheimer's disease** (see page 5),[70–73] **anorexia nervosa** (see page 77),[74–79] **attention deficit disorder** (see page 22), **benign prostatic hyperplasia** (see page 24),[80–86] **bladder infection** (see page 28), **cataracts** (see page 42), **diabetes** (see page 65),[87,88,89] Down's syndrome,[90,91,92] **eczema** (see page 78), **impotence** (see page 100),[93] inflammatory bowel disease (**ulcerative colitis** [see page 179] and **Crohn's disease** [see page 57]),[94–97] **macular degeneration** (see page 115),[98,99] **osteoporosis** (see page 136),[100] **periodontal disease** (see page 142), prostatitis,[101] **psoriasis** (see page 148), **tinnitus** (see page 178),[102,103] and **wound** (see page 123) and **burn** (see page 123) healing.[104,105,106]

WHAT IS THE SCIENTIFIC EVIDENCE FOR ZINC?

Colds

Numerous studies have evaluated the effects of zinc lozenges for colds. All but one found that zinc lozenges can significantly improve cold symptoms, as long as the right form of zinc is used (zinc gluconate or acetate).[107,108] For example, in a double-blind study, 100 nursing home workers with early cold symptoms received either zinc gluconate lozenges or placebo.[109] They took the lozenges until their cold symptoms abated. Overall, the workers who took zinc had fewer days of coughing (2.2 days, compared to 4 for the placebo group), sore throat (1 day versus 3), nasal drainage (4 days versus 7), and headache (2 days versus 3) than the placebo group.

Good results have been seen in several other double-blind studies,[110,111] including one that used zinc acetate and enrolled about 100 participants.[112]

A few studies found no benefit, but a close review of the evidence showed that these studies used forms of zinc lozenges that did not release virus-killing ions into the throat.[113] There has been only one study using the proper chemical form of zinc that did not find benefits, but a cherry flavoring added to the lozenges in that study might have interfered with ion release.[114]

Besides using zinc as a "virus killer," supplementation at nutritional dosages may also help reduce the frequency of colds by strengthening your overall health.

In a 2-year study of nursing home residents, participants given zinc and selenium developed illnesses much less frequently than those given placebo.[115] Of course, it isn't clear from this study which was more helpful, the zinc or the selenium. However, we do know that chronic zinc deficiency weakens the immune system,[116] and studies performed in developing countries using zinc alone have found benefits. For example, a 6-month double-blind placebo-controlled study of 609 preschool children in India found that zinc supplements reduced the rate of respiratory infections by 45%.[117] Nine other studies have also found zinc supplements helpful for preventing illness.[118]

Acne

Studies suggest that people with acne have lower-than-normal levels of zinc in their bodies.[119,120,121] This fact alone does not prove that taking zinc supplements will help acne, but several small double-blind studies involving a total of over 300 people have found generally positive results.

In one of these studies, 54 people were given either placebo or 135 mg of zinc as zinc sulfate daily. Zinc produced slight but measurable benefits.[122] Similar results have been seen in other studies using 90 to 135 mg of zinc daily.[123–127] In some studies, however, no benefits were seen.[128,129]

Two studies have compared zinc against a standard treatment for acne, the antibiotic tetracycline. One found that zinc was as effective as tetracycline,[130] but another found the antibiotic more effective.[131]

Keep in mind that the dosages of zinc used in these studies are rather high, and should be used only under a physician's supervision.

Sickle-Cell Anemia

Zinc may also be helpful in preventing "sickle-cell crisis" in individuals with sickle-cell anemia.[132] A double-blind placebo-controlled study treated 145 sickle-cell subjects with either 220 mg of zinc sulfate 3 times daily or placebo. During 18 months of treatment, the zinc-treated subjects had an average of 2.5 crises, compared to 5.3 for the placebo group. However, zinc didn't seem to reduce the severity of a crisis, as measured by the number of days spent in the hospital for each crisis.

Warning: Sickle-cell anemia is far too serious a condition to self-treat, and the relatively high dosages of zinc used in this study should be taken only under the supervision of a doctor (see Safety Issues).

Macular Degeneration

Macular degeneration is one of the most common causes of vision loss in the elderly. One double-blind study of 151 individuals followed for 1 to 2 years found that zinc supplements helped preserve vision.[133] However, another study of 112 individuals found no benefit.[134]

SAFETY ISSUES

Zinc seldom causes any immediate side effects other than occasional stomach upset, usually when it's taken on an empty stomach. Some forms do have an unpleasant metallic taste.

However, long-term use of zinc at dosages of 100 mg or more daily can cause a number of toxic effects, including severe copper deficiency, impaired immunity, heart problems, and anemia.[135,136,137] Unless a physician specifically advises you to take a higher dosage, you should stick to the nutritional dosage range described under Requirements/Sources.

Use of zinc can interfere with the absorption of penicillamine and antibiotics in the tetracycline or fluoroquinolone (Cipro, Floxin) families.[138–143]

The potassium-sparing diuretic amiloride was found to significantly reduce zinc excretion from the body.[144] This means that if you take zinc supplements at the same time as amiloride, zinc accumulation could occur. This could lead to toxic side effects. However, the potassium-sparing diuretic triamterene does not seem to cause this problem.[145]

⚠ INTERACTIONS YOU SHOULD KNOW ABOUT

If you are taking

- Medications that reduce stomach acid such as **Zantac (ranitidine)** or **Prilosec (omeprazole); zidovudine (AZT); ACE inhibitors; oral contraceptives; estrogen-replacement therapy; thiazide diuretics; calcium; copper;** or **iron:** You may need to take extra zinc.
- **Manganese, antacids, soy,** or antibiotics in the **fluoroquinolone** (e.g., **Cipro**, **Floxin**) or **tetracycline** families: It may be advisable to separate your doses of zinc and these substances by at least 2 hours.
- **Zinc supplements:** You should also take extra copper, and perhaps magnesium as well because zinc interferes with their absorption. Zinc interferes with iron absorption, too, but you shouldn't take iron supplements unless you know you are deficient.
- **Penicillamine:** You may need extra zinc; however, zinc interferes with penicillamine's absorption so it may be advisable to take zinc and penicillamine at least 2 hours apart.
- **Amiloride:** It could reduce zinc excretion from the body, leading to zinc accumulation, which could cause toxic side effects. Do not take zinc supplements unless advised by a physician.

LOOKING FOR REFERENCES?

Because of the large number of references for a project of this magnitude, we've placed all our research citations conveniently online at **www.TNP.com/references/NHB2/**. Just click on the condition, herb, or supplement for which you would like to see a citation and scroll down to the appropriate reference.

If you would prefer to receive an electronic copy of all the references in this book, please send an e-mail request to websupporthlth @primapub.com.

INDEX

Index

Visit Us at TNP.com

Index

Visit Us at TNP.com

Index

Visit Us at TNP.com

Index

Visit Us at TNP.com

Index

Visit Us at TNP.com

Index

Visit Us at TNP.com

Index

Visit Us at TNP.com

Index

Visit Us at TNP.com

Index

Visit Us at TNP.com

Index

Visit Us at TNP.com

Index

Visit Us at TNP.com

Index

Visit Us at TNP.com

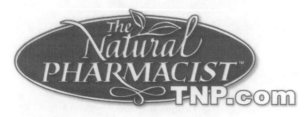

About the Authors

Steven Bratman, M.D., Medical Director and Senior Editor of The NATURAL PHARMACIST series of books, has many years of experience in the alternative medicine field. A graduate of the University of California at Davis, Medical School, he has also trained in herbology, nutrition, Chinese medicine, and other alternative therapies, and has worked closely with a wide variety of alternative practitioners. Dr. Bratman is both a strong proponent and vocal critic of alternative treatments, and he believes that alternative medicine has both strengths and weaknesses, just like conventional medicine. This even-handed critique has made him a trusted party on both sides of the debate.

His books include *The Alternative Medicine Ratings Guide: An Expert Panel Ranks the Best Alternative Treatments for Over 80 Conditions* (Prima Health, 1998), the professional text *Clinical Evaluation of Medicinal Herbs and Other Therapeutic Natural Products* (Prima Health, 1999), and the following titles in The NATURAL PHARMACIST series: *Your Complete Guide to Herbs* (Prima Health, 1999), *Your Complete Guide to Illnesses and Their Natural Remedies* (Prima Health, 1999), *Natural Health Bible, First Edition* (Prima Health, 1999), and *St. John's Wort and Depression* (Prima Health, 1999).

David J. Kroll, Ph.D., is a professor of pharmacology and toxicology at the University of Colorado School of Pharmacy and a consultant for pharmacists, physicians, and alternative practitioners on the indications and cautions for herbal medicine use. He received a degree in toxicology from the Philadelphia College of Pharmacy and Science and obtained his Ph.D. from the University of Florida College of Medicine.

Dr. Kroll has lectured widely and has published articles in a number of medical journals, abstracts, and newsletters. He is also a Series Editor for The NATURAL PHARMACIST series of books from Prima Health, and is co-author of both *Natural Health Bible, First Edition* and the professional text *Clinical Evaluation of Medicinal Herbs and Other Therapeutic Natural Products*.

Index

Visit Us at TNP.com